PROGRESS IN CLINICAL AND BIOLOGICAL RESEARCH

RECENT TITLES

Vol 206: **Genetic Toxicology of the Diet,** Ib Knudsen, *Editor*

Vol 207: **Monitoring of Occupational Genotoxicants,** Marja Sorsa, Hannu Norppa, *Editors*

Vol 208: **Risk and Reason: Risk Assessment in Relation to Environmental Mutagens and Carcinogens,** Per Oftedal, Anton Brøgger, *Editors*

Vol 209: **Genetic Toxicology of Environmental Chemicals,** Claes Ramel, Bo Lambert, Jan Magnusson, *Editors*. Published in two volumes: Part A: *Basic Principles and Mechanisms of Action.* Part B: *Genetic Effects and Applied Mutagenesis*

Vol 210: **Ionic Currents in Development,** Richard Nuccitelli, *Editor*

Vol 211: **Transfusion Medicine: Recent Technological Advances,** Kris Murawski, Frans Peetoom, *Editors*

Vol 212: **Cancer Metastasis: Experimental and Clinical Strategies,** D.R. Welch, B.K. Bhuyan, L.A. Liotta, *Editors*

Vol 213: **Plant Flavonoids in Biology and Medicine: Biochemical, Pharmacological, and Structure–Activity Relationships,** Vivian Cody, Elliott Middleton, Jr., Jeffrey B. Harborne, *Editors*

Vol 214: **Ethnic Differences in Reactions to Drugs and Xenobiotics,** Werner Kalow, H. Werner Goedde, Dharam P. Agarwal, *Editors*

Vol 215: **Megakaryocyte Development and Function,** Richard F. Levine, Neil Williams, Jack Levin, Bruce L. Evatt, *Editors*

Vol 216: **Advances in Cancer Control: Health Care Financing and Research,** Lee E. Mortenson, Paul F. Engstrom, Paul N. Anderson, *Editors*

Vol 217: **Progress in Developmental Biology,** Harold C. Slavkin, *Editor*. Published in two volumes.

Vol 218: **Evolutionary Perspective and the New Genetics,** Henry Gershowitz, Donald L. Rucknagel, Richard E. Tashian, *Editors*

Vol 219: **Recent Advances in Arterial Diseases: Atherosclerosis, Hypertension, and Vasospasm,** Thomas N. Tulenko, Robert H. Cox, *Editors*

Vol 220: **Safety and Health Aspects of Organic Solvents,** Vesa Riihimäki, Ulf Ulfvarson, *Editors*

Vol 221: **Developments in Bladder Cancer,** Louis Denis, Tadao Niijima, George Prout, Jr., Fritz Schröder, *Editors*

Vol 222: **Dietary Fat and Cancer,** Clement Ip, Diane F. Birt, Adrianne E. Rogers, Curtis Mettlin, *Editors*

Vol 223: **Cancer Drug Resistance,** Thomas C. Hall, *Editor*

Vol 224: **Transplantation: Approaches to Graft Rejection,** Harold T. Meryman, *Editor*

Vol 225: **Gonadotropin Down-Regulation in Gynecological Practice,** Rune Rolland, Dev R. Chadha, Wim N.P. Willemsen, *Editors*

Vol 226: **Cellular Endocrinology: Hormonal Control of Embryonic and Cellular Differentiation,** Ginette Serrero, Jun Hayashi, *Editors*

Please contact the publisher for information about previous titles in this series.

DIETARY FAT AND CANCER

DIETARY FAT AND CANCER

Editors

Clement Ip
Department of Breast Surgery
Roswell Park Memorial Institute
Buffalo, New York

Diane F. Birt
Eppley Institute for Research in Cancer
University of Nebraska Medical Center
Omaha, Nebraska

Adrianne E. Rogers
Department of Pathology
Boston University School of Medicine
Boston, Massachusetts

Curtis Mettlin
Department of Cancer Control and Epidemiology
Roswell Park Memorial Institute
Buffalo, New York

ALAN R. LISS, INC. • NEW YORK

Address all Inquiries to the Publisher
Alan R. Liss, Inc., 41 East 11th Street, New York, NY 10003

Library of Congress Cataloging-in-Publication Data

Dietary fat and cancer.

    (Progress in clinical and biological research;
v. 222)
    Includes bibliographies and index.
    1. Cancer—Nutritional aspects. 2. Lipids in
nutrition. 3. Fat—Physiological effect. 4. Carcino-
genesis. I. Ip, Clement. II. Series. [DNLM: 1. Dietary
Fats—adverse effects. 2. Neoplasms—etiology.
W1 PR668E v.222 / QZ 202 D5645]
RC268.45.D56 1986   616.99'4071   86-20014
ISBN 0-8451-5072-3

Contents

Contributors xi

Preface
Clement Ip xv

I. EPIDEMIOLOGICAL AND CLINICAL STUDIES ON DIETARY FAT AND CANCER

Methodological Issues in Epidemiologic Studies of Dietary Fat and Cancer
Curtis Mettlin 3

Dietary Fat and the Epidemiology of Breast Cancer
Anthony B. Miller 17

Body Size, Body Mass and Cancer of the Breast
F. de Waard 33

The Biochemical Epidemiology of Prostatic Carcinoma
David P. Rose 43

The Epidemiology of Colon Cancer and Dietary Fat
Laurence N. Kolonel and Loïc Le Marchand 69

Clinical Trials of Low Fat Diets and Breast Cancer Prevention
Carolyn K. Clifford, Ritva R. Butrum, Peter Greenwald, and Jerome W. Yates 93

Methodological Issues in Clinical Trials of Dietary Fat Reduction in Patients With Breast Dysplasia
N.F. Boyd, M. Cousins, M. Beaton, L. Han, and V. McGuire 117

II. FOOD FATS AND OILS: CONSUMPTION, PROPERTIES, AND REQUIREMENT

Levels and Sources of Fat in the U.S. Food Supply
Nancy R. Raper and Ruth M. Marston 127

Food Fats and Oils
J. Edward Hunter 153

Heated and Oxidized Fats
J. Craig Alexander 185

Nutritional and Functional Requirements for Essential Fatty Acids
Ralph T. Holman 211

III. EFFECTS OF DIETARY FAT ON CARCINOGENESIS IN LABORATORY ANIMALS

Experimental Studies on Dietary Fat and Cancer in Relation to Epidemiological Data
Kenneth K. Carroll 231

Introduction to the Effects of Neutral Fats and Fatty Acids on Carcinogenesis in Experimental Animals
Diane F. Birt 249

Chemically-Induced Mammary Gland Tumors in Rats: Modulation by Dietary Fat
Adrianne E. Rogers and Soon Y. Lee 255

Relevance of Trans Fatty Acids and Fish Oil in Animal Tumorigenesis Studies
Clement Ip, Margot M. Ip, and Paul Sylvester 283

Amount and Type of Dietary Fat and Colon Cancer: Animal Model Studies
Bandaru S. Reddy 295

Dietary Fat and Colon Cancer: Variable Results in Animal Models
Paul M. Newberne and Kathleen M. Nauss 311

Enhancement of Pancreatic Carcinogenesis by Dietary Fat in the Hamster and Rat Models
D.F. Birt and B.D. Roebuck 331

Oil Gavage Test-Compound Administration Effects in NTP Carcinogenesis-Toxicity Testing
Robert E. Landers, Michael J. Norvell, and Mark A. Bieber 357

IV. STUDIES OF INTERACTION OF FAT WITH OTHER NUTRITIONAL FACTORS IN EXPERIMENTAL CARCINOGENESIS

The Macronutrients in Experimental Carcinogenesis of the Breast, Colon, and Pancreas
Steven K. Clinton and Willard J. Visek 377

Fat–Protein Interaction, Defined 2-Generation Studies
E.J. Hawrylewicz 403

Cholesterol Conundrums: The Relationship Between Dietary and Serum Cholesterol in Colon Cancer
Selwyn A. Broitman 435

Fat, Lipotropes, Hypolipidemic Agents and Liver Cancer
Hisashi Shinozuka, Sikandar L. Katyal, and Mohan I.R. Perera 461

Effect of Dietary Calcium on the Toxicity of Bile Acid and Orally Administered Fat to Colonic Epithelium
R.P. Bird and W.R. Bruce 487

Fat, Calories and Fiber
David Kritchevsky 495

Role of Acute Caloric-Restriction in Murine Tumorigenesis
Paul W. Sylvester 517

V. CELLULAR AND OTHER MECHANISMS OF FAT EFFECTS ON CARCINOGENESIS

Metabolic Adaptations to Dietary Fats
Steven D. Clarke 531

Mechanisms of Dietary Fat Modulation of Tumorigenesis: Changes in Immune Response
Kent L. Erickson 555

Metabolic Activation of Carcinogens
Adelbert E. Wade and Suniti Dharwadkar 587

Effects of Lipids on Gap Junctionally-Mediated Intercellular Communication: Possible Role in the Promotion of Tumorigenesis by Dietary Fat
Charles F. Aylsworth 607

Interrelationship Between Dietary Fat and Endocrine Processes in Mammary Gland Tumorigenesis
Clifford W. Welsch 623

The Metabolism of the Intestinal Microflora and Its Relationship to Dietary Fat, Colon and Breast Cancer
Barry R. Goldin 655

Eicosanoids and Cancer
Rashida A. Karmali 687

Fatty Acid Growth Requirements of Normal and Neoplastic Mammary Epithelium
William R. Kidwell 699

Fatty Acid-Induced Modifications of Mouse Mammary Epithelium as Studied in an Organ and Cell Culture System
Nitin T. Telang 707

VI. POTENTIAL RESPONSES TO AND IMPACTS OF EPIDEMIOLOGICAL AND EXPERIMENTAL DATA ON DIETARY FAT AND CANCER

Dietary Guidelines
Thomas P. O'Connor and T. Colin Campbell 731

The Diet and Cancer Branch, NCI: Current Projects and Future Research Directions
Ritva R. Butrum, Elaine Lanza, and Carolyn K. Clifford 773

Cancer and Diet Interactions
Mark A. Bieber 789

Dietary Fat and Cancer: A Perspective From the Livestock and Meat Industry
Donald M. Kinsman and George D. Wilson 801

Changing Patterns in the Dairy Industry
Lois D. McBean, Emerita N. Alcantara, and Elwood W. Speckmann 815

Index 863

Contributors

Emerita N. Alcantara, National Dairy Council, Rosemont, IL 60018 **[815]**

J. Craig Alexander, Department of Nutritional Sciences, University of Guelph, Guelph, Ontario, Canada N1G 2W1 **[185]**

Charles F. Aylsworth, Department of Anatomy, Michigan State University, East Lansing, MI 48824-1101 **[607]**

M. Beaton, Ludwig Institute for Cancer Research, Toronto, Canada M4Y 1M4 **[117]**

Mark A. Bieber, Best Foods Research and Engineering Center, A Division of CPC International, Inc., Union, NJ 07083 **[357,789]**

R.P. Bird, Ludwig Institute for Cancer Research, Toronto Branch, Toronto, Ontario M4Y 1M4, Canada **[487]**

Diane F. Birt, Eppley Institute for Research in Cancer, University of Nebraska Medical Center, Omaha, NE 68105 **[249,331]**

N.F. Boyd, Ludwig Institute for Cancer Research, Toronto, Canada M4Y 1M4 **[117]**

Selwyn A. Broitman, Department of Microbiology and Pathology, Boston University School of Medicine, Boston, MA 02118 **[435]**

W.R. Bruce, Ludwig Institute for Cancer Research, Toronto Branch, Toronto, Ontario M4Y 1M4, Canada **[487]**

Ritva R. Butrum, Diet and Cancer Branch, Division of Cancer Prevention and Control, National Cancer Institute, Silver Spring, MD **[93,773]**

T. Colin Campbell, Division of Nutritional Sciences, Cornell University, Ithaca, NY 14853 **[731]**

Kenneth K. Carroll, Department of Biochemistry, University of Western Ontario, London, Ontario, Canada N6A 5C1 **[231]**

Steven D. Clarke, The Upjohn Company, Kalamazoo, MI 49001 **[531]**

Carolyn K. Clifford, Diet and Cancer Branch, Division of Cancer Prevention and Control, National Cancer Institute, Silver Spring, MD **[93,773]**

Steven K. Clinton, Department of Medicine, University of Chicago, Chicago, IL 60637 **[377]**

M. Cousins, Ludwig Institute for Cancer Research, Toronto, Canada M4Y 1M4 **[117]**

The number in brackets is the opening page number of the contributor's article.

F. de Waard, National Institute of
Public Health and Environmental
Hygiene, Bilthoven, The Netherlands
[33]

Suniti Dharwadkar, Department of
Pharmacology and Toxicology, College
of Pharmacy, University of Georgia,
Athens, GA 30602 **[587]**

Kent L. Erickson, Department of
Human Anatomy, University of
California, School of Medicine, Davis,
CA 95616 **[555]**

Barry R. Goldin, Department of
Medicine, Infectious Disease Division,
Tufts-New England Medical Center
Hospitals, Boston, MA 02111 **[655]**

Peter Greenwald, Division of Cancer
Prevention and Control, National
Cancer Institutes of Health, Bethesda,
MD 20892 **[93]**

L. Han, Ludwig Institute for Cancer
Research, Toronto, Canada M4Y 1M4
[117]

E.J. Hawrylewicz, Department of
Research, Mercy Hospital and Medical
Center, Chicago, IL 60616 **[403]**

Ralph T. Holman, Hormel Institute,
University of Minnesota, Austin, MN
55912 **[211]**

J. Edward Hunter, The Procter &
Gamble Company, Winton Hill
Technical Center, Cincinnati, OH 45224
[153]

Clement Ip, Department of Breast
Surgery, Roswell Park Memorial
Institute, Buffalo, NY 14263 **[xv, 283]**

Margot M. Ip, Grace Cancer Drug
Center, Roswell Park Memorial
Institute, Buffalo, NY 14263 **[283]**

Rashida A. Karmali, Department of
Nutrition, Rutgers University, New
Brunswick, NJ 08903; and Memorial
Sloan-Kettering Cancer Center, New
York, NY 10021 **[687]**

Sikandar L. Katyal, Department of
Pathology, University of Pittsburgh
School of Medicine, Pittsburgh, PA
15261 **[461]**

William R. Kidwell, Laboratory of
Tumor Immunology and Biology,
National Cancer Institute, Bethesda,
MD 20892 **[699]**

Donald M. Kinsman, Department of
Animal Sciences, University of
Connecticut, Storrs, CT 06268 **[801]**

Laurence N. Kolonel, Epidemiology
Program, Cancer Research Center,
University of Hawaii, Honolulu, HI
96813 **[69]**

David Kritchevsky, The Wistar
Institute of Anatomy and Biology,
Philadelphia, PA 19104 **[495]**

Robert E. Landers, Best Foods
Research and Engineering Center, A
Division of CPC International, Inc.,
Union, NJ 07083 **[357]**

Elaine Lanza, Diet and Cancer Branch,
Division of Cancer Prevention and
Control, National Cancer Institute,
Silver Spring, MD **[773]**

Soon Y. Lee, Department of Applied
Biological Sciences, Massachusetts
Institute of Technology, Cambridge, MA
02139 **[255]**

Loïc Le Marchand, Epidemiology
Program, Cancer Research Center,
University of Hawaii, Honolulu, HI
96813 **[69]**

Ruth M. Marston, Human Nutrition
Information Service, U.S. Department
of Agriculture, Hyattsville, MD 20782
[127]

Lois D. McBean, National Dairy Council, Rosemont, IL 60018 [815]

V. McGuire, Ludwig Institute for Cancer Research, Toronto, Canada M4Y 1M4 [117]

Curtis Mettlin, Roswell Park Memorial Institute, Buffalo, NY 14263 [3]

Anthony B. Miller, NCIC Epidemiology Unit, University of Toronto, Toronto, Ontario M5S 1A8, Canada [17]

Kathleen M. Nauss, Department of Applied Biological Sciences, Massachusetts Institute of Technology, Cambridge, MA 02139 [311]

Paul M. Newberne, Department of Applied Biological Sciences, Massachusetts Institute of Technology, Cambridge, MA 02139; and Department of Pathology, Boston University School of Medicine, Boston, MA 02118 [311]

Michael J. Norvell, Best Foods Research and Engineering Center, A Division of CPC International, Inc., Union, NJ 07083 [357]

Thomas P. O'Connor, Division of Nutritional Sciences, Cornell University, Ithaca, NY 14853 [731]

Mohan I.R. Perera, Department of Pathology, University of Pittsburgh School of Medicine, Pittsburgh, PA 15261 [461]

Nancy R. Raper, Human Nutrition Information Service, U.S. Department of Agriculture, Hyattsville, MD 20782 [127]

Bandaru S. Reddy, Division of Nutrition and Endocrinology, Naylor Dana Institute for Disease Prevention, Valhalla, NY 10595 [295]

B.D. Roebuck, Department of Pharmacology and Toxicology, Dartmouth Medical School, Hanover, NH 03756 [331]

Adrianne E. Rogers, Department of Pathology, Boston University School of Medicine, Boston, MA 02118 [255]

David P. Rose, American Health Foundation, Valhalla, NY 10595 [43]

Hisashi Shinozuka, Department of Pathology, University of Pittsburgh School of Medicine, Pittsburgh, PA 15261 [461]

Elwood W. Speckmann, National Dairy Council, Rosemont, IL 60018 [815]

Paul W. Sylvester, Grace Cancer Drug Center, Roswell Park Memorial Institute, Buffalo, NY 14263 [283,517]

Nitin T. Telang, Surgical Oncology Research Laboratory, Department of Surgery, Memorial Sloan-Kettering Cancer Center, New York, NY 10021 [707]

Willard J. Visek, University of Illinois College of Medicine, Urbana, IL 61801 [377]

Adelbert E. Wade, Department of Pharmacology and Toxicology, College of Pharmacy, University of Georgia, Athens, GA 30602 [587]

Clifford W. Welsch, Department of Anatomy, Michigan State University, East Lansing, MI 48824 [623]

George D. Wilson, American Meat Institute, Washington, DC 20007 [801]

Jerome W. Yates, Division of Cancer Prevention and Control, National Institutes of Health, Bethesda, MD 20892 [93]

Preface

This book is sponsored by the Organ Systems Coordinating Center, an external function of the Organ Systems Program of the National Cancer Institute. It is intended to be a comprehensive, state-of-the-art review of the subject focusing on solid tumors. Most of the epidemiological and experimental data on fat and cancer are centered on the breast and the colon, with limited but growing information on the pancreas and the prostate. In addition to data evaluation, the objectives of this publication are to gain some collective insight on future research direction and to assess the potential impact on dietary practices and on the food industries of evidence linking fat consumption and increased risk of tumor development.

On behalf of the editors, I would like to thank all the authors for their voluntary contributions in bringing this project to fruition. All the manuscripts were collected in the first four months of 1986; thus this book contains up-to-date information from different segments ranging from clinical intervention trials to laboratory investigations on nutrient interaction and mechanistic studies.

Special thanks are extended to Patricia Beers who has done an excellent job in handling correspondences to and inquiries from authors and in processing all the manuscripts.

Clement Ip, Ph.D.
Scientific Administrator
Breast Cancer Program

I. Epidemiological and Clinical Studies on Dietary Fat and Cancer

Dietary Fat and Cancer, pages 3–15
© 1986 Alan R. Liss, Inc.

METHODOLOGICAL ISSUES IN EPIDEMIOLOGIC STUDIES OF DIETARY
FAT AND CANCER

Curtis Mettlin, Ph.D.

Roswell Park Memorial Institute
666 Elm Street
Buffalo, New York 14263

INTRODUCTION

As several contributions to this section document,
dietary fat has been implicated, by hypothesis or by
evidence, in the etiology of several different types of
cancer. The cancers for which a role for dietary fat is
suspected include breast, colorectal, prostate, ovarian,
pancreatic and, cervical cancer. The papers which follow
will show that epidemiologic research has played a significant role in bringing this aspect of nutrition and cancer to
the forefront of scientific and public health interest.

Epidemiologic research alone has not, however, brought
about a resolution of the question of whether patterns of
dietary fat consumption represent an avoidable source of
cancer risk. One of the reasons that epidemiologic studies
have yielded inconclusive and, sometimes, mixed results may
be that there are methodological issues inherent to the
study of the dietary fat-cancer hypothesis.

To better understand how epidemiology might provide
some support for the hypothesis of an etiological role for
dietary fat while not always doing so, several
methodological problems in the field of fat and cancer will
be reviewed herein. These issues include:

1. Investigator assumptions concerning biological
processes of dietary carcinogenesis.

2. Whether the diseases in question have singular or multiple etiologies.

3. How the exposure to risk is distributed within and across populations.

4. Whether the research designs employed are appropriate to the research issues.

5. Whether confounding and interacting exposures are accounted for in research methodology.

6. Whether the measurement of population exposure to dietary fat is sufficiently sensitive.

7. Whether the impact of interventions to affect disease risk may be inferred and quantified accurately.

In this chapter, each of these issues will be examined and discussed with the goal of identifying potential sources of error in epidemiologic approaches to studying dietary fats and cancer. Perhaps unfairly to epidemiology, equal attention is not given to the strengths of the epidemiologic method. However, the value and need for studies of cancer risk and diet in human populations are well established.

ASSUMPTIONS REGARDING BIOLOGICAL PROCESSES

Among the criteria by which epidemiologists generally evaluate the correctness of their conclusions is that of "biological plausibility". The processes of disease causation inferred from epidemiologic data must, ultimately, conform to some reasonable understanding of the biology of the disease. Very often, the epidemiology of a condition will direct laboratory and clinical scientists toward areas of inquiry from which precise pathological mechanisms are identified.

More often, however, the basic approach of an epidemiologist to a disease casuation question is guided by assumptions the investigator must make regarding the likely, or possible, biological mechanisms which operate. Where essential features of the biological processes are unclear or in dispute, this may be reflected in uncertainty about the proper epidemiologic methods to apply.

For example, laboratory data suggest that dietary fat consumption may fit best as a promoter in the two-step model of carcinogenesis involving initiation and promotion. On the basis of this assumption concerning biological processes, some research has focused on dietary exposures recent to the onset of disease. Another model, however, suggests that, at least in the case of breast cancer, the critical biological events influenced by dietary fat may be intitating events occurring during young adulthood in maturing breast tissue. Research guided by this biological perspective obviously would be directed toward events quite distant from the actual onset of clinical disease and would require a different methodological model.

In a research environment where experimental data supports alternative or conflicting models of carcinogenesis, as it does in the case of dietary fat and cancer, the meaning and correctness of epidemiologic results will remain difficult to interpret. This points to the essential linkage necessary between progress in research by laboratory scientists and epidemiologists. The limits of epidemiologic methods are, in some part, a reflection of the limits of laboratory data.

SINGLE VS. MULTIPLE ETIOLOGIES

Most epidemiological studies of fat and cancer are based on the assumption that there may be a single etiology operating for the disease. Thus, entire populations of tumors are examined in association with common exposures. For example, the per capita fat consumption of nations are related to the total mortality experience of the countries or, the dietary histories of a consecutive series of patients admitted to a hospital are compared to some referent population.

This occurs in spite of the fact that we know that many of the diseases in question have multiple etiologies. Some breast cancer is known to result from radiation exposure, in mice it is known to be chemically inducible, there is ample evidence that hormone events related to pregnancy and menopause affect incidence and, familial cancer history accounts for some breast cancer occurrences. Colon cancer, similarly, is related in some instances to conditions such as familial polyposis and Gardner's syndrome, while other instances have different etiologies.   Boyle et al. (1985) recently have reviewed the descriptive epidemiology of colorectal cancer concluding that the world-wide patterns of incidence and mortality suggest that different etiologies operate for this disease in different regions.

It is possible that dietary fat may not be part of a single etiology of cancer but rather, a component of only some of the multiple etiologies for the disease.   This has obvious implications for the methodological approach to the question.   Studies of patient populations which might reflect multiple etiologies will be less likely to detect the effects of dietary fat than those which focus only on those groups of patients in which the fat-related etiology operates.   Smaller studies of select populations may have greater power than larger studies of heterogeneous tumor populations.

To date, researchers have made few attempts to focus their investigations on those sub-populations in which dietary fat plays the greatest role.   The limited instances in which this has been attempted include studies of dietary fat intake in women of the same menopausal status or of the same tumor histology.   Further efforts to delimit study populations to reduce the effects of multiple etiologies obscuring the role of dietary fat may lead to a better understanding of the personal or environmental circumstances which represent the greatest risk.

DISTRIBUTION OF EXPOSURE

The power of the epidemiologic method derives from the ability of the observer to identify circumstances in which the juxtapositioning of observations mimics an experiment. It is necessary to find such naturally occurring situations because the actual experimental induction of cancer in populations is not an acceptable alternative.   In many instances, it is not difficult to mimic the experimental method.   Often, two groups can be identified which appear to vary only with respect to some exposure and some disease outcome. In those situations, the difference in outcome reasonably may be attributed to the difference in exposure.

In the case of dietary fat, it has proven more difficult to identify such natural experiments.   There are few instances of different groups that differ in their exposure to dietary fat, and in little else. There is a greater tendency for populations to be homogeneous in their dietary fat consumption levels. On the other hand, when populations do vary in dietary fat intake, they tend also to vary greatly in a number of other relevant aspects. Greater variations in fat consumption are observable between nations or cultural groups than within nations or groups. When comparisons must span territorial or cultural boundaries, the ability to isolate the effect to differences in dietary habit is limited by the need to consider the many other differences between countries or cultures.

While the comparisons between dietary fat consumption in Japan and in the United States and the related differences in rates of colon, breast, and other cancers are striking, there are many other differences between Japan and its people and the United States and its population. Contrarywise, studies of a population or hospital-based series of patients and some matched control series, may increase the comparability of the groups but, reduce the contrast in exposure.

The impact of the varability, or lack of variability, of fat consumption within populations on the power of case-referent studies to detect the effects of dietary fat has been quantified by McKeown-Eyssen and Thomas (1985.) Essentially, studies in populations where there is greater uniformity in dietary practice must observe more subjects than where uniformity is less. The relative homogeneity of dietary fat consumption in groups, communities or regions may be the reason that some case-control investigations fail to detect that which appears more clear from cross-cultural or interational comparisons.

The nature of the distribution of exposure to dietary fat represents a real limitation to the ability of the epidemiologist to mimic the experiment. Where differences in exposure are greatest, confounding differences also are greatest. This implies that international or cross-cultural comparisons must attempt to account for the confounding effects of differences in exposure to other risks by multivariate statistical means. There are only a limited number of countries for which there are reliable food and mortality data and multivariate analysis can only be done to a very limited extent.

Studies within populations, on the other hand, must increase the number of observations made as a function of the degree of variablity in exposure. In culturally homogeneous communities, the sample size required to detect an effect may exceed the population of tumors available to study. To date, most case-control studies have not been planned with due respect to this issue and many have lacked adequate statistical power.

ADEQUACY OF RESEARCH DESIGN

Cancer and chronic diseases typically are the result of chronic processes. In the case of diet and cancer especially, the exposures to risk do not occur in an instant in time, but rather, across some potentially extensive interval. The cancers most often linked to dietary fat only begin to appear in middle age and accelerate in frequency in later decades of the lifespan. Because of this, epidemiologic research must be designed to associate long, and possibly low level, exposures with outcomes which may occur long after the onset of the exposure. Most often, this is attempted by retrospective designs such as by examining the lifetime dietary histories of cancer patients and control subjects.

Although there is some evidence that subjects can report past dietary habits with some validity (Byers et al, 1983) the possible interactions of events of the present and recall of the past are manifold. Subjects of different ages, when asked to recall dietary events at an earlier age, will be reflecting on different social and economic eras, persons of different current health status possibly will have perceptions of the past differently influenced by their present conditions and, persons of different life history may weigh different periods of their lives differently in aggregating their total dietary experience.

One alternative to the complexities associated with describing exposures retrospectively is to study the associations prospectively. Some groups have had their dietary habits documented in the past for epidemiologic or other purposes. These earlier observations can be related to subsequent disease experience. Prospective studies, however, typically fail to document changes in dietary habit which may have occurred in the interval between the initial observation and the disease outcome. Dietary fat intake is known to have increased throughout the first part of this century (McCall and Sanches, 1967) and the prospective design typically is insensitive to such changing patterns of exposure.

The third major epidemiologic approach, which has perhaps provided the greatest support to the dietary fat-cancer hypothesis, is the correlational study. Per capita consumption, and trends in fat consumption have been correlated to differences in disease risk of different populations or changes in disease rates across time.

The inadequacies of this research design have been cited elsewhere (Graham and Mettlin, 1979), the major problem being the fact that the populations being compared across space or time differ in so many respects other than their dietary habits. Even if other factors are considered, it remains difficult to factor in the lag between exposure and disease onset or the variability within the populations with respect to dietary habits. Although crude correlations between dietary fat and disease risk are often suggestive and supportive of experimental findings, this basic research design, considered alone, usually is not conclusive.

CONFOUNDING AND INTERACTION

As already has been indicated, the fact that dietary habits occur in association with other behaviors and traits which may affect risk challanges virtually all epidemiologic dietary studies. This inability to control for all possible causative factors is known as confounding. The accentuation or suppression of effects as a result of the joint occurrence of two or more factors is interaction. In the case of dietary fat, it occurs in two basic dimensions. Firstly, the role of dietary fat in cancer etiology may be masked by its association with non-dietary sources of risk. Secondly, it is possible also that the interrelationships among different macro and micronutrients affect the power of epidemiologic investigations of fats and cancer.

One example of confounding by non-dietary factors is illustrated by the potential role of social class. High levels of dietary fat intake are, in part, a product of affluence. When affluence is linked to another risk factor, such as in the case of breast cancer, delayed age of first childbirth, it becomes problematic whether the dietary habit, the childbearing practice or, some other feature of social status truly is responsible for the risk. This particular source of potential confounding has been documented in Italy (La Vecchia, 1986) and probably occurs elsewhere.

Non-dietary factors also may have interactive effects on risk. For example, dietary fat may have greater, or lesser, effect when it occurs in conjunction with other risk factors. The effects of dietary fat may vary according to the presence of family history of disease, the age of the individual, the presence of precursor lesions or, any of a number of possible other factors.

Confounding by dietary factors is the product of the fact that exposure to dietary fat does not vary independently of variations in other aspects of food intake. Diets rich in animal fat sources will tend to manifest lower vegetable intake. The attribution of risk specifically to the high fat content of the diet as opposed to the low vegetable intake is virtually impossible in such circumstances. Nutrient interaction also may occur. It is possible that dietary fat constitutes a risk only when it occurs in the presence or absence of some other dietary constituent.

While other examples of confounding and interaction abound, recent findings regarding the possible role of caloric intake vis a vis caloric expenditure in cancer risk are a pertinent illustration of the problem of confounding. High fat diets tend also to be high calorie diets. In the case of breast and colon cancer, low levels of physical activity have been related to higher risk of disease. (Frisch et al., 1985; Vena, 1985.) Thus, the role of fat in cancer etiology may be confounded by its association with energy balance.

MEASUREMENT SENSITIVITY

Some aspects of diet are measured more easily than are others. Nutrients that are found in a few foods in relatively constant amounts may be quantified more precisely than food attributes which occur in many different foods and food types in variable amounts. Unfortunately for the epidemiologist attempting to measure exposure to it, dietary fat may be consumed through many different food habits. In addition, the same food may vary in its fat content as a function of the means of its production and/or preparation.

The accuracy, reliability and validity of methods of dietary measurement in epidemiologic studies have been studied and commented upon extensively (Bazzarre and Yuhas, 1983; Lee et al., 1983.) One finding concerning the United States diet may suggest, however, that the measurement of dietary fat may be a problem of manageable proportions. Block (1985) has analyzed the National Health and Nutrition Examination Survey data to determine the principal food sources for several different nutrients. She found that 80% of the total fat consumption in the U.S. diet was attributable to just 24 food items. This may suggest that measurable variations in fat intake may be detected by something less than an examination of all of the many and varied sources of fat in the diet.

INTERVENTION METHODOLOGY

In light of extensive laboratory data and suggestive, but inconclusive, evidence from observational epidemiology, some feel that it is timely to move research in human populations forward by means of a more powerful research tool, the controlled intervention trial. Several randomized trials already are underway studying the roles of various micronutrients and chemopreventive agents in populations at risk of cancer. The expectation is, that by more closely approximating the experiment, more definitive data on the potential public health benefits of dietary change may result.

Although having several advantages over the case-control, cohort or, correlational study, intervention trials also have many unique difficulties. These have been summarized elsewhere (Magnus and Miller, 1980; Mettlin et al., 1986) and include problems relating to logistics, compliance, management of the control population, specificity of the intervention and, selectivity in subject recruitment.

The first of these, logistics, involves questions of

whether the resources, financial and manpower, are available to recruit and intervene upon the large populations over the long interval that would be required to discern significant effects. One approach to this problem is to focus attention upon persons at particularly high risk of disease to increase the number of disease events expected. The disadvantage of this approach is possibly that nutritional change may affect persons at high risk differently than persons of lesser risk and, the generalizability of the trial result to less than high risk populations will be unknown.

Achieving sufficient change in dietary habits in a large population and sustaining these changes across a long period of time represents another uncertainty with the intervention trial method. Simple behaviors, such as pill taking, may be introduced to a population with minimal instruction and may be monitored by several means. Achieving large reductions in dietary fat intake would require much more complex instruction involving issues of food selection, food preparation and, cooperation of family members. Monitoring changes would be subject to the limits of the sensitivity of diet measurement cited earlier.

Untreated populations, control groups, may require management and monitoring as well to insure that they do not, on their own, adopt the food habits being acquired by the intervention group. Unlike a drug trial, it would be difficult to provide a placebo to control subjects and it is uncertain how the different levels of attention provided to the treatment and control groups would affect their health behaviors.

As is the case with observational studies, the interrelated nature of the human diet will represent a significant obstacle to intervention trial approaches. Reduction of dietary fat may lead to caloric changes and the substitution of fat sources with other macronutrients, such as fiber. Whether subsequently observed changes in risk are attributable to the fat reduction or to the concomitant other changes in diet will be difficult to infer.

Some evidence indicates that persons who are interested in participating in intervention trials differ from others in a number of health related attitudes and behaviors (Mettlin, 1986.) Persons who join a trial with the belief that the dietary change being studied will be effective, may undertake other changes in health habits to help fulfill those expectations. Thus, the outcome of the trial may be as related to the motivations of the subjects as to the efficacy of the intervention.

SUMMARY

Every scientific discipline has unique methodological constraints. Each scientific discipline also has differing degrees of power to resolve different questions. The methods of epidemiology are not exempt from these generalizations. In this brief review, several categories of methodological problems in epidemiological studies of dietary fat and cancer have been cited. Other problems could have been discussed and, several more examples illustrating the occurrence of the problems in research could have been presented.

These problems notwithstanding, epidemiologic study of the association of dietary fat to cancer is an essential investigative tool in moving toward a better understanding of the public health impact of dietary fat. There are no known biological universals, and, as persuasive as data from animal models may be, extrapolation from the laboratory environment to human experience always is tentative. Laboratory methods require human validation before application to populations at risk of disease. Given the mutual dependency of epidemiologic studies and laboratory approaches, it is useful that the evidence from both realms be integrated and evaluated together as they are in this volume.

Finally, given the limitations of any single epidemiologic method applied to the topic, future progress in understanding the role of dietary fat in cancer cause and prevention must rely on the application of multiple methodologies. By this means, it may be possible to compare and contrast the findings from different approaches to yield insights which would not otherwise be achievable.

REFERENCES

Bazzarre TL, Yuhas JA (1983). Comparative evaluation of methods of collecting food intake data for cancer epidemiology studies. Nutr Cancer 5:201-214.

Block G, Dresser CM, Hartman AM, Carroll MD (1985). Nurient sources in the American diet: quantitative data from the NHANES II survey. Am J Epidemiol 122:27-40.

Byers T, Rosenthal R, Marshall J, Rzepka T, Cummings KM, Graham S (1983). Dietary history from the distant past: a methodological study. Nutr Cancer 5:69-77.

Boyle P, Zaridze DG, Smans M (1985). Descriptive epidemiology of colorectal cancer. Int J Cancer 36:9-18.

Frisch RE, Wyshal G, Albright NL, Albright TE, Schiff I, Jones KP, Witschi J, Shiang E, Koff E, Marguglio M (1985). Lower prevalence of breast cancer and cancers of the reproductive system among former college atheletes compared to non-atheletes. Br J Cancer 52:885-891.

Graham S, Mettlin C (1979). Diet and colon cancer. Am J Epidemiol 109:1-20.

La Vecchia C, Pampallona S (1986). Age at first birth, dietary pracices and breast cancer mortality in various Italian regions. Oncology 43:1-6.

Lee J, Kolonel LN, Hankin JH (1983). On establishing the interchangeability of different dietary-intake assessment methods used in studies of diet and cancer. Nutr Cancer 5:215-218.

Magnus K, Miller AB (1980). Controlled prophylactic trials in cancer. J Natl Cancer Instit 66:1196-1305.

McCall DC, Sanches A (1967). Trends in fat disappearance in the United States, 1909-1965 J Nutr 93:1-28.

McKeown-Eyssen GE, Thomas DC (1985). Sample size determination in case-control studies: the influence of the distribution of exposure. J Chron Dis 39:559-568.

Mettlin C (1986). Changing the public's health behaviors by

diet and chemopreventive interventions. in Meyskens F, Prasad K, Moon T (Eds.) Vitamins and Cancer. Humana Press.

Mettlin C, Cummings KM, Walsh D (1986). Risk factor and behavior correlates of willingness to participate in cancer prevention trials. Nutr Cancer 7:198-198.

Vena J, Graham S, Zielezny M, Swanson MK, Barnes RE, Nolan J (1985). Lifetime occupational exercise and colon cancer. Am J Epidemiol 122:357-365.

Dietary Fat and Cancer, pages 17–32
© 1986 Alan R. Liss, Inc.

DIETARY FAT AND THE EPIDEMIOLOGY OF BREAST CANCER

Anthony B. Miller

NCIC Epidemiology Unit
University of Toronto
Toronto, Ontario M5S 1A8, Canada

INTRODUCTION

Breast cancer is the number 1 ranking cancer in women in the world (Parkin et al., 1984). Breast cancer is well recognized as hormonally associated but diet for some time has been suspected as an important cause (Miller and Bulbrook, 1980; 1986). In particular, animal experimental studies have demonstrated that in the presence as well as the absence of mammary carcinogens, the incidence of mammary tumors in rats increases substantially with high fat diets, providing the diet contains a small amount of unsaturated fat (Carroll and Hopkins, 1979).

However, it is the purpose of this paper to consider the epidemiologic evidence associating high dietary fat intake with incidence and mortality from breast cancer. This evidence, though not conclusive, has been considered by at least one expert committee to justify recommending dietary guidelines that may reduce the incidence of breast and other cancers (Committee on diet, nutrition and cancer, 1982). I shall review this evidence under two broad headings, that from descriptive epidemiology and that from analytic epidemiology, and then consider the implications for further research and for breast cancer prevention.

DESCRIPTIVE EPIDEMIOLOGY

Various studies have suggested that changing environmental factors in a country can increase the incidence of breast cancer, for example in Iceland (Bjarnson et al., 1974) and Japan (Hirayama, 1977). Studies of migrants show the effects of acculturation, usually with a slow change in incidence of breast cancer over several generations (Buell, 1974). In Japanese migrants to California, however, the incidence of breast cancer in pre-menopausal women has now almost reached that of the Caucasian population (Dunn, 1977). Many aspects of lifestyle change with the acculturation to the host country which follows migration. However, dietary aspects of lifestyle are one of the most important, especially if the migrants are rapidly absorbed into the surrounding cultural milieu. This may be happening in Israel, where substantial changes are occurring in the rates of cancer in groups that have migrated there from Africa and Asia, together with a rise in the incidence in the Israeli born up to the levels experienced by those born in Europe and America (Steinitz, 1982). These changes are occurring almost as rapidly for breast cancer as they are for colo-rectal cancer, suggesting that some influences on breast cancer do not necessarily operate only in early life or adolescence, as had tended to be assumed from the changes following migration of the Japanese.

Some studies of special religious groups (Lyon et al, 1980) also suggest the influence of cultural or lifestyle factors on the etiology of breast cancer. Interestingly, some cohort studies of religious groups who entered orders or changed to a special group in adult life have not shown lower breast cancer rates than expected from the general population. This is true for Adventist women in California (Phillips et al, 1980), as well as members of strict religious orders in Britain who eschew or eat very little meat (Kinlen, 1982). This suggests that if dietary factors operated in these groups at all, they had to do so before adult life, or alternatively that the use of high fat dairy products in these groups in substitution for meat maintained a total fat intake little less than normal. Kinlen (1982) attempted to evaluate the latter in his study of nuns by making a crude estimate of dietary fat intake. He found no evidence of an association. Kinlen et al. (1983) also failed to find any indication of lower portions of breast cancer deaths, or for that matter deaths from cardiovascular disease, among members of a vegetarian society. Nevertheless, Moolgavkar et al. (1980) have shown that changes in incidence of breast cancer in different

populations can be related to changes in successive birth
cohorts, supporting the possibility that patterns
established in relatively early life are critical.

Somewhat more informative but still not conclusive have
been population correlation studies associating breast
cancer incidence and mortality with total dietary fat and
other nutrient intake. Such correlations have been noted
internationally (Drasar and Irving, 1973; Armstrong and
Doll, 1975; Carroll 1975; Knox, 1977) but also within Japan
(Hirayama, 1977). In the United States strong correlations
were noted with total fat, saturated and unsaturated fat and
fat of vegetable origin but not with animal fat (Enig et
al., 1978). Hirayama (1977) commented that dietary fat
intake appears to have shown the most striking increase of
all the nutritional changes that have been noted in Japan in
recent years. Gaskill et al. (1979) found a positive
correlation between breast cancer mortality and milk, table
fats, beef, calories, protein and fat, and a negative
correlation with egg consumption within the United States.
Only the association of milk and egg consumption remained
significant, however, when age of first marriage (as an
indicator of age at first birth) was controlled. These two
associations also persisted after controlling for other
demographic and dietary variables including intake of fat.
This study thus suggested a special role for dairy products
in the etiology of breast cancer. Hems (1978) found age-
standardized breast-cancer mortality rates for women of 41
countries during 1970-71 were positively correlated with
total fat, animal protein and animal calories, independently
of other components of diet for 1964-66. Differences in
childbearing appeared to contribute little to the variation
of breast cancer mortality rates between countries. (Hems
(1980) subsequently evaluated changes of breast cancer
mortality for women in England and Wales between 1911 and
1975 in relation to changes in the consumption of fat, sugar
and animal protein one to two decades earlier. The
association was strongest for fat and sugar intake one
decade earlier. The mortality changes were not related to
changes in child-bearing. He noted that the social class
gradient in breast cancer mortality almost disappeared
during the 1950's, rates declining for the upper classes but
increasing for the lower. These changes could have resulted
from the changes that occurred in the diet of the different
classes in the early 1940's.

Schrauzer (1976,1977) postulated an inverse relationship between mortality from breast and colon cancer and the consumption of cereals and seafoods, according to food consumption tables published by the Food and Agricultural Organization. There appeared to be a direct correlation between these cancers and a high intake of fat, sugar, and meat (Schrauzer, 1975). Schrauzer suggested that food consumption patterns reflected the selenium content of the diets consumed, and postulated a negative correlation between selenium intake of population groups and their mortality from cancer.

One of the difficulties of many of the studies performed to date, is a failure of the investigators to consider the effect of multiple variables, and their inter-relationships. In the past this was often due to the complexity of the required analytic procedures so that most analyses were conducted in the univariate mode. In addition, many of the available data sets were either too small, or contained too little information on many of the variables that should be considered, to permit such analyses. Gray et al. (1979) however attempted in a population type correlation analysis to evaluate the effect of total fat and animal protein consumption on breast cancer incidence and mortality rates internationally while controlling for height, weight and age at menarche. They found that a significant effect of the dietary variables persisted after controlling for the other factors. This suggests that although some of the effects of diet on breast cancer may be mediated through effects on risk factors such as height, weight and age at menarche, there would seem to be more direct effects as well.

In general, therefore, population correlation studies, especially at the international level, but to a lesser extent at the national level also, have been strongly supportive of an association between dietary fat and breast cancer. Such associations cannot prove causation, but they point the way to the need for further studies at the individual level. They may also provide stronger evidence in favour of the association than is possible at an individual level, as the variation between fat intake is greater between countries at different stages of development and with different cultural habits than may be seen between individuals within a country, where the diet may be relatively homogeneous.

ANALYTIC EPIDEMIOLOGY

Indirect evidence comes from the effect of certain risk factors for breast cancer, which are themselves probably nutritionally mediated. These are particularly weight, height (and the related indices of body mass dependent on height and weight) and age at menarche.

The role of obesity in increasing the risk of breast cancer, especially in post-menopausal women, has been fairly extensively reviewed (de Waard, 1982; Miller, 1985; Miller and Bulbrook, 1986). Although a few studies have been negative, most studies have shown an association of excess weight with post-menopausal breast cancer but not with breast cancer in pre-menopausal women. Some of the strongest evidence has come from a large case-control study in Israel (Lubin et al, 1985). However, no study has yet clarified whether the effect of obesity is secondary to high calorie intake, to relatively low energy expenditure or to high intake of other nutrients such as dietary fat. Nevertheless, as breast cancer in some studies has had, if anything, a stronger relationship to fat intake in pre-menopausal women than in post-menopausal women (Howe, 1985), excess weight would seem to be an additional factor over and above dietary fat intake.

Age at menarche is a risk factor for breast cancer, though the effect is relatively weak (Miller, 1978). Women with an early age at menarche, especially prior to the age of 12, have the highest risk. There is evidence that body weight and food intake are related to early estrus of rats (Frisch et al., 1975) supportive of the hypothesis that a critical body composition of fatness is essential for estrus in the rat, as it appears to be for age at menarche in the human female (Frisch and McArthur, 1975). Hence the effect of diet and nutrition on breast cancer could be at least partly through age at menarche (Miller and Bulbrook, 1980).

Petrakis et al. (1981) investigated nipple aspirates of breast fluid from nonpregnant healthy women. Cholesterol levels were found to be elevated above plasma levels and to increase with advancing age. Cholesterol epoxide, a carcinogen in animals, was detected in 7 of 17 women, most of whom had high levels of breast fluid cholesterol. Petrakis hypothesized that high dietary fat may increase the level of cholesterol in breast fluid with local derivation of carcinogenic substances such as cholesterol epoxide.

The presumably most conclusive evidence, should come from studies of diet and nutrition at the individual level, either of the case-control or cohort type. Difficulties with dietary methodology have tended to inhibit investigations of this type. So far preliminary results of only one cohort study has been reported but several case-control studies are contributory.

The earliest case-control study involved 77 breast cancer cases and controls (Phillips, 1975). The cases were discharged from 2 Adventist operated hospitals and the controls, where possible, comprised 2 for each case selected from hospitalized cases of hernia and osteoarthritis and a third from the general Seventh-day Adventist population. The food questions in the interview were designed to test the hypothesis that intake of high fat, low fiber or both are associated with risk for breast cancer. Five foods were associated with breast cancer; fried foods, fried potatoes, hard fat frying, dairy products except milk, white bread, with relative risks ranging from 1.6 to 2.6. That for fried potatoes was highest and highly significant.

The second was a case-control study in four areas of Canada (Eastern Townships area of Quebec, Toronto, Southern Manitoba and Sasketchewan) involving in all 400 newly diagnossed cases and 400 neighbourhood controls (Miller et al., 1978). Three different approaches to assessment of diet were used, a 24 hour recall, a 4 day diary and a detailed quantitative diet history. However, the results were derived from the diet history, as this gave a higher response than the diary from the controls, and was directed to a period 6 months prior to the time of interview, and thus prior to the point of diagnosis of the cases. In a preliminary report (Miller, 1977) results from a mean of the diary and diet history were given, which suggested an association with total fat intake. In the main report the mean nutrient intake as estimated by the dietary history alone for 6 nutrients (total calories, total fat, saturated fat, oleic acid, linoleic acid and cholesterol) was greater for the cases as a group than the controls though the differences were not statistically significant when the pre-menopausal and post-menopausal groups were considered independently. In a risk ratio analysis, the strongest association in the pre-menopausal group was for total fat with weaker associations for saturated fat and cholesterol. When the effect of each nutrient was controlled for the effect of the others, the association for total fat increased in strength while those for saturated fat and cholesterol diminished. In the post-menopausal group, the only consistent finding was for total fat intake. The risk ratios were low (1.6 for total fat in pre-menopausal women and 1.5 for post-menopausal women) and there was no evidence of a dose response relationship.

In a re-analysis of these data, Howe (1985) found that combining the data from the 24-hour recall and diet history (6 months before interview) resulted in increased strength of the association. He found increasing risk with increasing consumption of saturated fat, significant at the p = 0.02 level. The risk for estimated daily intake of saturated fat greater than 35g relative to less than 23g was 2.4 for all women, 5.9 for pre-menopausal women and 1.5 for post-menopausal women. The trend was highly significant in pre-menopausal but not significant in post-menopausal women.

Lubin et al. (1981) reported the results of a case-control study in Northern Alberta, Canada, involving 577 women age 30 to 80 with breast cancer interviewed in 1976-77, and 826 disease-free controls interviewed subsequently. The questionnaire included information on the frequency with which eight food items and milk and butter were usually consumed. The major sources of animal fat and animal protein were represented. Significant increasing trends of risk with more frequent consumption of beef, pork and sweet deserts were found. The relative risk for the highest consumption level of beef or pork compared to the lowest was 2.7. Elevated risks were also noted for the use of butter at the table and for frying with butter and margarine, as opposed to vegetable oils. Using standard portion sizes, estimates of consumption of animal fat were computed. Risk increased significantly with increasing indices of consumption of animal fat and animal protein, but not with cholesterol intake. The risk for the highest consumption level of animal fat or animal protein relative to the lowest was 1.8. Although the relative risk was higher in this study from beef/pork intake than estimated consumption of animal fat, the evidence on mechanisms from animal studies suggests that high fat intake is the relevant risk factor, meat consumption contributing to high risk because of high fat content.

Graham et al. (1982) reported the analysis of food frequency questionnaires administered to 2024 cases of breast cancer and 1463 hospital controls without cancer at Roswell Park Memorial Institute from 1958 to 1965. No association of breast cancer with estimated consumption of animal fat or other dietary factors was found. However this was a relatively brief questionnaire with estimates of fat consumption based on standard portion sizes and was not specifically designed to assess the fat hypothesis.

In an indirect attempt to assess the diet of women with breast cancer, Nomura et al. (1978) compared the diet of 86 Japanese men whose wives had developed breast cancer with that of the remaining 6774 men in Hawaii who had had dietary data collected in the Japan-Hawaii Cancer Study. They assumed that there is a similarity between the diet of husbands and wives. They found that the husbands of the cases consumed more beef or meat, butter/margarine/cheese, corn and weiners and less Japanese foods than the control spouses.

Preliminary findings from a case-control study in Hawaii have been reported (Kolonel et al., 1983). A positive association between breast cancer risk and the intake of dietary fat (particularly saturated fat) and animal protein in post-menopausal women, especially the Japanese, was noted. However, in a report on obesity including the case-control study population on whom dietary information was obtained in Israel, it was noted that an association with dietary fat intake had also been found (Lubin et al., 1985). The increased risk of breast cancer appeared among high fat, high animal protein consumers age 50+. No correlation between high fat, high animal protein consumption and overweight was found.

Hislop et al. (1985) used a food frequency questionnaire directed to current diet and to dietary practices in childhood in a case-control study in British Columbia, Canada. Although unable to determine nutrient intake, they found significant associations with current intake of fat associated foods, especially whole milk and beef, while increased risk was found for those who consumed visible fat on meat, both recently and in childhood.

Hirayama (1985) has been following a large cohort of Japanese men and women from whom dietary information was collected in the mid 1960s. Associations are now being seen of increased risk of breast cancer for those with daily consumption of meat (possibly due to higher fat consumption). This seems congruent with the increasing incidence and mortality from breast cancer being seen in Japan.

One possible mechanism for the effect of high fat diets in increaing the risk of breast cancer would be through changes in serum cholesterol and/or plasma lipids. However, a prospective study of women who have had such measurements failed to find evidence of an association (Hiatt et al., 1982). Nevertheless, if the relevant mechanism is dependent on the levels of fat in the intestine differences in cholesterol or blood lipids are not only likely to be minimal but irrelevant. Even so, a study of the incidence and mortality of cancer of the breast among women who had previously had total colectomy and terminal ileostomy, mostly for ulcerative colitis, or Crohn's disease, failed to find a lower incidence of breast cancer, though there was a slight deficiency of deaths from this cause (Rang et al., 1983). These findings suggest that, at least in adult life, the colon may not be involved in the etiology of breast cancer.

DISCUSSION

It is clear that a number of different sources of information support the association of diet, especially high fat in the diet, with risk of breast cancer. Although further epidemiological study is desirable to clarify the association, and experimental work to determine more precisely the mechanism, the increasing consistency of the evidence derived from the epidemiologic studies and the similar data derived from experimental studies, suggest that the association is causal. Indeed, some of this evidence, together with similar evidence relating to colo-rectal and other cancers, led a committee of the U.S. National Academy of Sciences (1982) to recommend attempts to achieve population reduction of dietary fat intake from the present level of 40% to 30% of available calories. This reduction seems achievable without a major disturbance in dietary habits, is unlikely to be hazardous and after a period, should result in a reduction in the incidence of breast and other fat-associated cancers. It is important that early action be taken to ensure that the population makes appropriate changes in their diet. If, as some of the migrant and other descriptive studies suggest, much of the effect of diet and nutrition in increasing the risk of breast cancer operates early in life, there could be a substantial delay before the full impact of primary prevention is seen in the population (Miller, 1983).

Some of the available case-control studies can be used to derive an estimate of the possible effect on risk of breast cancer of reduction in fat intake. Miller (1978) computed a population attributable risk of 27% for total fat intake on the basis of his case control study in Canada (Miller et al., 1978). From another study in Canada (Lubin et al., 1981) population attributable risks for intake of beef and pork intake can be computed. Dichotomizing the consumption of beef between the author's levels 4 and 5, and for pork between their levels 3 and 4, results in estimates of attributable risk of 27% and 26% respectively. Because of the imprecision of dietary methodology, such estimates are likely to be too low rather than too high (Jensen et al., 1984). Further they probably underestimate the eventual potential for prevention, as they relate to current intake rather than that in early life.

However, more discriminating data on the desirable level of fat intake that should be regarded as the optimum for human populations is still needed. We need to resolve in man the relative importance of different types of fat, particularly the possible opposed effects of unsaturated and saturated fats. We also need to determine the dose response for cancer induction for total, unsaturated and saturated fats. Thus we need to answer the question "At what level does further protection from (breast) cancer from lowering fat intake cease?" Does it cease at 30% or should we aim for 25% or even 20% or less? We also need to be concerned over the possibility that adverse effects on health, either through increased incidence of other cancer sites, unexpected effects on cardiovascular disease, etc., might offset the benefits derived by reducing the incidence of fat associated cancers.

Where is the evidence required likely to come from? The NAS Committee on Diet, Nutrition and Cancer (1983) made several recommendations for further research in this area. Further observational analytic epidemiologic studies are clearly needed, both of the case-control and cohort type. Case-control studies could profitably be performed in different populations with differing diets and breast cancer incidence. Cohort studies in which dietary data are collected well in advance of the diagnosis offer the advantage that the dietary information may well be collected at a more relevant time period to the natural history of the cancer, but also suffer from the disadvantages of less complete dietary information, expense, and long duration of follow-up required. One such study is now underway in Canada.

Pending the results of these observational studies, there are many who feel that carefully planned intervention studies of dietary factors that may prevent cancer induction should now be initiated in man. An alternative would be to promote more radical population dietary changes and then access trends in incidence and mortality. Essentially this was the approach used over smoking and lung cancer. However, apart from the long delay before an effect may be detectable, especially in the case of dietary fat and breast cancer, the strength of the association between dietary fat and breast cancer is so much weaker than in the case of smoking and lung cancer that many will remain unconvinced of the causal nature of the association without confirmation from an intervention trial. To moment such a trial on breast cancer and fat, will require detailed and repeated instruction in the ways to achieve a low fat diet. Although far from simple, some groups have already initiated pilot studies in this area and, in women who perceive themselves at high risk for breast cancer, have already achieved substantial success. Wynder and Cohen (1982) recommended an intervention study of fat reduction in women with stage 2 breast cancer, as there is some experimental evidence that supports such an approach in experimental animals. However, a follow-up of 300 of the cases in our case-control study of diet and breast cancer has failed to find any influence of fat on prognosis of breast cancer, though excess weight, and possibly particularly obesity, was associated with poor prognosis (Newman et al, 1986). This supports a suggestion by deWaard (1982) that weight reduction should be assessed as a means of improving prognosis in women with breast cancer. If intervention studies of reduction in fat intake in women at high risk for breast cancer do proceed they must be carefully planned. They should involve randomization of subjects to experimental and control groups whenever possible. Care will have to be taken to define high risk in a way relevant to the hypothesis under test. Thus it does not seem sensible to define this by, for example, family history. Rather, some attempt should be made to select women at risk by virtue of a high fat intake (Miller and Bulbrook, 1986). The intervention should also be carefully planned to avoid dilution. Thus care will have to be taken to ensure compliance with the recommended dietary changes in the study group but minimal dietary changes in the control group. To achieve will not be easy, especially if informed consent of all subjects is insisted upon and major public campaigns on diet and cancer are mounted. Further, the intervention will not have to be so complex that it would be impossible to use this as an approach to control breast cancer in the general population subsequently.

This is a formidable list of problems, but care taken in the design stage of a trial will bring dividends later. Further, there will be other benefits from such a trial, not least assessment of the impact of dietary modification on other fat associated cancers, especially if the woman's spouse is also followed, as inevitably there will be changes in his diet as a consequence of those practiced by his wife. Some will object to the idea of any trial because of doubts on whether the cost will justify such "risky" research. However, failing to mount a trial means that all we can do is to advise the public on the actions they should take and monitor the subsequent impact of changes in diet on the cancer rates in the population. Probably both approaches can be supported, yet as the need now is for firmer evidence to justify major shifts of diet in the population, the intervention trial approach would seem to be the most scientifically justifiable.

REFERENCES

Armstrong B, Doll R (1975). Environmental factors and cancer incidence and mortality in different countries, with special reference to dietary practices. Int J Cancer 15:617-631.
Bjarnson O, Day M, Snaedal G, Tulinius H (1974). The effect of year of birth on the breast cancer age incidence curve in Iceland. Int J Cancer 13:689-696.

Buell P (1974). Changing incidence of breast cancer in Japanese-American women. J Nat Cancer Inst 51:1479-1483.

Carroll KK (1975). Experimental evidence of dietary factors and hormone-dependent cancers. Cancer Res 35:3374-3383.

Carroll KK, Hopkins GJ (1979). Dietary polyunsaturated fat versus saturated fat in relation to mammary carcinogenesis. Lipids 14:155-158.

Committee on diet, nutrition and cancer (1982). Diet, nutrition and cancer. Assembly of Life Sciences, National Research Council. National Academy Press, Washington, D.C.

Committee on diet, nutrition, and cancer (1983). Diet, nutrition and cancer; Directions for research. Commission on Life Sciences, National Research Council. National Academy Press, Washington, D.C.

de Waard F (1982). Nutritional epidemiology of breast cancer: where are we now, and where are we going? Nutr Cancer 4:85-89.

Drasar BS, Irving D (1973). Environmental factors and cancer of the colon and breast. Brit J Cancer 27:167-172.

Dunn JE (1977). Breast cancer among American Japanese in the San Francisco Bay area. Nat Cancer Inst Mon 47:157-160.

Enig MG, Munn RJ, Kenney M (1978). Dietary fats and cancer trends - a critique. Fed Proc 37:2215-2220.

Frisch RE, Hegsted DM, Yoshinaga K (1975). Body weight and food intake at early estrus of rats on a high fat diet. Proc Nat Acad Sci, U.S.A. 72:4172-4176.

Frisch RE, McArthur J (1974). Menstrual cycles: Fatness as a determinant of minimum weight for height necessary for their maintenance or onset. Science 185:949-951.

Gaskill SP, McGuire WL, Osborne CK, Stern MP (1979). Breast cancer mortality and diet in the United States. Cancer Res 39:3628-3637.

Graham S, Marshall J, Mettlin C, Rzepka T, Nemoto T, Byers T (1982). Diet in the epidemiology of breast cancer. Am J Epidemiol 116:68-75.

Gray GE, Pike MC, Henderson BE (1979). Breast cancer incidence and mortality rates in different countries in relation to known factors and dietary practices. Brit J Cancer 39:1-7.

Hems G (1978). The contributions of diet and child bearing to breast cancer rates. Brit J Cancer 37: 974-982.

Hems G (1980). Associations between breast cancer mortality rates, child-bearing and diet in the United Kingdom. Brit J Cancer 41:429-437.

Hiatt RA, Friedman GD, Bawol RD, Ury HK (1982). Breast cancer and serum cholesterol. J Nat Cancer Inst 68:885-889.

Hirayama T (1977). Changing patterns of cancer in Japan with special reference to the decrease of stomach cancer mortality. In "Origins of Human Cancer". Cold Spring Harbor Laboratory, Cold Spring Harbor, N.Y., pp 55-75.

Hirayama T (1985). Personal communication.

Hislop TG, Coldman AJ, Bauer G, Kan L (1985). Childhood and recent eating patterns and risk of breast cancer. Cancer Detect Prev, in press.

Howe GR (1985). The use of polytomous dual response data to increase power in case control studies: an application to the association between dietary fat and breast cancer. J Chron Dis 38:663-670.

Jensen OM, Wahrendorf J, Rosenquist A, Geser A (1984). The reliability of questionnaire - derived historical dietary information and temporal stability of food habits in individuals. Am J Epidemiol 120:218-289.

Kinlen LJ (1982). Meat and fat consumption and cancer mortality: A study of strict religious orders in Britain. Lancet 1:946-949.

Kinlen LJ, Herman C, Smith PG (1983). A proportionate study of cancer mortality among members of a vegetarian society. Br J Cancer 48:355-361.

Knox EG (1977). Foods and diseases. Brit J Soc Prev Med 31:71-80.

Kolonel LN, Nomura AMY, Hinds MW, Hirohata T, Hankin JH, Lee J (1983). Role of diet in cancer incidence in Hawaii. Cancer Res 43:2397s-2402s.

Lubin F, Ruder AM, Wax Y, Modan B (1985). Overweight and changes in weight throughout adult life in breast cancer etiology. Am J Epidemiol 122:579-588.

Lubin JH, Burns PE, Blot WJ, Ziegler RG, Lees AW, Fraumeni JF (1981). Dietary factors and breast cancer risk. Int J Cancer 28:685-689.

Lyon JL, Gardner JW, West DW (1980). Cancer risk and life-style: Cancer among Mormons from 1967-1975. In Cairns J, Lyon JL, Skolnick M (eds): "Cancer Incidence in Defined Populations". Banbury Report 4. New York: Cold Spring Harbor Laboratory, Cold Spring Harbor, pp 3-27.

Miller AB (1977). Role of nutrition in the etiology of breast cancer. Cancer 39:2704-2708.

Miller AB (1978). An overview of hormone associated cancers. Cancer Res 38:3985-3990.

Miller AB (1983). Approaches to the control of breast cancer. In Rich MA, Hager JC and Furmanski P (eds): "Understanding Cancer. Clinical Laboratory Concepts," New York: Marcel Dekker, Inc., pp 3-25.

Miller AB (1985). Obesity and cancer. In Frankle RT, Dwyer J, Moragne L, Owen A (eds): "Dietary Treatment and Prevention of Obesity," London: John Libby, pp 155-166.

Miller AB, Bulbrook RD (1980). Special report: The epidemiology and etiology of breast cancer. New Engl J Med 303:1246-1248.

Miller AB, Bulbrook RD (1986). The epidemiology, etiology and prevention of breast cancer. Int J Cancer, in press.

Miller AB, Kelly A, Choi NW, Matthews V, Morgan RW, Munan L, Burch JD, Feather J, Howe GR, Jain M (1978). A study of diet and breast cancer. Am J Epidemiol 107:499-509.

Moolgavkar SH, Day NE, Stevens RG (1980). Two-stage model for carcinogenesis: Epidemiology of breast cancer in females. J Nat Cancer Inst 65:559-569.

Newman SC, Miller AB, Howe GR (1986). A study of the effect of weight and dietary fat on breast cancer survival time. Am J Epidemiol, in press.

Nomura A, Henderson BE, Lee J (1978). Breast cancer and diet among the Japanese in Hawaii. Am J Clin Nutr 31:2020-2025.

Parkin DM, Stjernsward J, Muir CS (1984). Estimates of the worldwide frequency of twelve major cancers. Bull World Hlth Org 62:163-182.

Petrakis NL, Gruenke LD, Craig JC (1981). Cholesterol and cholesterol epoxides in nipple aspirates of human breast fluid. Cancer Res 41:2563-2565.

Phillips RL (1975). Role of life-style and dietary habits in risk of cancer among Seventh-Day Adventists. Cancer Res 35:3513-3522.

Phillips RL, Garfinkel L, Kuzoma JW, Beeson WL, Lotz T, Brim B (1980). Mortality among California Seventh-Day Adventists for selected cancer sites. J Natl Cancer Inst 65:1097-1107.

Rang EH, Kinlen LJ, Herman-Taylor J (1983). A study of cancer of the breast and other sites in women after total colectomy and ileostomy for non-malignant disorders. Lancet 1:1014-1017.

Schrauzer GN (1975). Selenium and cancer. A review. Bioin Chem 5:275-281.

Schrauzer GN (1976). Cancer mortality correlation studies II. Regional associations of mortalities with the consumption of foods and other commodities. Med Hypoth 2:39.

Schrauzer GN, White DA, Schneider CJ (1977). Cancer mortality correlation studies III. Statistical associations with dietary selenium intakes. Bioin Chem, 7:23-34.

Steinitz R (1982). Cancer risks in immigrant populations in Israel. In Aoki K (ed): "Proceedings of the First UICC Conference on Cancer Prevention in Developing Countries," University of Nagoya Press, pp 363-381.

Wynder EL, Cohen L (1982). A rationale for dietary intervention in the treatment of postmenopausal breast cancer patients. Nutr Cancer 3:195-199.

Dietary Fat and Cancer, pages 33–41
© 1986 Alan R. Liss, Inc.

BODY SIZE, BODY MASS AND CANCER OF THE BREAST

by F.de Waard

National Institute of Public Health and
Environmental Hygiene, Bilthoven, The Netherlands

THE HYPOTHESIS

The French surgeon Paul Broca was probably the first to
note that there might be a relationship between body weight
and mammary cancer.

Our interest in this matter, which arose in the late
1950s, derived from an epidemiologic study of cancer of the
endometrium. While many gynecologists had observed an association between the incidence of this predominantly post-
menopausal cancer and the triad of obesity, hypertension
and decreased glucose tolerance, others had focused on the
possibility of a causal role being played by the unopposed
action of estrogens (Novak, 1954). We also postulated that
estrogen production from extra-ovarian sources might be
found in women possessing the above triad. While we were
sorting out which of the three clinical signs was the most
important variable in this respect, a paper by Desaive et
al. (1958) drew our attention to the existence of a bimodal
age distribution of breast cancer patients (corresponding
to 'Clemmesen's hook' in age-specific incidence curves);
they speculated that the two modes represented the peaks of
two frequency distributions, one of them premenopausal (with
the involvement of ovarian estrogens and the other postmenopausal (involving adrenal estrogens).

In synopsis, the background to our current thinking is
as follows: a case-control study (de Waard et al., 1964)
showed that overweight and high blood pressure were indeed
more prevalent in patients with breast cancer than in a

control population and that this association was confined
to those aged 50 or over. Moreover, by means of exfoliative
cytology, it was shown that the main determinant of estrogen
status in the postmenopausal female was overweight (de Waard
and Oettlé, 1965; de Waard and Baanders, 1969). These findings gained general acceptance after Poortman et al. (1973)
and MacDonald et al. (1978) had elucidated the biochemical
basis of extra-ovarian estrogen production.

Several papers published within the framework of Mac-
Mahon's international study confirmed an association between
body weight and breast cancer (Mirra et al., 1971; Lin et al.,
1971). At present, the literature consists of some 20 papers
on case-control studies, most of which report such a relationship in the postmenopausal period (for references see
de Waard 1982, 1986). In addition, similar findings have
been reported in a few cohort studies and population
screening projects.

When evaluating the effect of obesity on the risk of
breast cancer, it emerged that height was also a risk factor
(de Waard and Baanders, 1974; Lin et al., 1971). Since any
index of overweight is computed by correcting weight for
height, the degree of risk attached to obesity is highly
dependent on the relative importance of height itself as a
further determinant of the degree of risk. This problem not
only complicated the statistics, but also made us somewhat
uncertain whether the pathophysiologic mechanism relating
body weight to cancer of the breast was really dependent
upon estrogens. If body size (in terms of body surface area,
which is calculated from weight and height) were a better
anthropometric variable, one would have to consider other
biologic mechanisms.

A solution to this dilemma was provided by the discovery that the effect of height was present at all ages (de
Waard et al., 1977) whereas that of weight was restricted
to the postmenopausal age group. Since height is determined
at a young age its effect on breast cancer risk may be
related to the determinant of early menarche. Apparently
nutritional factors operating at puberty and adolescence
set the stage for neoplastic development in the mammary
gland.

Thus, height may be a marker of endocrine events which
contribute to early stages of malignant change. In contrast,

as we shall see, obesity probably acts very late in the carcinogenic process, viz., as a growth-enhancing factor on estrogen-sensitive cancer cells in the postmenopause, when the ovarian source of estrogen has dried up.

This notion developed when we analyzed estrogen-receptor status in cancers occurring in a population screened for cancer of the breast (de Waard et al., 1984). It was discovered that patients whose cancers contained estrogen receptors (E.R. +) were, on the average, heavier than their counterparts in the overall population of screened women. However, patients with cancers not containing receptors (E.R. -) were definitely leaner than their peers in the population from which they derived. These findings could be explained by assuming that relative weight determined the composition of a mix of E.R.positive and E.R. negative cells in a cancer.

Since our screening project was undertaken in a population aged 50 or over at the time of entry to the study, almost all breast cancer cases were postmenopausal. Thus, estrogen status depended heavily on the amount of adipose tissue as the main endogenous source of estrogen (the use of estrogenic drugs is less prevalent in the Netherlands than in the U.S.). We concluded that E.R.positive cancer cells were thriving in overweight women and constituted a majority of the cancer cells; on the other hand, in women without sufficient estrogen (the lean ones) E.R.positive cancer cells would not grow and divide so as to be overwhelmed by clones of E.R.negative cancer cells that multiplied independently from such stimulus (de Waard et al., 1981).

Such an explanation implied that overweight as a risk factor acts very late in the promotion of breast cancer, viz., as a growth enhancer. This notion fitted well with other observations, the most persuasive of which being that overweight is not only a risk factor but also a prognostic factor in the follow up of cancer of the mammary gland (e.g., Boyd et al., 1981). We were able to confirm the latter finding in a follow-up study of 907 breast cancer patients in the Netherlands (de Waard et al., 1985; see fig.1).

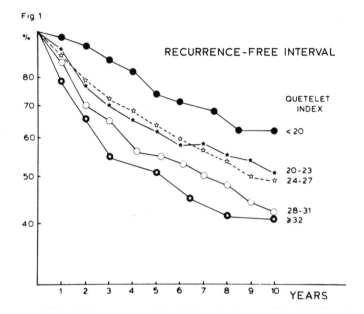

Fig.1 Recurrence-free interval (distant metastases), with respect to Quetelet's index of overweight, in 907 breast cancer patients in the Netherlands, initially treated in 1972-1974.

PROOF OF CAUSATION

In epidemiology a cause is defined as a factor which increases the incidence of the disease under study. The issue is whether we shall ever be in a position to prove scientifically that obesity is a cause of breast cancer.

The criteria for judgment are: consistency and strength of the association, biologic plausibility, time relation between cause and effect, and, finally, the effect of intervention.

The consistency of the association between weight (or overweight) and mammary cancer has been fair to good, with positive findings in about 20 out of 25 epidemiologic studies. Time relationships have been established through a few cohort studies in which increased body weight preceded the incidence of postmenopausal breast cancer.

The strength of the association on a world scale is moderate, with a smooth gradient of risk. The causal nature of the factor obesity seems distinctly possible in the light of endocrine mechanisms which focus on stimuli of extra-ovarian estrogens on hormone-sensitive breast cancer cells.

Final proof will have to come from an intervention study. Such a study would require a very large obese population to be randomized into an intervention group (weight reduction) and a control group; the incidence of mammary cancer would have to be monitored.

However, a study such as this does not look feasible. Apart from the costs involved, our experience suggests that, even with intense efforts, weight reduction in otherwise healthy women who are beyond their first bloom is a very difficult task (Baanders et al., 1984).

There is, however, an alternative method of intervention. Since it is probable that obesity acts only late in the natural history of breast cancer, weight reduction could be started after randomization of obese postmenopausal breast cancer patients (instead of obese otherwise healthy women), and the clinical occurrence of distant metastases could be taken as the outcome variable related to the growth rate of cancer untouched by surgery and/or radio-therapy.

Motivation for weight reduction might be stronger in obese cancer patients than in obese "healthy" women. If the study were to produce results in favor of the group advised to slim, one could interpret these in terms of interference with growth rates of estrogen-sensitive cancer cells. Slower growth of tumor cells in a preventive context would lead to the later appearance of a clinical cancer, which is synonymous with reduced incidence.

In discussing the feasibility of such a study it is often argued that weight reduction might change the cancers from a positive into a negative E.R. status, the latter having a worse prognosis. My response to such criticism is twofold: 1) Weight reduction does not lead to leanness, only to lesser degrees of obesity; 2) The change from

positive to negative E.R.status by means of clonal selection
implies a period when growth rates of E.R.positive cells
are much reduced. Such a reduction of growth rates would
probably compensate well for the difference in prognosis
between E.R.positive and E.R.negative tumors in a clinical
setting. After all, the latter difference is less than one
would expect from the observations of some clinicians (Adami
et al., 1985; Raemakers et al., 1985).

SPECIFIC PUBLIC HEALTH IMPACT OF OVERWEIGHT

The hypothesis that obesity is a risk factor for
breast cancer through its effect on endocrine status in
postmenopausal women has gained acceptance since its formulation some 20 years ago. Apart from the scientific evidence,
there is the question of how important overweight is in
terms of public health, with regard to the prevention of
breast cancer.

This question is more complex than one might think at
first glance. Although obesity is usually defined as heavi-
ness in relation to a given height, it is somewhat arbitrary as to where normal weight ends and overweight begins.
Standards have been derived mainly from American life
insurance data and these relate to total mortality in
Western society.

In the West the distribution of body weights among
women at risk of developing breast cancer is such that
those weighing less than 60 kilograms are taken as the
low risk reference group, with a relative risk of 1.0. With
such a standard the relative risk of breast cancer in the
heaviest subgroup does not usually exceed a factor of 2.
Therefore, the relative importance of obesity as a causative
factor in the etiology of breast cancer is not very impressive.

However, in Japan (which is often taken for comparison
when discussing the high incidence rates in North America
and N.W.Europe) more than one-third of women aged 50-59
were found to weigh less than 45 kilograms (de Waard et al.,
1977). Since the risk gradient of mammary cancer with
respect to weight was present within the 40-49 kg class as
well, the gradient of risk on a world scale is fourfold
rather than twofold.

More or less the same reasoning holds true for height. In the Dutch-Japanese comparison we found that body weight and height taken together could statistically 'explain' about half the difference in breast cancer incidence between the two countries.

There is a conceptual problem in that overweight is defined in terms of a weight/height ratio whereas in populations weight and height tend to vary in a parallel fashion. The latter phenomenon is most clearly seen in the Japanese migrants to Hawaii where the grandchildren (Sansei) of the migrants (Issei) are no less than 10 cm taller than their grandparents (Froehlig, 1970); their increase in weight will lead to only a modest change in their Quetelet index as they grow older. Still, the somatotype is changing dramatically and breast cancer follows closely in a cohort-wise fashion (de Waard, 1978).

Obesity is not the reason for the recent steep rise in the incidence of mammary cancer among second and third generation Americans of Japanese descent. Only some of these have reached the postmenopause , viz., the period when obesity exerts its specific effect. Apparently the early nutritional influences that determine both height and adolescent weight plus associated endocrine effects (such as age at menarche) set the stage for the development of breast cancer, which will be expressed clinically later in life.

REFERENCES

Adami HD, Lindgren A, Sällström J (1985). Prognostic implication of estrogen receptor content in breast cancer. Breast Cancer Res. Treatm. 5: 293-300.

Baanders-van Halewijn EA, Choy YN, van Uitert J, de Waard F, (1984). The Cordon study of weight reduction based on behaviour modification. Int. J. Obesity 8: 161-170.

Boyd NF, Campbell JE, Germanson T, Thomson DB, Sutherland DJ, Meakin JW. Body weight and prognosis in breast cancer. JNCI 67: 785-789 (1981).

Desaive P, Lavigne J, Adrianne A (1958). In: Proc. 2nd.Int. Symp.Mammary Cancer, Perugia, Italy. p. 37-51.

Froehlich JW. Migration and the plasticity of physique in the Japanese Americans of Hawaii. Am J Phys Anthropol 32: 429-442 (1970).

Lin TM, Chen KP, MacMahon B. Epidemiologic characteristics of cancer of the breast in Taiwan. Cancer (1971) 27: 1497-1504.

MacDonald PC, Edman CD, Hemsell DL, Porter JL, Siiteri PK. Effect of obesity on conversion of plasma androstenedione to estrone in postmenopausal women with and without endometrial cancer. Am J Obstet Gynecol 130: 448-453 (1978).

Mirra AP, Cole Ph, MacMahon B (1971). Breast cancer in an area of high parity, Sao Paulo, Brazil.Cancer Res. 31: 79-83.

Novak ER. Relationship of endometrial hyperplasia and adenocarcinoma of the uterine fundus. J Am Med Assoc 154: 217-220 (1954).

Poortman J, Thyssen JHH, Schwarz F (1973). Androgen production and conversion to estrogens in normal postmenopausal women and in selected breast cancer patients. J Clin Endocr 37: 101-109.

Raemakers JMM, Beex LVAM, Koenders AJM, Pieters GFFM, Smals AGH, Benraad ThJ, Kloppenborg PWC (1985). Disease-free interval and estrogen receptor activity in tumor tissue of patients with primary breast cancer: analysis after long-term follow up. Breast Cancer Res. Treatm. 6: 123-130.

De Waard F. Recent time trends in breast cancer incidence. Prev.Med. 7: 160-167 (1978).

De Waard F (1982). Nutritional etiology of breast cancer. Nutrition and Cancer 4: 85-89.

De Waard F (1986). Dietary fat and mammary cancer. Nutrition and Cancer, in press.

De Waard F, Baanders-van Halewijn EA, Huizinga J. The bimodal age distribution of patients with mammary carcinoma. Cancer 17: 141-151 (1964).

De Waard F, Oettle AG. A survey of postmenopausal estrus in Africa. Cancer 18: 450-459 (1965).

De Waard F, Baanders-van Halewijn EA. Cross-sectional data on estrogenic smears in postmenopausal women. Acta Cytol. 13: 675-678 (1969).

De Waard F, Baanders-van Halewijn EA (1974) A prospective

study in general practice on breast cancer risk in post-menopausal women. Int J Ca 14: 153-160.

De Waard F, Cornelis JP, Aoki K, Yoshida M. Breast cancer incidence according to weight and height in two cities of the Netherlands and in Aichi prefecture, Japan Cancer 40: 1269-1275 (1977).

De Waard F, Poortman J, Collette HJA. Relationship of weight to the promotion of breast cancer after menopause. Nutr. Cancer (1981) 2: 237-240.

De Waard F, Collette HJA, Rombach JJ, Baanders-van Halewijn EA, Honing C (1984). The DOM-project for the early detection of breast cancer, Utrecht, the Netherlands. J of chron dis 37: 1-44.

De Waard F, Van der Velden JW, De Does M (1985). De invloed van het relatieve lichaamsgewicht op de prognose van borst-kanker bij vrouwen (in Dutch, with summary in English). Ned.Tijdschr.v.Geneesk. 129: 454-459.

Dietary Fat and Cancer, pages 43–68
© 1986 Alan R. Liss, Inc.

THE BIOCHEMICAL EPIDEMIOLOGY OF PROSTATIC CARCINOMA

David P. Rose, M.D., Ph.D., D.Sc.

American Health Foundation

Valhalla, New York 10595

I.   INTRODUCTION

The biochemical epidemiology of prostate cancer as it is currently represented in the literature, comprises essentially case-control and population-based endocrine studies, and investigations concerned with dietary patterns.

Sex hormones have been implicated in the etiology of prostate cancer because of their requirement for normal and disordered growth, the clinical response of tumors to endocrine manipulation, the presence of steroid hormone receptors in some prostate cancer tissues, and the induction of prostatic tumors in experimental animals by prolonged administration of testosterone. Despite this supporting evidence, assays of serum hormones in prostate cancer patients have, as will be discussed, given generally disappointing results. One possible explanation is that altered circulating hormones in early adulthood may be involved directly or indirectly in the neoplastic process, and that this abnormality is not discernable in later life when hormone levels change as part of the aging process.

There is currently considerable interest in diet-hormonal relationships, not only as these may relate to prostate cancer risk, but also to their possible involvement in the etiology of the other sex hormone-related cancers· those of breast, endometrium and, possibly, ovary. High fat diets may influence hormone production metabolism, or bioactivity, or exert an indirect effect via, say, prostaglandin synthesis. Certainly, international comparisons show an association between animal fat consumption and the incidence of all four sex hormone-related cancers, and the limited amount of data available indicate that dietary fat influences circulating hormone levels.

In this chapter, we will review the evidence that dietary fat and hormones influence prostate cancer risk, and draw comparisons between this important cancer in men, and breast cancer in women.

II. INTERNATIONAL AND INTRANATIONAL VARIATIONS IN PROSTATIC CANCER RISK

In general, there is a good correlation between prostate and breast cancer mortality rates in different countries (Fig. 1). These are highest in northern Europe, and in countries with large population segments of northern European origin. Intermediate in rank are the southern European countries and those of Latin America, while the Far East shows the lowest mortality rates. A number of possible elements common to prostatic and breast cancer could explain these international differences; for example, genetic factors, varying levels of socio-economic and industrial development, and the influence of differing dietary practices between geographic areas. Yet, of the 28 countries in Fig. 1, the United Kingdom ranks first in breast cancer mortality rate, but only eighteenth in prostatic cancer mortality rate (12.1/100,000) occupying a position intermediate between Spain (12.8/100,000) and Venezuela (11.3/100,000). This could be interpreted as indicating that the common risk factor is present in the United Kingdom, but is favorably modified by another unidentified factor specific to prostate cancer.

"Latent carcinoma of the prostate" is a term introduced by Andrews (1949) to describe disease which can be diagnosed only by histological examination and

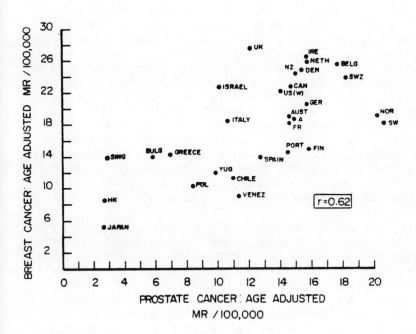

Fig. 1. Relationship between prostate and breast cancer mortality rates for 30 countries in 1978-79. UK = United Kingdom; VENZ = Venezuela; US(W) = United States (white); A = Austria; AUS = Australia; SWZ = Switzerland; SW = Sweden.

is consequently symptom-free. It is usually recognized at autopsy, or in prostates removed for the treatment of benign prostatic hyperplasia (BPH). While Japan has a relatively low incidence of clinically manifest prostatic carcinoma. and hence a low mortality rate, latent cancer is found at autopsy with about the same frequency in Japanese men as in white Americans (Wynder et al., 1971). Within the United States, prostatic cancer risk is particularly high among blacks, but still has a low incidence in African black males (Wynder et al., 1971). Jackson et al. (1977) compared the incidence rates of prostate cancer recognized among blacks at unselected consecutive autopsies in Nigeria and the United States. After age adjustment, the incidence rates of invasive disease per 1000 autopsies were 27.9 in Washington, DC, and 18.5 in Ibadan. The corresponding rates for micro ("latent")-carcinoma were about the same, at 23.5 and 25.5 per 1000 autopsies respectively. These observations, which have been confirmed and refined in other international comparisons (for example, Breslow et al., 1977) are consistent with the operation of an environmental factor in populations with high prostate cancer mortality rates which promotes the progression of pre-existing latent disease.

Several countries contain populations which permit comparisons to be made between ethnicity and prostatic cancer risk without the confounding influence of urban versus rural-related factors. This is true of Hawaii, where Haenszel and Kurihara (1968) showed that the mortality rate from prostatic cancer among Japanese-Americans in Hawaii was intermediate between the rates for Japanese in Japan and white males in the United States. Kolonel (1980) compared the patterns of cancer incidence for the Japanese, Chinese, Hawaiian and Filipino populations with those of whites on the United States mainland. Cancer of the prostate occurred with less frequency in all four ethnic groups. When taken alone, this difference might be explained by the relatively low level of industrialization in Hawaii compared with the continental United States. However, the white population of the islands shows the same high prostatic cancer risk as that of whites on the mainland. The observed ethnic differences are consistent with a role for diet in prostate cancer etiology; the white population of Hawaii consumes more beef and fat than the other ethnic groups.

III. DIETARY FAT AND PROSTATIC CANCER

Fat is probably the most extensively studied component of foods in relation to cancer risk. Indeed, the bulk of the evidence that diet impinges in any way on prostatic cancer risk relates to the consumption of fat.

Armstrong and Doll (1975) found that prostatic cancer deaths for 32 countries were highly correlated with total fat consumption. We found this to remain true for the 1978-79 data from 29 countries (r=0.61), although the relationship is really limited to animal fat (r=0.69), there being no association with fats from vegetable sources (r=-0.07). These analyses were made using cancer mortality statistics prepared by Kurihara et al. (1984), and the food balance sheets published for 1979-81 by the Food and Agriculture Organization of the United Nations (1984). Utilizing these same sources, we also found that there is a strong correlation between prostate cancer mortality rates and milk consumption in different countries (r=0.69), but a much weaker one for meats (r=0.39), and no association with eggs (r=0.01).

In Japan, there has been an increase in the incidence and mortality rates from both cancer of the prostate (Hirayama, 1979) and breast (Hirayama, 1978) over the past few decades. Kagawa (1978) pointed out that over this same period the Japanese diet became closer to that of the Western countries, with the result that there has been a pronounced increase in the consumption of animal fat and protein.

Similar changes in dietary practices and cancer incidence have taken place in Puerto Rico. While in the past fat intake was relatively low, by 1966 there was a pronounced increase in the per capita consumption of meat, eggs, fats and oils at all income levels (Fernandez, 1975). These altered food habits have been accompanied by a marked increase in the incidence of prostatic cancer (Waterhouse et al., 1976), although it remains substantially lower than in the United States (Martinez et al., 1975).

Approximately 50% of Seventh-Day Adventists in California are lacto-ovo-vegetarians, and virtually all abstain from pork products. This dietary practice, with its resulting approximately 25% reduction in fat intake, may explain, at least in part, the lower breast cancer mortality rate in Seventh-Day Adventists compared with the general population; their prostate cancer risk, however, does not show a corresponding reduction (Phillips, 1975). One explanation relates to the age at which dietary factors may modify the likelihood of developing prostatic cancer in later life. Approximately half of the Seventh-Day Adventists over 40 years of age are adult converts to the Church, and so any element of life-style which adversely affects cancer risk early in life may have already exerted its effect. This has been demonstrated for ischemic heart disease risk; Snowdon et al (1982) found that the risk of dying from ischemic heart disease among Seventh-Day Adventists baptized as children was only 71% of the risk for those baptized as adults.

In case-control studies, prostatic cancer risk has also been associated with diets high in animal fats, and with greater consumption of fatty meats, cheeses and creams and eggs (Schuman et al., 1977; Rotkin, 1977; Graham et al. 1983; Kolonel et al., 1983; Heshmat et al., 1985). Kolonel et al. (1981, 1983) are performing a study of diet and cancer risk in Hawaii. In their first report, food consumption data were analyzed for 4657 adults, 2293 of whom were males aged 45 years or older. The dietary interview provided information on the usual weekly intake of 83 food items selected to include the main sources (85-90% of total intake) of fat and protein. Special care was taken to obtain a reliable indication of the amounts of a given food consumed at each meal. The main ethnic groups resident in Hawaii -- Caucasian, Japanese, Chinese, Filipinos and Hawaiians -- were included in the survey, but were not evaluated separately in this preliminary report. Analysis of the data demonstrated that the population-based prostatic cancer incidence was positively correlated with age-adjusted daily consumption of animal (and saturated) fat.

The second report by Kolonel et al. (1983) included results from a prostatic cancer case-control study. For men less than 70 years of age, there was no statistically significant influence of dietary components on risk, but for older men there was a dose response-related risk associated with fat, notably saturated fat, consumption. This observation regarding age and risk was also made by Graham et al. (1983), but here the same trend for risk was present in men aged under 70 years although it failed to achieve statistical significance.

Mettlin (1980) reviewed the data generated by the Health and Nutrition Examination Survey (HANES) in the context of prostatic and esophageal cancer risk among American blacks. The results did not support an involvement of dietary fat in the development of these tumors. Indeed, black males of all ages tended to report less frequent consumption of fat and oils compared with whites. In the age group 18-44 years, 81% of blacks stated that they did so only once a day or less, largely in the form of butter or margerine, compared with 66% of white males. For older age groups, the difference was even more pronounced. Meat intake was about the same, while in the 18-44 year age group blacks did eat more eggs.

The case for a role for dietary fat in breast cancer etiology is supported by experiments with animal models (Carroll and Khor, 1970, 1971; Chan et al., 1977). Recently, Pollard and Luckert (1985) reported that feeding a high fat (20% corn oil wt/wt) diet accelerated the rate of development of prostate adenocarcinomas in testosterone-treated Lobund strain Wistar rats. There is an urgent need for the development of additional animal models and their application to studies of diet and prostatic carcinogenesis.

In breast cancer, there is at least some evidence to suggest that dietary fat alters hormone production levels (Rose, 1982). The mechanism may involve increased capacity for the aromatization of androstenedione, a C_{19} steroid, to form estrone. This transformation occurs predominantly in adipose tissue (Grodin et al., 1973), the conversion rate of androstenedione to estrone is positively correlated with body weight (MacDonald and Siiteri, 1974), and there are a number of reports that obesity is a risk factor for postmenopausal breast cancer (Rose, 1982). Several investigators have sought a similar relationship in prostatic cancer patients. Wynder et al. (1971) found no significant differences in body weight or height between 300 patients and 400 controls, and a more recent case-control study reached the same conclusion (Graham et al., 1983). Greenwald et al. (1974) performed a retrospective study of various physical characteristics in which data obtained from 268 male college students who eventually died of prostatic cancer were compared with those from 536 controls. No differences were found for height, weight, or ponderal index. Despite these negative results, Snowdon et al (1984) reported recently the results of a prospective study of 6,763 white male Seventh-Day Adventists who completed a dietary questionnaire in 1960. Obesity was found to be associated with an increased risk of fatal prostate cancer, and there was suggestive evidence for a relationship with milk, cheese, egg and meat consumption. When all four foods were combined, heavy intakes had a predicted relative risk of 3.6 for fatal prostate cancer. Obesity was also shown to be associated with increased prostate cancer risk in a cohort study performed by Lew and Garfinkel (1979), and in a third case-control study (Meikle et al., 1982). Thus, the relationship between obesity and prostate cancer is unclear at the present time. Clearly, this is an area which demands further investigation, together with appropriate endocrine studies.

IV. ENDOCRINOLOGY OF PROSTATIC CANCER

A.   Plasma Steroid Hormone Studies

1.   Normal Values and Controls

Most published studies of prostate cancer biochemical epidemiology involved the assay of hormones in plasma samples. The results have proven to be inconsistent and contradictory. One difficulty is the choice of suitable controls in case-control studies, and of exclusion criteria in population-based investigations of differing levels of prostate cancer risk.

Virtually all men over the age of 50 years have some degree of asymptomatic benign prostatic hyperplasia (BPH), a condition which has its own endocrine abnormalities. Some investigators have attempted to deal with the problem by comparing prostate cancer patients with younger male controls, but, unfortunately, plasma steroid levels change with increasing age. A number of studies showed that, with advancing age, there is an increase in plasma estrogens, a reduction in androgens, and an elevation in sex hormone-binding globulin (SHBG) which is a consequence of this altered estrogen/androgen ratio (Pirke and Doerr, 1973; Baker et al., 1976; Purifoy et al., 1981). In their "Normative Aging Study", Sparrow et al. (1980) did not find an increase in plasma estrogens with age. Likewise, in a carefully controlled study in which extrinsic and pathological factors which might affect serum steroid were excluded, Harman and Tistouras (1980) found not a decline, but an increase in plasma testosterone with age. These investigators deliberately studied a physically fit group of men, and avoided the potentially confounding influences of obesity, high alcohol consumption and medications.

Clearly, the question of control selection for plasma hormone assays in prostate cancer is extremely difficult. "Overscreening" of individuals for inclusion in high-risk versus low-risk population studies may exclude just those elements that are responsible for the difference in prostate cancer incidence rates. For example, we have seen that in some, but not all studies, obesity has been associated with increased prostate cancer risk, and that the conversion of androstenedione to estrone is positively correlated with body weight. Also, being overweight results in a reduction in plasma SHBG and a consequent increase in the unbound, biologically active, plasma estrogens (Siiteri et al., 1982). If these endocrine abnormalities are involved in prostate cancer etiology, they will not be recognized if overweight individuals are excluded from studies based on groups of men drawn from high-risk and low-risk populations.

Yet another problem, which applies with equal force to plasma hormone studies relative to breast cancer risk, is the selection of age range for endocrine evaluation. In the absence of any firm knowledge of the age at which hormones might influence future prostatic cancer development, the tendency has been to study disease-free men of similar age to most prostatic cancer patients when comparing high- and low-risk populations. However, some of the studies of sexuality and prostatic cancer risk (Krain et al., 1974; Greenwald et al., 1974; Mishina et al., 1985) would suggest the importance of hormonal variations much earlier in life.

2.   Case-Control Studies

Most investigators have determined serum or plasma testosterone, dihydrotestosterone (DHT) and estrogen levels. High, normal and low concentrations of testosterone have all been reported in prostatic cancer patients. Ghanadian et al. (1979) found a significantly higher serum testosterone concentration in their patients compared with healthy men of similar age who were free of urological symptoms. The mean serum DHT levels were similar, but nevertheless the best distinction between groups was still the T/DHT ratio. Ahluwalia et al. (1981), in a case-control study performed in the United States and Nigeria, found higher plasma testosterone levels in American blacks with prostatic cancer than in their control group, whereas in the Nigerians the reverse was true. Although statistically significant, the differences between cases and controls in this study were quite small. However, in another case-control study of blacks, this time in South Africa, plasma testosterone was also subnormal in prostatic cancer patients (Hill et al., 1982). A study from Romania, where the male population is at an intermediate level of risk in terms of international variation in incidence, involved the assay of seven different steroids in patients with prostatic cancer or BPH, and in age-matched healthy controls (Drafta et al. 1982). The plasma testosterone levels were elevated in carcinoma of the prostate, as was the T/DHT ratio, whereas DHT was increased with both these patients and those in benign disease.

These reports of elevated serum or plasma testosterone levels in prostatic cancer are at variance with other studies, which have shown either normal or subnormal concentrations. Two studies, one performed in

Germany (Bartsch et al. 1977) and the other in Wales (Harper et al., 1976), showed no difference in the plasma testosterone and DHT levels of prostatic cancer patients. Høisaeter et al. (1982) reported a tendency for the plasma testosterone levels of their patients to fall in the lower portion of the normal range regardless of disease stage. They did not, unfortunately, describe how they established their normal limits. Habib (1980) compared plasma testosterone and DHT levels in prostatic cancer patients with those of patients with BPH, and found no significant differences. This may, in any event, have been an inappropriate choice of controls; other investigators found the plasma DHT to be elevated in BPH (Horton et al., 1975; Ghanadian et al., 1977), and so a similar abnormality in the cancer patients would have been missed.

Zumoff et al. (1982), to avoid problems inherent in hormone assays of single samples, obtained blood through an indwelling venous catheter every 20 min. for 24 hr. This permitted the determination of 24 hr mean plasma concentrations of testosterone, DHT, and 11 other steroid or peptide hormones. It was found that whereas testosterone decreased with age in the controls, and DHT was unaffected, both steroids showed age-related increases in the cancer patients. The net result was that patients below 65 years of age showed significantly lower levels of testosterone and DHT than the controls below this age, whereas there were no differences for the older age groups. Although the under 65 years control group was considerably younger than the patients (mean ages were 42.6 and 60.0 years, respectively) this did not appear to have an adverse effect on the observed differences.

Rannikko and Adlercreutz (1983) compared patients with prostatic cancer or BPH with a younger group of healthy men (average age 49.4 years). A relatively young control group was selected to avoid confusion due to the inclusion of men with subclinical benign prostatic hyperplasia. In addition to the total testosterone, the biologically active free fraction and the SHBG concentration were assayed in this study. There were no differences in the plasma total testosterone concentration between the three groups, but the free testosterone was higher in the younger controls which was consistent with their lower SHBG levels. The prostatic cancer patients had a mean free testosterone level which appeared only slightly lower than that of the BPH group, although the difference was statistically significant. It is relevant to our earlier discussion of appropriate controls to note that the patients with prostatic disease were matched not only for age but for height and weight.

A number of investigators have reported abnormalities in the plasma estrogens of prostatic cancer patients, and here again there is some lack of consistency between studies. Høisaeter et al. (1982), in their study relating blood hormone concentration to prostatic cancer stage and grade, found that many of the estradiol levels were above the normal range. There was no relationship between estradiol concentration and grade, and when all patients were combined 24/93 (26%) showed elevated levels. In their study of prostatic cancer and BPH, Rannikko and Adlercreutz (1983) observed higher plasma estradiol levels in the non-cancerous disease than in the cancer patients or young controls; the latter groups showed no significant difference.

Ahluwalia et al. (1981) measured plasma estrone and estradiol in their study of American and Nigerian blacks. Only the plasma estrone showed abnormalities, with black prostatic cancer patients in the United States having higher levels than their controls. Zumoff et al. (1982), in their assessment of 24 hr mean plasma levels for 13 hormones or their metabolites, did not include estradiol. Plasma estrone levels were measured, were not influenced by age, and the 24 hr mean value was higher in the cancer patients (81 pg/ml) than in the controls (47 pg/ml).

In contrast to these observations, Drafta et al. (1982) found both plasma estradiol and estrone to be subnormal in prostatic cancer, and in BPH. They suggested that in both conditions there is an excessive production of testicular androgens with increased peripheral conversion of testosterone to DHT, and decreased aromatization of the C_{19} steroids to yield estrogens.

Finally, there are some investigators who found no abnormality in the plasma estrogen concentrations of
prostatic cancer patients (Harper et al., 1976; Bartsch
et al., 1977).

3. Populations at high risk

There have been only a few studies comparing plasma steroid hormone concentrations in populations at
different levels of risk for prostatic cancer. Two of
these took as a high risk population American blacks,
and compared their plasma hormone levels with those of
blacks in Africa.   Ahluwalia et al. (1981) obtained
single plasma samples for hormone assay from patients
in Washington, D.C. and Ibadan, Nigeria.   These patients, who were also employed as the controls for the
case-control study described earlier, were free of neoplastic, urological, or endocrine disease.   Plasma was
assayed for testosterone, DHT, estrone and estradiol,
and it was found that the Nigerians had considerably
lower levels of testosterone; plasma estrone concentrations were also significantly lower, but the difference
was not great. The authors suggested that the lower
testosterone and estrone levels in Nigerians might be
due to a relatively low activity of the 17-dehydrogen-
ase involved in the formation of both steroids.   The
possibility of low aromatase activity was rejected because plasma estradiol, formed by the aromatization of
testosterone, was normal.

The second study of black populations compared
healthy black South Africans and black Americans in the
age range 40-55 years (Hill et al., 1982).   This investigation involved a series of stimulation tests.
The levels of estradiol, estrone and androstenedione in
basal plasma samples were higher in the South African
blacks, but there was no difference in the testosterone
concentration. After human chorionic gonadotropin administration, the increases in plasma steroids were
similar in the two groups.

Several studies have demonstrated a familial risk
for prostatic cancer. Woolf (1960) found that deaths
among the fathers and brothers of 228 prostatic cancer

patients occurred at a rate three times that of the fathers and brothers of controls. The investigation was performed in Utah, and in part utilized the records of the Genealogical Society of the Mormon Church. In this, as in other family studies, consideration should be given to the confounding influence of a common life-style. As part of their extensive studies of familial cancer risk, Lynch et al. (1966) observed an aggregation of prostatic cancer occurring in 3 of 6 brothers, 2 of whom also had a second primary malignancy. Similar familial clusters have been reported by Krain (1974), and Schuman et al. (1977).

Meikle and Stanish (1982) found that there was a four-fold higher relative risk for the brothers of prostatic cancer patients compared with their brothers-in-law and the general male population. The cases had all been diagnosed before the age of 62 years. There were two groups of controls for the plasma hormone assays; one selected to correspond to the ages of the probands and their brothers, and the other of similar age range to the patients sons. It was found that the cancer cases and their brothers had significantly lower mean plasma testosterone levels than the corresponding controls, while the sons had lower levels of both testosterone and DHT than their control group. It is worth noting that the prostatic cancer patients in this study were all under 62 years of age, and that Zumoff et al. (1982) found low plasma testosterone and DHT levels only in their patients below the age of 65 years.

B. Prolactin and the Prostate

There is no doubt that prolactin has an important role in prostate endocrinology. Early experiments showed, for example, that the response of the prostate to testosterone is augmented by the simultaneous administration of prolactin in hypophysectomized rats (Grayhack, 1963) and, more recently, cell membrane prolactin receptors have been demonstrated in both rat (Aragona and Friesen, 1975; Kledzik et al., 1976; Keenan et al., 1979) and human (Keenan et al., 1979) prostate glands. In addition to normal human tissues, prolactin receptors occur in BPH and in some carcinomas (Keenan et al., 1979).

In spite of these findings, a number of investigators have reported normal levels of plasma prolactin in prostatic cancer patients (Hammond et al., 1977; Griffiths et al., 1979; Høisaeter et al., 1982; Rannikko and Adlercreutz, 1983), including the 24 hour mean concentrations (Zumoff et al., 1982). Giuliani et al. (1979) demonstrated an increased prolactin response to TRH stimulation in both prostatic cancer and BPH patients, and an abnormally prolonged response was observed in South African black prostatic cancer patients (Hill et al., 1982). However, these abnormalities could well be stress-mediated and a consequence of disease rather than being of etiologic significance.

C.   Prostatic Fluid

Prostatic fluid is the normal secretory product of acinar epithelial cells, and so is likely to be modified by biochemical events taking place within the gland (Anderson and Fair, 1976; Grayhack et al., 1977a and b). The failure of plasma hormone studies to produce consistent results in prostatic cancer patients, together with the recognition that the prostate gland is an active site of steroid metabolism and peptide hormone processing, prompted us to examine the hormone content of prostatic fluid.

In a preliminary study of prostate cancer patients and controls of similar age (Rose et al., 1984), both groups showed estradiol and estrone levels to be higher in prostatic fluid than in the serum, but some of the cancer patients also had elevated concentrations of estradiol in the fluid compared with the controls. - Testosterone levels were assayed in 28 controls and 10 cancer patients. While the concentrations were extremely low in the controls, 6 of the patients with prostate cancer had levels ranging from 73 to 550 ng/ml. In a single fluid sample, the testosterone concentration was 86 ng/100 ml, but the level of DHT was 1037 ng/100 ml; 76% and 71% respectively were in the unbound form. Prolactin levels were frequently higher in the prostatic fluids than in the corresponding sera and 5 of 19 patients had concentrations which exceeded those seen in the control group. There was no correlation between the prolactin and estradiol levels.

Obviously, a great deal has to be done before the metabolic implications of these results are understood. The high levels of estrogens in prostatic fluid compared with serum were unexpected. It seems unlikely that these were due to "trapping" of estrogen by the gland, but rather suggests the presence of aromatase for the metabolic conversion of testosterone to estradiol and androstenedione to estrone. The high DHT/T ratio presumably reflects high 5α-reductase activity relative to the further metabolism of DHT to 5α-androstanediols. Comparisons of the prostatic fluid DHT/T ratio in prostatic cancer, BPH and normal controls should be of interest. Like several other peptide hormones, prolactin becomes internalized by endocytosis, and internal binding sites have been demonstrated in the Golgi region of epithelial cells of the rat ventral prostate (Witorsch and Smith, 1977). The fate of prolactin once it has entered the prostatic cell is unknown. Our results indicate that immunoreactive molecules can enter the prostatic fluid, and in some preliminary, unpublished, experiments we have shown that this prolactin has retained its bioactivity, as judged by the Nb_2 rat lymphoma bioassay developed by Tanaka et al. (1980).

One of the problems attending the application of biochemical epidemiology is that it involves the analysis of samples from large numbers of individuals. While it is not possible to obtain tissue from apparently healthy males at high or low risk of prostate cancer, it is feasible to design a project utilizing prostatic fluid.

D.   Diet-Hormonal Interactions

A number of studies on the effect of diet on circulating hormones have been published which may be relevant to the biochemical epidemiology of prostate cancer. Most have compared either vegetarians with non-vegetarians, or have observed the effect of reducing dietary fat consumption on serum hormone levels.

Howie and Shultz (1985) studied 12 Seventh-Day Adventist lacto-ovo-vegetarians, 10 others who were omnivorous, and 8 non-Seventh-Day omnivores. Dietary intakes of energy, protein and saturated fat were not significantly different, although the vegetarians consumed more crude and dietary fiber than men in the other two groups, and 4-6% less of their total calories was derived from fat. The principal hormonal differences were significantly lower concentrations of estradiol and testosterone in plasma samples from the vegetarians. Also, there was an inverse relationship between fiber intakes and the plasma hormone levels. The differences in plasma steroid concentrations were not due to differences in body weight, but may be explained by altered enterohepatic recirculation resulting from the high fiber intake. Goldin et al. (1982), in a study of premenopausal women, found that vegetarians had higher fecal weights and an increased fecal excretion of estrogens. Urinary estriol excretion was lower in the vegetarians, and their plasma levels of estrone and estradiol were negatively correlated with fecal estrogen excretion.

Hill and Wynder (1979) transferred four healthy men from their regular omnivorous diet to a vegetarian one providing 25% calories from fat. Multiple blood samples were collected through an indwelling catheter before, and two weeks after initiating the dietary change. The vegetarian diet produced a decrease in plasma testosterone and in the normal nocturnal elevation in testosterone and prolactin levels; estrogens were not assayed in this study. These same investigators fed a typical Western diet containing 40% of calories from fat to healthy black South African men (who are at low prostate cancer risk) and demonstrated an increase in urinary estrogen and androgen excretion; feeding a vegetarian diet with 30% of calories from fat to black American men (high prostate cancer risk) caused a reduction in these urinary steroids (Hill et al., 1979).

The profound effect of a very low-fat diet, (less than 10% of calories), high-fiber, high-complex carbohydrate on serum estradiol levels in men was demonstrated by Rosenthal et al. (1985). The 21 patients, average age 51 years, had a history of coronary heart disease, hypertension, or diabetes. The diets were fed in a residential setting (Pritikin Longevity Center), and after 21 days serum estradiol levels were reduced from 47.2 ± 4.6 to 23.8 ± 2.5 pg/ml (mean $\pm$ SEM). Compliance was confirmed by decreases in serum cholesterol and triglycerides, but, unexpectedly, there was no change in serum testosterone.

The results of these five studies serve to demonstrate that diet does influence the circulating levels of hormones which are suspected of being involved in prostatic carcinogenesis. They also draw attention specifically to the roles of fat and fiber.

E.   Conclusions

Until recently, the evidence that dietary fat exerts an influence on prostate carcinogenesis was, perhaps, less persuasive than in the case of breast or colon. While international comparisons were compatible with such an effect, negative findings included the absence of a reduced prostate cancer risk in Seventh-Day Adventists, and no excess dietary fat consumption by American black males despite their extremely high risk for this cancer. Other problems were the lack of support from dietary studies using animal models, and of relevant data concerning dietary-hormone interactions.

The review presented here shows that this situation is currently in a state of flux. Population and case-control studies in the continental United States, Hawaii, and Puerto Rico, for example, support a promotional effect of high fat intakes in prostate cancer development, and the preliminary experiments performed by Pollard and Luckert (1985) are also indicative of such a mechanism in an animal model. Finally, endocrine studies in volunteers fed different diets, and of selected subpopulations are providing us with new insights as to how dietary fat and fiber may modify hormonal action.

As more investigators from many scientific disciplines become involved in studies of this important cancer, we can anticipate a rapid acceleration in our understanding of its etiology, and the contribution made by specific dietary and endocrine factors.

The author's own work on the biochemical epidemiology of prostate cancer is supported by grant CA39161 from the National Cancer Institute.

REFERENCES

Ahluwalia B, Jackson MA, Jones GW, Williams AO, Rao MS, Rajguru S (1981). Blood hormones profiles in prostate cancer patients in high-risk and low-risk populations. Cancer 48:2267-2273.

Anderson RU, Fair WR (1976). Physical and chemical determinations of prostatic secretion in benign hyperplasia, prostatitis, and adenocarcinoma. Invest Urol 14:137-140.

Andrews GS (1949). Latent carcinoma of the prostate. J Clin Pathol 2:197-208.

Aragona C, Friesen HG (1975). Specific prolactin binding sites in the prostate and testis of rats. Endocrinology 97:677-684.

Armstrong B, Doll R (1975). Environmental factors and cancer incidence and mortality in different countries, with special reference to dietary practices. Int J Cancer 15:617-631.

Baker HWG, Burger HG, deKretser M, Hudson B, O'Connor S, Wang C, Mirovics A, Court J, Dunlop M, Rennie GC (1976). Changes in the pituitary-testicular system with age. Clin Endocrinol 5:349-372.

Bartsch W, Horst H-J, Becker H, Nehse G (1977). Sex hormone binding globulin binding capacity, testosterone, 5α-dihydrotestosterone, oestradiol and prolactin in plasma of patients with prostatic carcinoma under various types of hormonal treatment. Act Endocrinol 85:650-664.

Breslow N, Chan CW, Dhom G, Drury RAB, Franks LM, Gellei B, Lee YS, Lundberg S, Sharke B, Sternby NH, Tulinius H (1977). Latent carcinoma of prostate at autopsy in seven areas. Int J Cancer 20: 680-688.

Carroll KK, Khor HT (1970). Effects of dietary fat and dose level of 7,12-dimethylbenz(a)anthracene on mammary tumor incidence in rats. Cancer Res 30: 2260-2264.

Carroll KK, Khor HT (1971). Effects of level and type of dietary fat on incidence of mammary tumors induced in female Sprague-Dawley rats by 7,2-dimethylbenz(a)anthracene. Lipids 6:415-420.

Chan P-C, Head JF, Cohen LA, Wynder EL (1977). Influence of dietary fat on the induction of mammary tumors by N-nitrosomethylurea: associated hormone changes and differences between Sprague-Dawley and F344 rats. J Natl Cancer Inst 59:1279-1283.

Drafta D, Proca E, Zamfir V, Schindler AE, Neacsu E, Stroe E (1982). Plasma steroids in benign prostatic hypertrophy and carcinoma of the prostate. J Steroid Biochem 17:689-693.

Fernandez NA (1975). Nutrition in Puerto Rico. Cancer Res 35:3272-3291.

Food and Agriculture Organization of the United Nations (1984). Food Balance Sheets, 1979-1981 Average. Rome.

Ghanadian R, Lewis JG, Chisholm GD, O'Donoghue EPN (1977). Serum dihydrotestosterone in patients with benign prostate hypertrophy. Br J Urol 59: 541-544.

Ghanadian R, Puah CM, O'Donoghue EPN (1979). Serum testosterone and dihydrotestosterone in carcinoma of the prostate. Br J Cancer 39:696-699.

Giuliani D, Pescatore D, Martorana G, Giberti C, Barreca T, Rolandi E (1979). Increased serum prolactin pituitary reserve in patients with prostatic neoplasms. Brit J Urol 51:390-392.

Goldin BR, Adlercreutz H, Gorbach SL, Warram JH, Dwyer JT, Swenson L, Woods MN (1982). Estrogen excretion patterns and plasma levels in vegetarian and omnivorous women. N Engl J Med 307:1542-1547.

Grayhack JT (1963). Pituitary factors influencing growth of the prostate. Natl Cancer Inst Monogr 12:189-199.

Grayhack JT, Wendel EF, Lee C, Oliver L (1977a). Analysis of prostatic fluid in prostatic disease. Cancer Treat Rep 61:205-210.

Grayhack JT, Wendel EF, Lee C, Oliver L, Cohen E (1977b). Lactate dehydrogenase isoenzymes in human prostatic fluid: an aid in recognition of malignancy? J Urol 118:204-208.

Graham S, Haughey B, Marshall J, Priore R, Byers T, Rzepka T, Mettlin C, Pontes JE (1983). Diet in the epidemiology of carcinoma of the prostate gland. J Natl Cancer Inst 70:687-692.

Greenwald P, Damon A, Kirms V, Polan AK (1974). Physical and demographic features of men before developing cancer of the prostate.J Natl Cancer Inst 53:341-346.

Griffiths K, Davies P, Harper ME, Peeling WB, Pierrepoint CG (1979). The etiology and endocrinology of prostatic cancer, in Endocrinology of Cancer, Vol II, Rose DP, ed, CRC Press, Boca Raton, 1-55.

Grodin JM, Siiteri PK, MacDonald PC (1973). Source of estrogen production in postmenopausal women. J Clin Endocrinol Metab 36:207-214.

Habib FK (1980). Evaluation of androgen metabolism studies in human prostate cancer-correlation with zinc levels. Prev Med 9:650-656.

Haenszel W, Kurihara M (1968). Studies of Japanese migrants. I. Mortality from cancer and other diseases among Japanese in the United States. J Natl Cancer Inst 40:43-68.

Hammond GL, Kontturi M, Maattala P, Puuka M, Vihko R (1977). Serum FSH, LH and prolactin in normal males and patients with prostatic diseases. Clin Endocrinol 7:129-135.

Harman SM, Tistouras PD (1980). Reproductive hormones in aging men. I. Measurement of sex steroids, basal luteinizing hormone, and Leydig cell response to human chorionic gonadotropin. J Clin Endocrinol Metab 51:35-40.

Harper ME, Peeling WB, Cowley T, Brownsey BG, Phillips MEA, Groom G, Fahmy DR, Griffiths K (1976). Plasma steroid and protein hormone concentrations in patients with prostatic carcinoma, before and during oestrogen therapy. Acta Endocrinol 81:409-426.

Heshmat MY, Kaul L, Kovi J et al (1985). Nutrition and prostate cancer: a case-control study. Prostate 6:7-17.

Hill P, Wynder EL (1979). Effect of a vegetarian diet and dexamethasone on plasma prolactin, testosterone and dehydroepiandrosterone in men and women. Cancer Lett 7:273-282.

Hill P, Wynder EL, Garbaczewski L, Garnes H, Walker ARP (1982). Response to luteinizing releasing hormone. thyrotrophic releasing hormone, and human chorionic gonadotrophin administration in healthy men at different risks for prostatic cancer and in prostatic cancer patients. Cancer Res 42:2074-2080.

Hirayama T (1978). Epidemiology of breast cancer with special reference to the role of diet. Prev Med 7:173-195.

Hirayama T (1979). Epidemiology of prostate cancer with special reference to the role of diet. Natl Cancer Inst Monogr 53:149-155.

Høisaeter PÅ, Haukaas S, Bakke A, Hoiem L, Segadal E, Thorsen T (1982). Blood hormone levels related to stages and grades of prostatic cancer. Prostate 3:375-381.

Horton R, Hsieh P, Barberia J, Pages L, Cosgrove M (1975). Altered blood androgens in elderly men with prostate hyperplasia. J Clin Endocrinol Metab 41:793-796.

Howie BJ, Shultz TD (1985). Dietary and hormonal interrelationships among vegetarian Seventh-Day Adventists and non-vegetarian men. Am J Clin Nutr 42:127-134.

Jackson MA, Ahluwalia BS, Herson J, Heshmat MY, Jackson AG, Jones GW, Kapoor SK, Kennedy J, Kovi J, Lucas AO, Nkposong EO, Olisa E, Williams AO (1977). Characterization of prostatic carcinoma among blacks: a continuation report. Cancer Treat Rep 61:167-172.

Kagawa Y (1978). Impact of westernization on the nutrition of Japanese: changes in physique, cancer, longevity and centenarians. Prev Med 7:205-217.

Keenan EJ, Kemp ED, Ramsey EE, Garrison LB, Pearse HD, Hodges CV (1979). Specific binding of prolactin by the prostate gland of the rat and man. J Urol 122:43-46.

Kledzik GS, Marshall S, Campbell GA, Gelato M, Meites J (1976). Effects of castration, testosterone, estradiol and prolactin on specific prolactin-binding activity in ventral prostate of male rats. Endocrinology 98:373-379.

Kolonel LN (1980). Cancer patterns for four ethnic groups in Hawaii. J Natl Cancer Inst 65:1127-1139, 1980.

Kolonel LN, Hankin JH, Lee J, Chu SY, Nomura AMY, Hinds MW (1981). Nutrient intakes in relation to cancer incidence in Hawaii. Brit J Cancer 44:332-339.

Kolonel LN, Nomura AMY, Hinds MW, Hirohata T, Hankin JH, Lee J (1983).Role of diet in cancer incidence in Hawaii. Cancer Res 43:2397s-2402s.

Krain LS (1974). Some epidemiologic variables in prostatic carcinoma in California. Prev Med 3:154-159.

Kurihara M, Aoki K, Tominaga S (1984). Cancer Mortality Statistics in the World. Univ Nagoya Press.

Lew EA, Garfinkel L (1979). Variations in mortality by weight among 750,000 men and women. J Chronic Dis 32:563-576.

Lynch HT, Larsen AL, Magnuson CW, Krush AJ (1966). Prostate carcinoma and multiple primary malignancies; study of a family and 109 consecutive prostate cancer patients. Cancer 19:1891-1897.

MacDonald PC, Siiteri PK (1974). The relationship between the extraglandular production of estrone and the occurrence of endometrial neoplasm. Gynecol Oncol 2:259-263.

Martinez I, Torres R, Frias Z (1975). Cancer incidence in the United States and Puerto Rico. Cancer Res 35:3265-3271.

Meikle AW, Stanish WM (1982). Familial prostatic cancer risk and low testosterone. J Clin Endocrinol Metab 54:1104-1108.

Meikle A, Stanish W, West D (1982). Abstracts of the American Public Health Association Meeting, Montreal, Canada, 30.

Mettlin C (1980). Nutritional habits of blacks and whites. Prev Med 9:601-606.

Mishina T, Watanabe H, Araki H, Nakao M (1985). Epidemiological study of prostatic cancer by matched-pair analysis. Prostate 6:423-436.

Phillips RL (1975). Role of lifestyle and dietary habits in risk of cancer among Seventh-Day Adventists. Cancer Res 35:3513-3522.

Pirke KM, Doerr P (1973). Age related changes and interrelationships between plasma testosterone, oestradiol and testosterone-binding globulin in normal adult males. Acta Endocrinol 74:792-800.

Pollard M, Luckert PH (1985). Promotional effects of testosterone and dietary fat on prostate carcinogenesis in genetically susceptible rats. Prostate 6:1-5.

Purifoy FE, Koopmans LH, Mayes DM (1981). Age differences in serum androgen levels in normal adult males. Hum Biol 53:499-511.

Rannikko S, Adlercreutz H (1983). Plasma estradiol, free testosterone, sex hormone binding globulin binding capacity, and prolactin in benign prostatic hyperplasia and prostatic cancer. Prostate 14:223-229.

Rose DP (1982). Diet, hormones and breast cancer, in Endocrinology of Cancer, Vol III, Rose DP, ed, CRC Press, Boca Raton, 94-111.

Rose DP, Laakso K. Sotarauta M, Wynder EL (1984). Hormone levels in prostatic fluid from healthy Finns and prostate cancer patients. Europ J Cancer Clin Oncol 20:1317-1319.

Rosenthal MB, Barnard RJ, Rose DP, Inkeles S, Hall J, Pritikin N (1985). Effects of a high-complex-carbohydrate, low-fat, low-cholesterol diet on levels of serum lipids and estradiol. Am J Med 78:23-27.

Rotkin ID (1977). Studies in the epidemiology of prostatic cancer: expanded sampling. Cancer Treat Rep 61:173-180.

Schuman LM, Mandel J, Blackard C, Bauer H, Scarlett J, McHugh R (1977). Epidemiologic study of prostatic cancer: Preliminary report. Cancer Treat Rep 61:181-186.

Siiteri PK, Murai JT, Hammond GL, Nisker JA, Raymoure WJ, Kuhn RW (1982). Rec Prog Horm Res 38:457-509.

Snowdon DA, Phillips RL, Choi W (1984). Diet, obesity, and risk of fatal prostate cancer. Am J Epidemiol 120:244-250.

Snowdon DA, Phillips RL, Kuzma JW (1982). Age at baptism into the Seventh-Day Adventist Church and risk of death due to ischemic heart disease -- A preliminary report, in Banbury Report 11, Hunt VR, Smith MK, Worth D, eds, Cold Spring Harbor Laboratory.

Sparrow D, Bosse R, Rowe JW (1980). The influence of age, alcohol consumption and body build on gonadal function in men. J Clin Endocrinol Metab 51:508-512.

Tanaka T, Shiu RPC, Gout PW, Beer CT, Noble RL, Friesen HG (1980). A new sensitive and specific bioassay for lactogenic hormones: measurement of prolactin and growth hormone in human serum. J Clin Endocrinol Metab 57:1058-1063.

Waterhouse J, Muir C, Correa P, Powell J (1976). Cancer Incidence in Five Continents, Vol III, IARC Scientific Publication No 15, International Agency for Research on Cancer, Lyon, France, 1-548.

Witorsch RJ, Smith JS (1977). Evidence for androgen-dependent intracellular binding of prolactin in rat ventral prostate gland. Endocrinology 101:929-938.

Woolf CM (1960). An investigation of the familial aspects of carcinoma of the prostate. Cancer 13:739-744.

Wynder EL, Mabuchi K, Whitmore WF Jr (1971). Epidemiology of cancer of the prostate. Cancer 28:344-360.

Zumoff B, Levin J, Strain GW, Rosenfeld RS, O'Connor J, Freed SZ, Kream J, Whitmore WS, Fukushima DK, Hellman L (1982). Abnormal levels of plasma hormones in men with prostate cancer: evidence toward a "two-disease" theory. Prostate 3:579-588.

Dietary Fat and Cancer, pages 69–91

THE EPIDEMIOLOGY OF COLON CANCER AND DIETARY FAT

Laurence N. Kolonel and Loïc Le Marchand

Epidemiology Program, Cancer Research
Center, University of Hawaii, Honolulu,
Hawaii 96813

INTRODUCTION

In this chapter, we review the epidemiologic literature
on fats in relation to colon cancer risk. We also assess
the human literature on biochemical measurements in fecal
materials, although most of this research is not strictly
epidemiological in design. Not included here is another
component of lipids, namely, cholesterol, which is reviewed
in a separate chapter so that the human and animal
literature can be discussed together.

EPIDEMIOLOGIC STUDIES BASED ON DIETARY ASSESSMENTS

A substantial number of studies have now examined the
relationship between dietary intake of fat and the risk for
colon cancer. However, most of these studies only
determined intake of a selection of high fat foods, or meats
specifically, which are only presumptive indicators of a fat
association. A second component of the diet which has been
implicated in colon cancer risk is fiber, and since dietary
fiber intake may modify any carcinogenic effect of dietary
fat, we will consider some of the fiber literature here as
well. Only a few studies have attempted to examine both fat
and fiber in the same analysis.

1. Correlational Studies

Correlational studies demonstrate associations between
the average exposure levels and the cancer rates in several

different populations. Such studies are generally viewed as among the weakest of epidemiologic approaches to etiologic research, because they cannot control for many important confounders, and they do not necessarily encompass the same sources of subjects for the exposure and outcome data (ecologic fallacy). However, because of dietary homogeneity within the single populations in which case-control and cohort studies are generally conducted, associations between dietary risk factors and cancer may actually be more readily identified in correlational analyses.

Fat intake has been correlated with colon cancer risk in several studies. Drasar and Irving (1973) examined per capita intakes in relation to colon cancer incidence in 37 countries and found a significant correlation between total fat (excluding oils and butter) and colon cancer. In a similar analysis, using both incidence and mortality data, Armstrong and Doll (1975) also found an association between total fat intake and this cancer site. Knox (1977) used a more selected set of 19 countries, and obtained data on per capita intake of a wide variety of foods but only a few nutrients (measured as caloric equivalents); he found a strong positive correlation of total fat, as well as total calories, with colon cancer mortality. A more recent analysis of mortality data by McKeown-Eyssen and Bright-See (1984), however, identified animal fat in particular as the most strongly correlated factor.

In contrast, Enstrom (1975) reported a lack of correlation between per capita fat consumption by state and colorectal cancer mortality in the U.S., as well as a lack of parallel between the two in secular trends or urban-rural gradients. Bingham et al. (1979) also found no significant correlation between fat intake and colon cancer mortality by region in Great Britain, and McMichael et al. (1979) found inconsistencies between trends for dietary fat intake and colon cancer mortality in the U.S., United Kingdom, Australia and New Zealand. Furthermore, Lyon and Sorenson (1978) noted that colon cancer incidence is substantially lower in Mormon and non-Mormon residents of Utah than in the U.S. as a whole, whereas fat intake differs little between Utah and the country overall. Kolonel et al. (1981, 1986a, 1986b) have noted similar discrepancies in Hawaii. For example, Caucasians and native Hawaiians have equally high fat intakes, yet the Hawaiians have a low incidence of colon cancer whereas the Caucasians have a very high incidence.

On the other hand, first generation Japanese migrants to Hawaii have somewhat lower fat intakes than the second generation, yet colon cancer incidence is equally high in both groups. Smith et al. (1985) also noted that colorectal cancer mortality is low and has been declining in New Zealand Maoris, whereas it is high and has been increasing in non-Maoris, despite similar dietary fat intakes in the two populations.

There is equally conflicting evidence on the association between intake of meats, possibly an indicator food for fat (especially animal fat) and colon cancer risk. Both Armstrong and Doll (1975) and Knox (1977) found even stronger support for a meat association than for fat, and Howell (1975), in a similar analysis, found a high correlation between meat consumption, especially beef and cattle but not chicken and pork, and colon cancer mortality in 37 countries. Hirayama (1979) reported a modest correlation between the proportion of daily meat consumers and mortality from colorectal cancer for 29 health center districts in Japan. In the analysis by McKeown-Eyssen and Bright-See (1984), which found a positive correlation between animal fat and colon cancer mortality, the association was largely due to red meats (but not just beef) in the diet. Non-supportive evidence for an association with meat comes from several of the same negative studies cited above for fat (Enstrom, 1975; Lyon and Sorenson, 1978; Bingham et al., 1979; McMichael et al., 1979). In addition, Kinlen (1982) reported that colorectal cancer mortality was no lower for non-meat eating or low-meat eating nuns in England and Wales than for the general population of those countries. Thus, the correlational literature on meat consumption and colon cancer risk does little to clarify the inconsistent literature on fat.

It is also of interest that in the reports by Drasar and Irving (1973), Armstrong and Doll (1975), and Knox (1977) animal protein was significantly correlated with colon cancer mortality, as one might expect given the associations with fat, which is largely from animal sources in most westernized countries. Although Knox found that the correlation was stronger with fat than with animal protein, Armstrong and Doll found that the association with animal protein was more impressive, in that it persisted in a partial correlation analysis controlling for fat whereas the association with fat was substantially reduced in a similar analysis controlling for animal protein.

Although dietary fiber is not the subject of this
review, one proposed mechanism for a protective role of this
dietary constituent is its effect on the stool concentration
of bile acids (Kritchevsky, 1985). Since fat consumption
influences bile acid production and biliary excretion, it
follows that the ability to demonstrate an association
between dietary fat intake and colon cancer risk may depend
on fiber consumption levels in populations as well.
Unfortunately, while several correlational studies have
examined the association between fiber intake and colon
cancer, some showing an inverse relationship (Howell, 1975;
Bingham et al., 1979; Powles and Williams, 1984;
McKeown-Eyssen and Bright-See, 1984; Bingham, et al., 1985)
and some not (Drasar and Irving, 1973; Lyon and Sorenson,
1978; Barker and Godfrey, 1984; Smith et al., 1985), none of
these examined the fat association in a restricted set of
populations with low fiber intake. Thus, another reason for
the lack of consistency in the correlational data on fat
could be related to this additional influence of dietary
fiber. In this regard, a report by Liu et al. (1979) is of
interest. In a partial correlation analysis, these
investigators found that initial associations of dietary fat
and fiber intake with colon cancer mortality were reduced to
non-significance after controlling for dietary cholesterol
consumption.

2. Case-Control Studies

In only one case-control study have the investigators
attempted to estimate actual fat intake levels in the study
subjects. This study was carried out by Miller and his
associates in Canada using a quantitative diet history
method. In an anlysis based on 348 colon cancer cases, 542
neighborhood controls individually matched on age, sex and
residence, and 535 hospital controls group-matched on age
and sex, they found an increased risk for colon cancer
associated with fat intake (saturated fat in particular) and
a dose-response gradient (relative risks of 2.0 and 2.5 for
the medium and high intake groups compared to the low).
Although the fat association was the strongest result, they
also found positive associations with total protein and
total caloric intake (Jain et al., 1980). When the same
data were analyzed for food items and food groups, no

individual foods stood out as major contributors to the fat relationship, thus supporting the interpretation that the relevant association was with fat itself, rather than certain foods incidentally high in fat content (Miller et al., 1983).

Several other investigators have compared cases and controls in terms of consumption of high fat foods. The results have been inconsistent. In an early study, based on 69 colon cancer cases, 307 hospital controls, and frequency of intake of a small selection of foods, Wynder et al. (1969) reported that the cases had a higher caloric and fat intake, though the data were not shown (cases did consume more milk). Dales et al. (1979) also recorded frequency of intake of selected foods in a case-control study among blacks in northern California. They found an increase in risk (not statistically significant but with a dose-respone gradient) for colon cancer associated with consumption of high-fat foods (based on 77 cases and 215 controls from both hospitalized patients and participants in a multiphasic health checkup program). This association was seen only in men, however. In a study similarly limited in food sources and quantification, Pickle et al. (1984) found a non-significant increase in risk for colon cancer (58 cases and 116 matched hospital controls) associated with consumption of several dietary fat sources. This result pertained particularly to those subjects of Bohemian ancestry in the study.

Other studies based on food-frequency data have been completely negative. Higginson (1966) reported on combined results for colon and rectum cases (207 colon and 133 rectum) and 1020 hospital controls. He found no significant case-control differences in intake of a variety of fat sources in the diets of the study subjects. Similarly, Modan et al. (1975) found no evidence for an association between consumption of high-fat foods and colon cancer, based on a study of 198 cases and matched controls (one surgical patient and one neighborhood resident) in Israel.

Several of these and other investigators have also reported on the association of meats specifically with colon cancer risk. Haenszel et al. (1973) found a significant association of the frequency of meat intake (especially beef) with large bowel cancer (colon and rectum combined) among Japanese subjects in Hawaii. In a study in Greece also based on food-frequency data, Manousos et al. (1983) found a positive association between meat intake (primarily beef and lamb) and colon cancer risk. The study by Pickle et al. (1984) also found a positive association between meat intake and colon cancer. On the other hand, even more studies failed to find evidence for a specific association of meat intake with colon cancer risk. These include the previously cited studies by Higginson (1966), Modan et al. (1975) and Dales et al. (1979), and studies by Haenszel et al. in Japan (1980) and Graham et al. in New York state (1978).

Although some of these same studies also looked at the intake of high-fiber foods, the results have been mixed. Inverse associations were reported by some investigators (Haenszel et al., 1973; Modan et al., 1975; Graham et al., 1978; Dales et al., 1979; Haenszel et al., 1980; Manousos et al., 1983) but not by others, including Miller and his co-workers who estimated actual intake of both total and crude fiber (Higginson, 1966; Jain et al., 1980; Miller et al., 1983; Pickle et al., 1984). Only two of these studies attempted to look at a possible modifying effect of fiber on the fat-cancer association, although Jain et al. (1980) used a multivariate analysis to control for one while examining the other. Dales et al. (1979) found that whereas the associations for fat and fiber were not statistically significant alone, when subjects with both a high-fat and low-fiber intake were examined, their colon cancer risk was significantly increased over that for subjects with a low-fat, high fiber intake (relative risk = 2.7). This result was apparent with each of their two types of control subjects, and fat and fiber appeared to show a synergistic interaction in their data. Findings from the study by Manousos et al. (1983) in Greece were similar. These investigators found independent risks for high consumption of certain meats (beef and lamb) and low consumption of certain vegetables (cabbage, lettuce and spinach). When intake of these items was combined for each subject into a risk score, they found that colon cancer risk was greatly increased for those subjects in the highest quintile, i.e. with high meat and low vegetable intake (relative risk = 8.0).

3. Cohort Studies

Five studies of colon cancer and dietary fat have been based on data from follow-up on large cohorts. None of these studies found evidence for a direct association between fat intake and cancer risk. In fact, Stemmermann et al. (1984) reported an inverse association for saturated fat, although there was no dose-response gradient. This analysis was based on 106 colon cancer cases after 15 years of follow-up on 7074 men of Japanese ancestry in Hawaii, and used 24-hour dietary recall data. The findings were strongest for cancers in the right colon, somewhat weaker for cancers in the sigmoid colon and not present for cancers in the transverse and rectosigmoid colon. In another study among Japanese, based on a very large prospective cohort in Japan (265,118 adults), Hirayama (1981) found a protective effect of meat consumption against colorectal cancer mortality. This effect was independent of socioeconomic status and the intake of green and yellow vegetables. In an earlier report, however (Hirayama, 1979), which included sex- and site-specific results, this protective effect was only apparent for male colon cancer cases.

Based on follow-up of 1954 men in the Western Electric cohort in Chicago, Garland et al. (1985) found no differences between men who developed colorectal cancer (49 cases), or colon cancer specifically (29 cases), and those who did not, with regard to percent of dietary calories from fat or animal protein, or mean caloric intake. Phillips and Snowden (1985) reported on colorectal cancer mortality in 25,493 Seventh Day Adventists who had been followed for 21 years. Dietary data were based on a self-administered questionnaire containing frequency of consumption information for 21 food items. There was no clear association between consumption of high fat foods and colon cancer risk, although in men only, overweight and use of cheese were positively associated with disease outcome. There was also a positive relationship between intake of eggs and colon cancer risk, including a dose-response gradient for both men and women. This specificity for eggs rather than multiple sources of dietary fat suggests a more likely effect of cholesterol in particular.

Using both mortality and morbidity as end points, Jensen et al. (1980) examined large bowel cancer occurrence in the spouses of 1716 cases of large bowel cancer in

Sweden. They found no evidence for an increased risk for large bowel cancer in the spouses. Other diseases putatively related to dietary fat (breast cancer, ischemic heart disease, gallbladder disease) were also not increased in the spouses. These findings could suggest that any effect of dietary fat must be related to exposure levels occurring prior to the time of marriage.

4. Assessment

Taken together, the results of the various epidemiologic studies of dietary fat and colon cancer do not offer clear support for the fat hypothesis. The only consistency in findings is that for all three study types there are almost as many studies showing as not showing an association. The dietary methodology in many of the studies was weak and, in some cases, could be deemed inadequate. Only one analytic study has yet assessed actual fat intake (Jain et al., 1980), and this study did find an association with saturated fat. Thus, it would be premature at this time to conclude that no relationship exists.

If a positive relationship between fat and colon cancer does exist, it is probably complex, involving other dietary influences, such as fiber or calcium intake (Garland et al., 1985; Lipkin and Newmark, 1985), which will need to be considered simultaneously in epidemiologic analyses. In this regard, it is notable that the studies by both Dales et al. (1979) and Manousos et al. (1983), which attempted to incorporate data for high-fiber foods, reported positive associations for high-fat foods and colon cancer.

HUMAN STUDIES BASED ON METABOLIC ASSESSMENTS

The possibility that diet plays a role in colon cancer pathogenesis has led investigators to suspect that foods might be a source of carcinogens within the lumen of the gut. Two main research avenues have been followed, based on the observation that fecal excretion of steroids and of mutagens is increased in persons consuming a Western high-fat diet.

1. Fecal Steroids and Colon Cancer

An hypothesis of great interest in the 1970's was that certain bile acids and neutral steroids might be transformed into carcinogens or co-carcinogens by anaerobic gut bacteria. This hypothesis, put forward by Hill and colleagues (1971), was based on observations made in the 1930's that these compounds are sterically similar to polycyclic aromatic hydrocarbons and that deoxycholic and cholic acids can be experimentally transformed into 3-methylcholanthrene. These transformations follow metabolic pathways which are known to occur naturally in the gut, such as those activated by certain clostridia with nuclear dehydrogenase activity. Indeed, the possibility of a carcinogenic effect for bile acids is supported by the observations that lithocholic acid is co-mutagenic in the Ames Test (Silverman and Andrews, 1977) and that it causes transformation of hamster embryo cells (Kelsey and Pienta, 1979).

To test this hypothesis in man, attempts have been made to determine whether (a) changes in the diet (in particular, increased fat intake) would alter fecal excretion of bile acids and cholesterol metabolites, as well as the composition of fecal microflora; and (b) differences in these fecal constituents occur between high and low risk populations (or individuals) for colon cancer.

a. Nutritional Studies. Antonis and Bersohn (1962) found that an increase from 15 to 40% in the proportion of calories from fat in the diet of 43 White and Bantu prisoners resulted in an increase in fecal excretion of neutral sterols and bile acids. The effect was greater with unsaturated fat. Increasing the fiber content of the diet produced bulkier stools containing a greater amount of fatty acids, bile acids and sterols. The effect on fecal sterol concentrations was not reported.

Cummings et al. (1978) observed that healthy volunteers placed on controlled diets containing successively high and low levels of animal fat showed a significant increase in fecal steroid excretion on the high fat diet. The bacterial flora, however, remained unaltered. Reddy et al. (1980a) in a study with similar but somewhat longer dietary regimens observed an increase in fecal microflora enzymic activity in addition to the increase in fecal steroid excretion.

To distinguish between the effect of fat and that of protein, Cummings et al. (1979) studied the fecal bile excretion of volunteers taking metabolically controlled diets with low and high animal protein content. The change in protein intake was without effect on fecal bile acid excretion. In a similarly designed study, Hentges et al. (1977) showed that animal protein also has little effect on the fecal bacterial profile.

The results of these nutritional studies, supported by some animal data (Reddy et al., 1977), suggest that high fat intake is associated with increased fecal excretion of neutral and acid steroids, and that the type of fat (saturated or unsaturated) has no specific effect on biliary and fecal bile acid excretion.

b. <u>Studies on Population Groups</u>. The studies of Hill and his colleagues (Hill et al., 1971; Crowther et al., 1976) on small groups of volunteers from populations with different risks for colon cancer (and different dietary fat intakes), including residents of England, Scotland, the United States, Uganda, Japan, India and Hong Kong, have shown strong correlations between colon cancer incidence rates, counts of fecal anaerobes (in particular, nuclear dehydrogenating clostridia) and fecal excretion of bile acids and cholesterol metabolites. However, the differences they found in fecal flora between groups with different colon cancer risks were not confirmed in the extensive studies conducted by Finegold et al. (1974;1975) and Moore and Holdeman (1974;1975). Although minor quantitative variations were present, organisms specific to high-, or low-risk groups were not observed by these authors. Finegold and Sutter (1978), and Hill (1981) later pointed out the limitations of traditional bacteriologic techniques to investigate the flora of the colonic lumen, the region probably most relevant to carcinogen production. It was then suggested that measurement of bacterial enzymic activity (e.g. β-glucuronidase, 7α-dehydroxylase activities) was of greater interest than taxonomic grouping of bacteria, as it indicates the functional capabilities of bacterial flora to produce putative carcinogenic compounds in the gut.

Reddy and Wynder (1973) investigated β-glucuronidase activity and fecal constituents of several different population groups: 17 American volunteers on a Western diet; 11 Seventh-Day Adventists on a meatless diet; 12 ovo-lacto vegetarians; 21 recently-arrived Japanese migrants to the U.S. on a Japanese diet; and 11 Chinese on a low-fat Chinese diet. β-glucuronidase activity was significantly higher, and the excretion of total and secondary bile acids was greater in the group of Americans on a Western diet than in the other groups. A similar study (Reddy et al., 1978a) in 20 American volunteers and in 15 Finns from Kuopio (a low risk population) showed greater fecal excretion of neutral sterols and of bacterial nuclear dehydrogenase activity among the Finns. However, the concentrations of these constituents were the same in the two groups. Conversely, the two populations excreted the same amount of secondary bile acids daily, but the concentration of fecal bile acids in the American subjects was 2.5 times that of the Finns, due to the greater stool output of the latter. This finding suggests that the role of bile acids may be physical (dilution) rather than biological. Similar studies on volunteers from New York, U.S.A., and Umea, Sweden, conducted by the same group (Domellof et al., 1982; Reddy et al., 1983) led to comparable results.

Another international study coordinated by the IARC (1977) compared dietary intake and fecal characteristics of random population samples from Kuopio (Finland) and Copenhagen (Denmark). This study failed to confirm the correlation between large-bowel cancer incidence and fecal steroid output or concentration. No difference was found in dietary fat, fecal excretion of neutral steroids, acid steroids or their metabolites. Higher intake of dietary fiber and milk in the low-incidence area (Kuopio) suggested possible protective effects, but apparently unrelated to mouth-anus transit-time.

This IARC study was later extended to urban and rural areas of both countries to include areas with intermediate colon cancer risks (Jensen et al., 1982). Daily fecal loss of bile acids was found to be identical in the 4 areas, but due to differences in fecal bulk, the fecal bile acid concentrations varied, showing a positive correlation with large-bowel cancer incidence. No significant difference was found for neutral steroids or for the ratio of anaerobic to aerobic bacteria. The average concentration of clostridia was similar in the 4 areas, but the proportion of nuclear dehydrogenating strains of clostridia was higher in Finland than in Denmark, a finding which is not in line with that of

Hill et al. (1971).

Fecal characteristics were also correlated with colon cancer incidence for two other ethnically similar but geographically separate populations (Japanese in Hawaii and Japanese in Akita, Japan) with markedly different colon cancer risks (Mower et al., 1979; Nomura et al., 1983). Hawaii Japanese had significantly higher fecal concentrations of deoxycholic acid, cholesterol and total animal steroids than did the subjects in Akita. However, the results for the other bile acids or neutral steroids were unremarkable or inconsistent with those of Hill et al.(1971), and Reddy and Wynder (1973). The authors pointed out that, unlike these previous studies, their sample was large (n=369) and randomly selected, and their results were adjusted for the confounding effects of age and sex. Finally, although the Japanese in Hawaii have 4 times as much cancer, the ratio of primary to secondary bile acids was similar in Hawaii and Akita, suggesting no gross difference in metabolism.

Recently, Nair, Turjam and their colleagues studied 168 randomly selected subjects matched on age, sex and marital status (and on milk usage and dairy-egg index, when applicable) from 4 populations with different risks for colon cancer: pure-vegetarian, lacto-ovo vegetarian, and non-vegetarian Seventh-Day Adventists (SDA); and a demographically comparable group from the general population (Turjman et al., 1984). The concentration of total bile acids was statistically different among the four dietary groups, with increasing values from SDA pure-vegetarians to general population non-vegetarians. The ratio of secondary to primary bile acids also differed among the groups, suggesting a positive correlation between the formation of secondary bile acids and population risk for developing colon cancer. Similarly, fecal cholesterol and its metabolites were found to be lower among vegetarians (Nair et al., 1984).

In summary, these correlation studies have failed to identify specific differences in fecal flora between high-, and low-risk populations and have been inconsistent in showing a correlation of colon cancer risk with fecal output, with concentrations of neutral and acid steroids, or with the degree of degradation of these fecal constituents. However, the possible protective effect of dietary fiber identified in these studies suggests that concentration rather than total output of fecal steroids might be relevant to the pathogenesis of colon cancer.

c. Studies on Colon Cancer Patients. Hill et al. (1975) compared fecal bile acids in 44 patients with colorectal cancer and 90 patients with other diseases. Eighty-two percent of the cases had bile acid concentration higher than an arbitrary level, compared to 17% of the controls. Similarly, 82% of the cases had nuclear dehydrogenating clostridia in their feces compared to 5% of the controls. Reddy and his colleagues (Reddy and Wynder, 1977; Mastromarino et al., 1976) determined fecal concentrations of neutral sterols and bile acids in 31 patients with colon cancer, 13 patients with adenomatous polyps, 9 patients with other digestive diseases and 34 American and Japanese healthy controls. Fecal concentrations of cholesterol and its metabolites, total and secondary bile acids, and 7 α-dehydroxylase and cholesterol dehydroxylase activities were higher in colon cancer cases and patients with adenomatous polyps compared to normal controls or patients with other digestive diseases. However, the ratio of primary to secondary bile acids was the same in colon cancer patients and American controls.

Several other investigators have compared fecal constituents of colon cancer cases and controls. The results have been inconsistent. Murray et al. (1980) studied 37 colorectal cancer patients and 36 surgical controls. Total fecal bile acid concentration was significantly higher for controls, whereas no difference was found for individual bile acids. Nuclear dehydrogenating clostridia were isolated from the feces of 64% of colorectal cancer patients and 15% of controls. Other studies have been completely negative. Moskovitz et al. (1979) reported on 15 patients with colonic adenocarcinoma, 23 healthy controls and 16 patients with nongastrointestinal cancer. No significant difference in the total bile acid and total neutral sterol concentations were found between the groups. Contrary to what was expected, coprostanol, coprostanone and lithocholic excretion was decreased in the colon cancer groups compared with controls. Similarly, Mudd et al. (1980) failed to demonstrate a higher fecal bile acid concentation in patients with ulcerative colitis (n=11), previously resected adenoma (n=20), or resected colorectal carcinoma (n=25), compared to healthy controls matched on age and sex. To determine whether the high levels of bile acids reported by some workers for untreated patients might be an effect of the lesion, these investigators studied prospectively a group of patients with symptoms suggestive of large bowel carcinoma. The 20 patients who ultimately were found to have colorectal carcinoma had, before treatment, fecal bile acid concentrations similar to control values, and the levels were not altered by subsequent resection.

In summary, results from case-control studies have been inconsistent, possibly because of the sampling limitations and the small size of certain of these studies and because of the difficulties in sorting out causal factors from metabolic side effects of the disease or its treatment. The latter problem is certainly minimized when patients with adenomatous polyps (generally considered as colon cancer precursors) are studied. However, the two studies which considered such patients also reported different results. Finally, when the ratio of fecal primary to secondary bile acids could be computed in the studies showing a positive association (Reddy and Wynder, 1977), the value of this ratio did not differ between cases and controls, suggesting no gross metabolic difference.

d. Related Hypotheses. Because of these inconsistencies in the results described above, the initial interest in the possibility that bile acids might be metabolized to carcinogens through desaturation of the steroid nucleus has been recently refocused on the promotional role of these acids observed in experimental studies (Reddy et al., 1978b; Cohen et al, 1980). This promotional effect may result from the irritative action of bile acids on the intestinal epithelium (Turjman et al., 1982; Deschner et al., 1981) since the compensatory proliferation of colonic epithelial cells could increase the opportunity for initiated cells to produce altered progeny, leading eventually to neoplasia.

Newmark et al. (1984) pointed out that not only free bile acids but other lipids present in even greater quantities in the colon, i.e., the fatty acids directly derived from dietary fat or from cellular and microbial debris in the gut, are highly irritating to the colon epithelium. These authors suggested that intraluminal calcium ions could reduce the potentially promoting effect of these compounds in the colon by converting them to insoluble calcium soaps. This hypothesis was supported by animal data indicating that the toxic effect on colonic epithelium of intrarectally administered deoxycholic acid can be prevented by a moderate increase in the dose of oral calcium (Wargovich et al., 1983), and by the inverse association between colorectal cancer incidence and dietary intakes of vitamin D and calcium in the Western Electric cohort study (Garland et al., 1985). Furthermore, Lipkin and Newmark (1985) have recently demonstrated that the increased proliferative activity of colonic epithelial cells observed in subjects at high risk for familial colonic cancer can be normalized by dietary calcium supplementation.

2. Fecal Mutagens and Colon Cancer

In the search for an etiologic link between a high fat diet and colon cancer, some consideration has been given to fecal mutagens as indicators of cancer risk. Ehrich et al. (1979) compared three South African populations with different colon cancer risks and observed that 19% of the fecal samples from urban white South-Africans (high risk population) were mutagenic, compared to only 2% for urban blacks and 0% for rural blacks. Reddy et al. (1980b) studied fecal mutagen activity among American volunteers on a Western diet, vegetarian Seventh-Day Adventists from New York and rural Finns from Kuopio. The percentage of samples showing mutagenic activity was significantly higher in the American volunteers on a Western diet compared to the Kuopio subjects from a low-risk area. None of the vegetarian Seventh-Day Adventists showed any mutagenic activity. Finally, Kuhnlein et al. (1981) compared fecal mutagen activity in non-vegetarians, ovo-lacto vegetarians, and pure vegetarians and observed significantly higher levels in non-vegetarians.

Two small case-control studies failed to show a significant association of fecal mutagens with adenomatous polyps in autopsy specimens (Correa et al., 1981) or with colon cancer in newly diagnosed patients (Bruce and Dion, 1980). Although further research is being conducted, preliminary results from nutritional studies have suggested that fat intake does not affect the excretion of the mutagen of bacterial origin isolated by Bruce and his colleagues (Bruce and Dion, 1980). However, the latter investigators did obtain reduction in mutagen levels by supplementation (in the nutritional range) with vitamin C, vitamin E or fiber.

Although fecal mutagens appear to be the product of bacterial action on feces and to be more frequently found in populations at high risk for colon cancer, their relationship to dietary fat remains uncertain.

CONCLUSIONS

As noted earlier, the epidemiologic evidence for dietary fat as a risk factor for colon cancer is inconsistent. Furthermore, the metabolic studies are equally divided and provide little clarification of the findings from the epidemiologic reports. Thus, at the present time, one cannot firmly conclude that dietary fat either promotes or has no effect on colon carcinogenesis in humans. The issue is unresolved. Several reasons for this ambiguous situation can be identified: 1) Dietary assessments have been weak in most epidemiologic studies reported up to now; 2) Many reports have paid minimal attention to the control of potential confounders; 3) Subjects used in most of the metabolic studies were not randomly selected and thus were probably not representative of their respective high- and low-risk population; and 4) Interactions between fat and other factors in the diet, which are likely to be important in the genesis of this cancer, have not been considered in most studies.

The needs for future research in this area are apparent from this general assessment, and include the following: 1) Additional case-control and cohort studies should be conducted; these studies should incorporate validated, quantitative dietary history methods for assessing intakes of fat, fiber and other nutrients, and should take advantage, where appropriate, of the availability of subjects with precursor lesions of colon cancer; 2) Such studies should also include analytic approaches that examine the interactive effects of several dietary factors, while simultaneously controlling for confounders; 3) Food composition data on the components of fiber in the diet are very much needed, in order to adequately incorporate this dietary constituent into future studies; 4) Newer hypotheses, such as those pertaining to the effects of dietary calcium, total caloric intake (with which fat consumption is highly correlated), and exercise should be tested in epidemiologic studies of various types; 5) Studies using validated biochemical markers of exposure to fats or other dietary factors should be pursued, although such markers have yet to be identified; 6) Past metabolic studies of fecal steroids have primarily attempted to explain a putative dietary fat etiology, but, because of the complexity of metabolic pathways and inattention to appropriate sampling procedures in many instances, these studies have not been particularly illuminating and the potential value of similar studies in the near future appears limited.

REFERENCES

Antonis A, Bersohn I (1962). The influence of diet on fecal lipids in South African White and Bantu prisoners. Am J Clin Nutr 11:143–155.
Armstrong B, Doll R (1975). Environmental factors and cancer incidence and mortality in different countries with special reference to dietary practices. Int J Cancer 15:617–631.
Barker DJP, Godfrey KM (1984). Geographical variations in the incidence of colorectal cancer in Britain. Br J Cancer 50:693–698.
Bingham SA, Williams DRR, Cole TJ, James WPT (1979). Dietary fiber and regional large-bowel cancer mortality in Britain. Br J Cancer 40:456–463.
Bingham SA, Williams DRR, Cummings JH (1985). Dietary fibre consumption in Britain: new estimates and their relation to large bowel cancer mortality. Br J Cancer 52:399–402.
Bruce WR, Dion PW (1980). Studies relating to a fecal mutagen. Am J Clin Nutr 33:2511–2512.
Cohen BI, Raicht RF, Deschner EE, Takahashi M, Sarwal AN, Fazzini E (1980). Effect of cholic acid feeding on N-methyl-N-nitrosourea induced colon tumors and cell kinetics in rats. J Natl Cancer Inst 64:573–578.
Correa P, Paschal J, Pizzolato P, Pelon W, Leslay DE (1981). Faecal mutagens and colorectal polyps: Preliminary report of an autopsy study. IN: Bruce WR, Correa P, Lipkin M, Tannenbaum SR, Wilkins TD (eds.). Banbury Report 7: Gastrointestinal cancer: Endogenous factors. Cold Spring Harbor, NY: Cold

Spring Harbor Laboratory, pp. 119-127.

Crowther JS, Drasar BS, Hill MJ, MacLennan R, Magnin D, Peach S, Teoh-Chan CH (1976). Faecal steroids and bacteria and large bowel cancer in Hong Kong by socio-economic groups. Br J Cancer 34:191-198.

Cummings JH, Hill MJ, Jivraj T, Houston H, Branch WJ, Jenkins DJA (1979). The effect of meat protein and dietary fiber on colonic function and metabolism. I. Changes in bowel habit, bile acid excretion, and calcium absorption. Am J Clin Nutr 32:2086-2093.

Cummings JH, Wiggins HS, Jenkins DJA, Houston H, Jivraj T, Drasar BS, Hill MJ (1978). Influence of diets high and low in animal fat on bowel habit, gastrointestinal transit time, fecal microflora, bile acid, and fat excretion. J Clin Invest 61:953-963.

Dales LG, Friedman GD, Ury HK, Grossman S, Williams SR (1979). A case-control study of relationships of diet and other traits to colorectal cancer in American Blacks. Am J Epidemiol 109:132-144.

Deschner EE, Cohen BI, Raicht RF (1981). Acute and chronic effects of dietary cholic acid on colonic epithelial cell proliferation. Digestion 21:290-296.

Domellof L, Darby L, Hanson D, Mathews L, Simi B, Reddy BS (1982). Fecal sterols and bacterial β-glucuronidase activity: a preliminary metabolic epidemiology study of healthy volunteers from Umea, Sweden, and Metropolitan New York. Nutr Cancer 4:120-127.

Drasar BS, Irving D (1973). Environmental factors and cancer of the colon and breast. Br J Cancer 27:167-172.

Ehrich M, Aswell JE, Van Tassell RL, Wilkins TD (1979). Mutagens in the feces of 3 South-African populations at different levels of risk for colon cancer. Mutation Res 64:231-240.

Enstrom JE (1975). Colorectal cancer and consumption of beef and fat. Br J Cancer 32:432-439.

Finegold SM, Sutter VL (1978). Fecal flora in different populations, with special reference to diet. Am J Clin Nutr 31:S116-S122.

Finegold S, Attebery HR, Sutter VL (1974). Effect of diet on human fecal flora: comparison of Japanese and American diets. Am J Clin Nutr 27:1456-1469.

Finegold S, Flora DJ, Attebery HR, Sutter VL (1975). Fecal bacteriology of colonic polyp patients and control patients. Cancer Res 35:3407-3417.

Garland C, Shekelle RB, Barrett-Connor E, Criqui MH, Rossof AH, Paul O (1985). Dietary vitamin D and calcium and risk of colorectal cancer: a 19-year prospective study in men. Lancet i:307-309.

Graham S, Dayal H, Swanson M, Mittelman A, Wilkinson G (1978). Diet in the epidemiology of cancer of the colon and rectum. J Natl Cancer Inst 61:709-714.

Haenszel W, Berg JW, Segi M, Kurihara M, Locke FB (1973). Large bowel cancer in Hawaiian Japanese. J Natl Cancer Inst 51:1765-1779.

Haenszel W, Locke FB, Segi M (1980). A case-control study of large bowel cancer in Japan. J Natl Cancer Inst 64:17-22.

Hentges DJ, Maier BR, Burton GC, Flynn MA, Tsutakawa RK (1977). Effect of a high-beef diet on the fecal bacterial flora of humans. Cancer Res 37:568-571.

Higginson J (1966). Etiological factors in gastrointestinal cancer in man. J Natl Cancer Inst 37:527-545.

Hill MJ (1981). Diet and the human intestinal flora. Cancer Res 41:3778-3780.

Hill MJ, Drasar BS, Aries V, Growther JS, Hawksworth G, Williams REO (1971). Bacteria and aetiology of cancer of large bowel. Lancet i:95-100.

Hill MJ, Drasar BS, Williams REO (1975). Faecal bile-acids and clostridia in patients with cancer of the large bowel. Lancet i:535-539.

Hirayama T (1979). Diet and cancer. Nutr Cancer 1:67-81.

Hirayama T (1981). A large-scale cohort study on the relationship between diet and selected cancers of digestive organs. IN: Bruce WR, Correa P, Lipkin M, Tannenbaum SR, Wilkins TD (eds.). Banbury Report 7: Gastrointestinal cancer: Endogneous factors. Cold Spring Harbor, NY: Cold Spring Harbor Laboratory, pp. 409-429.

Howell MA (1975). Diet as an etiological factor in the development of cancers of the colon and rectum. J Chron Dis 28:67-80.

International Agency for Research on Cancer Intestinal Microecology Group (1977). Dietary fibre, transit-time, faecal bacteria, steroids and colon cancer in two Scandinavian populations. Lancet ii:207-211.

Jain M, Cook GM, Davis FG, Grace MG, Howe GR, Miller AB (1980). A case-control study of diet and colo-rectal cancer. Int J Cancer 26:757–768.

Jensen OM, MacLennan R, Wahrendorf J (on behalf of the IARC large bowel cancer group) (1982). Diet, bowel function, fecal characteristics, and large bowel cancer in Denmark and Finland. Nutr Cancer 4:5–19.

Jensen OM, Sigtryggsson P, Nguyen-Dinh X, Bolander AM, Vercelli M, MacLennan R (1980). Large bowel cancer in married couples in Sweden. Lancet i:1161–1163.

Kelsey MI, Pienta RJ (1979). Transformation of hamster embryo cells by cholesterol- -epoxide and lithocholic acid. Cancer Lett 6:143–149.

Kinlen LJ (1982). Meat and fat consumption and cancer mortality: A study of strict religious orders in Britain. Lancet i:946–949.

Knox EG (1977). Foods and diseases. Br J Prev Soc Med 31:71–80.

Kolonel LN, Hankin JH, Nomura AMY, Chu SY (1981). Dietary fat intake and cancer incidence among five ethnic groups in Hawaii. Cancer Res 41:3727–3728.

Kolonel LN, Hankin JH, Nomura AMY, Hinds MW (1986a). Studies of nutrients and their relationship to cancer in the multiethnic population of Hawaii. Natl Cancer Inst Monogr. (in press).

Kolonel LN, Hankin JH, Nomura AMY (1986b). Multiethnic studies of diet, nutrition and cancer in Hawaii. Proceedings of the XVI International Symposium of the Princess Takamatsu Cancer Research Fund (in press).

Kritchevsky D (1985). Dietary fiber and cancer. Nutr Cancer 6:213–219.

Kuhnlein U, Bergstrom D, Kuhnlein H (1981)., Mutagens in feces from vegetarians and non-vegetarians. Mutation Res 85:1–12.

Lipkin M, Newmark H (1985). Effect of added dietary calcium on colonic epithelial-cell proliferation in subjects at high risk for familial colonic cancer. N Engl J Med 313:1381–1384.

Liu K, Moss D, Persky V, Stamler J, Garside D, Soltero I (1979). Dietary cholesterol, fat, and fibre, and colon cancer mortality. An analysis of international data. Lancet ii:782–785.

Lyon JL, Sorenson W (1978). Colon cancer in a low-risk population. Am J Clin Nutr 31:S227–S230.

Manousos O, Day NE, Trichopoulos D, Gerovassilis F, Tzonou A, Polychronopoulou A (1983). Diet and colorectal cancer: a case-control study in Greece. Int J Cancer 32:1–5.

Mastromarino A, Reddy BS, Wynder EL (1976). Metabolic epidemiology of colon cancer: enzymic activity of fecal flora. Am J Clin Nutr 29:1455-1460.

McKeown-Eyssen GE, Bright-See E (1984). Dietary factors in colon cancer: International relationships. Nutr Cancer 6:160-170.

McMichael AJ, Potter JD, Hetzel BS (1979). Time trends in colo-rectal cancer mortality in relation to food and alcohol consumption: United States, United Kingdom, Australia and New Zealand. Int J Epidemiol 8:295-303.

Miller AB, Howe GR, Jain M, Craib KJP, Harrison L (1983). Food items and food groups as risk factors in a case-control study of diet and colo-rectal cancer. Int J Cancer 32:155-161.

Modan B, Barell V, Lubin F, Modan M, Greenberg RA, Graham S (1975). Low-fiber intake as an etiological factor in cancer of the colon. J Natl Cancer Inst 55:15-18.

Moore WEC, Holdeman LV (1974). Human fecal flora: the normal flora of 20 Japanese-Hawaiians. Appl Microbiol 27:961-979.

Moore WEC, Holdeman LV (1975). Discussion of current bacteriological investigations of the relationships between intestinal flora, diet, and colon cancer. Cancer Res 35:3418-3420.

Moskovitz M, White C, Barnett RN, Stevens S, Russell E, Vargo D, Floch MH (1979). Diet, fecal bile acids, and neutral sterols in carcinoma of the colon. Dig Dis Sci 24:746-751.

Mower HF, Ray RM, Shoff R, Stemmermann GN, Nomura AMY, Glober GA, Kamiyama S, Shimada A, Yamakawa H (1979). Fecal bile acids in two Japanese populations with different colon cancer risks. Cancer Res 39: 328-331.

Mudd DG, McKelvey STD, Norwood W, Elmore DT, Roy A (1980). Faecal bile acid concentrations of patients with carcinoma or increased risk of carcinoma in the large bowel. Gut 21:587-590.

Murray WR, Blackwood A, Trotter JM, Calman KC, MacKay C (1980). Faecal bile acids and clostridia in the aetiology of colorectal cancer. Br J Cancer 41:923-928.

Nair PP, Turjman N, Goodman GT, Guidry C, Calkins BM (1984). Diet, nutrition intake, and metabolism in populations at high and low risk for colon cancer.

Metabolism of neutral sterols. Am J Clin Nutr 40: 931–936.

Newmark HL, Wargovich MJ, Bruce WR (1984). Colon cancer and dietary fat, phosphate and calcium: A hypothesis. J Natl Cancer Inst 72:1323–1325.

Nomura AMY, Wilkins TD, Kamiyama S, Heilbrun LK, Shimada A, Stemmermann GN, Mower HF (1983). Fecal neutral steroids in two Japanese populations with different colon cancer risks. Cancer Res 43:1910–1913.

Phillips RL, Snowdon DA (1985). Dietary relationships with fatal colorectal cancer among Seventh-Day Adventists. J Natl Cancer Inst 74:307–317.

Pickle LW, Greene MH, Ziegler RG, Toledo A, Hoover R, Lynch HT, Fraumeni JF (1984). Colorectal cancer in rural Nebraska. Cancer Res 44:363–369.

Powles JW, Williams DRR (1984). Trends in bowel cancer in selected countries in relation to wartime changes in flour milling. Nutr Cancer 6:40–48.

Reddy BS, Wynder EL (1973). Large-bowel carcinogenesis: Fecal constituents of populations with diverse incidence rates of colon cancer. J Natl Cancer Inst 50:1437–1442.

Reddy BS, Wynder EL (1977). Metabolic epidemology of colon cancer. Fecal bile acids and neutral sterols in colon cancer patients and patients with adenomatous polyps. Cancer 39:2533–2539.

Reddy BS, Ekelund G, Bohe M, Engle A, Domellof L (1983). Metabolic epidemiology of colon cancer: Dietary pattern and fecal sterol concentrations of three populations. Nutr Cancer 5:34–40.

Reddy BS, Hanson B, Mangat S, Mathews L, Sbaschnig M, Sharma C, Simi B (1980a). Effect of high-fat, high-beef diet and of mode of cooking of beef in the diet on fecal baterial enzymes and fecal bile acids and neutral sterols. J Nutr 110:1880–1887.

Reddy BS, Hedges AR, Laakso K, Wynder EL (1978a). Metabolic epidemiology of large bowel cancer. Fecal bulk and constituents of high-risk North American and low-risk Finnish population. Cancer 42:2832–2838.

Reddy BS, Mangat S, Sheinfil A, Weisburger JH, Wynder EL (1977). Effect of type and amount of dietary fat and 1,2-dimethylhydrazine on biliary bile acids, fecal bile acids, and neutral sterols in rats. Cancer Res 37:2132–2137.

Reddy BS, Sharma C, Darby L, Laakso K, Wynder EL (1980b). Metabolic epidemiology of large bowel cancer.

Fecal mutagens in high- and low-risk populations for
colon cancer. Mutation Res 72:511-522.

Reddy BS, Weisburger JH, Wynder EL (1978b). Mechanisms
of tumor promotion and co-carcinogenesis. IN: Slaga
TJ, Sivak A, Boutwell RK (eds.): "Carcinogenesis",
vol. 2, New York:Raven Press, pp. 453-464.

Silverman SJ, Andrews AW (1977). Bile acids: co-mutagenic
activity in the Salmonella-mammalian-microsome
mutagenicity test. J Natl Cancer Inst 59:1557-1559.

Smith AH, Pearce NE, Joseph JG (1985). Major colorectal
cancer aetiological hypotheses DO NOT explain
mortality trends among Maori and non-Maori New
Zealanders. Int J Epidemiol 14:79-85.

Stemmermann GN, Nomura AMY, Heilbrun LK (1984). Dietary
fat and the risk of colorectal cancer. Cancer Res
44:4633-37.

Turjman N, Goodman GT, Jaeger B, Nair PP (1984). Diet,
nutrition intake, and metabolism in populations at
high and low risk for colon cancer. Metabolism of
bile acids. Am J Clin Nutr 40:937-941.

Turjman N, Jacob C, Bhagavan M, Wityk N (1982). Effect
of lithocholic acid on incorporation of thymidine
into DNA of proliferating rat colon epithelial cells.
Fed Proc 41:884.

Wargovich MJ, Eng VWS, Newmark HL, Bruce WR (1983).
Calcium ameliorates the toxic effect of deoxycholic
acid on colonic epithelium. Carcinogenesis
4:1205-1207.

Wynder EL, Kajitani T, Ishikawa S, Dodo H, Takano A
(1969). Environmental factors of cancer of the colon
and rectum. II. Japanese Epidemiological Data.
Cancer 23:1210-1220.

Dietary Fat and Cancer, pages 93-115
© 1986 Alan R. Liss, Inc.

CLINICAL TRIALS OF LOW FAT DIETS AND BREAST CANCER PREVENTION

Carolyn K. Clifford, Ritva R. Butrum,
Peter Greenwald and Jerome W. Yates
Division of Cancer Prevention and Control, National
Cancer Institute, National Institutes of Health
Bethesda, Maryland 20892

INTRODUCTION

The National Cancer Institute (NCI) has initiated two national collaborative trials to determine the ability of low fat diets to prevent or reduce breast cancer incidence. This chapter reviews developments which led up to these studies and outlines their purpose, design and scope. These two multi-institution randomized clinical trials are known as 1) Women's Health Trial, a Phase III trial of a low fat diet to prevent breast cancer in women at increased risk, and 2) Nutrition Adjuvant Study, a Phase III trial of a low fat diet to prevent recurrence in women surgically treated for stage II breast cancer. Feasibility studies for both trials are currently in progress. The decision to undertake full-scale trials awaits the results of the feasibility studies and review by the NCI and its advisory boards.

OVERVIEW OF NCI CANCER PREVENTION AND CONTROL PROGRAM

In continuous efforts to reduce cancer incidence, morbidity and mortality, the National Cancer Institute has recently embarked on a research and resources development program which emphasizes coordinated and innovative approaches to cancer prevention and control. National cancer control objectives are being established to guide NCI cancer control efforts toward the specific goal of reducing cancer mortality by 50 percent by the year 2000.

Cancer control is defined as the reduction of cancer incidence, morbidity, and mortality through an orderly sequence from research on interventions and their impact in defined populations to the broad systematic application of the research results (Greenwald and Cullen, 1985). Cancer control research studies are classified into five phases which represent the orderly progression noted above. These are I) hypothesis development, II) methods development and testing, III) controlled intervention trials to establish cause-and-effect relationships, IV) research in defined populations, and V) demonstration and implementation studies.

Within the NCI, the Division of Cancer Prevention and Control has primary responsibility to plan, develop, and direct cancer prevention and cancer control programs. In 1982, the Division's research objectives were revised and new program directions were developed. The emphasis of these programs is on research studies to identify, evaluate and implement techniques and approaches for prevention and early detection of cancer. Current directions for the cancer prevention and control program indicate that research efforts should give priority to cancers causing the greatest morbidity and mortality, cancers for which substantial risk has been associated with environmental factors, and cancers for which effective actions are available.

Scientific knowledge from etiologic research provides the primary basis for cancer prevention. Cancer prevention, as defined, is applied research to systematically test or introduce a specific intervention aimed at having a measurable impact on an important cancer. The purpose of the intervention is to reduce cancer incidence with subsequent reduction in morbidity and mortality rates in populations.

Recently, the cancer prevention program has emphasized research efforts in the development and implementation of clinical trials as a systematic, multidisciplinary approach to cancer prevention. One of the programmatic thrusts in the cancer prevention program is to reduce cancer incidence or progression through applied research in the area of diet and nutrition. Accordingly, the NCI currently is supporting feasibility studies for two Phase III controlled intervention trials to test the efficacy of low fat diets in the prevention of breast cancer. The rationale, experimental design, and intervention approaches of these trials are described herein.

TRIAL DEVELOPMENT PROCESS

Controlled intervention trials, when feasible, represent an integral part of the effective bridge between basic knowledge and the application of research results to cancer prevention. Although costly and often complex, well-designed randomized controlled trials can provide the most definitive evidence of the efficacy of an intervention for human populations. Multi-institution trials are often necessary if adequate numbers of trial participants are to be achieved.

In the development of a decision process for cancer prevention trials, the NCI reviewed previous approaches used by the National Heart, Lung, and Blood Institute. Levy and Sondik (1978) outlined four key factors which should be balanced in the clinical trial decision process. These include: 1) state of the science, 2) feasibility of the trial, 3) potential impact, and 4) ethical considerations. Another important consideration is the practical timing of a randomized trial. There is a period of time during which sufficient research evidence exists to merit testing the proposed intervention, but before the proposed intervention is widely accepted or rejected as being beneficial unless tested.

The process of developing cancer prevention trials is structured around three major decision points by which the NCI commits resources to plan the trial, conduct the trial, and terminate the trial. In the decision-making process, the Institute uses its well established management structure which is centrally involved in any major funding decision (Figure 1). The National Cancer Advisory Board (NCAB) is responsible for advising the Director of the NCI. The NCAB has an overview of the National Cancer Program efforts and is the advisory body that provides the final review of all NCI grant applications. The NCI Executive Committee, composed of senior NCI staff, serves as an advisory group to the Director concerning planning and coordination of NCI program activities. Within the NCI, the four divisions that have programmatic responsibilities have chartered Boards of Scientific Counselors (BSCs). The BSCs provide expert

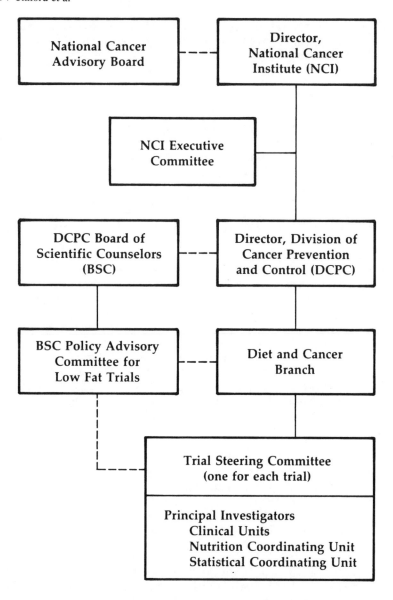

Figure 1

Management and Advisory Structure for Low Fat Trials to Prevent Breast Cancer

advice to the Director, NCI and to the director of each division on matters pertaining to scientific programming policy. The Board of Scientific Counselors also advises the Director on matters related to the progress of the programs of the Division. This is accomplished by examining projects through the concept review mechanism, furnishing advice on policies and planning, and evaluating the ongoing activities.

The concepts for the two clinical trials of a low fat diet to prevent or reduce breast cancer were presented to the Division of Cancer Prevention and Control, Board of Scientific Counselors in January 1983. The rationale and feasibility of the proposed trials, as well as several study design options were discussed. Board members expressed concern about several aspects of the trial including assumptions for estimating sample size, ability of women to adopt and comply with the proposed low fat diet, whether such a diet would be nutritionally adequate, and whether the dietary change could be accurately documented for research purposes. Also of concern was that, as the American diet undergoes subtle but important changes over a period of years, the control subjects might approach the experimental group in dietary habits thus interfering with evaluation of the basic hypothesis. On the other hand, Board members acknowledged the importance and potential impact of the trials. Breast cancer is the most common cancer among women in the United States and affects approximately one of every 11 women. Both epidemiological studies and experimental studies support the importance of dietary factors in breast cancer incidence and mortality and are suggestive of causality. Despite the cost, in relation to the importance of the possible endpoints, these trials would make a major contribution to knowledge of breast cancer etiology and progression.

The BSC was favorable to this type of prevention program initiative and voted conditional approval of the concepts for both trials. The conditions to be satisified for each trial were that both information from a feasibility study and the trial design would be presented to the Board for review before proceeding to a large-scale trial. Funding was approved by the National Cancer Advisory Board with the same conditions as recommended by the Board of Scientific Counselors.

In August 1983, the Division of Cancer Prevention and Control issued Requests for Applications (RFA) for cooperative agreements to support participation in "A Phase III Trial of a Low Fat Diet in Women with Stage II Breast Cancer", and in November 1983, an RFA was issued for cooperative agreements to support participation in "A Phase III Trial of a Low Fat Diet in Women at Increased Risk for Breast Cancer".

Applications were reviewed according to the NIH grant application review process. In the initial peer review process, applications are reviewed and evaluated on the basis of scientific merit with assignment of priority scores. A series of NCI programmatic reviews follows: Division Directors, Board of Scientific Counselors, NCI Executive Committee, and National Cancer Advisory Board. These reviews consider the results of the initial peer review, the availability of Institute funds, and the contribution that the proposed research would make to the Institute's mission.

Both trials are supported through the cooperative agreement mechanism. With this type of grant, substantial programmatic involvement is anticipated, and an assistance relationship exists between the National Cancer Institute and the principal investigators for the implementation and conduct of these trials. There is NCI involvement with regard to: 1) development of the protocol, 2) monitoring adherence to the protocol, 3) monitoring of the safety of the trial participants, and 4) coordination of the trial. The principal investigators have primary responsibility for the development and conduct of the trials and will identify, enroll and follow participants using common protocols developed jointly by the investigators and NCI.

For each trial, awards were made in three categories: 1) a statistical coordinating unit with primary responsibility for statistical design, data collection, management and analysis; 2) a nutrition coordinating unit responsible for dietary assessment and monitoring, nutrient analysis of dietary records, nutrition intervention protocols, and instructional material for clinical nutritionists and study subjects; and 3) clinical units responsible for enrollment of women into the trial and implementation of study protocols.

Both trials established a Steering Committee of study

investigators and various planning subcommittees including quality control, nutritional and behavioral intervention, design and analysis, and publications. Each Steering Committee proposed the final study design and developed policies for the investigators and management of the study.

A Policy Advisory Committee was established as a senior advisory committee to the Director of the Division of Cancer Prevention and Control and to the Division's Board of Scientific Counselors. The Policy Advisory Committee consists of members from the Board of Scientific Counselors, as well as individuals external to the Board, and is responsible for periodically reviewing the progress and providing policy guidance to the operation of each trial. This Policy Advisory Committee has primary responsibility for reviewing the feasibility study and making a recommendation to the Board of Scientific Counselors on whether to continue, modify, or stop the trial. This recommendation will be given further consideration by the Board of Scientific Counselors whose recommendation will be presented to the NCI Executive Committee and the National Cancer Advisory Board, both of which will participate in the final decision on whether to proceed to a full-scale trial.

EPIDEMIOLOGICAL AND EXPERIMENTAL BACKGROUND

A prerequisite to cancer prevention research is scientific evidence of an etiologic association with a potential intervention. In planning for diet and cancer prevention research studies, the NCI commissioned the National Research Council to conduct a comprehensive review of the available scientific literature on diet and cancer and make recommendations for possible future research directions (Committee on Diet, Nutrition and Cancer, 1982, 1983). The Committee concluded that the epidemiological and experimental evidence is consistent and most suggestive for a causal relationship between high fat intake and occurrence of breast cancer. The conclusion is based on several types of studies supporting the importance of dietary factors in breast cancer incidence and mortality: descriptive epidemiological studies, correlation studies, evaluation of nutrition-mediated risk factors, case-control and cohort studies. Additional supporting evidence was derived from experimental studies in laboratory animals.

The National Cancer Institute and its advisory boards also assessed the level of association between dietary fat and breast cancer occurrence, using the five epidemiologic criteria for causality previously developed and applied in smoking research (Surgeon General's Report, 1982). These criteria included: 1) consistency of the association, 2) strength of the association, 3) specificity of the association, 4) temporal relationship of the association, and 5) coherence of the association. Based on this assessment of existing epidemiologic and laboratory data, the NCI concluded that the evidence is strong enough to warrant implementation of clinical trials on breast cancer prevention using a low fat diet as the intervention. The evidence for the role of diet in the etiology of breast cancer is briefly summarized.

Breast cancer is the leading cause of cancer morbidity and mortality in North American women. Although this cancer is hormone-associated (MacMahon et al., 1973), the hypothesis that breast cancer risk is associated with dietary factors has attracted much interest (Wynder et al., 1976; Wynder, 1980; Kakar and Henderson, 1985).

Descriptive epidemiological studies have shown large international variations in breast cancer incidence and suggest that cultural factors or lifestyle, especially diet, influence the etiology of this disease (Armstrong and Doll, 1975; Doll and Peto, 1981; Wynder and Hirayama, 1977). Breast cancer incidence is much higher in North America, Western Europe, Australia and New Zealand than in Asia and Africa.

International correlation studies (Armstrong and Doll, 1975; Carroll, 1975; Drasar and Irving, 1973; Hems, 1978; Knox, 1977; Hirayama, 1978; Enig et al., 1978; Kolonel et al., 1981) of breast cancer incidence and mortality with various dietary factors have shown a positive correlation with per capita intake of total fat, animal protein, total protein and total calories. The strongest and most consistent positive association was per capita intake of total fat.

Further evidence suggesting that cultural or lifestyle factors are associated with breast cancer is provided from studies on populations who have undergone a lifestyle change through migration, industralization or wartime experience.

Migrant studies suggest that differences in breast cancer incidence and mortality are due largely to environmental factors rather than racial or genetic factors (Haenszel, 1961; Buell, 1973; Dunn, 1977; Kolonel et al., 1981). Studies of migrant populations from a country with a low incidence to a country with a high incidence of breast cancer show that the populations acquire the rates of their host country. The incidence of breast cancer increases coincident with increased fat intake. Japan is an industrialized country where breast cancer incidence is still low, but mortality and morbidity rates are steadily increasing as the Japanese lifestyle becomes more westernized, accompanied by a two-fold increase in dietary fat intake (Hirayama, 1978). At the onset of World War II, there was a marked reduction in breast cancer mortality and intake of fat, meat and sugar in England and Wales, with significant correlations being maximal for a diet breast cancer mortality reduction 12 years later (Ingram, 1981).

Nutrition-mediated factors that affect the risk of breast cancer include weight, height and body mass (de Waard, 1975; de Waard and Baandersvan Halewijn, 1974; de Waard et al., 1977) and age at menarche (MacMahon et al., 1973; Miller, 1978). A positive association between obesity and risk of breast cancer has been reported by some investigators (Hirayama, 1978; de Waard, 1975) but not by others (Adami et al., 1977; Wynder et al., 1978). Another study (Gray et al., 1979) showed breast cancer incidence and mortality rates were correlated with total fat, even after controlling for other breast cancer risk factors. This suggests that, while some effects of diet and breast cancer may be mediated by effects on anthropometric risk factors, there may also be more direct effects.

Several observations suggest that nutritional factors, especially dietary fat, may provide promotional stimuli for the development and progression of breast cancer (Wynder et al., 1976; Wynder and Cohen, 1982). Survival rates are significantly higher in Japanese breast cancer patients compared to U.S. patients, even after controlling for stage at diagnosis, tumor size, histology and medical care (Wynder et al. 1963; Morrison et al., 1976, 1977; Nemoto et al., 1977; Ward-Hinds et al., 1982). Dietary differences between the two countries have been suggested as a possible explanation for the different survival rates (Wynder, 1980). The differences in survival are greater for post-menopausal

women than for pre-menopausal women (Sakamoto et al., 1979)
and overweight breast cancer patients have a greater chance
of early recurrence and shorter survival than do non-obese
patients (Donegan et al., 1978; Tartter et al., 1981; Abe
et al., 1976; Boyd et al., 1981). These observations are
consistent with the demographic and correlation evidence
that dietary fat is associated with an increase in the
incidence of breast cancer.

Three case-control studies support the suggested causal
association of fat intake with breast cancer risk. In a
study (Phillips, 1975) of 77 breast cancer cases and matched
controls among California Seventh Day Adventists, there was
a direct association between frequency of consumption of
high fat foods and breast cancer. Miller et al. (1978)
reported a weak direct association between total fat
consumption and breast cancer in both pre-menopausal and
post-menopausal women in a study of 400 cases and 400
matched controls in Canada. Another Canadian study (Lubin
et al., 1981) which involved 577 breast cancer cases and
826 controls, found significant increasing trends in relative
risk with more frequent consumption of red meat, pork and
sweet desserts. An analysis of mean daily nutrient intake
supported a link between breast cancer and consumption of
animal fat and protein. Another case-control study (Graham
et al., 1982) reported no significant link of breast cancer
with dietary factors.

In a prospective study (Nomura et al., 1978), the
dietary records of Japanese men whose spouses had breast
cancer were compared with another group whose wives did not
develop the disease, based on the assumption that dietary
patterns of husbands and wives are similar. The breast
cancer spouses consumed more fats, meats and cheese and
less Japanese food.

Laboratory animal studies provide strong support for an
association between dietary fat and breast cancer. Numerous
studies in different strains of mice and rats have shown
that high fat diets enhance spontaneous mammary tumors
(Tannenbaum, 1942) as well as those induced by several
types of initiators of carcinogenesis. These include
chemically-induced (Carroll and Khor, 1970; Chan et al.,
1977; Hopkins and Carroll, 1979), transplantable (Hillyard
and Abraham, 1979) and radiation induced mammary tumors
(Silverman et al., 1980). Dietary fat affects the promo-

tional rather than the initiating stages of mammary tumor-igenesis (Carroll and Khor, 1975). Tumor enhancement is greater when high fat diets are fed after administration of the carcinogen. Within ranges, the promoting effect is proportional to both quantity and duration of fat intake (Dao and Chan, 1983). The total concentration rather than the type of fat is more effective in promoting mammary tumorigenesis, once a minimum essential fatty acid require-ment has been met (Carroll, 1980). The promotional effect of fat cannot be explained on the basis of the high calorie density of fat since the same effect occurs in pair-fed animals. Moreover, most experiments comparing high and low fat diets have used isocaloric diets and shown little difference in growth rates (Carroll, 1980). Dietary fat reduction, even late in carcinogenesis, can reduce tumor incidence (Davidson and Carroll, 1982). Restriction of calorie intake reduces the promotional effect (Tannenbaum, 1945; Kritchevsky et al., 1984).

There are well recognized limitations in epidemiologi-cal research on the relationship of diet to breast cancer. For example, the methods for assessing exposure may be of varying adequacy. Per capita intakes of foods and nutrients are based on food disappearance data and may not represent actual consumption. Eating patterns of a population may not be representative of the diet of women who develop breast cancer. The choice of controls in case-control studies also may present limitations. Despite these inherent limitations and those of experimental animals studies, the current knowlege of the etiology of breast cancer supports the role of dietary risk factors, particularly the level of total dietary fat. The central question which remains unresolved is how much of a role does dietary fat play. To address this question, controlled dietary intervention trials will be required. In such an endeavor, practical issues may be as important as theoretical considerations.

OBJECTIVES AND SCOPE OF FEASIBILITY STUDIES

The feasibility studies for both trials will consider factors such as:

o   Of eligible women invited, how many agree to parti-
     cipate?

o   For those enrolled, what are the rates of drop-ins

(control group adopts a low fat diet) and drop-outs (intervention group returns to usual diet)?

o What is the dietary fat intake in the control and the intervention group at various time points?

o Are there any unanticipated adverse effects?

The feasibility studies will provide an opportunity to 1) demonstrate that women can be recruited from high-risk breast cancer populations to undertake a rather stringent dietary regimen; 2) demonstrate that the dietary intervention can substantially reduce the level of fat intake in women over a 6-month period; 3) develop and test forms, methods, procedures, and organization, that will be required to implement a long-term full-scale trial; 4) estimate the number of potentially eligible women accessible to the clinical units; and 5) estimate the costs of required personnel and other necessary costs to achieve the dietary intervention objectives for use in planning a full-scale trial. Due to the short time frame, the feasibility studies will provide essentially no information about the ability of recruited women to maintain a low fat diet over the long-term or the endpoints of the full-scale trials.

WOMEN'S HEALTH TRIAL

The primary hypothesis to be tested is whether a low fat diet (20% of calories from fat), compared to the customary American diet (approximately 40% of calories from fat) will significantly reduce the incidence of breast cancer among women at increased risk of the disease.

Recruitment and Screening

Recruitment into the feasibility study began at three clinical units (Table 1) in March 1985 with an enrollment goal of 300 women. Women eligible for participation are identified from registered cohorts of women, age 45-69, and characterized as to their risk factors for breast cancer and their interest in participating in periodic followup for early detection of breast cancer. Eligibility criteria include 1) two or more first- or second-degree female relatives with a history of breast cancer or 2) more than one of the following characteristics: a) history of benign breast disease documented by two or more surgical biopsies,

b) history of unilateral breast cancer in one first- or second-degree female relative, c) nulliparous or parous with first full-term delivery at age 30 or older, d) single surgical biopsy with atypical epithelial hyperplasia.

TABLE 1. Participants in Feasibility Study for the Women's Health Trial

Principal Investigator	Institution	Unit
Ross L. Prentice, Ph.D.	Fred Hutchinson Cancer Research Center	Statistical
Sherwood L. Gorbach, M.D.	New England Medical Center	Nutrition
Maureen M. Henderson, M.D.	Fred Hutchinson Cancer Research Center	Clinical
William Insull, Jr., M.D.	Baylor College of Medicine	Clinical
Myron Moskowitz, M.D.	University of Cincinnati	Clinical

Potentially eligible women are recruited primarily from a cohort of women who had previously participated in the Breast Cancer Detection Demonstration Project and from health maintenance organization cohorts. Various techniques are used to solicit voluntary participation, the most common being to send an introductory letter. The women are informed of the randomized nature of the trial.

Further screening for eligibility will be conducted by scheduling clinic visits. At these visits, the purpose and scope of the trial and requirements for participation are explained in detail. Women who sign the informed consent form will be invited to continue the eligibility screening which includes 1) breast examination, 2) instruction on breast self-examination, 3) mammography, 4) height and weight measurement, 5) 4-day diet record, 6) food frequency questionnaire and other questionnaires on health history and habits. Eligibility will be further determined on the basis of reviewing the questionnaires and an assessment of willingness and ability to adhere to the proposed intervention program.

Reasons for exclusion include body weight greater than 50% above ideal weight, refusal to sign consent form, medical conditions (e.g., cancer, alcohol dependence, lipid-lowering medication), not interested in trial participation, characterized as potentially unreliable or noncompliant, currently following a low fat diet (less than 35% of calories from fat) or lacto-ovovegetarian diet, or 50% or more of meals eaten outside the home.

Randomization

After eligibility and willingness to enter the trial have been established, the women will be randomized into either the nutrition intervention group or the control group. Allocation to the nutrition intervention group or the control group will be stratified by clinical unit in the ratio of 3 nutrition intervention to 2 control women.

Intervention

Women in the control group will not be offered a nutrition intervention program since the general strategy adopted for this group was minimum interference with customary diets while collecting nutritional data considered necessary for appropriate comparison with the nutrition intervention group. If needed, participants in the control group will be provided basic nutrition principles for maintaining nutritionally adequate diets with no emphasis placed on modification of dietary fat. The control group will be invited to return for a 6-month followup visit, at which time a 4-day food record is submitted and body weight recorded.

The intervention program for the nutrition intervention group is a nutrition education and counseling approach aimed at providing the women with skills necessary to make a permanent lifestyle change to a low fat eating plan (20% of calories from fat). The general strategy incorporates teaching nutrition skills, self-monitoring techniques, behavior modification techniques, and group support systems. Common protocols, data forms, educational materials, a nutritionist's manual and a participant's manual were developed, and training workshops for nutritionists were conducted to establish uniformity in methods and procedures for the intervention program.

Nutrition instruction and counseling will be conducted primarily in group sessions held weekly for the first 8 weeks of intervention, followed by biweekly sessions through-out the remainder of the 6-month intervention period for the feasibility study. Individual sessions are scheduled for developing an individualized low fat eating plan and for a 3- and 6-month followup visit.

The low fat eating plan developed for an individual participant is based on information obtained from the 4-day food record, food frequency questionnaire and other nutritional information collected at baseline. In adapting the low fat eating plan, consideration will be given to amounts and combinations of foods ordinarily eaten, between-meal snacks and food preparation methods. Low fat eating plans are based on conventional foods and designed to be adequate for the essential nutrients.

A fat scoring system was devised as a self-monitoring tool for the participant and to provide rapid feedback to the participant and nutritionist for monitoring the progress and effectiveness of the intervention program. Dietary adherence will be monitored by 4-day food records collected at the 3- and 6-month followup visits. In addition, body weight will be recorded at the 6-month visit. Serum cholesterol, determined at baseline and at 6 months on the intervention program, will be used to evaluate the effectiveness of this objective biochemical measure in monitoring adherence to the low fat eating plan.

Sample Size

It is estimated that a study population of 30,000 women with a followup period of 8-10 years would be required to obtain a statistically reliable test of the hypothesis. The endpoint is occurrence of histologically diagnosed breast cancer.

NUTRITION ADJUVANT STUDY

The primary hypothesis to be tested is whether a low fat diet (15% of calories from fat) compared to the usual American diet (approximately 40% of calories from fat) can significantly reduce recurrence rate and prolong disease-free survival and overall survival in post-menopausal women surgically treated for stage II breast cancer.

Recruitment and Screening

Recruitment for the feasibility study began in September 1985 at 8 clinical units (Table 2) with an enrollment goal of 250 women. Potentially eligible women are identified through breast cancer patient logs maintained by oncologists and surgeons at the clinical units and/or practicing physicians and surgeons in the local medical community.

TABLE 2. Participants in Feasibility Study for the Nutrition Adjuvant Study

Principal Investigator	Institution	Unit
Robert M. Elashoff, Ph.D.	University of California, LA	Statistical
I. Marilyn Buzzard, Ph.D.	University of Minnesota	Nutrition
George L. Blackburn, M.D., Ph.D.	New England Deaconess Hospital	Clinical
Rowan T. Chlebowski, M.D., Ph.D.	Harbor-UCLA Medical Center	Clinical
Bernard Fisher, M.D.	University of Pittsburgh	Clinical
William Insull, Jr., M.D.	Baylor College of Medicine	Clinical
Peter R. Jochimsen, M.D.	University of Iowa Hospitals	Clinical
Daniel W. Nixon, M.D.	Emory University	Clinical
Edward F. Scanlon, M.D.	Illinois Cancer Council	Clinical
Ernst L. Wynder, M.D.	American Health Foundation	Clinical

Initial screening for eligibility is by review of the patient's medical history, surgery and pathology reports. Eligibility criteria requires diagnosis of stage II breast cancer treated by 1) modified radical mastectomy, 2) total mastectomy, or 3) segmental mastectomy with post-operative radiotherapy. For purposes of this trial, stage II breast cancer is characterized as a tumor more than 2 cm but not more than 5 cm in its greatest dimension and at least one axillary lymph node considered to contain growth. An early issue in patient selection concerned the choice of adjuvant chemotherapy and the range of adjuvant chemotherapy options which would be acceptable in this multi-institution trial. In keeping with a September 1985 NIH Consensus Conference on Adjuvant Chemotherapy for Breast Cancer, it was decided to use Tamoxifen, a relative nontoxic hormonal therapy. All trial particpants will receive Tamoxifen (20 mg/day) for two years, with treatment to begin within 60 days post-mastectomy.

Potentially eligible women, age 50-75, are contacted and informed of the purpose and scope of the trial and requirements for participation are explained in detail. The women are also informed of the randomized nature of the trial and the possibility of being assigned to a long-term followup study.

Participants will be selected through a series of screening visits. Women who are interested in participating in the trial and who sign the consent form will be invited to a series of three pre-randomization nutrition screening visits which begin approximately 4 weeks postsurgery. The purpose of these visits is to collect baseline nutritional data and to assess the woman's willingness and ability to complete data collection forms and adhere to the proposed intervention program. During a 4-week nutrition run-in-period the following will be obtained: 1) diet history, 2) health habits and history questionnaire, 3) 4-day food record, 4) 24-hour telephone recall, 5) anthropometric data, and 6) blood sample. In addition, a pre-study oncology visit will be scheduled and include: physical examination, chest x-ray, pap smear and mammography.

Reasons for exclusion include prior therapy for breast cancer including chemotherapy, immunotherapy and/or hormonal therapy; interval between mastectomy and eligibility deter-mination exceeds 120 days; refusal to sign consent form; not interested in participation; nonmalignant systemic disease (e.g., Type I diabetes; cardiovascular, renal, or hepatic disorders) which prevents prescription of a low fat diet; body weight less than 85% or greater than 50% of ideal weight; characterized as potentially unreliable or noncompliant; expected geographic mobility; not accessible by telephone; baseline dietary fat intake less than 30% of calories from fat.

Randomization

After eligibility and willingness to enter the trial have been established, the women will be equally randomized into either the intensive intervention group (low fat diet) or the nonintensive intervention group (usual diet). Allocation to intensive intervention group or nonintensive intervention group will be stratified by clinical unit, the number of histological positive axillary lymph nodes, and estrogen receptor status.

Intervention

Women in the nonintensive intervention group are expected to maintain their usual diet (approximately 40% of calories from fat). Nutrition education materials and counseling will emphasize nutritionally adequate diets. Individual followup visits are scheduled at 3-month intervals. It is anticipated that any attempts by participants in this group to reduce fat intake will be minimally successful without professional assistance and a planned intervention strategy.

The intervention program for the intensive intervention group is aimed to reduce fat intake to 15% of total calories while maintaining a nutritionally adequate diet. The intervention strategies are based on education, goal setting, evaluation and feedback, including participant self-monitoring, incentives and rewards. The major approach to intensive intervention will be a step-by-step approach to dietary change based on the needs and abilities of the individual participant. A low fat eating plan will be developed based on information obtained from the diet history and other nutritional information collected at baseline. Individual counseling sessions will be conducted at least biweekly during the first 3 months of intervention and then monthly during the remainder of the feasibility study. A fat scoring system was devised as a self-monitoring tool for the participant. To establish uniformity in methods and procedures, common protocols, educational materials for nutritionists and participants, and data forms were developed and training workshops held for the nutritionists.

Dietary adherence will be monitored in both groups by 4-day food records, 24-hour recalls, and anthropometric measurements collected at 3- and 6-month followup visits in the feasibility study. In addition, blood samples will be collected and analyzed for several biochemical parameters including serum lipoprotein and total cholesterol, plasma phospholipid fatty acid profiles and hormones. The biochemical parameters will be compared with nutrient intake data to evaluate their potential use in monitoring compliance to the low fat diet.

Sample Size

It is estimated that a study population of 2,000 women with a followup period of 5 years would be required to obtain a statistically reliable test of the hypothesis. The endpoints are disease-free survival time and overall survival time.

CONCLUSION

Feasibility studies are currently in progress for two clinical trials to determine whether a preventive program directed at the reduction of dietary fat intake to less than 20% of calories will significantly reduce the incidence or recurrence and mortality from breast cancer. Based on assessment of the feasibility studies, a decision will then be made on whether to proceed to full-scale trials. The National Cancer Institute and its advisory boards believe the rationales are strong and the clinical trials, if feasible, deserve high priority.

REFERENCES

Abe R, Kumagai W, Kimura M, Hirosaki A, Nakamura T (1976). Biological characteristics of breast cancer in obesity. Tohoku J Exp Med 120: 351-359.

Adami HO, Rimsten A, Stenkvist B, Vegelius J (1977). Influence of height, weight and obesity on risk of breast cancer in an unselected Swedish population. Br J Cancer 36:787-792.

Armstrong B, Doll P (1975). Environmental factors and cancer incidence and mortality in different countries, with special reference to dietary practices. Intl J Cancer 15:617-631.

Boyd NF, Campbell JE, Germanson T, Thompson DB, Sutherland DJ, Meakin JW (1981). Body weight and prognosis in breast cancer. J Natl Cancer Inst 67:785-789.

Buell P (1973). Changing incidence of breast cancer in Japanese American women. J Natl Cancer Inst 51:1479-1483.

Carroll KK (1975). Experimental evidence of dietary factors and hormone-dependent cancers. Cancer Res 35:3374-3383.

Carroll KK (1980). Influence of diet on mammary cancer. Nutr Cancer 2:232-236.

Carroll KK, Khor HT (1970). Effects of dietary fat and dose level of 7,12dimethylbenz(a)anthracene on mammary incidence in rats. Cancer Res 30:2260-2264.

Carroll KK, Khor HT (1975). Dietary fat in relation to tumorigenesis. Prog Biochem Pharmacol 10:308-353.

Chan PC, Head, JF, Cohen LA, Wynder EL (1977). Influence of dietary fat on the induction of rat mammary tumors by N-nitrosomethylurea: associated hormone changes and differences between Sprague-Dawley and F344 rats. J Natl Cancer Inst 59:1279-1283.

Consensus Conference (1985). Adjuvant chemotherapy for breast cancer. JAMA 254:3461-3463.

Dao TL, Chan PC (1983). Effect of duration of high fat intake on enhancement of mammary carcinogenesis in rats. J Natl Cancer Inst 71:201-205.

Davidson MB, Carroll KK (1982). Inhibitory effect of a fat-free diet on mammary carcinogenesis in rats. Nutr Cancer 3:207-215.

de Waard F (1975). Breast cancer incidence and nutritional status with particular reference to body weight and height. Cancer Res 35:33513356.

de Waard F, Baanders-van Halewijn EA (1974). A prospective study in general practice on breast cancer risk in post-menopausal women. Intl J Cancer 14:153-160.

de Waard F, Cornelis JP, Aoki K, Yoshida M (1977). Breast cancer incidence according to weight and height in two cities of the Netherlands and in Aichi prefecture, Japan. Cancer 40:1269-1275.

Doll R, Peto R (1981). The causes of cancer: quantitative estimates of avoidable risks of cancer in the United States today. J Natl Cancer Inst 66:1191-1308.

Donegan WL, Hartz AJ, Rimm AA (1978). The association of body weight with recurrent cancer of the breast. Cancer 41:1590-1594.

Drasar BS, Irving D (1973). Environmental factors of cancer of the colon and breast. Br J Cancer 27:167-172.

Dunn J (1977). Breast cancer among American Japanese in the San Francisco Bay Area. Natl Cancer Inst Monogr 47:157-160.

Enig MG, Munn RJ, Keeney M (1978). Dietary fat and cancer trends--a critique. Fed Proc 37:2215-2220.

Graham S, Marshall J, Mettlin C, Rzepka T, Nemoto T, Byers T (1982). Diet in the epidemiology of breast cancer. Am J Epidemiol 116:68-75.

Gray GE, Pike MC, Henderson BE (1979). Breast cancer incidence and mortality rates in different countries in relation to known risk factors and dietary practices. Br J Cancer 39:1-7.

Greenwald P, Cullen JW (1985). The new emphasis in cancer control. J Natl Cancer Inst 74:543-551.

Haenszel W (1961). Cancer mortality among the foreign-born in the United States. J Natl Cancer Inst 26:37-132.

Hems G (1978). The contributions of diet and child-bearing to breast cancer rates. Br J Cancer 37:974-982.

Hillyard LA, Abraham S (1979). Effect of dietary poly-unsaturated fatty acids on growth of mammary adenocarcinomas in mice and rats. Cancer Res 39:4430-4437.

Hirayama T (1978). Epidemiology of breast cancer with special reference to the role of diet. Preventive Med 7:173-195.

Hopkins GJ, Carroll KK (1979). Relationship between amount and type of dietary fat in promotion of mammary carcino-genesis induced by 7,12dimethylbenz(a)anthracene. J Natl Cancer Inst 62:1009-1012.

Ingram DM (1981). Trends in diet and breast cancer mortality in England and Wales 1928-1977. Nutr Cancer 3:75-80.

Kakar F, Henderson M (1985). Diet and breast cancer. Clin Nutr 4:119-130.

Knox EG (1977). Foods and diseases. Br J Prev Soc Med 31:71-80.

Kolonel LN, Hankin JH, Lee J, Chu SY, Nomura AMY, Ward-Hinds MW (1981). Nutrient intakes in relation to cancer incidence in Hawaii. Br J Cancer 44:332-339.

Kritchevsky D, Weber MM, Klurfeld, DM (1984). Dietary fat versus caloric content initiation and promotion of DMBA-induced mammary tumorigenesis in rats. Cancer Res 44:3174-3177.

Levy RI, Sondik EJ (1978). Decision-making in planning large-scale comparative studies. Ann NY Acad Sci 304:441-447.

Lubin JH, Burns PE, Blot WJ, Ziegler RG, Lees AW, Fraumeni JF (1981). Dietary factors and breast cancer risk. Intl J Cancer 28:685-689.

MacMahon B, Cole P, Brown J (1973). Etiology of human breast cancer: a review. J Natl Cancer Inst 50:21-42.

Miller AB (1978). An overview of hormone-associated cancers. Cancer Res 38:3985-3990.

Miller AB, Kelly A, Choi NW, Matthews V, Morgan RW, Muran L, Burch JD, Feather J, Howe GR, Jain M (1978). A study of diet and breast cancer. Am J Epid 107:499-509.

Morrison AS, Lowe CR, MacMahon B, Ravnihar B, Yuasa S (1977). Incidence, risk factors and survival in breast cancer: report on five years of follow-up observation. Europ J Cancer 13:209-214.

Morrison AS, Lowe CR, MacMahon B, Ravnihar B, Yuassa S (1976). Some international differences in treatment and survival in breast cancer. Intl J Cancer 18:269-273.

National Research Council (1982). Diet, Nutrition, and Cancer. Committee on Diet, Nutrition and Cancer, Assembly of Life Sciences, National Academy Press. Washington, DC.

National Research Council (1983). Diet, Nutrition, and Cancer: Directions for Research. Committee on Diet, Nutrition and Cancer, Assembly of Life Sciences, National Academy Press. Washington, D.C.

Nemoto T, Tominago T, Chamberlain A, Iwasa, Z, Koyama H, Hama M, Bross I, Dao T (1977). Differences in breast cancer between Japan and the United States. J Natl Cancer Inst 58:193-197.

Nomura A, Henderson BE, Lee J (1978). Breast cancer and diet among the Japanese in Hawaii. Am J Clin Nutr 31: 2020-2025.

Office of Smoking and Health (1982). The health consequences of smoking: cancer, a report of the Surgeon General. US Govt Print Off, Washington, DC.

Phillips RL (1975). Role of lifestyle and dietary habits in risk of cancer among Seventh Day Adventists. Cancer Res 35:3513-3522.

Sakamoto G, Sugamo H, Hartman WH (1979). Comparative clinico-pathological study of breast cancer among Japanese and American females. Jap J Cancer Clin 25:161-170.

Silverman J, Shellabarger CJ, Holtzman S, Stone JP, Weisburger JH (1980). Effect of dietary fat on x-ray induced mammary cancer in Sprague-Dawley rats. J Natl Cancer Inst 64:631-634.

Tannenbaum A (1942). The genesis and growth of tumors: III. Effect of a high fat diet. Cancer Res 2:468-475.

Tannebaum A (1945). The dependence of tumor formation on the composition of the calorie-restricted diet as well as on the degree of restriction. Cancer Res 5:616-625.

Tartter PI, Papatestas AE, Ioannovich J, Mulvihill MN, Lesnick G, Aufses AH (1981). Cholesterol and obesity as prognostic factors in breast cancer. Cancer 47:2222-2227.

Ward-Hinds M, Kolonel LN, Nomura AMY, Lee J (1982). Stage-specific breast cancer incidence rates by age among Japanese and Caucasian women in Hawaii (1960-1979). Br J Cancer 45:118-123.

Wynder EL (1980). Dietary factors related to breast cancer. Cancer 46:899-904.

Wynder EL, Cohen LA (1982). A rationale for dietary intervention in the treatment of post-menopausal breast cancer patients. Nutr Cancer 3:195-199.

Wynder EL, Hirayama T (1977). Comparative epidemiology of cancers of the United States and Japan. Prev Med 6:567-594.

Wynder EL, Kajitani T, Kuno K, Lucas J, Depalo A, Farrow J (1963). A comparison of survival rates between American and Japanese patients with breast cancer. Surg Gynecol Obstet 117:196-200.

Wynder EL, MacCormick F, Hill P, Cohen LA, Chan PC, Weisburger JH (1976). Nutrition and the etiology and prevention of breast cancer. Cancer Detection and Prevention 1:293-310.

Wynder EL, MacCormick FA, Stellman SD (1978) The epidemiology of breast cancer in 785 United States Caucasian women. Cancer 41: 2341-2354.

Dietary Fat and Cancer, pages 117–124
© 1986 Alan R. Liss, Inc.

METHODOLOGICAL ISSUES IN CLINICAL TRIALS OF DIETARY FAT
REDUCTION IN PATIENTS WITH BREAST DYSPLASIA

Boyd NF, Cousins M, Beaton M, Han L, McGuire V

Ludwig Institute for Cancer Research

9 Earl St., Toronto, Canada M4Y 1M4

I INTRODUCTION

Considerable evidence, described elsewhere in this volume, suggests that dietary fat consumption may be related
to the development of breast cancer. This evidence is derived from epidemiological observations and from abundant
animal experimental data. There is however little information available about the effects of dietary fat on human
breast epithelial tissues. Such information could provide
important insights into the ways in which fat consumption
may be related to cancer risk and could lead to the development of preventive strategies.

We have elected initially to study the effects of dietary fat on the breast by examining the influence of dietary
fat reduction on the radiological manifestations of breast
dysplasia. Breast dysplasia has been shown by several investigators to be a risk factor for the development of
breast cancer (Carlile T et al.1985;Wolfe JN,1976abc 1977)
and to be associated with the histologic changes that also
confer increased risk of breast cancer (Bright R et al.1985;
Wellings SR 1978).

The initial goals of the study were to determine if it
was feasible to carry out a clinical trial of dietary fat
reduction in patients with breast dysplasia and to assess
compliance with a reduced fat diet. Preliminary results of
these aspects of the trial, based upon an experience with
174 subjects, have already been published (Boyd NF et al.
1984) and detailed final results will be given elsewhere.

In this chapter, we will discuss some of the methodological issues that have arisen during the course of this study. These issues are likely to have a bearing on other dietary intervention studies. They concern the feasibility of such studies, the recruitment and enrollment of subjects, the promotion and assessment of dietary compliance and the measurement of outcome.

II Patients and Methods

General Method. The general method employed in this study was to recruit women with mammographically demonstrated breast dysplasia from the breast diagnostic clinic at Women's College Hospital, and to allocate them randomly to receive one of two types of dietary advice. A group of controls was given general advice about maintaining a healthy diet according to Canada's Food Guide, but were not counselled to change the composition of their diets. The average fat intake of this group was 40% of calories. A second group of subjects was given advice and education about reducing dietary fat intake to 15% of total calories. In both groups, breast dysplasia was assessed mammographically one year after randomization and the appearances compared with the changes.

Patient Population. Subjects were eligible for the study if they were aged at least 30 years and had been examined by mammography within 3 months of entry and found to have at least 50% of the breast volume occupied by the radiological changes of dysplasia. Subjects were excluded if they were pregnant or breast feeding, or if they were taking a medically prescribed diet.

After explanation of the study, subjects who gave signed consent visited the study dietician for an initial dietary evaluation (see below).

To date, 269 patients have entered the study. The mean age of the patients was 51 years and most were Caucasian.

III   Feasibility

We have assessed the feasibility of dietary inter-

vention studies of this type by maintaining a log of all
patients eligible for the study seen in the Women's College
Hospital Breast Unit since the study began, and determining
the proportion of eligible patients who agreed to enter the
study and gave signed consent to undergo randomization.
Sixty-one percent of all eligible patients entered the
study, clearly indicating that the study is feasible from
the point of view of recruitment.

IV   Maintenance of Patients After Entry, Drop-Outs, and
      the Influence of Screening

Recruitment, however, is only one aspect of the
feasibility of dietary intervention studies. To test
adequately hypotheses concerning the effects of dietary
fat on the breast dietary changes must be maintained for
a substantial period of time. We have adopted two
approaches to entering patients into the study that have
had a striking influence on the maintenance of subjects in
the study. These are described below in the sequence in
which they were deployed, referred to as the Initial and
Modified procedures.

Initial procedure. The research assistant contacted
eligible patients by telephone, explained the purposes of
the study and arranged to meet those patients who were
interested in entering. The procedures to be followed
were reviewed and patient's questions answered. Patients
who agreed to enter the study signed informed consent and
were instructed in maintaining food records. Each subject's
diet was assessed initially by a 3 day food record, food
frequency questionnaire, and one day diet recall. Subsequently, in patients allocated to the study group, the procedures to promote compliance that are described were then
followed. Patients in the intervention group were then seen
at intervals of one month for a year. Patients in the
control group were seen once every 4 months for a year.

With these procedures (Table 1) 47 of 227 randomized
subjects (20.7%) dropped out of the study, 32 in intervention group and 15 in control group. More than 50% of drop-
outs took place at the time of randomization, before the
dietary intervention had been taught.

Modified procedure. In an attempt to reduce the
number of subjects dropping out of the study we introduced
a screening period before randomization. During this time
subjects were taught to maintain dietary records of food
intake over at least 6 days and asked to keep at least 2
appointments with the dieticians before being randomized.
This procedure allowed the subjects time to evaluate the
commitment involved in the study, and also enabled the
dieticians to ensure that subjects knew how to maintain
dietary records of appropriate quality before they entered
the study.

Consent was obtained and randomization carried out
only after these procedures had been successfully completed. If a subject had not learned to maintain suitable
food records within this period of time, but still wished
to enter the study, further instruction was given until
record-keeping improved to the point where the subject
could enter the study.

To date, 47 subjects have entered the study after this
period of initial screening (25 study and 22 control).
Three subjects (6%) have dropped out, 2 from the control
group and 1 from the study group.

Table 1

Drop Outs and the Influence of Screening Before
Randomization

Time of Drop Out	No Screening		Screening	
	Total	Dropout(%)	Total	Dropout(%)
Randomization	227	22 (10%)	47	1 (2%)
1-4 months	205	17 (8%)	41	2 (5%)
4-8 months	188	8 (4%)	27	0 (0%)
8-12 months	180	0 -	20	2 (10%)

V   Promotion and Assessment of Compliance

Table 2 summarizes the procedures used to promote
dietary compliance. After the initial assessment of each
subject's diet by means of a three-day food record, food
history, food frequency questionnaire, and a one-day diet
recall, an individual isocaloric diet prescription was

prepared for each subject in the intervention group. As far as possible this prescription was based on the individual's own food preferences and practices.

In addition, subjects in the intervention group were given a number of dietary aids. These included dietetic scales to weigh food, an extensive food guide giving information about shopping for and cooking reduced fat meals and a list of food exchanges for fats.

Table 2

Procedures to Promote Compliance

Individual Diet Prescription
Close Follow-up
Food Guide
Shopping Guide
Recipes

Subjects in the intervention group were seen each month for 1 year, and controls were seen every 4 months for a year. At each visit, subjects in both groups provided food records. The nutrient analysis of these records was the principal method used to assess dietary compliance.

In the absence of other established methods for the assessment of compliance with a reduced fat diet, we have also employed several biochemical measures with the objective of comparing these with the subject's food intake as assessed by food records. These measures are summarized in Table 3. Duplicate meals have also been collected from volunteers in both intervention and control groups and chemically analyzed. The preliminary results, shown in Table 4, show large differences between the groups in the intake of fat and carbohydrate.

Table 3

Comparison of Methods of Assessing Compliance

Fasting Blood	Lipoprotein Profile, Vitamins
24 hr. Urine	Methylhistidine, Malonaldehyde
Faecal	Fat, Lignin
Food Records	Duplicate Meals

Table 4

Chemical Analysis of Duplicate Meals

	Intervention	Control	T	P
N	21	18		
Calories	1418	1434	-0.05	0.96
Fat G.	27	47	-4.14	0.0004
Fat & Cals	17	30	-5.4	0.0001
Cho G.	226	182	2.40	0.02
Cho & Cals.	63	51	4.49	0.0001

VI   Assessment of Outcome

The outcome measure to be employed in this trial is a comparison of breast dysplasia, as assessed mammographically, at the beginning of the trial and one year later. This comparison is complicated by sources of variation in mammographic images that arise from differences in radiologic technique, film processing and breast compression, as well as from the subjective nature of radiologic image interpretation.

To overcome these problems an image analysis system has been developed by Dr. Martin Yaffe at the Ontario Cancer Institute. This system can digitize the optical density that is associated with dysplasia in the mammographic image and display the data as histograms or cumulative distribution functions. This process both makes the mammographic information quantitative and facilitates the statistical comparison of paired images.

VII   Assessment of Dietary Practices after Leaving the Study

To determine whether taking part in a study of this type has a persistent effect on the dietary practices of the participants we have carried out a preliminary assessment of the dietary intake of subjects who have completed the study.

From the 125 subjects who had completed the study between 1 and 3 years previously we selected at random 40 women. This random selection of subjects was stratified according to their mean intake of fat consumption, as assessed by food records maintained during the time they were in the trial.

Subjects selected in this way were contacted by telephone and asked to take part in a follow-up study in which they provided food records over 3 assigned days and a blood sample for measurement of serum cholesterol.

Thirty-six agreed to participate and 29 actually returned completed food records. The preliminary analysis of the food records shows that subjects in the intervention group continue to consume substantially less dietary fat than they did at entry to the study, although somewhat more than they consumed during the period of dietary intervention. Further, the fall in serum cholesterol observed in the group during the period of dietary intervention was sustained. The subjects who had been in the control group showed no change in dietary fat intake and a slight rise in serum cholesterol.

Additional information from a larger number of subjects is obviously required before firm conclusions can be drawn, but these preliminary data suggest that relatively short periods of intensive dietary change may be followed by dietary modification over a prolonged interval.

VIII   Conclusions

Our results to date clearly indicate that studies of dietary intervention involving a substantial reduction in dietary fat are feasible, and that satisfactory compliance can be obtained. The patient population that we have studied is however, symptomatic and may therefore be more receptive than the general population to a clinical trial of this type.

A simple preliminary screening of subjects, in which they are asked to carry out some of the procedures to be followed in the study, has apparently lead to a dramatic reduction in the number of drop-outs.

Preliminary evidence indicates that subjects who have

reduced dietary fat in this trial may continue to consume
less fat after leaving the study than they did at entry.

REFERENCES

Boyd NF, Cousins ML, Bayliss SE, Fish ED, Fishnell E, Bruce
WR (1984) Diet and breast diesease: Evidence for the
feasibility of a clinical trial involving a major reduction in dietary fat. In: A study of diet and breast
dysplasia. Lawrence Earl Baum Assoc. Inc., New Jersey.
Bright R, Morrison A, Brisson J, Burstein N (1985). Relationship between mammographic image and histology in
women who have benign breast biopsy. American J Epidemiology 122:3; 516.
Carlile T, Thompson DJ, Whitehead J, et al. (1985). Breast
cancer prediction and the Wolfe classification of mammo-
grams. JAMA 254:1050-1053.
Committee for the Revision of the Dietary Standard of Canada,
(1983) "Recommended Nutrient Intakes for Canadians" Health
Protection Branch, Department of National Health and
Welfare.
Wellings SR, Wolfe JN (1978). Correlative studies of the
histological and radiographic appearance of the breast
parenchyma. Radiology 129:299-306.
Wolfe JN (1976a). Breast patterns as an index of risk for
developing breast cancer. Am J Roentgenol 126:1130-1139.
Wolfe JN (1976b). Risk for breast cancer development
determined by mammographic parenchymal pattern. Cancer
37:2486-2492.
Wolfe JN (1977). Risk of developing breast cancer determined by mammography. In: Wolfe JN, ed. Breast cancer.
New York: Liss, 233-238.
Wolfe JN (1976c). Breast parenchymal patterns and their
changes with age. Radiology 121:545-552.

II. Food Fats and Oils: Consumption, Properties, and Requirement

Dietary Fat and Cancer, pages 127–152
© 1986 Alan R. Liss, Inc.

LEVELS AND SOURCES OF FAT IN THE U.S. FOOD SUPPLY

Nancy R. Raper and Ruth M. Marston

Human Nutrition Information Service
U.S. Department of Agriculture
Hyattsville, Maryland 20782

Interest in the fat content of the American diet and how it has changed over the years has increased because of the growing understanding of the relationship of dietary fat and health. USDA estimates each year the per capita quantities of foods in the national food supply and the daily quantities of nutrients provided by these foods. A consistent methodology is employed to develop estimates of food and nutrient levels in the U.S. food supply for each year dating from a base period of 1909-13. These annual estimates of the nutrient content of the U.S. food supply are the only means of monitoring year to year changes in the American diet over the past decades. This chapter reports estimates of the amounts, types, and sources of fat in the U.S. food supply.

Food supply data are useful in assessing trends in food consumption and nutrient levels in the American diet since early in this century. Food supply data do not indicate actual use of food by households or intake of food by individuals; nor do they account for variations in the distribution of food among individuals. Food consumption surveys, such as those conducted periodically by USDA, provide these types of data (U.S. Department of Agriculture, Human Nutrition Information Service, 1983, 1984, 1985).

The per capita amounts of foods in the food supply are published by the Economic Research Service of USDA (U.S. Department of Agriculture, Economic Research Service, 1968, 1982, 1983, 1984, 1985). These data are sometimes referred to as disappearance data because they are derived by subtracting data on exports, military use, year-end inventories and nonfood use from data on imports and beginning-of-the-year inventories. Consumption is measured of approximately 350 basic foods before they are combined with other foods. Because of the complexity of the system, foods are not measured at the same level in the marketing system. For example, eggs and fresh produce are measured at the farm level; meat, at the slaughter level; and flour, at the milled level. Processed fruits and juices, vegetables, and potatoes are measured after processed, that is, canned, frozen and dehydrated. Estimates of all foods are converted from the weights of measurement to retail equivalent weights. No measure is made of losses in food and nutrients that occur after consumption is measured. Food consumption estimates include inedible food components (such as bones, rinds, and pits), food used by pets, unused leftovers, spoiled food and waste incurred in processing and marketing.

Nutrient levels in the U.S. food supply are estimated by USDA's Human Nutrition Information Service (HNIS) from the annual per capita quantities of foods consumed and from appropriate food composition data. Estimates of nutrients are based on food composition data which exclude inedible food components, such as bones, rinds, peelings, and pits. The nutritive value of foods is based on published tables (Haytowitz and Matthews, 1984; Posati and Orr, 1976; Posati, 1979; Reaves and Weihrauch, 1979; Watt and Merrill, 1963) and on unpublished information provided by HNIS's Nutrient Data Research Branch. The nutrient content of some foods has changed during this century because of changes in growing and marketing practices. These changes are taken into consideration when sufficient reliable data are available. Otherwise, the most recent food composition data are used. Levels of nutrients in the food supply include estimates of quantities of nutrients added to foods in enrichment and fortification. These estimates are based on enrichment standards and on periodic surveys of industry conducted for USDA by the Bureau of Census. Additional information on the methodology for determining per capita nutrient levels has been published (U.S. Department of Agriculture, Economic Research Service, 1965).

Using these procedures, changes in the level and sources of fat in the U.S. food supply reflect changes in

both the quantity and fat content of food use over time.
The per capita quantities of foods which are the major
sources of fat in the food supply are summarized in an
Appendix to this chapter.   Fat in the food supply includes
fat from all sources--fat naturally present in foods such
as meats, dairy products, and nuts; fat used in cooking or
as table spreads; and fat used in the manufacture of food
products such as baked goods, salad dressings, and potato
chips.   Because estimates do not account for losses that
occur after use is estimated, the food supply reflects more
fat and other nutrients than are actually ingested.   For
example, some fat used for frying in commercial establishments and in the home is discarded, but the amount is not
known.

LEVELS OF FAT

The amount of fat in the food supply increased by
one-third between 1909-13 and 1984, from 124 grams per
capita per day to 166 grams (Figure 1).   The gain in fat
did not occur as a steady upward increase throughout the
years.   Between 1909-13 and 1925-29, the fat level rose
11 grams to 135 grams per capita per day.   Most of the
increase during the period was due to gains from use of
fats and oils--edible oils, shortening, and lard.   During
the next 10 years (1925-29 to 1935-39), the fat level
declined slightly (2 grams) because of somewhat lower
levels of food consumption during the Depression.   In the
decade that followed (1935-39 to 1947-49), the fat level
increased 8 grams to 141 grams per capita per day.   Increased use of meat, dairy products, margarine, and lard
was largely responsible for the increase.   During the next
20 years (1947-49 to 1967-69), the fat level increased 16
grams to 157 grams per capita per day.   The increase during
this period was due to gains from use of edible oils, meat,
and margarine.   Between 1967-69 and 1975, the fat level
decreased by 5 grams to 152 grams per capita per day,
reflecting less use of lard and pork.   In the next 10 years
(1975-1984), fat increased 14 grams to 166 grams per capita
per day, mainly due to gains from shortening and edible
beef fat.

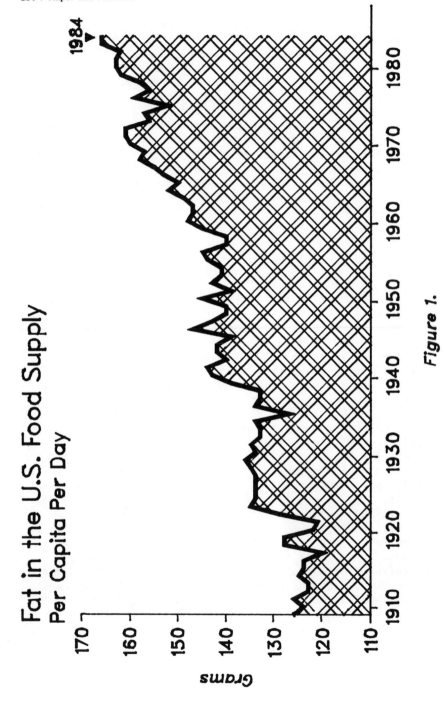

Fat in the U.S. Food Supply
Per Capita Per Day

Figure 1.

FOOD ENERGY FROM FAT

The food energy or Calorie level of the food supply is determined by the amount of fat, as well as carbohydrate and protein. The energy level of the food supply fluctuated throughout the century, reaching a low of 3,080 Calories in 1957 and a high of 3,460 Calories in 1928. The level was 3,450 Calories in 1984. Since 1960, the energy level fluctuated upward, due in part to the increasing level of fat in the food supply. The share of Calories derived from fat increased from 32 percent in 1909-13 to 43 percent in 1984 (Figure 2). Conversely, the proportion derived from carbohydrate decreased from 56 to 46 percent between 1909-13 and 1984. Protein accounted for a relatively constant 11 or 12 percent of calories throughout the century.

Sources of Food Energy in the U.S. Food Supply[a]

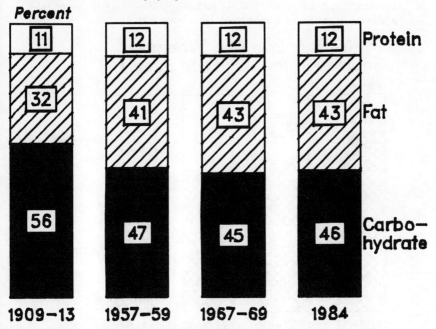

Percent

	Protein
11	12	12	12
32	41	43	43	Fat
56	47	45	46	Carbo-hydrate
1909-13	1957-59	1967-69	1984

[a]Components may not add to total due to rounding.

Figure 2.

SOURCES OF FAT

Animal and Vegetable Sources

The gain in the level of fat in the food supply was due to an increase in fat from vegetable sources. Fat from vegetable sources more than tripled, from 21 grams per capita per day in 1909-13 to 70 grams in 1984, reflecting increased use of margarine, vegetable shortenings, and edible oils. Vegetable sources accounted for 42 percent of the fat in the 1984 food supply, compared with 17 percent in 1909-13 (Figure 3).

Although the increase in fat in the food supply is due to vegetable sources, animal sources have always provided the largest proportion. The quantity of fat from animal sources declined only 7 grams between 1909-13 and 1984, from 103 to 96 grams per capita per day. However, its proportionate contribution to the total fat in the food supply declined from 83 to 58 percent, due to the marked increase in fat from vegetable sources.

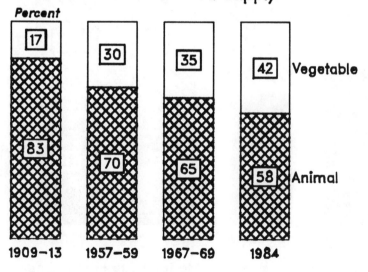

Fat from Animal and Vegetable Sources in the U.S. Food Supply

Percent

| 1909-13 | 1957-59 | 1967-69 | 1984 |

Vegetable: 17 / 30 / 35 / 42

Animal: 83 / 70 / 65 / 58

Figure 3.

Food Group Sources

    Three food groups--fats and oils; meat, poultry, and
fish; and dairy products--provided about 90 percent of the
fat in the food supply over the past 75 years. The amount
of fat provided by the fats and oils group and the meat,
poultry and fish group increased and the amount provided by
the dairy products group was about the same in 1984 as in
1909-13. However, the proportions of fat provided by the
groups have changed (Table 1). In 1909-13, the fats and
oils group and the meat, poultry, and fish group each
accounted for 37 percent of the fat in the food supply,
while the dairy products group contributed 15 percent. By
1925-29, the fats and oils group was the leading source of
fat, a position which it has maintained throughout the
years. In contrast, the share of fat from the meat,
poultry, and fish group and the dairy products group
fluctuated downward throughout the century. In 1984, the
proportionate contribution of fat from the fats and oils
group was 44 percent; the meat, poultry, and fish group,
34 percent; and the dairy products group, 12 percent.

Table 1. Level and Sources of Fat by Major Food Groups in
the U.S. Food Supply

Year	Total	Meat, poultry, fish	Fats, oils	Dairy products	Other [a/] foods
	grams/ capita/ day	---------------percent---------------			
1909-13	124	37	37	15	11
1925-29	135	33	40	15	12
1935-39	133	30	42	16	12
1947-49	141	33	37	18	12
1957-59	142	34	40	15	11
1967-69	157	37	40	13	10
1975	152	35	43	12	10
1980	163	36	44	11	9
1984	166	34	44	12	10

[a/] Includes eggs; dry beans, peas, nuts and soy products;
    potatoes; vegetables; fruits; grain products; sugars;
    spices; and miscellaneous.

Fats and oils group. Fat from the fats and oils group
increased from 46 to 73 grams per capita per day between
1909-13 and 1984, a 59 percent gain (Table 2). The fats
and oils group includes butter, margarine, shortening,
lard, edible beef fat, and edible oils. Over the past
75 years, increased use of edible oils, margarine, shortening and edible beef fat were responsible for the increase
in fat from this group. Edible oils accounted for about
one-half of the gain and margarine, shortening and edible
beef fat for the other half. Shifts also occurred in the
share of fat provided by foods within the group. Over the
years, margarine and shortening replaced butter and lard as
sources of fat.

Margarine replaced butter as a source of fat, reflecting a trend toward greater use of vegetable sources of
fats. Butter was the major source of fat in the fats and
oils group in 1909-13, providing 38 percent of the fat.
In contrast, margarine provided only 3 percent. Use of
margarine increased during the 1940's due to a number of
factors--its relatively low price compared with butter,
improvements in quality, the repeal of antimargarine laws,
and the substitution of margarine for butter during World
War II (Kromer, 1974). By 1957-59, the contributions of
fat from margarine and butter were 16 and 15 percent,
respectively. Between 1957-59 and 1975, margarine continued to account for about 16 or 17 percent of the fat,
but by 1984, it accounted for only 14 percent, reflecting
decreased use of margarine and increased use of shortening
and oils. The share of fat provided by butter was halved
from 15 to 7 percent between 1957-59 and 1984. Although
use of margarine increased over the years, use of butter
declined even more. Therefore, the total amount of fat
from these two table spreads declined 24 percent between
1909-13 and 1984.

A shift in use of the cooking fats--lard and shorten-
ing--occurred over the past 75 years. Lard accounted for
32 percent of the fat in 1909-13, but only 4 percent in
1984. In contrast, the share of fat from shortening
increased from 23 to 36 percent between 1909-13 and 1984.

Direct use of lard, such as for baking or frying,
fluctuated between 10 and 14 pounds per capita until the
mid-1950's. Since then, use declined substantially and was
only 2 pounds per capita in 1984. In contrast, indirect

Table 2. Fats and Oils Group: Contribution of Fat by Components

Year	Total	Table spreads		Cooking fats			Edible oils
		Butter	Margarine a/	Shortening a/	Lard b/	Edible beef fat c/	
	grams/capita/day	--percent--					
1909-13	46	38	3	23	32		4
1925-29	54	33	5	22	29		11
1935-39	56	31	5	26	24		14
1947-49	53	20	11	23	29		17
1957-59	56	15	16	25	20		24
1967-69	63	9	17	32	11		31
1975	65	7	17	32	6		38
1980	71	6	16	32	5	2	39
1984	73	7	14	36	4	3	36

a/ Includes small amounts of lard and beef fat.
b/ Direct use; excludes use in some margarine and shortening.
c/ Direct use; excludes use in some margarine and shortening. Data available beginning in 1979.

use of lard as an ingredient in some margarine and shortening increased from less than 1/2 to more than 1 pound per
capita between 1909-13 and 1984. Over the past 75 years,
total fat from use of lard declined from 15 to 4 grams per
capita per day.

Shortening more than doubled in use in the past 75
years. Per capita use of shortening, including small
amounts of lard and edible beef fat used in its manufacture,
increased from 8 to 21 pounds between 1909-13 and 1984,
rising almost steadily after the late 1950's. In 1984, the
proportion of fat which shortening provided from the fats
and oils group was equal to that from edible oils--36
percent.

Data on direct use of edible beef fat are only available dating from 1979. Direct use of this fat increased
from 1/2 to slightly less than 2 pounds per capita in the
last 5 years, primarily reflecting its use in deep-frying
by the restaurant industry. In 1984, direct use of edible
beef fat accounted for 3 percent of the fat from the fats
and oils group. Indirect use of edible beef fat as an
ingredient in shortening and margarine also increased, from
1 to 3-1/2 pounds per capita between 1909-13 and 1984,
providing 6 percent of the fat from the fats and oils group
in 1984.

Edible oils are mainly used as salad and cooking oils.
However, small amounts are used in the production of other
products, such as toppings and cream substitutes. Use of
edible oils increased from less than 2 pounds to 11 pounds
per capita between 1909-13 and 1957-59. Thereafter, they
were the leading source of fat in the fats and oils group.
Use doubled by 1975 but increased more slowly thereafter.
In 1984, edible oils accounted for 36 percent of the fat
from the fats and oils group. The increase in use of
edible oils reflects several factors--new and improved
methods of processing; the phenomenal growth of the fast-
food industry featuring foods cooked in oil; increased use
of convenience foods, many of which are fried in oil or
contain added oil; and a preference by consumers for liquid
oils instead of solid fats (Kromer, 1973, 1974).

Meat, poultry, and fish group. During the past 75
years, fat from the meat, poultry, and fish group increased
24 percent, from 46 grams to 57 grams per capita per day

(Table 3). Despite this increase, the meat, poultry, and fish group accounted for a smaller share of fat in the food supply in 1984, 34 percent, compared with 37 percent in 1909-13--primarily because of the increased share provided by the fats and oils group.

Table 3. Meat, Poultry, and Fish Group: Contribution of Fat by Components

Year	Total	Beef	Pork	Other meat	Poultry	Fish
	grams/ capita/ day	------------------percent------------------				
1909-13	46	25	60	7	5	3
1925-29	44	21	65	7	5	2
1935-39	39	24	60	8	5	3
1947-49	47	24	62	6	6	2
1957-59	48	29	55	6	7	3
1967-69	58	32	52	4	10	2
1975	53	38	44	4	11	3
1980	59	30	53	2	13	2
1984	57	32	49	3	14	2

Over the years, pork was the leading source of fat among the foods in the meat, poultry, and fish group. The amount of fat from use of pork was the same in 1909-13 and in 1984, 28 grams per capita per day. However, the share of fat contributed by pork declined from 60 to 49 percent between 1909-13 and 1984, primarily because the percentage of fat contributed by beef and poultry increased as use of these foods increased. Use of pork, which fluctuated considerably over the past 75 years, reached a low of about 51 pounds in 1975 when use of beef was near a record high. Consequently, the share of fat from pork was lowest in 1975--44 percent. However, use of pork increased to 62 pounds in 1984, and its share of fat from this group increased to 49 percent.

Beef ranked second as a source of fat in the meat, poultry, and fish group, providing 32 percent in 1984

compared with 38 percent in 1975 (nearly a peak year for
beef use) and 25 percent in 1909-13. The amount of fat
from beef increased 56 percent between 1909-13 and 1984.
Use of beef fluctuated over the years, ranging between
37 and 59 pounds per capita until the early 1950's. Thereafter, use rose almost steadily to a peak of 94 pounds per
capita in 1976, but declined to 79 pounds in 1984.

Other meats--veal, lamb and mutton, edible offals, and
game--provided 3 percent of the fat from the meat, poultry,
and fish group in 1984, down from 7 percent in 1909-13.
Although use of veal, lamb, and mutton has always been low
compared with use of beef and pork, it has declined substantially over the years, and was 3 pounds per capita in
1984. Use of edible offals fluctuated between approximately
9 and 11 pounds per capita for most of the past 75 years.

The share of the fat provided by poultry almost tripled,
from 5 percent in 1909-13 to 14 percent in 1984. Use of
chicken, by far the largest component of poultry, varied
between 13 and 23 pounds per capita over the first half of
the century. Between 1950 and 1984, use rose almost steadily
from 21 to 56 pounds per capita.

Fish accounted for 2 to 3 percent of the fat in the
meat, poultry, and fish group over the years. Use--as well
as the fat content of fish and shellfish--are relatively
low compared with meats and poultry.

Dairy products group. The dairy products group provided almost the same level of fat in 1984, 20 grams per
capita per day, as in 1909-13, 18 grams (Table 4). However, the share of fat in the food supply from the dairy
products group declined from 15 to 12 percent over the past
75 years. Both the amount and share of fat from this group
increased until the late 1940's, as use of dairy products
rose to a peak level. Beginning in the 1950's, shifts
occurred in the use of products within the group which
resulted in a decline in fat from this group.

Whole milk was the leading source of fat throughout
most of the past 75 years. The share of fat from whole
milk fluctuated between 60 and 55 percent between 1909-13
and 1957-59 but declined to 28 percent in 1984. Use of
whole milk decreased steadily after the mid-1950's. Other
kinds of fluid milk--especially lowfat and skim (U.S.

Table 4. Dairy Products Group: Contribution of Fat by Components

Year	Total	Whole milk	Skim and lowfat milks, yogurt	Cream a/	Processed b/ milks	Frozen c/ desserts	Cheese
	grams/capita/day	----------------------------percent----------------------------					
1909-13	18	60	1	24	4	2	9
1925-29	21	55	1	23	6	6	9
1935-39	22	55	1	20	8	6	10
1947-49	25	57	1	13	8	10	11
1957-59	22	57	1	9	8	11	14
1967-69	19	52	4	6	5	13	20
1975	19	41	8	6	3	14	28
1980	18	34	10	6	3	13	34
1984	20	28	11	7	3	12	39

a/ Includes cream, milk-cream mixtures, sour cream and dips and eggnog.
b/ Includes canned and dry milks and whey.
c/ Includes ice cream and other milk-based desserts.

Department of Agriculture, Human Nutrition Information Service, 1985)--and perhaps other beverages such as soft drinks appear to have replaced some of the whole milk consumption. The decline in whole milk consumption may also reflect the decline in the proportion of young children in the population as the baby-boom generation grew older. The smaller share of fat from whole milk also reflected the substantial gain from increased use of cheese.

Despite a low fat content, the skim and lowfat milk and yogurt category increased its share of fat from 1 to 11 percent between 1909-13 and 1984. Products included in this category are skim, 1-and 2- percent fat milks, flavored lowfat milk, buttermilk, and yogurt. Use of products in this category declined to a record low of 24 pounds per capita by the late 50's. Since then, use increased to a peak of 106 pounds per capita by 1984. The upward trend in use of these products may be due to consumer concern about calories and fat in the diet.

Cheese was the leading source of fat among dairy products by 1984, when it accounted for 39 percent of the fat from dairy products. Cheese provided 9 percent of the fat from dairy products early in the century. Between 1909-13 and 1984, per capita use of cheese (including cottage cheese) rose from 5 to 26 pounds per year. Most of the increase in the proportionate contribution of fat from cheese occurred since 1957-59.

Frozen desserts contributed 12 percent of the fat in the dairy products group in 1984, compared with 2 percent in 1909-13. Most of the gain in fat from this group occurred prior to 1947-49, reflecting the increased availability of home refrigeration. Creams, which include light and heavy cream, half and half, sour cream and dips and eggnog, ranked second as a source of fat in the dairy products group between 1909-13 and 1947-49. However, the share of fat from cream during this time declined 11 percentage points, from 24 to 13 percent, and declined to 7 percent by 1984. The share of fat from processed milks-- canned and dry milks and whey--increased from 4 to 8 percent between 1909-13 and 1947-49, but declined to 3 percent by 1984.

Other food groups. All other food groups--eggs, dry beans, peas, nuts and soy products, fruits, vegetables, grain products, and miscellaneous foods--together accounted for 9 to 12 percent of the fat in the food supply (Table 1). Despite their relatively high use, potatoes, fruits, and vegetables accounted for less than 1 percent of the fat in the food supply because of their low fat content. Use of grains declined over the years. Consequently, the share of fat in the food supply provided by grains declined from 4 to 1 percent between 1909-13 and 1984. Eggs accounted for about 4 percent of the fat in the food supply in 1909-13, but in 1984, they accounted for about 2 percent. In contrast, the proportion of fat from the dry beans, peas, nuts, and soy products group rose from 2 to 4 percent between 1909-13 and 1984. Nuts, particularly peanuts, are the chief source of fat in this group.

LEVELS OF FATTY ACIDS

Changes in the level and sources of fat in the food supply over the past 75 years affected the fatty acid content. Estimated levels for total saturated fatty acids (TSFA), oleic acid, and linoleic acid reflect the shift from animal to vegetable sources of fats.

Between 1909-13 and 1984, the level of TSFA increased 10 percent, from 52 to 57 grams per capita per day (Table 5). However, the proportion of total fat accounted for by TSFA declined from 42 to 35 percent during this period. Levels for two of the unsaturated fatty acids--oleic and linoleic--were also higher in 1984 than at the beginning of the century. Oleic acid increased 39 percent, from 46 to 64 grams per capita per day, but represented about the same proportion of total fat in 1984 as in 1909-13--37 or 38 percent. The amount of fat from linoleic acid more than doubled from 9 to 26 grams per capita per day and accounted for 15 percent of the fat in 1984 compared with 7 percent in 1909-13.

FOOD ENERGY FROM FATTY ACIDS

Changes in fatty acids levels of the food supply affected the proportionate share of calories from each (Table 6). TSFA accounted for roughly the same share in 1984 as in 1909-13--14 or 15 percent. Over the same period, the share of calories from oleic acid increased

from 12 to 17 percent and the share from linoleic acid
increased from 2 to 7 percent.

Table 5. Selected Fatty Acids in the U.S. Food Supply

Year	Satu-rated	Oleic	Lin-oleic	Satu-rated	Oleic	Lin-oleic
	---grams/capita/day--			-------percent-------		
1909-13	52	46	9	42	37	7
1925-29	56	50	11	42	37	8
1935-39	56	50	12	42	37	9
1947-49	57	53	14	40	38	10
1957-59	56	54	16	40	38	11
1967-69	59	60	20	37	38	13
1975	53	60	23	35	39	15
1980	56	62	26	34	38	16
1984	57	64	26	35	38	15

Table 6. Food Energy Contributed by Selected Fatty Acids
in the U.S. Food Supply

Year	Saturated	Oleic	Linoleic
	------------percent------------		
1909-13	14	12	2
1925-29	15	13	3
1935-39	15	14	3
1947-49	16	15	4
1957-59	16	16	5
1967-69	16	17	6
1975	15	17	6
1980	15	17	7
1984	15	17	7

SOURCES OF FATTY ACIDS

Food Group Sources for Total Saturated Fatty Acids

The fats and oils group was the leading source of TSFA between 1909-13 and 1957-59, with contributions ranging between 34 and 41 percent of the total (Table 7). However, the meat, poultry, and fish group was the leading source by 1967-69, accounting for 39 percent of the total TSFA. The dairy products group provided about the same share (21 or 22 percent) of TSFA in 1984 and in 1909-13. However, this group provided a larger share in 1947-49--27 percent--when use of dairy products was at near peak levels.

Among the fats and oils, animal fats--butter and lard (direct use)--were the leading sources of TSFA between 1909-13 and 1947-49. However, as total use of these products declined, their contribution of TSFA from the fats and oils group also declined from 82 percent in 1909-13 to 22 percent in 1984. Direct use of beef fat, first reported in 1979, provided 6 percent of the TSFA in the fats and oils group in 1984. In contrast, the contribution of TSFA in the fats and oils group from margarine, shortening, and other edible oils increased from 18 to 73 percent between 1909-13 and 1984, as use of these fats increased. They became the leading source of TSFA in the fats and oils group in 1957-59.

Within the meat, poultry, and fish group, pork was the leading source of TSFA for most years and beef ranked second. In 1909-13, pork provided 54 percent of the TSFA in the group, but its share declined to 44 percent in 1984. On the other hand, beef accounted for 32 percent in 1909-13 and 41 percent in 1984. TSFA in the meat, poultry, fish group from beef was highest, 48 percent, in the mid-1970's, when use of beef was at record high levels and use of pork was at near record low levels. The share of TSFA in the group from other meats (veal, lamb, mutton, and offals) declined from 9 to 3 percent between 1909-13 and 1984, while the share from poultry increased from 4 to 11 percent. Fish accounted for only 1 to 2 percent of the TSFA throughout the past 75 years.

Among the dairy products, whole milk was the leading source of TSFA until 1984 when cheese became the main

Table 7. Fatty Acids Contributed by Major Food Groups in the U.S. Food Supply

Year	Saturated			Oleic			Linoleic		
	Meat, poultry, fish	Dairy products	Fats, oils	Meat, poultry, fish	Dairy products	Fats, oils	Meat, poultry, fish	Dairy products	Fats, oils
	--percent--								
1909-13	34	22	39	43	10	40	32	4	40
1925-29	30	23	40	38	10	43	25	4	50
1935-39	28	24	41	34	11	46	22	4	54
1947-49	32	27	34	38	12	41	22	4	57
1957-59	33	24	35	38	10	43	19	3	63
1967-69	39	21	34	41	8	42	19	2	67
1975	40	22	31	38	8	46	14	2	73
1980	40	20	33	40	7	45	16	2	74
1984	38	21	34	38	7	46	16	2	72

contributor. The proportion of TSFA in the dairy group from whole milk declined from 60 to 28 percent between 1909-13 and 1984, while the share from cheese increased from 9 to 39 percent during the same period. The share of TSFA in the group from creams declined from 24 to 7 percent between 1909-13 and 1984. In contrast, the share from skim and lowfat milks increased from 2 to 10 percent, and the contribution from frozen desserts increased from 2 to 13 percent. Processed milks provided roughly the same small proportion of saturated fatty acids from the dairy group in 1984 (3 percent) as in 1909-13 (4 percent).

Food Group Sources for Oleic Acid

The fats and oils group was the leading source of oleic acid for most of the past 75 years. However, the meat, poultry, and fish group was the chief source in 1909-13. The share of oleic acid from the fats and oils group fluctuated from 40 to 46 percent between 1909-13 and 1984 while the share from the meat, poultry, and fish group varied from 34 to 43 percent. The proportion from dairy products declined from 10 percent in 1909-13 to 7 percent in 1984.

Among the fats and oils, lard and shortening contributed almost equal shares of oleic acid in 1909-13--33 and 36 percent, respectively--and butter accounted for 24 percent. However, the proportion from lard and butter each declined to 4 percent by 1984, while that from shortening increased to 47 percent. The contribution of oleic acid in the fats and oils group from edible oils increased from 3 to 28 percent between 1909-13 and 1984.

Within the meat, poultry, and fish group, pork was the chief source of oleic acid, although its share fluctuated downward from 64 to 52 percent between 1909-13 and 1984. In contrast, the share from beef increased from 26 to 34 percent and the share from poultry rose from 4 to 12 percent.

Among the dairy products, the share of oleic acid from whole milk declined from 61 to 29 percent between 1909-13 and 1984; the share from skim and lowfat milks increased from 1 to 11 percent; and the share from cheese rose from 9 to 37 percent, reflecting the shift from whole to lowfat milks and the substantial increase in use of cheese.

Food Group Sources for Linoleic Acid

The fats and oils group was the major source of
linoleic acid throughout the century. Its contribution
of linoleic acid increased from 40 to 72 percent between
1909-13 and 1984. In contrast, the share of linoleic acid
from the meat, poultry, and fish group decreased from 32 to
16 percent during that period. Dairy products provided a
much smaller share of linoleic acid, 4 percent in 1909-13
and 2 percent in 1984.

The marked increase in use of vegetable fats over the
years has been the most important factor in the increase in
the level of linoleic acid in the food supply. Within the
fats and oils group, the share of linoleic acid from edible
oils rose from 22 to 62 percent between 1909-13 and 1984.
The proportion from margarine, although small compared with
that from edible oils, also increased from 5 to 19 percent
between 1909-13 and 1984. In contrast, the proportion of
linoleic acid from lard (direct use) declined sharply from
42 to 1 percent, and the share from butter declined from
11 to 1 percent over the past 75 years.

Pork and poultry are the major sources of linoleic
acid in the meat, poultry, and fish group, accounting for
55 and 40 percent, respectively, in 1984 compared with
76 and 13 percent in 1909-13.

CHOLESTEROL

The cholesterol level of the food supply in 1984,
481 mg per capita per day, was lower than the level at
the beginning of the century, 502 mg (Table 8). The
cholesterol level fluctuated considerably over the years,
reaching its lowest level of 459 mg per capita per day in
1917 and again in 1935. The peak level of 589 mg occurred
in 1945.

SOURCES OF CHOLESTEROL

Eggs are the major source of cholesterol in the food
supply, accounting for 41 percent of the total in 1984
compared with 45 percent in 1909-13. The quantity of
cholesterol from eggs was highest in 1951 when use of eggs

was at a peak. The proportion of cholesterol from the meat, poultry, and fish group (the second largest source) increased from 28 to 40 percent between 1909-13 and 1984. Pork was the major source of cholesterol in the meat, poultry, and fish group until 1957-59, but beef was the major source between 1957-59 and 1984, reflecting increased use. The proportion of cholesterol from edible offals, which include liver and other organ meats used mostly in the manufacture of luncheon meats and sausages, declined throughout the years.

Table 8. Cholesterol Contributed by Major Food Groups in the U.S. Food Supply

Year	Total	Eggs	Meat, poultry, fish	Dairy products	Fats, oils
	grams/ capita/ day		-----------------percent-----------------		
1909-13	502	45	28	14	13
1925-29	519	47	25	15	13
1935-39	484	45	25	17	13
1947-49	570	50	25	17	8
1957-59	548	49	29	15	7
1967-69	524	46	35	14	5
1975	479	44	38	14	4
1980	484	43	39	13	5
1984	481	41	40	14	5

The proportion of cholesterol in the food supply from dairy products varied between 14 and 17 percent. Although use of whole milk declined, it remained the major source of cholesterol among the dairy products until 1983 when cheese became the leading source. In 1984, cheese provided 36 percent of the cholesterol from dairy products and whole milk, 33 percent.

The proportion of cholesterol in the food supply from fats and oils declined from 13 to 8 percent between 1909-13

and 1947-49 and continued downward to 5 percent in 1984.
Decreased use of butter and lard were primarily responsible.
Despite decreased use from 18 to 5 pounds per capita,
butter still provided more than half of the cholesterol and
remained the leading source among the fats and oils group.
Lard's share of cholesterol in the fats and oils group also
decreased from 22 to 16 percent between 1909-13 and 1984,
reflecting substantially decreased use. In contrast, the
share of cholesterol from edible beef fat increased from
2 to 28 percent during the same period, surpassing lard in
the early 1980's. Direct use of edible beef fat, reported
since 1979, was a major factor in this trend.

SUMMARY

     The amount of fat in the U.S. food supply increased
one-third between 1909-13 and 1984, from 124 grams to 166
grams per capita per day. Also, the proportion of food
energy provided by fat increased from 32 to 43 percent.

     The gain in fat in the food supply was due to an
increase in fat from vegetable sources. The share of fat
from vegetable sources increased from 17 to 42 percent
between 1909-13 and 1984. Although animal fats provided
the largest share of fat, their proportionate contribution
declined from 83 to 58 percent between 1909-13 and 1984.

     Three food groups--fats and oils; meat, poultry, and
fish; and dairy products--provided about 90 percent of the
fat in the food supply throughout the past 75 years. However, the shares of fat provided by these groups changed.
The share from the fats and oils group increased from 37
to 44 percent between 1909-13 and 1984, while the share
from the meat, poultry, and fish group declined from 37 to
34 percent, and the share from the dairy products group
declined from 15 to 12 percent.

     Fat from the fats and oils group increased 59 percent
between 1909-13 and 1984. Most of the gain in fat from
this group was due to increased use of edible oils. Margarine replaced much of the butter and shortening replaced
much of the lard as sources of fat.

     Fat from the meat, poultry, and fish group increased
24 percent between 1909-13 and 1984. Pork accounted for

the largest proportion of fat from this group and beef
ranked second. The share of fat from poultry, although
much smaller than either pork or beef, almost tripled.

Fat from dairy products was about the same in 1984 as
in 1909-13. Cheese was the leading source of fat from dairy
products by 1984. Until recent years, whole milk was the
leading source, although its share declined substantially
after the late 1950's. Despite their low fat content, the
share of fat from skim and lowfat milks increased as use
increased, particularly in the past 25 years. The proportion
of fat provided by frozen desserts increased over the years,
while that from creams decreased.

Among the fatty acids in the food supply, the quantity
of TSFA increased by 10 percent between 1909-13 and 1984.
Quantities of oleic and linoleic acid increased by 39 and
189 percent, respectively, between 1909-13 and 1984. Higher
levels for these two fatty acids reflect increased use of
vegetable fats. Consequently, the proportion of fat accounted for by these fatty acids also changed. In 1909-13,
TSFA accounted for 42 percent of the fat in the food supply;
oleic acid, 37 percent; and linoleic acid, 7 percent. By
1984, these proportions had changed to 35 percent, 38 percent, and 15 percent, respectively.

The cholesterol level of the food supply in 1984--
481 mg per capita per day-- was lower than in 1909-13,
502 mg. Levels fluctuated considerably over the years.
Eggs are the major source of cholesterol. The meat,
poultry, and fish group ranks as the second largest source.
The share of cholesterol from dairy products was the same
in 1984 as in 1909-13, while the share from the fats and
oils group declined.

REFERENCES

Haytowitz DB, Matthews RH (1984). "Composition of Foods:
   Vegetable and Vegetable Products; Raw, Processed,
   Prepared." USDA Agriculture Handbook No 8-11.
Kromer GW (1973). Food fat consumption: More now and in
   the future. Speech presented at the Symposium on Fats
   and Carbohydrates in Processed Foods, American Medical
   Association, Chicago, Illinois, Oct 1, 1973.

Kromer GW (1974). US food fat consumption trends. In Kromer GW, Gazelle SA (eds): "Fats and Oils Situation," USDA, Economic Research Service: FOS-272: pp 16-32.

Posati LP, Orr ML (1976). "Composition of Foods: Dairy and Eggs Products; Raw, Processed, Prepared." USDA Agriculture Handbook No 8-1.

Posati LP (1979). "Composition of Foods: Poultry Products; Raw, Processed, Prepared." USDA Agriculture Handbook No 8-5.

Reaves JB III, Weihrauch JL (1979). "Composition of Foods: Fats and Oils; Raw, Processed, Prepared." USDA Agriculture Handbook No 8-4.

USDA, Economic Research Service (1965). US Food Consumption - Sources of Data and Trends. USDA Stat Bull 364.

USDA, Economic Research Service (1968). Food Consumption, Prices and Expenditures. Agric Econ Rept 138: Tables 8-30.

USDA, Economic Research Service (1982). Food Consumption, Prices and Expenditures. USDA Stat Bull 694: Tables 4-26.

USDA, Economic Research Service (1983). Food Consumption, Prices and Expenditures. USDA Stat Bull 702: Tables 4-26.

USDA, Economic Research Service (1984). Food Consumption, Prices and Expenditures. USDA Stat Bull 713: Tables 6-27.

USDA, Economic Research Service (1985). Food Consumption, Prices and Expenditures. USDA Stat Bull 736: Tables 6-32.

USDA, Human Nutrition Information Service (1983). Food Consumption: Households in the United States, Seasons and Year 1977-78. NFCS 1977-78, Report No H-6.

USDA, Human Nutrition Information Service (1984). Nutrient Intakes: Individuals in 48 States, Year 1977-78. NFCS 1977-78, Report No I-2.

USDA, Human Nutrition Information Service (1985). CSFII: Women 19-50 Years and Their Children 1-5 Years, 1-Day, 1985. NFCS, CSFII, Report No 85-1.

Watt BK, Merrill AL (1963). "Composition of Foods; Raw, Processed, Prepared." Agriculture Handbook No 8.

APPENDIX

Consumption of Selected Foods, Pounds Per Capita a/

Year	Meat, Poultry, and Fish						Dairy Products d/				
	Beef	Pork	Other meats b/	Poultry	Fish c/	Total	Fluid milks and cream	Processed milks	Ice cream and frozen desserts	Cheese	Total
1909-13	53.9	61.8	25.7	17.5	12.4	171.3	331.2	7.3	2.3	4.8	345.6
1925-29	43.1	63.1	22.8	16.6	12.9	158.5	337.6	15.7	9.9	5.7	368.9
1935-39	43.9	52.4	23.7	16.2	12.1	148.3	329.6	21.8	10.3	7.1	368.8
1947-49	51.8	63.6	25.8	22.4	11.6	175.2	358.7	29.5	20.2	9.5	417.9
1957-59	62.9	58.5	22.7	33.9	13.1	191.1	337.0	25.3	24.7	12.5	399.5
1967-69	80.7	60.6	19.9	45.8	14.7	221.7	281.6	19.2	28.5	15.1	344.4
1975	87.9	50.7	17.9	49.0	16.5	222.0	266.7	14.0	28.7	19.0	328.4
1980	76.5	68.3	14.9	61.0	16.9	237.6	249.6	12.8	26.4	22.1	310.9
1984	78.6	61.7	14.9	67.5	17.7	240.4	243.4	13.3	27.1	25.9	309.7

| Year | Fats and oils [d] | | | | | | | Eggs |
	Butter	Margarine [e]	Lard [f]	Short-ening [e]	Edible beef fat [f]	Edible oils	Total	
1909–13	17.6	1.4	11.8	8.4		1.5	40.7	37.4
1925–29	18.0	2.4	12.6	9.6		5.2	47.8	40.5
1935–39	17.0	2.9	11.0	11.8		6.5	49.2	36.4
1947–49	10.6	5.6	12.4	9.6		7.3	45.5	47.3
1957–59	8.2	8.9	9.3	11.4		10.8	48.6	45.2
1967–69	5.5	10.6	5.3	16.4		15.8	53.6	40.0
1975	4.7	11.0	2.8	17.0		19.9	55.4	35.2
1980	4.5	11.3	2.6	18.2	1.1	22.5	60.2	34.6
1984	5.0	10.4	2.1	21.3	1.7	21.1	61.6	33.0

a/ Adapted from data published by the Economic Research Service of USDA in Food Consumption, Prices, and Expenditures, Agricultural Economic Report No. 138, and Statistical Bulletin Nos. 696, 702, 713, and 736.

b/ Includes game, offal, veal, lamb, and mutton.

c/ Includes game fish.

d/ Product weight.

e/ Includes small amounts of lard and beef fat.

f/ Direct use; excludes use in some margarine and shortening. Data available for edible beef fat beginning in 1979.

Dietary Fat and Cancer, pages 153–184
© 1986 Alan R. Liss, Inc.

FOOD FATS AND OILS

J. Edward Hunter
The Procter & Gamble Company
Winton Hill Technical Center
6071 Center Hill Road
Cincinnati, Ohio 45224

I. IMPORTANCE OF FATS

Fats and oils have long been recognized as
essential nutrients for both humans and animals. They
provide the most concentrated source of energy of any
foodstuff, they are components of membranes of all living
cells, they supply essential fatty acids (the principal one
being linoleic acid, one precursor for important hormones,
the prostaglandins), and they act as carriers for the fat-
soluble vitamins A, D, E, and K. Fats also provide
desirable flavors and textures to many foods and give more
of a feeling of satiety after a meal than do proteins or
carbohydrates.

Fats and oils are present in varying amounts in many
foods. The principal sources of fat in the diet are meats,
dairy products, poultry, fish, nuts, and vegetable fats and
oils. Most vegetables and fruits consumed as such contain
only small amounts of fat. Overall, fats and oils provide
about 43% of the available calories in the current U.S.
diet.

II. WHAT IS A FAT?

Fats and oils are predominantly triesters of fatty
acids and glycerol, commonly called "triglycerides." They
are insoluble in water but soluble in most organic
solvents. They have lower densities than water and at
normal room temperatures range in consistency from liquids

to solid appearing substances. When solid appearing, they
are referred to as "fats" and when liquid they are called
"oils." Here the term "fat" will be applied to both liquid
and solid appearing fats or oils.

The term "lipids" embraces a variety of chemical
substances. In addition to triglycerides, it also includes
mono- and diglycerides, phosphatides, cerebrosides,
sterols, terpenes, fatty alcohols, fatty acids, fat-soluble
vitamins, and other substances.

The oils and fats most frequently used in the U.S. for
salad and cooking oils, shortenings, margarines, and salad
dressings include coconut, corn, cottonseed, lard, olive,
palm, palm kernel, peanut, safflower, soybean, sunflower,
and tallow. Specialized vegetable oils of lesser
availability in the U.S. include sesame, rice bran, walnut,
shea nut, illipe, and sal. More detailed information on
the use of some of these oils in specific products is
provided in Section VIII. Additional information on most
aspects of fats and oils may be found in Swern, ed., 1979
and 1982.

III. CHEMICAL COMPOSITION OF FATS

Triglycerides normally represent over 95% of the
weight of most food fats and oils. The minor components
include mono- and diglycerides, free fatty acids,
phosphatides, sterols, fatty alcohols, fat-soluble
vitamins, and other substances.

A. The Major Component--Triglycerides

A triglyceride is composed of glycerol and three fatty
acids. When all of the fatty acids in a triglyceride are
identical, it is termed a "simple" triglyceride. The most
common forms, however, are the "mixed" triglycerides in
which two or three kinds of fatty acid moieties are present
in the molecule. Illustrations of typical simple and mixed
triglyceride molecular structures are shown below.
R_1COO, R_2COO, and R_3COO represent the different fatty
acid moieties as they are esterified with the glycerol
moiety ($HOCH_2$--$CHOH$--CH_2OH).

$$R_1\text{--COO--}CH_2$$
$$R_1\text{--COO--}CH$$
$$R_1\text{--COO--}CH_2$$

$$R_1\text{--COO--}CH_2$$
$$R_2\text{--COO--}CH$$
$$R_3\text{--COO--}CH_2$$

Simple Triglyceride   Mixed Triglyceride

The fatty acids in a triglyceride define the properties of the molecule and are discussed in greater detail in Section IV.

B. The Minor Components

Mono- and Diglycerides. Mono- and diglycerides are the mono- and diesters of fatty acids with glycerol. Typical generalized structural formulas follow:

$$R_1\text{--COO--}CH_2$$
$$HO\text{--}CH$$
$$HO\text{--}CH_2$$

$$HO\text{--}CH_2$$
$$R_1\text{--COO--}CH$$
$$HO\text{--}CH_2$$

$$R_2\text{--COO--}CH_2$$
$$R_1\text{--COO--}CH$$
$$HO\text{--}CH_2$$

$$R_2\text{--COO--}CH_2$$
$$HO\text{--}CH$$
$$R_1\text{--COO--}CH_2$$

1-Mono-   2-Mono-   1,2-Diglyceride 1,3-Diglyceride
 glyceride   glyceride

Mono- and diglycerides are important as emulsifiers and are used frequently in foods for this purpose. They are prepared commercially by the reaction of glycerol with triglycerides or by the esterification of glycerol with fatty acids. Mono- and diglycerides are formed in the intestinal tract as the result of the normal digestion of triglycerides. They are found also in minor amounts in both animal and vegetable oils.

Free Fatty Acids. As the name suggests, free fatty acids are the uncombined fatty acids present in a fat. Some unrefined oils may contain as much as several percent free fatty acids. The levels of free fatty acids are reduced in the refining process discussed in Section VI. Refined fats and oils ready for use as foods usually have free fatty acid content on the order of a few hundredths of one percent.

Phosphatides. Phosphatides consist of polyhydric alcohols (usually glycerol), combined with fatty acids, phosphoric acid, and a nitrogen-containing compound. Lecithin and cephalin are common phosphatides found in edible fats. In lecithin, the nitrogen base is choline and in cephalin, hydroxyethylamine. For all practical purposes, refining removes the phosphatides from the fat or oil.

Sterols. Sterols are a class of substances containing the common steroid nucleus plus an 8 to 10 carbon atom side chain and an alcohol group. Although sterols are found in both animal fats and vegetable oils, there is a substantial difference biologically between those occurring in animal fats and those present in vegetable oils. Cholesterol is the primary animal fat sterol and is found in vegetable oils in trace amounts. Vegetable oil sterols collectively are termed "phytosterols." Sitosterol and stigmasterol are the best known vegetable oil sterols. The type and amount of vegetable oil sterols vary with the source of the oil.

Fatty Alcohols. Long chain alcohols are of little importance in most edible fats. A small amount esterified with fatty acids is present in waxes found in some vegetable oils. Larger quantities are found in some marine oils.

Tocopherols. Tocopherols are important minor constituents of most vegetable fats. They serve as antioxidants to retard rancidity and as sources of an essential nutrient, vitamin E. Among tocopherols, alpha-tocopherol has the highest vitamin E activity and the lowest antioxidant activity. The antioxidant activities of other tocopherols in decreasing order are as follows: gamma, delta, beta, and alpha. Tocopherols, naturally occurring in most vegetable fats, may be partially removed by processing, and they are not present in animal fats. Antioxidants commonly are added after processing to restore rancidity retardation in the finished product.

Carotenoids and Chlorophyll. Carotenoids are coloring materials occurring naturally in fats and oils. Most range in color from yellow to deep red. Chlorophyll is the green coloring matter of plants which plays an essential part in the photosynthetic process. At times,

the chlorophyll content of oils is increased and the oils
may be tinged green. This has no effect on oil quality.
The levels of most of these color bodies are reduced during
the normal processing of oils to give them acceptable
color, flavor, and stability.

Vitamins. Generally speaking, most fats and oils are
not good sources of vitamins other than vitamin E. The fat-
soluble vitamins A and D sometimes are added to foods which
contain fat, such as margarine and milk, because these
foods serve as good carriers.

IV. FATTY ACIDS

A. General

Triglycerides are comprised predominantly of fatty
acids present in the form of esters of glycerol. One
hundred grams of fat will yield approximately 95 grams of
fatty acids. Both the physical and chemical
characteristics of fats are influenced greatly by the kinds
and proportions of component fatty acids and the way in
which these are positioned on the glycerol moiety.
Variations in these characteristics result from the
physiological requirements of the plant or animal producing
them.

The predominant fatty acids are saturated and
unsaturated straight aliphatic chains with an even number
of carbon atoms and a single carboxyl group as illustrated
in the general structural formula for a saturated fatty
acid given below:

$$CH_3--(CH_2)_x-------COOH$$

aliphatic chain   carboxyl group

A number of minor acids are present in edible oils
including small amounts of branched chain, cyclic, and odd
number straight chain acids.

B. Classification of Fatty Acids

Fatty acids occurring in edible fats and oils are

classified according to their degree of saturation.

Saturated Fatty Acids. Those containing only single carbon-to-carbon bonds are termed "saturated" and are the least reactive chemically. In Table 1 are listed the saturated fatty acids of practical interest. All but acetic occur naturally in fats. The principal fat sources of the naturally occurring saturated fatty acids are included in the table. The melting point of saturated fatty acids increases with chain length. Decanoic and longer chain acids are solids at normal room temperatures.

TABLE 1

SATURATED FATTY ACIDS

Systematic Name	Common Name	No. of Carbon Atoms*	Typical Fat Source
Ethanoic	Acetic	2	–
Butanoic	Butyric	4	Butterfat
Hexanoic	Caproic	6	Butterfat
Octanoic	Caprylic	8	Coconut oil
Decanoic	Capric	10	Coconut oil
Dodecanoic	Lauric	12	Coconut oil
Tetradecanoic	Myristic	14	Butterfat, coconut oil
Hexadecanoic	Palmitic	16	Most fats and oils
Octadecanoic	Stearic	18	Most fats and oils
Eicosanoic	Arachidic	20	Lard, peanut oil
Docosanoic	Behenic	22	Peanut oil

*A number of saturated odd and even chain acids are present in trace quantities in many fats and oils.

Unsaturated Fatty Acids. Fatty acids containing one or more carbon-to-carbon double bonds are termed "unsaturated." The saturated and unsaturated linkages are illustrated below:

```
      H    H              H    H
      |    |              |    |
  --  C---C  --       --  C = C  --
      |    |
      H    H
```

Saturated	Unsaturated
Bond	Bond

When the fatty acid contains one double bond it is called "monounsaturated" or "monoenoic." If it contains more than one double bond, it is called "polyunsaturated" or "polyenoic."

In the Geneva system of nomenclature, the carbons in a fatty acid chain are numbered consecutively from the end of the chain, considering as number 1, the carbon of the carboxyl group. By convention, a specific bond in a chain is identified by the lower number of the two carbons which it joins. In oleic acid (cis-9-octadecenoic acid), for example, the double bond is between the ninth and tenth carbon atoms. When two fatty acids are identical except for the position of the double bond, they are referred to as positional isomers. Fatty acid isomers are discussed at greater length in subparagraph C of this section.

Table 2 lists some of the unsaturated fatty acids found in edible fats and oils and typical sources of each. Oleic acid is the fatty acid that occurs most frequently in nature.

TABLE 2

SOME UNSATURATED FATTY ACIDS IN FOOD FATS AND OILS

Systematic Name	Common Name	No. of Double Bonds*	No. of Carbon Atoms	Typical Fat Source
9-Decenoic	Caproleic	1	10	Butterfat
9-Dodecenoic	Lauroleic	1	12	Butterfat
9-Tetradecenoic	Myristoleic	1	14	Butterfat
9-Hexadecenoic	Palmitoleic	1	16	Fish oils
9-Octadecenoic	Oleic	1	18	Most fats oils
9-Octadecenoic	Elaidic	1	18	Butterfat, beef fat
11-Octadecenoic	Vaccenic	1	18	Butterfat, beef fat
9,12-Octadecadienoic	Linoleic	2	18	Most veget. oils
9,12,15-Octadecatrienoic	Linolenic	3	18	Soybean oi canola oi
9-Eicosenoic	Gadoleic	1	20	Fish oils
5,8,11,14-Eicosatetra- enoic	Arachidonic	4	20	Lard
5,8,11,14,17-Eicosapen- taenoic	-	5	20	Fish oils
13-Docosenoic	Erucic	1	22	Rapeseed o
4,7,10,13,16,19-Doco- sahexaenoic	-	6	22	Fish oils

*All double bonds are in the cis configuration except for elaidic acid and vaccenic acid which are trans.

Because of the presence of double bonds, unsaturated fatty acids are more reactive chemically than are saturated acids. This reactivity increases as the number of double bonds increases. Although double bonds normally occur in a nonconjugated position, they can occur in a conjugated position (alternating with a single bond) as illustrated below:

```
   H   H   H   H            H   H   H   H   H
   |   |   |   |            |   |   |   |   |
-- C = C - C = C --      -- C = C - C - C = C --
                                     |
                                     H

    Conjugated                  Nonconjugated
```

With the bonds in a conjugated position, there is a further
increase in certain types of chemical reactivity. For
example, fats are much more subject to polymerization when
bonds are in the conjugated position.

   Polyunsaturated Fatty Acids. Of the polyunsaturated
fatty acids, linoleic, linolenic, and arachidonic acids
containing respectively two, three, and four double bonds
are of most interest. The nutritional importance of these
fatty acids is discussed in Section V, Part C. Vegetable
oils are the principal sources of linoleic and linolenic
acids. Arachidonic acid is found in small amounts in lard
which also contains about 10% of linoleic acid. Fish oils
contain large quantities of a variety of longer chain fatty
acids having three or more double bonds.

C. Isomerism of Unsaturated Fatty Acids

   Isomers are two or more substances that are composed
of the same elements combined in the same proportions but
differing in molecular structure. The two important types
of isomerism among fatty acids are geometric and
positional.

   Geometric Isomerism. Unsaturated fatty acids can
exist in either the cis or trans form depending on the
configuration of the hydrogen atoms attached to the carbon
atoms joined by the double bonds. If the hydrogen atoms
are on the same side of the carbon chain, the arrangement
is called cis, and if the hydrogen atoms are on opposite
sides of the carbon chain, the arrangement is called
trans, as shown by the following diagrams:

```
     H   H   H   H              H   H           H
     |   |   |   |              |   |           |
  -- C - C = C - C --       -- C - C = C - C --
     |           |              |       |   |
     H           H              H       H   H


           cis                       trans
```

Elaidic and oleic acids are geometric isomers; in the
former the double bond is in the trans configuration and in
the latter, in the cis configuration.

Positional Isomerism. In this case, the location of the double bond differs among the isomers. Petroselinic acid, which is present in parsleyseed oil, is cis-6-octadecenoic acid and a positional isomer of oleic acid, cis-9-octadecenoic acid. Vaccenic acid, which is a minor acid in tallow and butterfat, is trans-11-octadecenoic acid and is both a positional and geometric isomer of oleic acid.

The position of the double bonds affects the melting point of the fatty acid to a limited extent. Processing such as hydrogenation can cause shifts in the location of double bonds in the fatty acid chains as well as cis-trans isomerization.

The number of positional and geometric isomers increases with the number of double bonds. For example, with two double bonds, the following four geometric isomers are possible: cis-cis, cis-trans, trans-cis, and trans-trans. Trans-trans dienes, however, are present in only trace amounts in partially hydrogenated fats and thus are insignificant in the human food supply. The geometric configuration has an appreciable effect upon the melting point of the fatty acid.

Generally speaking, cis isomers are those naturally occurring in food fats and oils. Although small amounts of trans isomers occur in fats from ruminants, most trans isomers result from the hydrogenation of fats and oils.

A considerable amount of research effort has indicated that trans isomers are metabolized in a manner similar to cis isomers. A recent report prepared by a special committee of scientists formed by the Life Sciences Research Office of the Federation of American Societies for Experimental Biology concluded that available scientific information suggests little reason for concern with the safety of dietary trans fatty acids both at their present and expected levels of consumption and at present and expected levels of consumption of dietary linoleic acid (Senti, ed., 1985).

V. NUTRITIONAL ASPECTS OF FATS AND OILS

A. General

Fats are a principal and essential constituent of the human diet along with carbohydrates and proteins. Fats are a major source of energy, supplying about 9 kcal per gram compared to about 4 kcal per gram from protein and carbohydrate. In calorie deficient situations, fats together with carbohydrates spare protein and improve growth rates. Some fatty foods are sources of fat-soluble vitamins, and the ingestion of fat improves the absorption of these vitamins regardless of their source. Fats are vital to a palatable and well-rounded diet and provide the essential fatty acids linoleic and linolenic acids.

B. Metabolism of Fats and Oils

In the intestinal tract, dietary triglycerides are hydrolyzed to 2-monoglycerides and free fatty acids. These digestion products, together with bile salts, then form a micelle which moves to the epithelial cell membrane. There the fatty acids and the monoglycerides are absorbed into the cell and the bile acid is retained in the lumen. From 95 to 100% of most dietary fats are absorbed. In the intestinal wall, the monoglycerides and free fatty acids are recombined to form triglycerides. If the chain length of the fatty acids has twelve or fewer carbon atoms, as in the case of the "medium chain length triglycerides," these acids are transported via the portal blood to the liver where they are metabolized rapidly. Triglycerides containing fatty acids having a chain length of more than twelve carbon atoms are transported via the lymphatics. These triglycerides, whether coming from the diet or from endogenous sources, are transported in the blood as lipoproteins. The triglycerides are stored in the adipose tissue until they are needed for energy. The amount of fat stored depends on the caloric balance of the whole organism. Excess calories, regardless of whether they are in the form of fat, carbohydrate, or protein, are stored as fat. Consequently an appreciable portion of the dietary carbohydrate and some protein are converted to fat. The body can make saturated and monounsaturated fatty acids by modifying other fatty acids or by de novo synthesis from carbohydrate and protein. However, certain polyunsaturated fatty acids, such as linoleic acid, cannot be made by the body and must be supplied in the diet.

Fat is mobilized from adipose tissue into the blood as

free fatty acids. These complex with blood proteins and
are distributed throughout the organism. The oxidation of
free fatty acids is a major source of energy for the body.
It has been known for many years that all of the usual
dietary fats are of equal caloric value. The establishment
of the common pathway of beta-oxidation by way of acetate,
regardless of whether a fatty acid is saturated,
monounsaturated, or polyunsaturated and whether the double
bonds are cis or trans, explains this equivalence in
caloric value.

C. Essential Fatty Acids

In the early 1930's work was done demonstrating the
essentiality of the long chain polyunsaturated fatty acids,
linoleic and arachidonic acids, for growth and good skin
and hair quality in rats. There are current indications
that linolenic acid is an essential fatty acid for humans
as well. Linoleic and linolenic acids are termed
"essential" because they cannot be synthesized by the body
and must be supplied in the diet. Arachidonic acid,
however, can be synthesized by the body from dietary
linoleic acid. Sometimes arachidonic acid is considered an
essential fatty acid because it is an essential component
of membranes and a precursor of a group of hormone-like
compounds called prostaglandins, thromboxanes, and
prostacyclins which are important in the regulation of
widely diverse physiological processes. Linolenic acid is
also a precursor of a special group of prostaglandins. The
dietary fatty acids that can function as essential fatty
acids must have a particular chemical structure, namely,
double bonds in the cis configuration and in specific
positions (carbons 6 and 9 or 3,6, and 9 from the methyl
end of the molecule) on the carbon chain.

In infants the requirement for these essential fatty
acids has been demonstrated clearly. While the minimum
requirement has not been determined for adults, there is no
doubt that they are essential nutrients. The American diet
provides at least the minimum essential fatty acid
requirement. According to the Food and Nutrition Board's
"Recommended Dietary Allowances" (9th edition, 1980), the
amount of dietary linoleic acid necessary to prevent
essential fatty acid deficiency in several animal species
and also in man is 1 to 2% of dietary calories. However

for much of the general population, 3% of calories as
linoleic acid is considered to be a more satisfactory
minimum intake.

D. Fat Level in the Diet

Although considerable animal, clinical, and
epidemiological research has been done in recent years in
an effort to define the optimum level of fat in the diet,
there is still no complete agreement as to what this level
should be. Based on total food disappearance information,
it is estimated that about 43% of the calories in the food
that U.S. families use comes from all sources of fat in the
diet (Marston and Welsh, 1984). Discarded foods, such as
fats that have been used for frying and fats trimmed from
meats, decrease this percentage appreciably. To lower this
level of fat in the diet significantly below 43% of
calories requires care in the selection of foods and
particularly in the selection of meats and dairy foods.
Most health authorities agree that in diets where weight
control is important, care must be taken not only to
maintain a balanced diet but also to avoid excessive intake
of fats and oils.

VI. PROCESSING

A. General

Food fats and oils are derived from oilseed and animal
sources. Animal fats are generally heat rendered from
animal tissues to separate them from protein and other
naturally occurring materials. Rendering may be either
with dry heat or with steam. Rendering and processing of
meat fats is conducted in USDA inspected plants. Vegetable
fats are obtained by the extraction or the expression of
the oil from the oilseed source. Historically, cold or hot
expression methods were used. These methods have been
replaced with solvent extraction methods which give a
better oil yield. In this process the oil is extracted
from the oilseed by hexane and the hexane is then separated
from the oil, recovered, and reused. Because of its high
volatility, no hexane residue remains in the finished oil
after processing.

The fats and oils obtained directly from rendering or from the extraction of the oilseeds are termed "crude" fats and oils. Crude fats and oils contain varying but relatively small amounts of naturally occurring nonglyceride materials that are removed through a series of processing steps. For example, soybean oil may contain small amounts of protein, free fatty acids, and phosphatides which must be removed through subsequent processing to produce the desired shortening and oil products. Similarly, meat fats may contain some free fatty acids, water, and protein which must be removed.

It should be pointed out, however, that not all of the nonglyceride materials are undesirable elements. Tocopherols, for example, perform the important function of protecting the oils from oxidation and provide vitamin E. Processing is carried out in such a way as to control retention of these substances (Hunter, 1981).

Hydrogenation is employed frequently to improve the keeping qualities of fats and oils and to provide increased usefulness by imparting a semi-solid consistency to the fat for many food applications. It is agreed by most nutritionists and food technologists that the modern processing of edible fats and oils is the single factor most responsible for upgrading the quality of the fat consumed in the U.S. diet today.

B. Refining

The process of refining generally is performed on vegetable oils to reduce the free fatty acid content and to remove other gross impurities such as phosphatides, proteinaceous, and mucilagenous substances. Meat fats, however, usually are not refined. By far the most important and widespread method of refining is by treatment of the fat or oil with an alkali solution. This results in a large reduction of free fatty acids through their conversion into water-soluble soaps. Phosphatides, proteinaceous, and mucilagenous substances are soluble in the oil only in an anhydrous form and upon hydrating with the caustic or other refining solution are readily separated. Oils low in phosphatide content (palm and coconut) may be steam stripped (i.e., steam refined) of free fatty acids.

C. Bleaching

The term "bleaching" refers to the treatment that is given to remove color producing substances and to further purify the fat or oil. Normally bleaching is accomplished after the oil has been refined. The usual method of bleaching is by adsorption of the color producing substances on an adsorbent material. Acid-activated bleaching earth or clay, sometimes called bentonite, is the adsorbent material that has been used most extensively. This substance consists primarily of hydrated aluminum silicate. Activated carbon also is used as a bleaching adsorbent to a limited extent.

D. Deodorization

Deodorization is the treatment of fats and oils to remove trace constituents that give rise to undesirable flavors and odors. Normally this is accomplished after refining and bleaching.

The deodorization of fats and oils is simply a removal of the relatively volatile components from the fat or oil using live steam. This is feasible because of the great differences in volatility between the substances that give flavors and odors to fats and oils and the triglycerides. Normally deodorization is carried out under vacuum to facilitate the removal of the volatile substances, to avoid undue hydrolysis of the fat, and to make the most efficient use of the steam. Deodorization does not have any significant effect upon the fatty acid composition of the fat or oil. In the case of vegetable oils, sufficient tocopherols remain in the finished oils after deodorization to provide stability.

E. Fractionation (Including Winterization)

The most widely practiced form of fractionation is that of crystallization wherein a mixture of triglycerides is separated into two or more different melting fractions based on solubility at a given temperature. The term "dry fractionation" frequently is used to describe fractionation processes such as winterization or pressing. Winterization is a process whereby a small quantity of higher melting triglycerides is crystallized and removed from edible oils by filtration to avoid clouding of the liquid fractions at refrigeration temperatures. Originally this processing was applied to cottonseed oil by subjecting the oil to ambient winter temperatures, hence the term "winterization." Today cottonseed oil is chilled using refrigeration and the practice has been extended to other vegetable oils.

Pressing is a fractionation process sometimes used to separate a small amount of liquid oil from a larger quantity of solid fat. The process squeezes or "presses" the liquid oil from the solid fat by means of hydraulic pressure. This process is used commercially to produce hard butters from fats such as palm kernel oil and coconut oil.

Solvent fractionation is the term used to describe a process for the crystallization of a desired fraction from a mixture of triglycerides dissolved in a suitable solvent. Fractions may be selectively crystallized at different temperatures after which the fractions are separated and the solvent removed. Solvent fractionation is practiced commercially to produce hard butters, specialty oils, and some salad oils from a wide array of edible oils.

F. Hydrogenation

Hydrogenation is the process by which hydrogen is added directly to points of unsaturation in the fatty acids. Hydrogenation of fats has developed as a result of the need (1) to convert liquid oils to the semi-solid form for greater utility in certain food uses and (2) to increase the stability of the fat or oil to oxidative rancidity.

Hydrogenation is an extremely important process so far as our food supply is concerned, because this processing is necessary in order to impart the desired stability to many edible oil products. The level of linolenic acid present in some oils such as soybean oil is reduced in order for the oils to have acceptable properties in many food applications. Hydrogenation is a practical way to impart this stability. The importance of this processing is further understood when it is recognized that soybean oil now provides about 75% of the total visible fat (excluding butter) in the U.S. diet (Bunch and Hazera, 1984).

In the process of hydrogenation, oil is combined with hydrogen gas at a suitable temperature and pressure in the presence of a catalyst. The catalyst most widely used is nickel supported on an inert carrier which is removed from the fat after the hydrogenation processing is completed. Under these conditions, the gaseous hydrogen reacts with the double bonds of the unsaturated fatty acids.

The hydrogenation process is easily controlled and can be stopped at any desired point. As hydrogenation progresses, there is a gradual increase in the melting point of the fat or oil. If the hydrogenation of cottonseed or soybean oil, for example, is stopped after only a small amount of hydrogenation has taken place, the oils remain liquid. Further hydrogenation can produce soft, but solid appearing fats, which still contain appreciable amounts of polyunsaturated fatty acids. This degree of hydrogenation is employed frequently in the preparation of vegetable oils for shortening and margarine. If an oil is hydrogenated completely, the double bonds are eliminated entirely and the resulting product is a hard brittle solid at room temperature. Most oils used for shortenings, margarines, and many salad and cooking oils are partially hydrogenated.

The hydrogenation conditions can be varied by the manufacturer to meet physical and chemical characteristics desired in the finished product. This is achieved through the selection of the proper temperature, pressure, time, catalyst, and starting oils. Both positional and geometric (trans) isomers are formed to some extent during hydrogenation, the amounts depending on the conditions employed.

Biological hydrogenation of polyunsaturated fatty acids occurs in some animal organisms, particularly in ruminants. This accounts for the creation of some trans isomers such as those that occur in the tissues and milk of ruminants. It is known that these result from the biohydrogenation of unsaturated fatty acids by rumen bacterial action.

G. Interesterification

Another process used in the manufacture of shortening permits a rearrangement or a redistribution of the fatty acids on the glycerol fragment of the molecule. This process, referred to as interesterification, is accomplished by catalytic methods at relatively low temperature. Under some conditions the fatty acids are distributed in a more random manner than they were present originally. Other conditions permit the rearrangement process to control the fatty acid distribution to an extent that allows further modification of shortening properties to be obtained. The rearrangement process does not change the degree of unsaturation or the isomeric state of the fatty acids as they transfer in their entirety from one position to another.

Lard in its natural state possesses a very narrow temperature range over which it has good consistency for practical use in the kitchen. At slightly above normal room temperature, ordinary lard becomes somewhat softer than desirable, and at temperatures slightly lower, it becomes somewhat firmer than is desirable. Molecularly rearranged lard shortenings have a satisfactory consistency over a much wider temperature range.

Rearranged lard and vegetable fats may be processed together in the manufacture of some types of shortening. Hydrogenation may be used in conjunction with rearrangement and may either precede or follow it. Thus, the shortening manufacturer has the means to impart a wide range of properties to products.

H. Esterification

For the most part, fatty acids are present in nature in the form of esters (triglycerides) and are consumed as such. When consumed and digested, fats are hydrolyzed initially to diglycerides and monoglycerides which are also esters. Carried to completion, these esters are hydrolyzed to glycerol and fatty acids. In the reverse process, esterification, an alcohol such as glycerol is reacted with an acid such as a fatty acid to form esters such as mono-, di-, and triglycerides. In an alternative esterification process, called alcoholysis, an alcohol such as glycerol is reacted with fat or oil to produce esters such as mono- and diglycerides. Using the foregoing esterification processes, edible acids, fats, and oils can be reacted with edible alcohols to produce useful food ingredients such as emulsifiers.

I. Emulsifiers

Many foods are processed and/or consumed as emulsions, which are dispersions of immiscible liquids such as water and oil, e.g., milk, mayonnaise, ice cream, icings, and sausage. Emulsifiers either present naturally in one or more of the ingredients or added separately provide emulsion stability. Lack of stability results in separation of the oil and water phases. Some emulsifiers also provide valuable functional attributes in addition to emulsification. These include aeration, starch and protein complexing, hydration, crystal modification, solubilization, and dispersion. Some common food emulsifiers are mono-/diglycerides, polyglycerol esters, propylene glycol esters, acetylated mono-/diglycerides, succinylated mono-/diglycerides, lactylated propylene glycol esters, sorbitan esters, ethoxylated mono-/ diglycerides, ethoxylated sorbitan esters, lecithin, lipoproteins, and gums. Typical examples of emulsifiers and the characteristics they impart to food are listed in Table 3.

TABLE 3

EMULSIFIERS AND THEIR FUNCTIONAL CHARACTERISTICS
IN PROCESSED FOODS

Emulsifier	Characteristic	Processed Food
Lecithin	Viscosity control and wetting	Confectionary coating
Mono-/diglycerides	Emulsification of water in oil	Margarine
	Anti-staling or softening	Bread
Lactylated mono-/ diglycerides	Aeration	Cake batter
Oxystearin or polyglycerol ester	Crystallization inhibitor	Salad Oil
Polyglycerol ester	Crystallization promoter	Sugar syrup

Emulsifiers are sanctioned for use by the Food and
Drug Administration. This agency provides guidelines for
industry usage as GRAS or regulated food additives.

J. Additives and Processing Aids

Manufacturers may add low levels of food approved
additives to fats and oils to protect their quality in
processing, storage, handling, and shipping of finished
products. This insures quality maintenance from time of
production to time of consumption. When addition provides
a technical effect in the end-use product, the material
added is considered a direct additive. Such usage must
comply with FDA regulations governing levels, mode of
addition, and product labeling. Typical examples of
industry practice are listed in Table 4.

TABLE 4

SOME DIRECT FOOD ADDITIVES USED IN FATS AND OILS

Additive	Effect Provided
Tocopherols Butylated hydroxyanisole (BHA) Butylated hydroxytoluene (BHT) Tertiary butylhydroquinone (TBHQ)	Antioxidant, retards oxidative rancidity
Carotene (pro-vitamin A)	Color additive, enhances color of finished foods
Methyl silicone (Dimethylpoly- siloxane)	Inhibits foaming of fats and oils during frying
Diacetyl	Provides buttery odor and flavor to fats and oils
Citric acid Phosphoric acid EDTA	Metal chelating agents, prevent metal- catalyzed oxidative breakdown

When addition is made to achieve a technical effect during processing, shipping, or storage followed by removal or reduction to an insignificant level, the material added is considered to be a processing aid. Typical examples of processing aids and provided effects are listed in Table 5. Use of processing aids also must comply with federal regulations which specify good manufacturing practices and acceptable residual levels.

TABLE 5

SOME PROCESSING AIDS USED IN
MANUFACTURING EDIBLE FATS AND OILS

Aid	Effect	Mode of Removal
Nickel catalyst	Hydrogen initiator	Post bleach and filtration
Sodium methoxide	Rearrangement catalyst	Water or acid neutralization, filtration, and deodorization
Mineral acids ⎫ Citric acid ⎬	Refining acids, metal chelators	Neutralization with base, filtration, or water washing
Acetone ⎫ Hexane ⎮ Isopropanol ⎬ 2-Nitropropane ⎭	Crystallization media for fractionation of fats and oils	Solvent stripping and deodorization
Nitrogen	Oxygen replacement	Diffusion
Polyglycerol esters ⎫ Oxystearin ⎬	Crystallization modification	Filtration

VII. REACTIONS OF FATS AND OILS

A. Hydrolysis of Fats

Like other esters, glycerides can be hydrolyzed readily. Partial hydrolysis of triglycerides will yield mono- and diglycerides and fatty acids. When the hydrolysis is carried to completion with water alone in the presence of an acidic catalyst, the mono-, di-, and triglycerides will hydrolyze to yield glycerol and fatty acids. With aqueous sodium hydroxide, glycerol and the sodium salts of the component fatty acids (soaps) are obtained. In the digestive tracts of humans and animals and in bacteria, fats are hydrolyzed by enzymes (lipases). Lipolytic enzymes present in some crude fats and oils are deactivated by the temperatures used in oil processing, so enzymatic hydrolysis does not occur in finished fats and oils.

B. Oxidation of Fats

Autoxidation. Of particular interest in the food field is the process of oxidation induced by air at room temperature referred to as "autoxidation." Ordinarily, this is a slow process which occurs only to a limited degree. In autoxidation, oxygen reacts with unsaturated fatty acids. Initially, peroxides are formed which in turn break down to hydrocarbons, ketones, aldehydes, and smaller amounts of epoxides and alcohols.

The result of the autoxidation of fats and oils is the development of objectionable tastes and odors characteristic of the condition known as "oxidative fat rancidity." Some fats resist this change to a remarkable extent while others are more susceptible depending on the degree of unsaturation, the presence of antioxidants, and other factors. The presence of light, for example, increases the rate of oxidation.

When rancidity has progressed significantly, it is apparent from the taste and odor. Expert tasters are able to detect the development of rancidity in its early stages. The peroxide value determination, if used judiciously, may be helpful in measuring the degree of oxidative rancidity in the fat. The stability of a fat or oil may be predicted to some degree by the active oxygen method (AOM).

It has been found that oxidatively abused fats can complicate nutritional and biochemical studies in animals in that they can affect food consumption under ad libitum feeding conditions and reduce the vitamin content of the food. If the diet has become unpalatable due to excessive oxidation of the fat component and is not accepted by the animal, the lack of growth of the animal may be due to its unwillingness to consume the experimental diet. Thus, the experimental results might be attributed unwittingly to the type of fat or other nutrient being studied rather than to the condition of the ration. Knowing the oxidative condition of unsaturated fats is of extreme importance in biochemical and nutritional studies with animals.

Oxidation at Higher Temperatures. Although the rate of oxidation is greatly accelerated at higher temperatures, oxidative reactions which occur at higher temperatures may not follow precisely the same routes and mechanisms as the reactions at room temperatures. Thus, differences in the stability of fats and oils often become more apparent when the fats are used for frying or slow baking. The more unsaturated the fat or oil, the greater will be its susceptibility to oxidative rancidity. Predominantly unsaturated oils such as soybean, cottonseed, or corn oil are less stable than a predominantly saturated oil such as coconut oil, for example. Soybean oil contains appreciable quantities of linolenic acid, a fatty acid with three double bonds. Frequently partial hydrogenation is employed in the processing of soybean oil to minimize the content of linolenic acid and thereby increase the stability of the oil.

C. Polymerization of Fats

All commonly used fats and particularly those high in polyunsaturated fatty acids tend to form polymers when heated under extreme conditions of temperature and time. Under normal processing and cooking conditions, these are formed in insignificant quantities. Although the mechanism of such polymer formation is not understood completely, it is believed that polymers are formed either by direct linkage of carbon to carbon atoms or by oxygen bridges. When an appreciable amount of polymer is present, there is a marked increase in viscosity. Animal studies have shown that any polymers that may be present in a fat or oil are absorbed poorly from the intestinal tract and are excreted as such in the feces.

D. Reactions During Heating and Cooking

Considerable work has been done studying the effects of elevated temperatures upon the composition and biological quality of edible fats and oils (Artman, 1969). Much of this work has been done with temperatures and other conditions which simulated those experienced in commercial deep frying operations such as in restaurants or food processing establishments. Other studies, however, have exposed the foods to exaggerated conditions that are

unrealistic and not indicative of actual use conditions.
Under these latter conditions, some substances are formed
in small amounts that when isolated and fed at concentrated
amounts can be shown to be toxic to laboratory animals.

The practical significance of these observations was
defined more clearly in a two-year animal feeding study by
Nolen et al., 1967. This work showed that animals
consuming used frying fats as the sole source of fat in the
diet throughout their life span thrived equally as well as
control animals consuming the same fat that had not been
subjected to frying conditions. Clark et al., 1978, also
have reviewed the nutritional aspects of heated fats.

Unsaturated fatty acids are subject to chemical
reactions (oxidation, polymerization, hydrolysis) which can
occur particularly during deep fat frying. The extent of
these reactions, which may be reflected as a decrease in
iodine value of the fat, depends largely on the frying
conditions, principally the temperature, aeration, and
duration. The composition of a frying fat also may be
affected by the kind of food being fried. For example,
when frying high fat foods such as chicken, fat will be
rendered and blended with the frying fat and some frying
fat will be absorbed by the food. In this manner the fatty
acid composition of the frying fat will change considerably
as frying progresses. Since absorption of fat by the fried
food may be extensive, it is often necessary to replenish
the fryer with fresh fat. This replenishment with fresh
fat tends to dilute overall compositional changes of the
fat during prolonged frying. Frying conditions do not,
however, saturate the unsaturated fatty acids, although the
ratio of saturated to unsaturated fatty acids will change
due to some polymerization of unsaturated fatty acids.

It is the usual practice to discard frying fat when
(1) prolonged frying causes excessive foaming of the hot
fat, (2) the fat tends to smoke excessively, usually from
the prolonged frying with low fat turnover, or (3) an
undesirable flavor or dark color develops. Any or all of
these qualities associated with the fat can decrease the
quality of the fried food.

The "smoke," "flash," and "fire points" of a fatty
material are standard measures of its thermal stability

when heated in contact with air. The smoke point is the
temperature at which the smoking is first detected in a
laboratory apparatus protected from drafts and provided
with special illumination. The temperature at which the
fat smokes freely is usually somewhat higher. The flash
point is the temperature at which the volatile products are
evolved at such a rate that they are capable of being
ignited but not capable of supporting combustion. The fire
point is the temperature at which the volatile products
will support continued combustion. For typical fats with a
free fatty acid content of about 0.05%, the smoke, flash,
and fire points are around 420°, 620°, and 680°F,
respectively. The degree of unsaturation of an oil has
little, if any, effect on its smoke, flash, or fire
points. Oils containing fatty acids of low molecular
weight such as coconut oil, however, have lower smoke,
flash, and fire points than other animal or vegetable fats
of comparable free fatty acid content.

VIII. PRODUCTS PREPARED FROM FATS AND OILS

A. General

A wide variety of products based on edible fats and
oils is available to the consuming public. Shortenings,
margarines, butter, salad and cooking oils, mayonnaise,
salad dressing, French dressing, Italian and other
specialty salad dressings, and confectioners' coatings are
some of the widely available products that are based
entirely on fats and oils or contain fat or oil as a
principal ingredient. Many of these products also are sold
in commercial quantities to food processors, snack food
manufacturers, bakeries, restaurants, and institutions.

Dietary fats have been categorized into what are termed
"visible" and "invisible" sources of fat. Visible fats are
defined for statistical reporting purposes as those that
have been isolated from animal tissues, oilseeds, or
vegetable sources, and are used in such products as
shortenings, margarine, and salad oil. These fats and oils
comprise about 43% of the total fat available for
consumption in the U.S. diet. Invisible fats are those
that have not been isolated from the animal tissues,
oilseeds, or vegetable sources, and are consumed as part of
the animal tissues or the vegetables in the diet. Examples

include fats consumed in meats, fish, poultry, eggs, and dairy products. Fats in these foods comprise the remaining 57% of the fat available for consumption in the U.S. diet.

B. Salad and Cooking Oils

Salad and cooking oils are prepared from vegetable oils that usually are refined, bleached, deodorized, and sometimes lightly hydrogenated. Soybean, cottonseed, and corn oil are the principal oils sold in this form, although peanut, safflower, sunflower, and olive oil also are used. When soybean oil is processed into salad oils and mayonnaise, a refined, bleached, and deodorized oil often is suitable. This is because under the usual conditions of handling and storage, the linolenic acid naturally present in the oil is not highly susceptible to oxidation which might produce undesirable odors and flavors in the oil. If soybean oil is intended for use as both a salad and cooking oil, some manufacturers employ light hydrogenation to assure the desired stability. However, in recent years improved refining, bleaching, and deodorization processes has enabled some manufacturers to produce oils suitable for cooking that have had no hydrogenation processing.

C. Shortenings (Baking and Frying Fats)

Shortenings are fats used in the preparation of many foods. Because they impart a "short" or tender quality to baked goods, they are called shortenings. For many years, lard and other animal fats were the principal edible fats used in shortenings in this country, but during the last third of the nineteenth century large quantities of cottonseed oil became available as a by-product from the growing of cotton. Many types of vegetable oils including soybean, cottonseed, corn, safflower, sunflower, and palm can be used in shortening products. Soybeans, not grown to any appreciable extent in this country until after 1930, are now by far our most important source of oil.

Hydrogenated shortenings may be made from a single hydrogenated fat, but usually they are made from a blend of two or more hydrogenated fats. The conditions and extent of hydrogenation may be varied for each to achieve the characteristics desired. Thus, in the manufacture of hydrogenated shortenings, considerable flexibility is possible providing a wide choice of finished product characteristics. Until 1961, most hydrogenated household vegetable shortenings were processed under conditions that substantially reduced the polyunsaturate content of the fats to levels ranging from 5 to 12%. These products had excellent consumer acceptance and were noted for their high degree of stability. Since 1961, most manufacturers of household vegetable shortenings have produced these products with substantially higher levels of polyunsaturated fatty acids in response to research findings which suggested the advisability of a greater intake of these fatty acids. These shortenings typically contain 22 to 32% polyunsaturated fatty acids.

Lard and other animal fats and mixtures of animal and vegetable fats also are used in shortening. Mixtures of animal and vegetable fats frequently are hydrogenated to some extent to obtain the physical characteristics desired. Lard is used extensively in some commercial applications such as the baking of pastry and bread.

Some shortening manufacturers market liquid shortening products that are based upon liquid or lightly hydrogenated liquid vegetable oils. These products usually have polynsaturated fatty acid contents ranging from 20 to 50%. These products also have had usage in some commercial baking and frying applications.

D. Hard Butters (Cocoa Butter Replacers, Substitutes, and Extenders)

Hard butters are fats which exhibit high solids content at room temperature (70 to 80°F) but which melt rapidly at body temperature (98.6°F). Cocoa butter, the fat present in chocolate, is a hard butter. Some vegetable fats, such as cocoa butter, have hard butter properties in their natural state; but most vegetable fats and oils, including soybean, cottonseed, coconut, palm, palm kernel, shea, and sal, must be modified by processing to achieve hard butter characteristics. Typical processing to derive hard butter properties includes one or more of the following steps: blending of oils, interesterification, fractional crystallization, and hydrogenation. Hard butters are used to formulate a variety of convenience foods such as nondairy toppings, coffee whiteners, mellorines, party dips, and confectioners' coatings.

E. Margarine

Margarines are fatty foods prepared by blending fats and/or oils with other ingredients such as water and/or milk products, suitable edible proteins, salt, flavoring and coloring materials, and vitamins A and D. By federal regulation, margarine must contain at least 80% fat. The margarine industry also produces reduced calorie (or diet, imitation) margarines containing 40% fat and spreads containing 50 to 60% fat.

Margarines are molded and distributed in quarter and one-pound stick forms. Many manufacturers also produce soft margarines which are sold in half and one-pound tubs. To a lesser extent these tub margarine formulations are also sold as whipped and diet products. Some manufacturers produce margarines in fluid form to provide additional convenience. The fats used in margarine may be from either vegetable or animal origin although vegetable oils are used more widely.

The fat in margarine may be prepared from a single hydrogenated fat, from two or more hydrogenated fats, or from a blend of hydrogenated fat(s) and unhydrogenated oil(s). This offers the manufacturer a wide range of compositional flexibility. Like shortening manufacturers, vegetable margarine producers have, since about 1959, marketed products with substantially higher levels of polyunsaturated fatty acids. Margarine fats and oils usually contain about 14 to 44% polyunsaturated fatty acids.

F. Butter

Butter must contain not less than 80% by weight of butterfat. The butterfat in the product serves as a plastic matrix enclosing an aqueous phase consisting of water, casein, minerals, and other soluble milk solids. These solids usually constitute about 1% of the weight of the butter. Frequently salt is added at levels from 1.5 to 3.0% of the weight of the product. Butter is an important

source of vitamin A, and to a lesser extent, of vitamin D.
Butterfat, like other fats and oils, is comprised of
triglycerides, but is characterized by the fact that a
substantial portion of the fatty acids is relatively short
chain saturated acids.

G. Dressings for Food

Mayonnaise and Salad Dressing. Mayonnaise and salad
dressing are emulsified, semi-solid fatty foods that by
federal regulation must contain not less than 65% and 30%
vegetable oil, respectively, and dried whole eggs or egg
yolks. Salt, sugar, spices, seasoning, vinegar, lemon
juice, and other ingredients complete these products.

Pourable-Type Dressings. The pourable dressings may
be two phase or the emulsified viscous type. There is a
great variety of products available of varying
compositions, including a wide range in their oil content.
Italian, French, and Roquefort types are representative of
this class. A federal standard for French dressing
requires a vegetable oil content of not less than 35%.
Some other ingredients that may be used in the preparation
of the pourable dressings are salt, sugar, emulsifiers,
spices, seasonings, and acidifying agents, such as vinegar,
citric acid, lemon or lime juice.

Reduced Calorie Dressings. One result of the current
interest in weight control in the U.S. has been the
introduction of reduced calorie food products. To qualify
as "reduced calorie," the product must contain at least one
third fewer calories than the conventional product. In the
case of reduced calorie salad dressings, for example, the
reduced calorie product contains less oil and/or
carbohydrate and more water than conventional salad
dressings.

H. Toppings, Coffee Whiteners, Confectioners' Coatings,
    and Other Formulated Foods

The use of vegetable fats in a variety of convenience
foods such as nondairy toppings, coffee whiteners, and
party dips, as well as confectioners' coatings for soft
cakes and candy, is increasing. Historically, cocoa

butter, palm kernel oil, and hydrogenated coconut oil have been used extensively because of their physical characteristics. There is now a trend toward the greater use of modified domestic oils.

I. Lipids for Special Nutritional Applications

In recent years special lipids referred to as "medium chain triglycerides" (MCT) containing C_6 to C_{12} saturated fatty acids have been used in particular clinical applications (Babayan, 1981). Certain modifications of MCT are soluble in both oil and water systems and are utilized more rapidly than conventional fats and oils containing C_{16} and C_{18} fatty acids. Whereas conventional fats and oils are absorbed slowly and transported via the lymphatic system, MCT are absorbed relatively quickly and transported via the portal system. Because of their unique ability to pass through the intestinal epithelium directly into the portal system, MCT have become the standard lipid used in the treatment of various fat malabsorption syndromes. Other MCT applications include their use as rapidly available energy sources for patients with intestinal resection or short bowel syndrome and for premature infants. In certain liquid formula diets and intravenous fluids, MCT may be combined in varying proportions with corn oil, soybean oil, or safflower oil.

ACKNOWLEDGMENT: Information for this chapter was selected from the booklet Food Fats and Oils prepared by the Technical Committee of the Institute of Shortening and Edible Oils, Inc., Washington, D.C., November 1982, and is used here with permission of the Institute of Shortening and Edible Oils, Inc.

References

1. Artman NR (1969). The chemical and biological properties of heated and oxidized fats. Adv Lipid Res 7:245-330.

2. Babayan VK (1981). Medium chain length fatty acid esters and their medical and nutritional applications. J Am Oil Chem Soc 58:49A-51A.

3. Bunch K, Hazera J (1984). Fats and oils: consumers use more, but different kinds. National Food Rev 26:18-21.

4. Clark WL, Nagle NE, Eder BD, Weiss TJ (1978). Nutritional aspects of frying fats--an overview. J Am Oil Chem Soc, Abstract #91, 55:244A.

5. Food and Nutrition Board, National Research Council (1980). "Recommended Dietary Allowances," 9th edition, Washington, DC: National Academy of Sciences, pp.34-35.

6. Hunter JE (1981). Nutritional consequences of processing soybean oil. J Am Oil Chem Soc 58:283-287.

7. Marston RM, Welsh SO (1984). Nutrient content of the U.S. food supply, 1982. National Food Rev 25:7-13.

8. Nolen GA, Alexander JC, Artman NR (1967). Long term rat feeding study with used frying fats. J Nutr 93:337-347.

9. Senti FR, ed. (1985). "Health Aspects of Dietary Trans Fatty Acids." Bethesda, MD: Life Sciences Research Office, Federation of American Societies for Experimental Biology.

10. Swern D, ed. (1979 and 1982). "Bailey's Industrial Oil and Fat Products," Volumes 1 and 2, 4th edition. New York: John Wiley & Sons.

Dietary Fat and Cancer, pages 185-209
© 1986 Alan R. Liss, Inc.

HEATED AND OXIDIZED FATS

J. Craig Alexander

Department of Nutritional Sciences, University of
Guelph, Guelph, Ontario, Canada N1G 2W1

INTRODUCTION

The common unsaturated fatty acid components of food
fats, particularly oleate, linoleate, linolenate and arachidonate are susceptible to oxidation on exposure to oxygen.
Peroxides form by the action of air and light, but at higher
temperatures, longer times of exposure, and more unsaturation, there is a greater degree of susceptibility and an
increased rate of oxidation. The reactions proceed by a
free-radical chain mechanism, that involves initiation, pro-
pagation, and termination (Gray, 1978). With unsaturated
fatty acids, hydrogen on a carbon next to a double bond is
labile, and removal of the labile hydrogen produces a free
radical. The initial reaction products of fatty acids with
oxygen are hydroperoxides, followed by more complex derivatives as indicated in Fig. 1 adapted from Fritsch (1981).
Specific details on the formation of cyclic peroxides and
malonaldehyde (MA) from polyunsaturated fatty acids in animal tissues have been outlined (Halliwell and Gutteridge,
1985).

When meats and fish are exposed to the intense heat of
the flame of a charcoal broiler, and the fat is pyrolyzed,
polycyclic aromatic hydrocarbons (PAH) are produced in the
food (Suess, 1976). Also, the thermal oxidation of fats
during deep-fat frying is the consequence of a complex
series of reactions and changes that produce numerous decomposition products (Chang et al., 1978; Selke et al., 1980;
Frankel et al., 1984). Continued acceptability of fat for
frying foods depends on the amount of deterioration. In
many restaurants, the fat is kept hot for extended periods
at about $180^{o}C$ while exposed to food ingredients, moisture
and air. The fried foods absorb this heated fat and it

becomes part of the consumer's diet (Alexander, 1978). The
sensory, functional, and nutritional qualities of the used
fats are altered and may decline so that wholesome foods can
no longer be prepared. When nutritional quality declines,
and toxic substances accumulate in the fat, there is justi-
fied concern about what effects heated and oxidized fat
derivatives might have on the consumer.

EVALUATING DETERIORATION OF FATS

Some measure of deterioration of frying fat should
enable the operator to determine when to change it in the
fryer, and thus avoid an excessive buildup of potentially

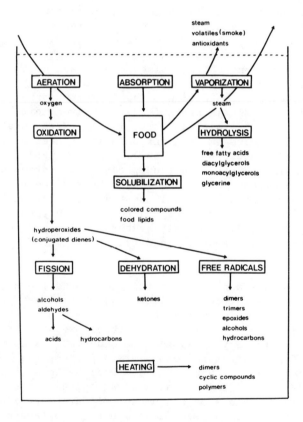

Figure 1. Changes that occur during deep-fat frying. (From
Fritsch CW (1981). J Am Oil Chem Soc 58:272-274)

harmful oxidative derivatives. Determination of total polar materials has received considerable interest (Freeman, 1974; Billek et al., 1978; Guhr and Waibel, 1979). On the basis of rat feeding experiments, Billek (1979) estimated that a frying oil should be regarded as deteriorated and unfit for human consumption if it contains 30% of polar components, as estimated by column chromatography with silica gel. Another method for estimating the oxidation of heated fats is by monitoring changes in dielectric constants (Fritsch et al., 1979). Oxidation increases the dielectric constant of oils through introduction of polar groups. The dielectric constants of frying fats increased linearly with heating time, and the increases were greater when potatoes were fried than when the fat was heated alone. When correlations were obtained between instrument readings and a number of other analyses, total polar lipids gave the best agreement with the readings (TABLE 1).

TABLE 1. Correlation Between Change in Dielectric Constant and Other Analyses of Fats Deteriorated Both by Frying Potatoes and by Heating Without Frying

Analysis	Number of samples	Correlation coefficient
Total polar materials	24	.991
Decrease in iodine value	18	.947
Color	24	.785
Peroxide value	24	.773
Diene content	24	.745
Free fatty acids	24	.569

(From Fritsch CW (1981). J Am Oil Chem Soc 58:272-274)

In addition to column chromatography of polar components, and dielectric constant measurements, gas liquid chromatography of triacylglycerol dimers has been evaluated for assessment of used frying oils (Paradis and Nawar, 1981). For heated fat samples from a large commercial frying operation (TABLE 2), a local restaurant (TABLE 3), and laboratory heated corn oil (TABLE 4) the three methods correlated well with elapsed time. Each responded to the

TABLE 2. Analysis of Samples of Fat from a Large Commercial Frying Operation

Days frying chicken parts	Silica gel column (% polar compounds)	GLC (% dimer)	Dielectric constant (sensor reading)
0	3.2	0	0.7
6	7.4	0	1.0
13	10.4	0	1.4
22	15.4	0.4	2.2

(From Paradis AJ, Nawar WW (1981). J Food Sci 46:449-451)

TABLE 3. Analysis of Samples from a Local Restaurant

Days frying	Silica gel column (% polar compounds)	GLC (% dimer)	Dielectric constant (sensor reading)
Control	3	0	0
3	11	0.1	0.7
4	12	0.2	1.0
7	41	3.0	5.6

development of polar material in the heated fats. The GLC method which is specific for triacylglycerol dimers was judged to be most useful.

Other techniques for measuring the peroxidative deterioration of fats containing polyunsaturated fatty acids have been used. Since peroxidation is accompanied by the utilization of oxygen in the formation of peroxy radicals, measurement of the rate of its uptake with an oxygen-electrode is a useful index (Halliwell and Gutteridge, 1985). Oxidation of unsaturated fatty acids results in the formation of conjugated dienes which absorb ultraviolet light and can be detected in the wavelength range 230-235 nm (Girotti, 1985). Small amounts of MA are produced during peroxidation, and it will react in the thiobarbituric acid (TBA) test with

TABLE 4. Comparison of Three Methods for Testing Corn Oil
Continuously Heated at 185°C

Hours at 185°C	Silica gel column (% polar compounds)	GLC (% dimer)	Dielectric constant (sensor value)
0	0.8	0	0
48	16.9	1.2	1.8
52	20.0	1.3	2.4
72	23.6	2.1	2.9
120	27.8	3.2	3.7
144	32.9	3.7	4.3
216	65.8	6.1	Offscale

the formation of a pink color that can be measured spectro-
photometrically at 532 nm. Since the TBA test measures decomposition of peroxides during the assay, a trace of iron
salts is needed to stimulate the conversion (Girotti, 1985).
Useful procedures to assess deterioration   of food fats due
to deep-fat frying include the peroxide value (A.O.C.S.,
1973), carbonyl value (Bhalerao et al., 1961; Yoshida and
Alexander, 1983a), iodine value (A.O.C.S., 1983), and lipase
hydrolysis (Mattson and Volpenhein, 1961; Yoshida and
Alexander, 1984). Due to the complex mixture of products
generated by peroxidizing lipids, thin layer chromatographic
methods have been valuable in separating certain species
(Ouette, 1965; Yoshida and Alexander,1983b). Recently, high
pressure liquid chromatography has been applied (Porter et
al., 1980).

CHEMICAL DERIVATIVES

Chemical constituents formed during frying with fats or
laboratory heating at comparable temperatures with aeration
have been reviewed (Chang et al., 1978; Selke et al., 1980).
It is convenient to divide the large number of compounds
produced into two categories: volatile and non-volatile
products. Of the approximately 220 volatile products identified, many vaporize during the frying operation, but some
remain to give flavor to the food.· Chemically the volatile

products are diverse, including (a) acidic species of saturated and unsaturated fatty acids of various chain lengths,
and (b) nonacidic species of saturated and unsaturated hydrocarbons, esters, alcohols, aldehydes, ketones, lactones
and aromatic compounds.

In studies of heated fat derivatives, much emphasis has
been placed on thermal oxidation of linoleic acid (Selke et
al., 1980; Henderson et al., 1980). This can be attributed
to its relatively high susceptibility to oxidation compared
with monoene or saturated isologues, and its much greater
abundance in edible fats and oils than the more reactive
linolenic acid.

More recently, studies have been carried out on the
oxidative decomposition of linolenate at elevated temperatures (Lomanno and Nawar, 1982), and it was found to produce
fewer volatile decomposition products than oleate or linoleate. A possible explanation for the smaller number of
derivatives may be that linolenates have a greater tendency
to form polymeric products.

The non-volatile products formed from thermal oxidation
of fats also are numerous and varied (Artman and Alexander,
1968; Artman, 1969; Chang et al., 1978; Porter et al., 1984).
Included are epoxides, hydroxyl and carbonyl-containing substances, alkoxy-substituted unsaturated esters, cyclic hydrocarbons, and conjugated diene ketones. Cyclic monomers,
derived from the intramolecular condensation of polyunsaturated fatty acids, have received special attention because
of their relatively toxic effects when fed to laboratory
animals (Michael et al., 1966; Michael, 1966; Meltzer et
al., 1981). The most common monomers are 18-carbon cyclic
diene disubstituted fatty acids (Iwaoka and Perkins, 1978).

Dimers, trimers and polymers in thermally oxidized fats
have been recognized for many years (Michael et al.,1966;
Perkins, 1967; Artman, 1969; Perkins and Wantland, 1973) and
may be linked through C-C bonds, C-O bonds or ether groups
(Williamson, 1953, Chang and Kummerow, 1953; O'Neill, 1954;
Ohfuji and Kaneda, 1973; Paulose and Chang, 1973).

Dienals, when oxidized, produce MA, a product of peroxidative fat metabolism formed in animal tissues deficient
in antioxidants (Shamberger et al., 1974). PAH are organic
compounds with two or more benzene rings (Lo and Sandi,

1978). More than 100 of these compounds are present in the environment, but only 5 have induced cancer in laboratory animals from oral administration (National Research Council, 1982). Extreme heat during processing and cooking promotes increased levels of PAH in our foods (Howard and Fazio, 1980).

NUTRITIONAL CONSIDERATIONS

The nutritive properties of a fat can be impaired by thermal oxidation as indicated by its nutritional evaluation using test animals as a model. Several criteria for assessing heated fat toxicity have been employed (Simko et al., 1963; Kaunitz et al., 1965; Risser et al., 1966; Thompson et al., 1967; Alexander, 1983).

Early work in the field involved feeding fats that had undergone quite severe damage by heat and oxidation. Animals fed these products invariably exhibited both morphological and biochemical changes (Dugan, 1969). Fat depots of rats that had received oxidized soybean oil had relatively high levels of fat oxidation products and decreased levels of polyunsaturated fatty acids (Degkwitz and Lang, 1962). Tappel (1973) reported lipid peroxidation damage to cell components as a result of oxidative deterioration of polyunsaturated fatty acids in rat diets. He suggested that the effects could be reduced with increased amounts of dietary antioxidants. Rats fed thermally oxidized soybean oil had increased levels of linoleate in liver lipids when extra tocopherol was added to their diet (Kajimoto and Yoshida, 1972). Also, with inadequate dietary vitamin E for rats (Privett and Cortesi, 1972), unsaturated fats stored at room temperature oxidized sufficiently to reduce body weight and organ size, and produce TBA-reacting substances in the tissues of the animals fed the fats. A primary function of tocopherols is to stabilize cellular and subcellular membranes by preventing peroxidative damage to structural fatty acids (Tappel, 1972; McCay et al., 1972). No obvious deleterious effects have resulted from long-term consumption of fatty acid isomers. Nevertheless, with animal studies (Alexander, 1981) transoctadecenoic acid changed the concentrations of the phospholipid classes in the liver lipids of rats, and interfered with conversion of the essential n-6 series of fatty acids to higher members. Compared to oleic acid, elaidic acid was preferentially incorporated into phospholipids instead of triacylglycerols, and also was concentrated in lipoprotein fractions (Guo and Alexander, 1978).

Evidence indicates that secondary oxidation products such as monomeric and dimeric compounds, rather than peroxides, are the principal factors in acute adverse biological effects seen with thermally oxidized fats. Paik et al. (1976) dosed mice with methyl linoleate hydroperoxides or autoxidized methyl linoleate containing secondary oxidation products. Tissue congestion, fatty degeneration, and necrosis correlated with the type of material fed, and mortality was 50% and 100%, respectively. Histopathological observations helped them to conclude that low molecular weight compounds containing carbonyl groups were involved. Animals given thermally oxidized fats in their diet, with low levels of vitamins and a fixed protein concentration (Hemans et al., 1973) responded poorly compared to those which received fresh fats and the same amounts of vitamins. Extra dietary protein helped to counteract the heated fat effects. Many of the early studies were complicated by improper protection of the diet and led to vitamin deficiencies in the test animals (Alexander, 1966), and it was found that frequent diet preparation and feeding, along with refrigeration, were beneficial. Long-term rat feeding studies with fats used for frying to the point of foaming in a restaurant-type operation showed suppression of growth rate, but few other effects (Nolen et al., 1967). Distillable non-urea-adductable fractions (DNUA) isolated from these used fats were toxic due to the concentration of secondary oxidation products.

Low erucic acid rapeseed oil (LEAR) and lard (Gabriel et al., 1977), and corn oil and olive oil (Gabriel et al., 1978) were heated at $180^{\circ}C$ with aeration for 72 hr. The fatty acids were converted to ethyl esters, and vacuum distillation was used to isolate the volatile fraction of each of the thermally oxidized fats. The distillates were fed to rats for 28 days as 15% of the diet. Body weights were depressed by the heated lard fraction, and both heated LEAR and lard fractions increased heart weights and heart total lipids. Organs selected for histopathological examination and the pertinent anatomical structures were:

```
Heart  - myocardial nuclei
       - nuclei of vascular media and endothelium
       - interstitial  tissue and myofibers
Liver  - hepatocellular nuclei
       - hepatocellular cytoplasm
```

```
                   - Kupffer and endothelial cells
         Kidney - glomeruli
                - tubules
                - vessels and interstitial tissues
```

Types of lesions found in the tissue sections were graded as to incidence and severity on a scale from zero for normal to three for necrotic tissue.

Evaluation (Table 5) showed that heated LEAR damaged the heart, liver, and kidneys, whereas heated lard was most injurious to the liver and kidneys. Results for heated corn oil and heated olive oil (Table 5) showed severe lesions in the liver and kidneys for the latter. The relatively greater toxicity of heated olive oil was due in part to a higher oleic: linoleic acid ratio and to higher tocopherol content of corn oil (Gabriel et al., 1978).

TABLE 5. Histological Scores for Organs of Rats Fed Different Dietary Fats

		Histological scores		
		Heart	Liver	Kidneys
LEAR	- Fresh	0.75	0.84	0.68
	DEOF	2.01	2.12	1.75
LARD	- Fresh	0.42	0.29	0.18
	DEOF	1.31	1.95	2.43
CORN OIL	- Fresh	0	0	0
	DEFF	0	0	0
	DEOF	0	0	0
OLIVE OIL	- Fresh	0	0	0
	DEFF	0.49	0	0
	DEOF	0.81	2.21	1.48

LEAR - Low erucic acid rapeseed oil.
DEOF - Distillable ethyl esters of oxidized fat.
DEFF - Distillable ethyl esters of fresh fat.
(From Gabriel HG, Alexander, JC, Valli VE (1977). Can J Comp Med 41:98-106, and (1978). Lipids 13:49-55)

Heart cells in culture, exposed to DNUA from thermally oxidized corn oil or olive oil (Bird and Alexander, 1978), took up more exogenous $1\text{-}^{14}C$-palmitic acid and incorporated more into the cell triacylglycerol fraction than did those exposed to fresh fats. Less radioactivity was deposited in the phospholipid fraction. There were lower concentrations of linoleic and arachidonic acids in the phospholipids, and a much higher level of arachidonic acid in the triacylglycerols (Bird and Alexander, 1979). Intracellular lipid accumulation, increased cytoplasmic vacuolation, mitotic aberrations, pyknotic cells and decreased mitosis also were observed (Bird et al., 1981). There were greater effects with heated olive oil, and the results indicate that oxidized fat components interfere physically and biochemically with normal cell functions resulting in pathological changes. Other studies have shown that some of the toxic effects of oxidized fats (increased red blood cell hemolysis, and low levels of linoleic acid in the liver, kidneys and testes) can be reduced by extra vitamin E in the diet (Yoshida and Kajimoto, 1974; Kajimoto et al., 1975).

Rat heart cell cultures were used to study the influence of two antioxidants, vitamin E and ascorbyl palmitate on biological effects of thermally oxidized fats (Bird and Alexander, 1981). Fatty acids from heated corn oil (100 μg per ml medium) depressed the mitotic index, caused lipid accumulation and increased the number of pyknotic nuclei in the cells. Addition of vitamin E (10 μg per ml medium) counteracted these changes, but a similar amount of ascorbyl palmitate had little effect. Nevertheless, both antioxidants increased the amount of arachidonic acid in cells where the level was depressed by treatment with heated fat.

OXIDIZED FATS, MUTAGENS AND CANCER

Epidemiologic studies have indicated that dietary practices, particularly a decrease in high fat foods should reduce the risk of cancer of the colon and breast (National Research Council, 1982). Much of this fat has been exposed to oxygen and heat during cooking and frying which results in many oxidized derivatives (Porter et al., 1984; Halliwell and Gutteridge, 1985). Laboratory studies of cooked foods are beginning to reveal a variety of mutagens and possible carcinogens (Ames, 1983). Because of the importance of genetic factors in the origin of cancer, any substance

capable of reacting with DNA and producing chemical changes
leading to expression of oncogenes could be a potential
carcinogen (Halliwell and Gutteridge, 1985). Based on this
assumption, most mutagens should be suspected of being carcinogenic and vice versa unless proven otherwise (National
Research Council, 1982).

About 50% of human cancers may have correlation with
food and its constituents (Wynder and Gori, 1977). Among
these, highly unsaturated dietary lipids tend to raise the
unsaturation of structural lipids as well, and this should
increase the rate of initiation of random free-radical reactions within the organism (Harman, 1982). Large amounts
of ingested fat also would increase the lipid peroxidation
as the quantity of lipid in the blood and tissues is raised.
Oxidized food fats already containing peroxides and other
derivatives (Chang et al., 1978; Porter et al., 1984) would
promote the formation of more free radicals. Adequate dietary vitamin E to prevent an overt deficiency should reduce
these adverse effects, but some biological degradation would
take place. Female C3H mice fed a readily peroxidizable
diet (20% menhaden oil) had a shorter life span compared to
those given a more saturated fat (20% lard) due to an increased incidence of mammary carcinoma (Harman, 1971). The
significant correlation in 23 countries between the consumption of fats and oils for cooking and the death rates from
malignant neoplasms in persons over 55 may be related to
lipid peroxidation (Lea, 1966).

Beef grilled over charcoal produces benzo[a]pyrene
(BaP) and other PAH compounds when pyrolyzed fat drips from
the meat onto the hot coals (Lijinsky and Shubik, 1964). In
this regard BaP has been used repeatedly as a quantitative
index of chemical carcinogens in foods (Doremire et al.,
1979). Its accumulation is directly related to the concentration of fat being heated. The possible contribution due
to pyrolysis of the fat which drips from meat was assessed
in fatty, charcoal-broiled ribs purchased from a restaurant
(Lijinsky and Shubik, 1965). Analysis showed the following
compounds in μg/kg: anthracene, 7.1; anthanthrene, 1.1;
benzanthracene, 3.6; benzoperylene, 4.7; BaP, 10.5; BeP,
7.5; chrysene, 2.2; coronene, 4.2; fluoranthene, 49; phenan-
threne, 58; perylene, 1.5 and pyrene, 42. The major dietary
sources of PAH are probably from broiling and smoking of
foods, and roasting of coffee (Howard and Fazio, 1980). The
concentration of carcinogenic PAH in raw sausage was 1.5

μg/kg (Fabian, 1968). After pan frying, charcoal grilling, grilling over pine cones or infrared cooking the concentrations were 7.4, 54.8, 88.5 and 0.17 μg/kg respectively. Since the levels of a number of PAH including BaP increased markedly after grilling, it was concluded that carcinogenic PAH are formed with pyrolysis of the fat, and enter the food with the smoke.

A PAH carcinogenic risk has existed ever since man began to cook and fry foods in fats. Lipid oxidation products and related substances promoted by application of heat during deep-fat frying and charcoal broiling are impossible to avoid. However, the concentrations of some substances can be reduced by altered processing and cooking methods (Gray and Morton, 1981). Examples are charcoal broiling at lower temperatures, with reduced fat content in the meat, and avoidance of direct contact of the meat and fat with the flame.

Carcinogenicity of BaP in animal species has been well documented (Huggins and Yang, 1962; Chu and Malmgren, 1965; Rigdon and Neal, 1969). Human cancers have multifactorial environmental causes stemming mainly from lifestyle habits including dietary practices (Weisburger and Wynder, 1984). Genotoxic carcinogens as nutritional factors may be found in pickled, salted, and smoked foods, and may be responsible for gastric cancer. Vitamins C and E, selenium and other antioxidants are effective inhibitors. Other types of genotoxic carcinogens are mutagenic chemicals found in broiled and fried foods, and these may be involved in cancer of the colon, breast, and prostate. Promoting effects associated with a high level of dietary fat (much of which has been exposed to cooking and frying temperatures) are dose-dependent, and provided the insult is not too far advanced, reversible.

The enzymatic oxidation of BaP to 6-hydroxybenzo[a]-pyrene occurs via the cation free-radical in vivo (Mason, 1982). The electrophilic BaP cation free-radical reacts with nitrogenous compounds such as purines, nucleosides and DNA (Wilk and Girke, 1972). Also, aromatic compounds undergo electrophilic attack by aromatic hydrocarbon cation radicals to form dimers and tetramers. Possibly, a reaction between antioxidants and polycyclic hydrocarbon cation radicals may account for the decrease in polycyclic hydrocarbon-induced tumors obtained when animals are treated with antioxidants (Krzywanska and Piekarski, 1977).

There is some epidemiological evidence concerning the relationship between ingestion of PAH-contaminated food and cancer in humans. For example, there is a report of an increased incidence of stomach cancer in West Hungary where home-smoked meats contain much higher BaP levels than smoked food consumed in other parts of the country (Soos, 1980). This and some other limited evidence does not confirm an association between dietary PAH and gastrointestinal tract cancer because N-nitroso compounds may have been involved. However, there is no doubt that in animals, oral PAH substances are carcinogenic.

A large increase in per capita consumption of french-fried potatoes is part of a trend towards more food products being crisped by exposure to heated fats. Compounds resulting from the frying and broiling of meat and fish have proved to be mutagenic in laboratory tests, and must be regarded as potential contributors to carcinogenesis (National Research Council, 1982). In one study (Higginson, 1966) there was an association reported between more frequent consumption of fried foods and greater use of animal fats by those with gastric cancer than for controls. In a case-control study (Phillips, 1975) involving 77 breast cancer cases and 77 controls, hard fat used for frying, and fried foods including fried potatoes were found to be associated with breast cancer.

Retinoids in foods are components of the lipid fraction, and associated with the acylglycerols. When food fats are oxidized by exposure to oxygen and heat, there is considerable oxidative destruction of the highly unsaturated retinoids. Some protection is afforded by natural or synthetic antioxidants. The substantial loss of these fat-soluble nutrients (vitamin A and its precursors) may be of significance in some cases of cancer risk (Mettlin and Graham, 1979; Mettlin et al., 1979). Retinoids suppress malignant transformations in cultured cells (Sporn and Newton, 1979) which indicates a protective effect. They also have decreased the incidence of cancer in experimental animals exposed to known carcinogens. Likewise, retinoids have been shown to antagonize the action of tumor promotors (Boatwell and Verma, 1979). In a retrospective study, Wald et al. (1980) obtained blood from healthy people and stored it for a number of years before analysis for retinol. By observing cancer incidence among the subjects, it was shown that persons with high blood retinol had a lower risk of

developing cancer. There has been some speculation about
how β-carotene might function in reducing cancer risk. It
may be related to the endogenous suppression of carcinogenesis by its action of quenching singlet oxygen (Wolf, 1982).
In this regard, plants probably protect themselves against
the damaging oxidative effects of singlet oxygen by producing large amounts of β-carotene (Linder, 1985).

Oxidized dietary fats have been administered to experimental animals to study the development of tumors since
Morris et al. (1943) reported gastric adenomas in old rats
fed rancid fats. In view of the possible carcinogenic
effects of organic peroxides and epoxides produced in heated
cooking fats, epoxidated fats and lipoperoxides were tested
in C57 mice (Kotin and Falk, 1963). Epoxides from soybean
oil and butyl-9,10-epoxystearate gave positive results in
groups of 50 mice. They produced subcutaneous sarcomas and
pulmonary adenomas in 3-10% of the animals over a period of
17-24 months. Diets containing 10% unheated or heated sunflower oil were fed to male rats for extended periods
(Vysheslavova, 1968). No tumors developed in the control
animals over 44 months. Those fed heated fat (190°C for 35
hr) had malignant tumors in 8/50 surviving animals from the
original 97.

Female guinea pigs (144/4 groups) were injected into
the wall of the stomach with 0.1 ml unheated fat (from the
peritoneal cavity of normal animals), preheated fat (180°C
for 30 min), unheated fat + 0.9 mg 3-methylcholanthrene (MC)
or preheated fat + MC (Zaldivar, 1969). Those treated with
unheated fat showed only local non-specific inflammatory
changes, whereas proliferating gastric lesions were found in
50% of those treated with preheated fat, 47% treated with
unheated fat + MC and 49% treated with preheated fat + MC
within 240 days. Nonurea adducts (NUA) were prepared from
fresh and heated hydrogenated vegetable fat and corn oil
(O'Gara et al., 1969). When these NUA materials were injected intramuscularly into newborn H1H rats, the authors
stated that the induction of sarcomas at the site indicated
the presence of a carcinogen in the heated fats.

In Japan a Prefecture (Akita) with a high rate of
stomach cancer was compared with one (Iwate) with a low rate
(Michioka et al., 1980). Cooked foods from 26 and 36 households respectively were randomly sampled. Acetone-soluble
fractions of crude fat and water-soluble fractions were

prepared and examined for mutagenicity by the Ames' test using Salmonella typhimurium strains. Mutagenicity was observed only in the acetone-soluble fractions, and was positive in 54% for Akita and 15% for Iwate. Regional stomach cancer mortalities reflected this difference in positive response rate in the Ames' technique. Lean pork was pan-broiled in Sweden at various temperatures between 100 and 290°C in an open frying pan (Overvik et al., 1984). The heated fat was extracted from the crust with organic solvents, and mutagenic activity was assayed with Ames' Salmonella test. Largest amounts of activity were detected in samples pan-broiled at 200-290°C, and the values were about 10 times higher than expected based on previous reports. Potent bacterial mutagens such as PAH are formed in meat during frying, and since these mutagens are consumed by humans, and are carcinogenic in rodents, their mechanism of formation is being studied (Barnes and Weisburger, 1984). A low concentration of corn oil (5-10%) enhanced mutagen formation more than lard, and higher concentrations (20%) doubled the amounts. At high temperatures lipid decomposition may contribute precursors for mutagen formation. Since supplementation with glycine and glucose doubled the mutagenic activity, glycerol may account for the enhancing effect of heated fat. These reactions are catalyzed by iron released through denaturation of the heme proteins of the meat.

Effects of variations in frying conditions on the formation of mutagens in deep-fat fried foods have been reported. Criteria included long periods, high temperatures, and repeated reuse of the frying oil (Taylor et al., 1983). Based on repetitive frying experiments, mutagen formation was by far the greatest with fish fillets among foods tested. However, no mutagenic activity was found in the oil after repetitive frying of fish fillets, onion rings or French fried potatoes.

Diet appears to be connected with cancer of the breast, colon and prostate (Huttunen, 1982). High cooking temperatures may enhance the formation of mutagens and carcinogens from natural nutrients. Cancer of the stomach is common in populations who smoke and fry their foods, and thermally oxidized fat could be an important factor. Colon cancer incidence and mortality vary geographically, and the environmental difference between low-risk and high-risk countries appears related to diet (Weisburger et al., 1981). In order

for colon cancer to occur, both initiators (mutagens produced during the frying and broiling of meats and fish) and
a promoter (high fat diet) may be required. Variations in
these factors can alter the incidence of colon cancer. The
level of total dietary fat controls the amount of biosynthetic bile acids in the gut which have promoting activity. In
contrast, more dietary fiber from cereal grains increases
the stool bulk, and lowers the cancer risk (Weisburger,
1981).

Malonaldehyde is a product of lipid peroxidation formed
in variable concentrations in foods as a result of oxidative
decomposition of highly unsaturated fatty acids, and is a
putative carcinogen in mice. In view of this, the relationship between cooking methods and the production of MA was
studied (Newburg and Concon, 1980). In hamburgers pan-fried
at moderate temperatures, the MA content increased 41-55%;
frying at higher temperatures (shorter cooking times) produced smaller increases. Microwave cooking increased concentrations by only 15%. In contrast, cooking chicken by
microwave, conventional oven, deep-fat frying, and broiling
increased MA concentrations by 60, 55, 18, and 22-fold
respectively. Appreciable amounts of MA also were found in
smoked trout, canned chicken broth, bouillon cubes, and
cheese depending on cooking conditions. Surveys (Shamberger
et al. 1977; Siu and Draper, 1978) confirmed the presence of
MA in supermarket samples of meat, poultry and fish. MA
produced a high incidence of liver tumors when applied to
the back skin of mice at a rate of 12 mg/day for 7-9 wk
(Shamberger et al., 1974). Its reactivity toward amino
groups can result in interactions with the nitrogenous bases
of DNA (Reiss et al., 1972) and inhibition of RNA and protein synthesis (Bird and Draper, 1980). Lipofuscin accumulates during aging in all mammalian species and has been
associated with lipid peroxidation (Demopoulos et al., 1980;
Harman, 1982). Fluorescent products in this age pigment are
thought to be formed by MA (a major end product of dietary
fat oxidation) cross-linking lipids and proteins (Tappel,
1980). Lipofuscin formation is inversely correlated with
longevity (Sohal, 1981). Adequate vitamin E in the diet is
an important protective factor (Halliwell and Gutteridge,
1985).

Bacon slices and the separated lean and fat components
were fried, and the pan residues and the trapped cooking
vapors analyzed for N-nitrosamines, some of which are well-

known carcinogens. The fat produced about 9 times more nitrosamines than the lean, with the largest proportions being recovered from the cooking vapors (Mottram et al., 1977). However, when the lean was cooked in corn oil, the yield of nitrosamines was increased greatly. It was concluded that non-polar lipid creates an environment conducive to nitrosamine formation during heating. There is evidence that ascorbic acid may inhibit the formation of nitrosamines (Correa et al., 1975).

CONCLUSIONS

Food fats exposed to oxygen and heat produce many chemical derivatives, including peroxides, epoxides, aldehydes, ketones, cyclic monomers, dimers, and polycyclic aromatic hydrocarbons. Feeding studies with experimental animals reveal that polar concentrates of heated fat components may cause substantial pathological injury to organ tissues. Also, high levels of oxidized dietary fats should advance the rate of formation of free radicals within body cells. Polycyclic aromatic hydrocarbons and some other heated-fat derivatives have been shown to be related to an increased incidence of malignant neoplasia in animal models, and there is epidemiological evidence indicating a correlation between dietary PAH intake in humans and cancer of the stomach, breast, prostate and colon. The susceptibility of cells to damage caused by reactions with metabolites of oxygen, such as free radicals, may be modified by dietary retinoids, vitamin E and selenium. Lipid peroxides may serve as efficient oxidants of a variety of chemical initiators of carcinogenesis that require oxidation to an active form, and therefore could function as promoters. Current data are not sufficient to quantitate the contribution of diet to cancer risk, therefore more specific laboratory studies are needed with polar constituents of heated and oxidized fats.

ACKNOWLEDGMENTS

Financial support was provided by the Natural Sciences and Engineering Research Council of Canada, and the Ontario Ministry of Agriculture and Food.

REFERENCES

A.O.C.S. (1973). Official method Cd 8-53. In Link WE (ed): "Official Methods and Recommended Practices of the American Oil Chemists' Society," Champaign, IL.

A.O.C.S. (1983). Official method Cd 1-25. In Walker RC (ed): "Official Methods and Recommended Practices of the American Oil Chemists' Society," Champaign, IL.

Alexander JC (1966). Effect of diet handling on nutritional studies with used frying fats. Lipids 1:254-257.

Alexander JC (1978). Biological effects due to changes in fats during heating. J Am Oil Chem Soc 55:711-717.

Alexander JC (1981). Chemical and biological properties related to toxicity of heated fats. J Toxicol Environ Health 7:125-138.

Alexander JC (1983). Biological properties of heated fats. In Finley JW, Schwass DE (eds): "Xenobiotics in Foods and Feeds." Washington, DC: American Chemical Society, pp 129-148.

Ames, BN (1983). Dietary carcinogens and anticarcinogens. Science 221:1256-1264.

Artman NR (1969). The chemical and biological properties of heated and oxidized fats. In Paoletti R, Kritchevsky D (eds): "Advances in Lipid Research," Vol. 7. New York: Academic Press, pp 245-330.

Artman NR, Alexander JC (1968). Characterization of some heated fat components. J Am Oil Chem Soc 45:643-648.

Barnes WS, Weisburger JH (1984). Formation and inhibition of mutagens during frying of beef and relationship to fat content. Proc Annu Meet Am Assoc Cancer Res 25:102.

Bhalerao VR, Andres JG, Kummerow FA (1961). A method for determining the carbonyl value in thermally oxidized fats. J Am Oil Chem Soc 38:689-691.

Billek G (1979). Heated oils: Chemistry and nutritional aspects. Nutr Metab 24:200-210.

Billek G, Guhr G, Waibel J (1978). Quality assessment of used frying fats: A comparison of four methods. J Am Oil Chem Soc 55:728-733.

Bird RP, Alexander JC (1978). Uptake and utilization of 1-^{14}C-palmitic acid by heart cells treated with fresh or thermally oxidized fats. Lipids 13:809-813.

Bird RP, Alexander JC (1979). Fatty acid composition of heart cells exposed to thermally oxidized fats. Lipids 14:836-841.

Bird RP, Alexander JC (1981). Effects of vitamin E and ascorbyl palmitate on cultured myocardial cells exposed to oxidized fats. J Toxicol Environ Health 7:59-67.

Bird RP, Draper HH (1980). Effect of malonaldehyde on cultured mammalian cells: Growth, morphology and synthesis of macromolecules. J Toxicol Environ Health 6:811-823.

Bird RP, Basrur PK, Alexander, JC (1981). Cytotoxicity of thermally oxidized fats. In Vitro 17:397-404.

Boatwell RK, Verma AK (1979). Effects of vitamin A and related retinoids on the biochemical process linked to carcinogenesis. Pure Appl Chem 51:857-866.

Chang SS, Kummerow FA (1953). The isolation and characterization of the polymers formed during the autoxidation of ethyl linoleate. J Am Oil Chem Soc 30:403-407.

Chang SS, Peterson RJ, Ho CT (1978). Chemical reactions involved in the deep-fat frying of foods. J Am Oil Chem Soc 55:718-727.

Chu EW, Malmgren RA (1965). An inhibitory effect of vitamin A on the induction of tumors of forestomach and cervix in Syrian hamster by carcinogenic polycyclic hydrocarbons. Cancer Res 25:884-895.

Correa P, Haenszel W, Cuello C, Tannenbaum S, Archer M (1975). A model for gastric cancer epidemiology. Lancet 2:58-60.

Degkwitz E, Lang K (1962). Changes in the body fat of rats subsequent to feeding with autoxidized soybean oils. Fette Seifen Anstrichm 64:893-900.

Demopoulos HB, Pietronnigro DD, Flamm ES, Seligman ML (1980). The possible role of free-radical reactions in carcinogenesis. J Environ Pathol Toxicol 3:273-303.

Doremire ME, Harmon GE, Pratt DE (1979). A research note. 3,4-benzopyrene in charcoal grilled meats. J Food Sci 44:622-623.

Dugan LR (1969). Processing and other stress effects on the nutritive value of lipids. In Bourne GH (ed): "World Review of Nutrition and Dietetics." New York: S. Karger, pp 181-205.

Fabian B (1968). Carcinogenic substances in edible fats and oils. V. Studies of sausage after different methods of cooking. Arch Hyg Bakteriol 152:251-254.

Frankel EN, Smith LM, Hamblin CL, Creveling RK, Clifford AJ (1984). Occurrence of cyclic fatty acid monomers in frying oils used for fast foods. J Am Oil Chem Soc 61:87-90.

Freeman IP (1974). A thin layer chromatography method for following oxidation of frying oils. Chem Ind 15:623-624.

Fritsch CW (1981). Measurement of frying fat deterioration:

A brief review. J Am Oil Chem Soc 58:272-274.

Fritsch CW, Egberg DE, Magnuson JS (1979). Changes in dielectric constant as a measure of the decomposition of frying fats. J Am Oil Chem Soc 56:746-752.

Gabriel HG, Alexander JC, Valli VE (1977). Biochemical and histological effects of feeding thermally oxidized rapeseed oil and lard to rats. Can J Comp Med 41:98-106.

Gabriel HG, Alexander JC, Valli VE (1978). Nutritional and metabolic studies of distillable fractions from fresh and thermally oxidized corn oil and olive oil. Lipids 13:49-55.

Girotti AW (1985). Hypothesis paper: Mechanisms of lipid peroxidation. J Free Rad Biol Med 1:87-95.

Gray JI (1978). Measurement of lipid oxidation: A review. J Am Oil Chem Soc 55:539-546.

Gray JI, Morton ID (1981). Some toxic compounds produced in food by cooking and processing. J Hum Nutr 35:5-23.

Guhr G, Waibel J (1979). Chromatographic methods for the determination of the decomposition of frying fats. Fette Seifen Anstrichm 81:511-519.

Guo LS, Alexander JC (1978). Incorporation of $10-^{14}C$-oleic acid or $10-^{14}C$-elaidic acid into lipids of liver, adrenal and plasma lipoproteins of normal and essential fatty acid-deficient rats. Can Inst Food Sci Technol J 11:169-172.

Halliwell B, Gutteridge JMC (1985). "Free Radicals in Biology and Medicine." Oxford: Clarendon Press.

Harman D (1971). Free radical theory of aging: Effect of the amount and degree of unsaturation of dietary fat on mortality rate. J Gerontol 26:451-457.

Harman D (1982). The free-radical theory of aging. In Pryor WA (ed): "Free Radicals in Biology," Vol. 5. New York: Academic Press, pp 255-275.

Hemans C, Kummerow FA, Perkins EG (1973). Influence of protein and vitamin levels on the nutritional value of heated fats for rats. J Nutr 103:1665-1672.

Henderson SK, Witchwoot A, Nawar WW (1980). The autoxidation of linoleates at elevated temperatures. J Am Oil Chem Soc 57:409-413.

Higginson J (1966). Etiological factors in gastrointestinal cancer in man. J Natl Cancer Inst 37:527-545.

Howard JW, Fazio T (1980). Review of polycyclic aromatic hydrocarbons in foods. Analytical methodology and reported findings of polycyclic aromatic hydrocarbons in foods. J Assoc Off Anal Chem 63:1077-1104.

Huggins C, Yang NC (1962). Induction and extinction of mammary cancer. Science 137:257-262.

Huttunen J (1982). Diet and cancer. Duodecim 98:1761-1772.

Iwaoka WT, Perkins EG (1978). Metabolism and lipogenic effects of the cyclic monomers of methyl linoleate in the rat. J Am Oil Chem Soc 55:734-738.

Kajimoto G, Yoshida H (1972). Toxic character of rancid oil. XI. Effect of tocopherol on the nutritive value of thermally oxidized oil. Yukagaku 21:307-313.

Kajimoto G, Yoshida H, Shibahara A (1975). Toxic character of rancid oil. XVI. Comparison of the nutritive value between thermally oxidized oil and tocopherol-free fresh oil. Yukagaku 24:511-517.

Kaunitz H, Johnson RE, Pegus L (1965). A long-term nutritional study with fresh and mildly oxidized vegetable fats. J Am Oil Chem Soc 42:770-774.

Kotin P, Falk HL (1963). Organic peroxides, hydrogen peroxide, epoxides and neoplasia. Radiat Res 3:193-211.

Krzywanska E, Piekarski L (1977). Benzo[a]pyrene free-radicals formation in the presence of butylated hydroxyanisole and their importance in carcinogenesis. Neoplasma 24:395-400.

Lea AJ (1966). Dietary factors associated with death rates from certain neoplasms in man. Lancet 2:332-333.

Lijinsky W, Shubik P (1964). Benzo[a]pyrene and other polynuclear hydrocarbons in charcoal broiled meat. Science 145:53-55.

Lijinsky W, Shubik P (1975). Polynuclear hydrocarbon carcinogens in cooked meat and smoked food. Ind Med Surg 34:152-154.

Linder MC (1985). Nutrition and cancer prevention. In Linder MC (ed): "Nutritional Biochemistry and Metabolism with Clinical Applications," New York: Elsevier, pp 347-368.

Lo MT, Sandi E (1978). Polycyclic aromatic hydrocarbons (polynuclears) in foods. Residue Rev 69:35-86.

Lomanno SS, Nawar WW (1982). Effect of heating temperature and time on the volatile oxidative decomposition of linolenate. J Food Sci 47:744-746, 752.

Mason RP (1982). Free-radical intermediates in the metabolism of toxic chemicals. In Pryor WA (ed): "Free Radicals in Biology," Vol. 5. New York: Academic Press, pp 161-222.

Mattson FH, Volpenhein RA (1961). The use of pancreatic lipase for determining the distribution of fatty acids in partial and complete glycerides. J Lipid Res 2:58-62.

McCay PB, Pfeifer PM, Stepe WH (1972). Vitamin E protection of membrane lipids during electron transport functions.

In Kayden HJ, Nair PP (eds): "Vitamin E and its Role in Cellular Metabolism," Vol. 203. New York: Annals of New York Academy of Sciences, pp 62-73.

Meltzer JB, Frankel EN, Bessler TR, Perkins EG (1981). Analysis of thermally abused soybean oils for cyclic monomers. J Am Oil Chem Soc 58:779-784.

Mettlin C, Graham S (1979). Dietary risk factors in human bladder cancer. Am J Epidemiol 110:255-263.

Mettlin C, Graham S, Swanson M (1979). Vitamin A and lung cancer. J Natl Cancer Inst 62:1435-1438.

Michael WR (1966). Thermal reactions of methyl linoleate. III. Characterization of C_{18} cyclic esters. Lipids 1:365-368.

Michael WR, Alexander JC, Artman NR (1966). Thermal reactions of methyl linoleate. I. Heating conditions, isolation techniques, biological studies and chemical changes. Lipids 1:353-358.

Michioka O, Kudo K, Kamiyama S (1980). Comparison of dietary mutagenicity between two populations with different stomach cancer mortalities. Proc. Japanese Cancer Assoc Tokyo, 39th Meeting.

Morris HP, Larsen CD, Lippincott JW (1943). Effects of feeding heated lard to rats with histological description of the lesions observed. J Natl Cancer Inst 4:285-303.

Mottram DS, Patterson RL, Edwards RA, Gough TA (1977). The preferential formation of volatile N-nitrosamines in the fat of fried bacon. J Food Sci Agr 28:1025-1029.

National Research Council (1982). "Diet,Nutrition and Cancer." Washington, DC: National Academy Press.

Newburg DS, Concon JM (1980). Malonaldehyde concentrations in food are affected by cooking conditions. J Food Sci 45:1681-1683, 1687.

Nolen GA, Alexander JC, Artman NR (1967). Long-term rat feeding study with used frying fats. J Nutr 93:337-348.

O'Gara RW, Stewart L, Brown J, Hueper WC (1969). Carcinogenicity of heated fats and fat fractions. J Natl Cancer Inst 42:275-287.

Ohfuji T, Kaneda T (1973). Characterization of toxic compounds in thermally oxidized oil. Lipids 8:353-359.

O'Neill LA (1954). The autoxidation of drying oils. Chem Ind (London) 1954:384-387.

Ouette K (1965). Identification of some lipid peroxides by thin layer chromatography. J Lipid Res 6:449-454.

Overvik E, Nilsson, L, Fredholm L, Levin O, Nord CE, Gustafsson JA (1984). High mutagenic activity formed in pan-broiled pork. Mutat Res 135:149-57.

Paik TH, Hochino T, Kaneda T (1976). Toxicity of autoxidized oils. V. Histopathological studies on mice administered autoxidized oils (acute toxicity). Eiyo to Syokuro 29:85-94.

Paradis AJ, Nawar WW (1981). Evaluation of new methods for the assessment of used frying oils. J Food Sci 46:449-451.

Paulose MM, Chang SS (1973). Chemical reactions involved in deep-fat frying of foods. VI. Characterization of non-volatile decomposition products of trilinolein. J Am Oil Chem Soc 50:147-154.

Perkins EG (1967). Formation of non-volatile decomposition products in heated fats and oils. Food Technol 21:125-130.

Perkins EG, Wantland LR (1973). Characterization of non-volatile compounds formed during thermal oxidation of 1-linoleyl-2,3-distearin. III. Evidence for presence of dimeric fatty acids. J Am Oil Chem Soc 50:459-461.

Phillips RL (1975). Role of life-style and dietary habits in risk of cancer among Seventh-Day Adventists. Cancer Res 35:3513-3522.

Porter NA, Lehman LS, Wujek DG, Gross PM (1984). Oxidation mechanisms of polyunsaturated fatty acids. In Bors W, Saran M, Tait D (eds): "Oxygen Radicals in Chemistry and Biology," Berlin: Walter de Gruyter, pp 235-247.

Porter NA, Wolf RA, Weenen H (1980). The free radical oxidation of polyunsaturated lecithins. Lipids 15:163-167.

Privett OS, Cortesi R (1972). Observation on the role of vitamin E in the toxicity of oxidized fats. Lipids 7:780-787.

Reiss U, Tappel AL, Chio KS (1972). DNA-malonaldehyde reaction: Formation of fluorescent products. Biochem Biophys Res Commun 48:921-926.

Rigdon RH, Neal J (1969). Relationship of leukemia to lung and stomach tumors in mice fed benzo[a]pyrene. Proc Soc Exp Biol Med 130:146-148.

Risser N, Kummerow FA, Perkins EG (1966). Metabolism of fats. III. Absorption of hydroxy acid via the lymph. Proc Soc Exp Biol Med 121:294-298.

Selke E, Rohwedder WK, Dutton HJ (1980). Volatile components from trilinolein heated in air. J Am Oil Chem Soc 57:25-30.

Shamberger RJ, Andreone TL, Willis CE (1974). Antioxidants and cancer. IV. Initiating activity of malonaldehyde as a carcinogen. J Natl Cancer Inst 53:1771-1773.

Shamberger RJ, Shamberger BA, Willis CE (1977). Malonaldehyde content of food. J Nutr 107:1404-1409.

Simko V, Bucko A, Babala J, Ondreicka R (1963). Chemical and physical changes induced in food fats during the process of heating, and their effect on the histological picture of guinea pig organs. Nutr Dieta 6:91-105.

Siu GM, Draper HH (1978). A survey of the malonaldehyde content of retail meats and fish. J Food Sci 43:1147-1149.

Sohal RS (1981). Metabolic rate, aging, and lipofuscin accumulation. In Sohal RS (ed): "Age Pigments," Amsterdam: Elsevier/North Holland, pp 303-316.

Soos K (1980). The occurrence of carcinogenic polycyclic hydrocarbons in foodstuffs in Hungary. Arch Toxicol Suppl 4:446-448.

Sporn MB, Newton DL (1979). Chemoprevention of cancer with retinoids. Fed Proc 38:2528-2534.

Suess MJ (1976). The environmental load and cycle of polycyclic aromatic hydrocarbons. Sci Total Environ 6:239-250.

Tappel AL (1972). Vitamin E and free radical peroxidation of lipids. In Kayden HJ, Nair PP (eds): "Vitamin E and its Role in Cellular Metabolism," Vol. 203. New York: Annals of New York Academy of Sciences, pp 12-28.

Tappel AL (1973). Lipid peroxidation damage to cell components. Fed Proc 32:1870-1874.

Tappel AL (1980). Measurement of and protection from in vivo lipid peroxidation. In Pryor WA (ed): "Free Radicals in Biology," Vol. 4. New York: Academic Press, pp 1-47.

Taylor SL, Berg CM, Shoptaugh NH, Traisman E (1983). Mutagen formation in deep-fat fried foods as a function of frying conditions. J Am Oil Chem Soc 60:576-580.

Thompson JA, Paulose MM, Reddy BR, Krishnamurthy RG, Chang SS (1967). A limited survey of fats and oils commercially used for deep-fat frying. Food Technol 21:405-407.

Vysheslavova M (1968). Carcinogenic effects of overheated fats. Vopr Pitan 27:63-68.

Wald N, Idle M, Boreham J, Bailey A (1980). Low serum-vitamin A and subsequent risk of cancer - Preliminary results of a prospective study. Lancet 2:813-815.

Weisburger JH (1981). On the causes and prevention of gastrointestinal cancer. Gastroenterol 80:1313.

Weisburger JH, Wynder EL (1984). The role of genotoxic carcinogens and of promoters in carcinogenesis and in human cancer causation. Acta Pharmacol Toxicol 2:53-58.

Weisburger JH, Spingarn NE, Wang YY, Vuolo LL (1981).

Assessment of the role of mutagens and endogenous factors in large bowel cancer. Cancer Bull 33:124-129.

Wilk M, Girke W (1972). Reactions between benzo[a]pyrene and nucleases by one-electron oxidation. J Natl Cancer Inst 49:1585-1597.

Williamson L (1953). The thermal decomposition of methyl linoleate hydroperoxide. J Appl Chem. 3:301-307.

Wolf G (1982). Is dietary β-carotene an anti-cancer agent? Nutr Rev 40:257-261.

Wynder EL, Gori GB (1977). Contribution of the environment to cancer incidence: An epidemiologic exercise. J Natl Cancer Inst 58:825-832.

Yoshida H, Alexander JC (1983a). Enzymatic hydrolysis of fractionated products from oils thermally oxidized in the laboratory. Lipids 18:402-407.

Yoshida H, Alexander JC (1983b). Enzymatic hydrolysis in vitro of thermally oxidized sunflower oil. Lipids 18:611-616.

Yoshida H, Alexander JC (1984). Changes in the structure of soybean triacylglycerols due to heat. Lipids 19:589-593.

Yoshida H, Kajimoto G (1974). Toxic character of rancid oil. XIV. Effect of tocopherol on phospholipids in rat tissues fed thermally oxidized oils. Yukagaku 23:375-379.

Zaldivar R (1969). Experimental cancer induction in guinea pigs by heated and non-heated fats in combination with methyl-cholanthrene. Arch Hyg Bakteriol 153:211-219.

Dietary Fat and Cancer, pages 211–228
© 1986 Alan R. Liss, Inc.

NUTRITIONAL AND FUNCTIONAL
REQUIREMENTS FOR ESSENTIAL FATTY ACIDS

Ralph T. Holman

Hormel Institute,
University of Minnesota,
Austin, Minnesota 55912

STRUCTURAL REQUIREMENTS FOR ESSENTIAL FATTY ACIDS

The essentiality of polyunsaturated fatty acids was
first indicated by nutritional studies revealing that
dietary fats contain an essential growth-promoting factor
not due to fat-soluble vitamins but traceable to the fatty
acid fraction (Burr and Burr, 1929). The following year
they reported that the activity was traceable to linoleic
acid, and perhaps to linolenic acid (Burr and Burr, 1930).
The first report appeared in the same volume in which a
prestigious nutrition laboratory reported that fats had no
special nutritional value aside from their caloric content
and their fat-soluble vitamins (McAmis, et al., 1929).
Thus, the essentiality of polyunsaturated fatty acids (PUFA)
was controversial from the beginning. The field has been
extremely active, and the literature covering the first 40
years has been reviewed for essential fatty acid (EFA)
deficiency (Holman, 1971) and for biological activities of
EFA (Holman, 1971a).

Two families of essential PUFA are known to have
physiological functions. The linoleic acid family,
including arachidonic acid, all have the terminal double
bond 6 carbon atoms from the terminal (ω) methyl group of
the fatty acid. These acids are all metabolically derived
from linoleic acid (9,12-18:2 or 18:2ω6) by desaturation and
chain-elongation reactions between the existing unsaturation
and the carboxyl group, and all have the ω6 structure. The
linolenic acid family of PUFA are similarly related to each

METABOLISM OF PUFA IN LIVER

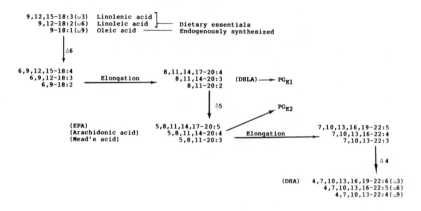

Figure 1. Metabolism of polyunsaturated fatty acids.

other, and are derived by the same reactions from linolenic acid (9,12,15-18:3 or 18:3ω3). These two families of PUFA are known to have functions related to their occurrence in the essential structural lipids in biologically active membranes, and to their conversion by enzymatic oxidation reactions to highly biologically active prostaglandins, prostacyclins, thromboxanes, leukotrienes and other active products of oxidation. The metabolism of the two families of essential PUFA is shown in Figure 1 with that of oleic acid.

Non-essential PUFA also occur naturally. Oleic acid (9-18:1 or 18:1ω9) can be desaturated and chain-elongated to form a series of ω9 PUFA (Mead, 1971). These PUFA are normally present as minor components in animal tissue lipids, but when dietary supply of EFA is low, these nonessential ω9 PUFA increase in proportion, and may become major components in overt EFA deficiency. In fact, 20:3ω9 is a very useful indicator of the severity of EFA deficiency. The metabolism of the oleic acid family of PUFA is included in the diagram in Figure 1. Palmitoleic acid also undergoes the same series of reactions to produce a family of ω7 PUFA, which are of lesser abundance than are the ω9 PUFA. The 20:4ω7, an isomer of arachidonic acid, can be detected in EFA deficiency. Because these four metabolic sequences are performed by the same enzymatic systems, the several substrates are competitive, and other acyl groups can act as inhibitors at each step. In deficiency, the nonessential PUFA are competitive with the diminished supplies of essential ω6 and ω3 PUFA and are incorporated into tissue lipids such as phospholipids (PL) to become components in biologically active membranes, in substitution for the ω6 and ω3 PUFA normally found.

The properties of the membranes are modulated by the kind and quantity of PUFA present. The many isomeric 18:1 acids occurring in partially hydrogenated vegetable oils are likewise competitive with essential PUFA and may be converted to yet other PUFA of unnatural structure (Holman and Mahfouz, 1982). Odd chain PUFA have been found in certain fish oils, and their metabolism has been studied (Schlenk, 1971). Their role or essentiality is not yet understood. Unusual isomers and homologs of PUFA have been synthesized, tested for essentiality and found to have little or no activity (Holman, 1971a). Essentiality seems confined largely to even-chained homologs and those isomers in which the unsaturation is all cis, methylene-interrupted and with either ω6 or ω3 terminal structure.

The members of the linolenic (ω3), linoleic (ω6) and oleic (ω9) acids are shown in Figure 1. The products formed from each of these precursors are all unique. There is no metabolic crossover between the ω3, ω6 and ω9 PUFA in animals. There is metabolic competition between these families of acids, and the ability to compete is ω3 > ω6 > ω9 (Holman, 1964). Isomeric 18:1 acids likewise are competitive in these reactions, and they inhibit the metabolism of linoleic acid to arachidonic acid (Hill, et al., 1982).

The biologically active oxidative products formed from individual PUFA of different structures are likewise all unique, and their biological functions are also modified by differences in their structures. From only three precursors 15 unique PUFA are formed, as is shown in Figure 1. If each of these were subject to conversion to a prostaglandin, a thromboxane, a prostacyclin and a leukotriene, 60 possible biologically active regulators of metabolism could be formed, not to mention all the intermediates in the biosynthesis of each of these. Thus, modulation of the composition of tissue PUFA by nutritional means has complex effects upon metabolic regulation.

NUTRITIONAL DEFICIENCIES OF PUFA

Deficiency of linoleic acid was the first EFA deficiency induced experimentally, and it has been studied exhaustively (Holman, 1971). The classic EFA deficiency (Burr and Burr, 1929) induced by fat-free diet, or by diets free of EFA but containing saturated or monounsaturated fat leads to weight loss, excessive loss of body water by evaporation, scaly skin and tail, kidney malfunction, fatty liver, poor reproduction, shortened lifespan and a variety of other physiological symptoms. Classic dermatitis of linoleic acid deficiency in rats is shown in Figure 2.

Linoleic acid has been demonstrated to be required also by humans. The classic work of Hansen demonstrated the dietary need of infants for linoleic acid, and he found that with low intake, infants developed dermatitis which could be cured by linoleate or arachidonate (Hansen, et al., 1963). The induction of dermatitis in humans when they were given total parenteral nutrition without fat has been studied thoroughly and the changes in PUFA of tissue lipids found are parallel to those found in experimental animals. The abnormal PUFA profiles of serum PL, kidney PL and liver PL from a very serious case of EFA deficiency are shown in Figure 3 in comparison to normal values for serum PL shown in black. The data show that the three tissues have very similar profiles which differ very significantly from the profile for normal serum phospholipids (PL).

Linolenic acid has been demonstrated to be less effective than linoleic acid in stimulating growth at comparable levels of intake. Arachidonic acid was more effective than either in this function. For each of these acids fed singly, maximum growth was attained by intake at about 1% of energy, but the maximum weight attained was in the order arachidonate > linoleate > linolenate. With respect to prevention of dermatitis, the efficacies were in the same order, but linolenate did not completely eliminate the dermatitis even at high intakes (Mohrhauer and Holman, 1963).

Weight gain and dermatitis are not specific measures of linoleate or linolenate, for they are affected by very many other factors. The most specific measures of these two

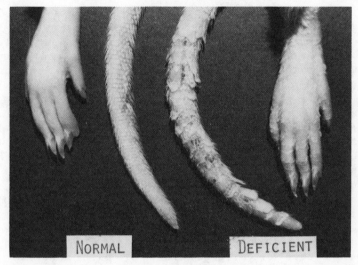

Figure 2. Dermatitis of linoleate deficiency in the rat.

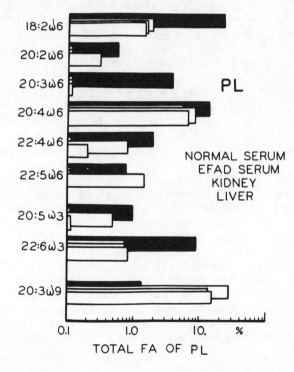

Figure 3. Profiles of tissue PL in linoleate deficiency.

acids are the longer chain, more highly unsaturated fatty acids which are produced from them in normal metabolism. The best assay of linoleate intake is the measurement of the ω6 acids formed from it, and the best assay of linolenate intake is the ω3 acids formed from it. This approach has been used to describe the dose-response phenomena between dietary supplements of pure linoleate, linolenate and arachidonate esters and ω6 and ω3 PUFA in tissue lipids (Mohrhauer and Holman, 1963). The same approach was extended to a study of gamma-linolenic acid (18:3ω6) (Garcia and Holman, 1965). Combinations of pure dietary PUFA have also been studied. The effects of variable intake of 18:3ω3 with constant intake of 18:2ω6(Mohrhauer and Holman, 1963), variable intake of 18:2ω6 acid with constant intake of 18:3ω3 (Rahm and Holman, 1964) and variable intake of 18:3ω3 with constant intake of 20:4ω6 (Holman, 1964) have been studied with pure esters to assess interactions among PUFA. The effects of triglycerides of pure monoenoic acids (Mohrhauer, et al., 1967) and of saturated fatty acids (Mohrhauer and Holman, 1967) upon the metabolism of linoleic acid have also been determined. These studies showed that monoenoic and saturated fatty acids have inhibitory effects upon conversion of linoleic to arachidonic acids, although these effects are less than the effects of the ω3 and ω6 PUFA upon each other (Holman, 1964).

The interactive behavior of all dietary fatty acids has been assessed via analytical studies relating the fatty acid composition of the diet to the fatty acid composition of tissue lipids. These studies employed the natural situation involving dietary fats, and the relationships were revealed by statistical methods (Caster, et al., 1966). There were high direct diet-tissue correlations among the ω6 acids and among the ω3 acids, and the levels of certain saturated and monounsaturated fatty acids in the diet had measurable effects upon those correlations. Equations were derived which permit estimate of intake of 18:3ω3, 18:2ω6 and saturated acids from analysis of the tissue lipids. Conversely the content of tissue 14:0, 18:1, 20:3ω9, 18:3, 20:5ω3, 22:5ω3 and 22:6ω3 can be estimated from the fatty acid composition of the diet. This study showed that when mixed fats containing many fatty acids are ingested, the interactions between the fatty acids of the acyl pool affect the composition of tissue lipids. The relationships between

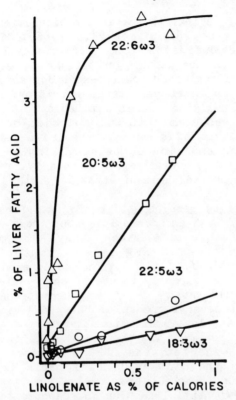

Figure 4. Relationship between dietary intake of linolenate and the concentration of ω3 acids in liver lipid.

dietary linolenate and liver ω3 PUFA deduced from this study are shown in Figure 4.

The essentiality of linolenic acid has been suspected since the discovery of the essentiality of linoleic acid. Only recently have the evidences for a function of the ω3 fatty acids accumulated. Many attempts have been made to induce linolenate deficiency and to precipitate abnormalities associated with it, but with little success (Tinoco, 1983). The abundance of ω3 PUFA in lipids of nervous and ocular tissues has led to the conjecture that they must function in these tissues. The evidence for this postulate is now appearing, and the field is becoming very active. Deficiency of ω3 acids induced nutritionally in monkeys has been associated with loss of visual function (Neuringer, et al., 1986). Similar association of ω3 acids with function of retinal tissue at the biochemical level has been recently made (Bazan, et al., 1986). One case of linolenic acid deficiency has been described. As a consequence of an accidental gunshot wound, a 6 year old girl underwent a series of bowel resections and repair, and was maintained on total parenteral nutrition. During one period when an emulsion low in linolenic acid and high in linoleic acid was administered, episodes of neuropathy occurred. Analysis of serum PL revealed a paucity of ω3 acids. When an emulsion containing linolenic acid was given, the ω3 acids were restored toward normal and the neuropathy disappeared (Holman, et al., 1982).

The quantified requirement for EFA was first estimated from observing growth and dermatitis, but these are affected by numerous factors other than PUFA. The most direct response to intake of EFA is the content of their metabolites in tissue lipids. The dose-response studies discussed above led directly to use of those data as a basis of setting requirements. The first such approach resulted from a study of several groups of rats receiving different fats and different levels of fats. Arrangement of the data versus dietary treatment was confusing until the content of diene, triene, and tetraene PUFA in tissue lipids was plotted versus the dietary linoleic acid intake. The tetraenoic acids (arachidonic acid) of heart lipids rose sharply in an exponential fashion in response to increasing dietary linoleate, and the trienoic acids (20:3ω9) dropped precipitously. In an effort to reduce these effects to one parameter, the triene/tetraene ratio was made, and it was found to reach a low, relatively constant value at an intake of linoleate equal to approximately 1% of calories (Holman, 1960). Using the method of alkaline isomerization for measurement of PUFA, the ratio was considered to be normal if it were less than 0.4.

When gas chromatography was introduced, many of the individual PUFA became measurable, and the 20:3ω9/20:4ω6 ratio was used to advantage. With the new methodology, it became apparent that, at least with human serum lipids, the upper limit of normalcy needed revision downward to about 0.2. With improved capillary gas chromatography and more precise measurement this value may be revised even lower. At the present time, it appears that setting a precise lower limit is straining at gnats, for the concept of the ratio needs revision in favor of better measures of response. The triene/tetraene ratio is affected by more than the dietary linoleate. Variations in dietary linolenic acid and other PUFA affect the biosynthesis of $20:3\omega9$ and $20:4\omega6$, and the ratio is now too simplistic for use as more than a rule of thumb. In our laboratory, we consider the total chromatogram and examine the data for total $\omega6$ acids, total metabolites of $18:2\omega6$, total $\omega3$ acids, total metabolites of $18:3\omega3$, products of 6-desaturation, products of 5-desaturation, products of 4-desaturation, products of elongation to C_{20}, products of elongation to C_{22}, and product/precursor ratios for key metabolic reactions. The preliminary evaluation of the complex and voluminous data is now done by computer. The pattern of PUFA is not only a measure of the dietary intake, but it can reveal metabolic abnormalities.

The dose-response curves, whether obtained by measured doses of pure fatty acid esters or by feeding mixtures of natural fats and oils, are all exponential curves which rise (or fall) in asymptotic fashion toward limiting values. Thus, infinite dose levels would induce maximum (or minimum) values. The asymptotic value is not achievable in practice, and is not the nutrient requirement. The "half-change" value for intake is a characteristic of exponential curves, and any point can be defined in terms of the half-change value, I:

$$\text{Minimum nutrient requirement:} \quad MNR = n\,I$$

The value of $n = 1.7$ was set by analogy to the requirements for thiamin and vitamin C which were also set from measurable, exponential biochemical responses for which n was found to be near this value. The value, $n = 1.7$, corresponds to about 70% of total change at asymptotic value, and gives estimates of MNR very close to those deduced from the triene/tetraene ratio and from physical changes in EFA deficiency.

This approach has been applied to data relating linoleate intake to several fatty acids in several tissues of rats of both sexes, and the data are summarized in a review of the biological activities of PUFA (Holman, 1971). As might be expected, different metabolic criteria require different intakes of EFA to achieve 70% of maximum response. Nearly all are below the 1 to 2% of calories arrived at by triene/tetraene ratios. The exceptions relate to $18:2\omega6$ deposition in tissue lipids and to $18:0$ which accompanies it in phospholipids. Deposition of a high level of linoleate may be desirable, but it is not a minimum requirement.

The sequel to setting a nutrient requirement is the need to assay nutritive status with respect to that standard. The same data and the same relationships derived from them, relating dietary intake to PUFA composition of tissue lipids may be used to solve for dietary intake when tissue PUFA values are known. Appropriate equations for estimating linoleate intake for rats, swine, chickens, dogs and guinea pigs have been derived (Holman, 1971). The earliest studies were made with measurement of PUFA by alkaline isomerization, and those equations are now obsolete. Some studies have been made with gas chromatography, and those equations are still useful. The only estimates we have for man and infants were made using alkaline isomerization, based on data from the very early studies of Hansen and his students (Hansen, et al., 1963). Alkaline isomerization, used to deduce relationships for infants (Holman, Caster and Wiese, 1964) and adult males (Holman, Caster and Wiese, 1964a) is now obsolete, and gas chromatographic data cannot appropriately be used with the equations. Thus, there is now no assay for EFA status of humans. The early data of Hansen, et al. included some instances of EFA deficiency innocently induced by the then common use of diluted skim milk and sugar for infant feeding. Similar data cannot now be ethically obtained, and any estimate derived in the future must be based upon linoleate intakes above the minimum nutrient requirement. With the emerging knowledge that PUFA deficiencies are rather common, the need for a quantitative assay of linoleate intake is soon critical.

Assay of EFA status of humans is, for the present, best done by analysis of PUFA pattern in serum lipids using gas chromatography. This laboratory has gathered a large computerized data base of packed column GLC analyses of serum PL, cholesteryl esters (CE), triglycerides (TG) and free or non-esterified fatty acids (FA) from control individuals (Holman, et al., 1979). In addition, studies of several diseases have provided a variety of PUFA patterns which differ significantly from normal. Recently, a data base obtained by the more discriminating and precise capillary GLC analysis (Johnson, et al., 1985) has been begun with normal and diseased humans. The analyses are done either on serum or plasma, and upon all four gross lipid classes, if possible. The best single analysis of EFA status is the PUFA pattern of serum PL, for this lipid class is richest in PUFA, it is the principal lipid component of membranes, and it responds to changes in dietary EFA most dramatically. The analyses of the other lipid classes provide additional and confirmatory information. The data are preferably expressed as % of total fatty acids of the lipid. The reason for this is that the properties of tissue membranes are influenced by the proportions of various types of fatty acids in their lipids, and because serum lipids reflect the EFA status of tissue lipids (Paulsrud, et al., 1972). The proportions of PUFA within lipids therefore are more indicative of function of membranes than are the concentrations of PUFA in the total aqueous space.

FACTORS AFFECTING EFA REQUIREMENT

Many conditions or deficiencies may have a bearing on the utilization of PUFA. Starvation, inanition, hormonal imbalances, genetic abnormalities, intake of non-essential fatty acids, imbalance of essential nutrients and disease all cause changes of metabolism and changes in lipid and fatty acid patterns within the homeostatic range of PUFA composition. These subjects have been reviewed (Holman, 1971, 1986). The abnormal patterns imply modified requirements for PUFA, and potential correction by nutritional means. Attempts in that direction have not been made yet, except with linoleate and linolenate.

EFA deficiencies in humans have been induced by long term total parenteral nutrition without fat (Paulsrud, et al., 1972), chronic malnutrition (Holman, et al., 1981), anorexia nervosa (Adams, et al., 1986), all of which involve restriction of EFA intake. Diabetes induced by streptozotocin (Holman, et al., 1983), and hypothyroidism induced by thiouracil (Holman, 1960) disturb PUFA patterns by hormonal imbalances. Achrodermatitis enteropathica (Cash and Berger, 1969), Sjogren-Larsson Syndrome (Hernell, et al., 1982), multisystem neuronal degeneration (Dyck, et al., 1981), cystic fibrosis (Lloyd-Still, et al., 1981), a hepato-pancreato-renal syndrome (Lindahl, et al., unpublished) and Prader-Willi Syndrome of obesity (Nelson, et al., 1981) are all genetically induced diseases which disturb the PUFA pattern. In Reye's Syndrome a paucity of PUFA in serum PL and a ten-fold enhancement of PUFA in non-esterified FA have been observed, suggesting that viral infection may trigger uncontrolled lipolysis by phospholipase A_2 (Ogburn, et al., 1982). Cirrhosis is accompanied by a highly significant distortion of PUFA pattern, notably a deficiency of arachidonate (Johnson et al., 1985).

Nutritional imbalances involving fatty acids are long known to affect the PUFA. Low intakes of linoleic and linolenic acids lead to gross tissue deficiencies of the ω6 and ω3 acids derived from them (Rieckehoff, et al., 1949). Excesses of non-essential fatty acids such as saturated acids (Mohrhauer and Holman, 1967), monoenoic acids (Mohrhauer, et al., 1967), and isomeric unsaturated acids (Hill, et al., 1982) affect fatty acid pattern of tissue lipids. Excessive intake of cholesterol (Holman and Peifer, 1960) and administration of hypercholesterolemic agents (Holman, 1971) accelerate the onset of dermatitis of EFA deficiency, and hypolipidemic agents induce abnormal PUFA patterns (unpublished). We postulate that excessive intake and transport of non-essential fat or cholesterol necessitate the mobilization of PUFA from tissues for synthesis of the PL necessary for their transport, leading to a relative deficiency of EFA.

Protein deficiency has a strong influence upon PUFA pattern. We have observed that, in any group of EFA deficient rats, those that grow the most also develop the most severe dermatitis. Therefore, a study of the effect of protein intake upon growth, dermatitis and PUFA pattern of tissue lipids was undertaken (Hill and Holman, 1980). Groups of rats were fed an EFA-deficient diet to limit growth and induce dermal symptoms, and were given levels of protein ranging from 5% to 40% of the diet to induce different rates of growth. The growth rate increased with the protein intake, and so did the dermal score, as far as 30% protein. The content of 20:3ω9 decreased, and the 20:4ω6 increased with increasing protein level. When the PUFA profiles of a protein deficient group were compared with the optimum group as control, several significant differences were observed in both liver and heart. The 18:2ω6, 18:3ω6, 20:2ω6, 20:4ω6, 22:5ω6 and 22:6ω3 were significantly less, but the 22:4ω6, 20:5ω3 and 20:3ω9 were significantly higher in a protein deficient group than in the control. These data are shown in Figure 5.

This phenomenon may be more related to the diminished growth than to the protein level. This is suggested from

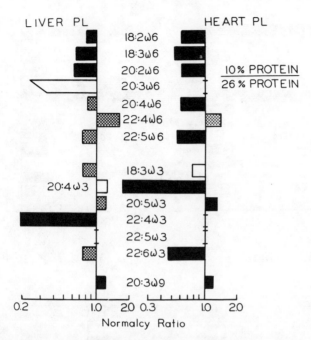

Figure 5. PUFA profiles in protein deficient rats.

two studies with other nutrient deficiencies. The effect of zinc deficiency upon PUFA metabolism was studied with groups given low zinc diet fed ad libitum, normal zinc diet fed ad libitum and the normal zinc diet pair-fed to the low zinc group. Significant differences in profile were found between the low and normal zinc groups, but not between the low zinc group and the normal zinc group pair-fed to it. Thus, the difference in profile induced by zinc deficiency is really not traceable to lack of zinc, but to lack of growth (Kramer et al., 1984). A very similar phenomenon was found with biotin deficiency (Kramer et al., 1984a). Obviously, assessment of effects of other nutrients upon PUFA patterns should be done with pair-fed controls.

PUFA PROFILES IN HUMAN DISEASE

Our survey of several human diseases for aberrations in PUFA pattern has revealed that many diseases do involve abnormal PUFA metabolism. Each disease profile is unique, but several have important features in common. The abnormal PUFA profiles have been published in detail in the original

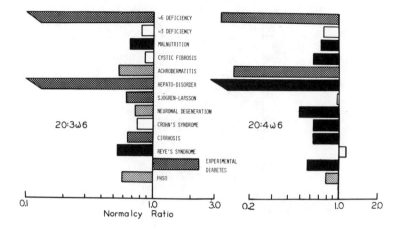

Figure 6. Normalcy ratios for 20:3ω6 and 20:4ω6 in diseases.

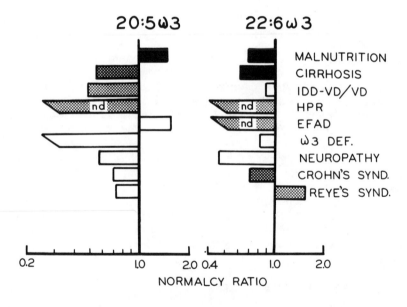

Figure 7. Normalcy ratios for 20:5ω3 and 22:6ω3 in malnutrition, cirrhosis, insulin-dependent diabetes and vascular disease, hepato-pancreato-renal syndrome, EFA deficiency, linolenate deficiency, multisystem neuropathy, Crohn's disease and Reye's syndrome.

references, but some similarities are worth summarizing here. Almost all the diseases studied had some statistically significant abnormalities in individual PUFA when compared with normal controls. Of these, deficiencies of $20:3\omega6$, $20:4\omega6$, $20:5\omega6$ and $22:6\omega3$ were common to several diseases. In Figure 6 the bars indicate the normalcy ratios (observed value/control value) for dihomogammalinolenic ($20:3\omega6$) and arachidonic ($20:4\omega6$) acids in serum PL in several physiological states, nutritional treatments and diseases. Arachidonic acid deficiency is the most common, and it is frequently accompanied by deficiency of $20:3_\omega6$.

Two $\omega3$ PUFA are also often abnormal in serum PL in disease states, as is indicated in Figure 7. Chronic malnutrition is accompanied by statistically significant elevation of $20:5\omega6$ and decreased $22:6\omega3$. It appears that diseases often disturb PUFA metabolism, and the attendant effects upon production of prostanoids and other autocoids may explain some of the elements of the syndromes.

Thus far the study of the effects of cancer upon the PUFA patterns of tissues has not received serious study. The link between dietary fat and cancer has been made and, indeed, is the motivation for the writing of this book. Our studies indicate that growth influences the pattern of PUFA in tissues, and the rapid growth of neoplastic tissue may also induce abnormal PUFA profiles. In our studies of other diseases, the probability of aberration of PUFA in a disease has been high, and on this probability alone, it appears that this may be a fruitful area for investigation with respect to cancer.

ACKNOWLEDGEMENTS

The author's research summarized in this report was supported in part by NIH Grant 04514, by Program Project Grant HLB 08214 and by the Hormel Foundation.

REFERENCES

Adams CE, Holman RT, Erdman JW, Nelson RA, Jaskiewicz JA, Johnson SB, Grater SJE (1986). Plasma Fatty Acid Profile in Patients with Anorexia Nervosa. Am J Clin Nutr (in press)
Bazan NG, Reddy TS, Bazan HEP, Birkle DL (1986). Metabolism of Arachidonic and Docosahexaenoic Acids in the Retina.

Prog Lipid Res 25: (in press)

Burr GO, Burr MM (1929) A New Deficiency Disease Produced by the Rigid Exclusion of Fat from the Diet. J Biol Chem 82: 345-367

Burr GO, Burr MM (1930) On the Nature and Role of the Fatty Acids Essential in Nutrition. J Biol Chem 86:587-621

Cash R, Berger CK (1969). Acrodermatitis Enteropathica: Defective Metabolism of Unsaturated Fatty Acids. J Pediat 74:717-729

Caster WO, Mohrhauer H, Holman RT (1966). Effects of Twelve Common Fatty Acids in the Diet Upon the Composition of Liver Lipid in the Rat. J Nutr 89:217-225

Dyck PJ, Yao JK, Knickerbocker DE, Holman RT, Gomez MR, Hayles AB, Lambert EH (1981). Multisystem Neuronal Degeneration Hepatosplenomegaly and Adrenocortical Deficiency Associated with Reduced Tisssue Arachidonic Acid. Neurology 31:925-34

Garcia PT, Holman RT (1965). Competitive Inhibitions in the Metabolism of Polyunsaturated Fatty Acids Studied via the Composition of the Phospholipids, Triglycerides and Cholesteryl Esters of Rat Tissues. J Am Oil Chem Soc 42:1137-1141

Hansen AE, Wiese HF, Boelsche AN, Haggard ME, Adam DJD, Davis H (1963). Role of Linoleic Acid in Infant Nutrition Clinical and Chemical Study of 428 Infants fed on Milk Mixtures Varying in Kind and Amount of Fat. Pediatrics 31:171-192

Hernell O, Holmgren G, Jagell SF, Johnson SB, Holman RT (1982). Suspected Faulty Essential Fatty Acid Metabolism in Sjogren-Larsson Syndrome. Pediatr Res 16:45-49

Hill EG, Holman RT (1980). Effect of Dietary Protein Level upon Essential Fatty Acid Deficiency. J Nutr 110:1057-1060

Hill EG, Johnson SB, Lawson LD, Mahfouz MM, Holman RT (1982) Perturbation of the Metabolism of Essential Fatty Acids by Dietary Partially Hydrogenated Vegetable Oil. Proc Natl Acad Sci USA 79:953-957

Holman RT (1960). The Ratio of Trienoic:Tetraenoic Acids in Tissue Lipids as a Measure of Essential Fatty Acid Requirement. J Nutr 70:405-410

Holman RT (1960a). The Lipids in Relation to Atherosclerosis. Am J Clin Nutr 8:95-103

Holman RT (1964). Nutritional and Metabolic Interrelationships between Fatty Acids. Fed Proc 23:1062-1067

Holman RT (1971). Essential Fatty Acid Deficiency. Prog Chem Fats Other Lipids 9:279-348

Holman RT (1971a). Biological Activities of and Requirements for Polyunsaturated Acids. Prog Chem Fats Other Lipids

9:611-682

Holman RT (1986). Control of Polyunsaturated Acids in Tissue Lipids. J Am Coll Nutr (in press)

Holman RT, Johnson SB, Gerrard JM, Mauer SM, Kupcho-Sandberg, Brown DM (1983). Arachidonic Acid Deficiency in Streptozotocin Induced Diabetes. Proc Natl Acad Sci USA 80:2375-2379

Holman RT, Johnson SB, Hatch TF (1982). A Case of Human Linolenic Acid Deficiency Involving Neurological Abnormalities. Am J Clin Nutr 35:617-623

Holman RT, Johnson SB, Mercuri O, Itarte HJ, Rodrigo MA, DeTomas ME (1981). Essential Fatty Acid Deficiency in Malnourished Children. Am J Clin Nutr 34:1534-1539

Holman RT, Mahfouz MM (1981). Cis and Trans Octadecenoic Acids as Precursors of Polyunsaturated Acids. Prog Lipid Res 20:151-156

Holman RT, Peifer JJ (1960). Acceleration of Essential Fatty Acid Deficiency by Dietary Cholesterol. J Nutr 70:411-417

Holman RT, Smythe L, Johnson S (1979). Effect of Sex and Age on Fatty Acid Composition of Human Serum Lipids. Am J Clin Nutr 32:2390-2399

Johnson SB, Gordon E, McClain C, Low G, Holman RT (1985). Abnormal Polyunsaturated Fatty Acid Patterns of Serum Lipids in Alcoholism and Cirrhosis: Arachidonic Acid Deficiency in Cirrhosis. Proc Natl Acad Sci USA 82:1815-1818

Kramer TR, Briske-Anderson M, Johnson SB, Holman RT (1984). Influence of Reduced Food Intake on Polyunsaturated Fatty Acid Metabolism in Zinc-Deficient Rats. J Nutr 114:1224-1230

Kramer TR, Briske-Anderson M, Johnson SB, Holman RT (1984a). Effects of Biotin Deficiency on Polyunsaturated Fatty Acid Metabolism in Rats. J Nutr 114:2047-2052

Lloyd-Still JD, Johnson SB, Holman RT (1981). Essential Fatty Acid Status in Cystic Fibrosis and the Effects of Safflower Oil Supplementation. Am J Clin Nutr 34:1-7

McAmis AJ, Anderson WE, Mendel LB (1929). Growth of Rats on "Fat-free" Diets. J Biol Chem 82:247-262

Mead JF (1971). The Metabolism of the Polyunsaturated Fatty Acids. Prog Chem Fats Other Lipids 9:159-192

Mohrhauer H, Holman, RT (1963). The Effect of Dose Level of Essential Fatty Acids upon Fatty Acid Composition of the Rat Liver. J Lipid Res 4:151-159

Mohrhauer H, Holman RT (1963a). Effect of Linolenic Acid upon the Metabolism of Linoleic Acid. J Nutr 81:67-74

Mohrhauer H, Holman RT (1967). Metabolism of Linoleic Acid in Relation to Dietary Saturated Fatty Acids in the Rat.

J Nutr 91:528-534

Mohrhauer H, Rahm JJ, Seufert J, Holman RT (1967). Metabolism of Linoleic Acid in Relation to Dietary Monoenoic Fatty Acids in the Rat. J Nutr 91:521-527

Nelson RA, Huse DM, Holman RT, Kimbrough BO, Wahner HW, Callaway CW, Hayles AB (1981). Nutrition, Metabolism, Body Composition and Response to the Ketogenic Diet in Prader-Willi Syndrome. In Holm VA, Pipes PL (eds): "The Prader-Willi Syndrome" Baltimore: Univ Park Press, pp 105-120

Neuringer M, Connor WE, Lin DS, Barstad L, Luck S (1986). Biochemical and Functional Effects of Prenatal and Post-natal ω3 Fatty Acid Deficiency on Retina and Brain in Rhesus Monkeys. Proc Natl Acad Sci USA 83: (in press)

Ogburn PL, Sharp H, Lloyd-Still JD, Johnson SB, Holman RT (1982). Abnormal Polyunsaturated Fatty Acid Patterns of Serum Lipids in Reye's Syndrome. Proc Natl Acad Sci USA 79:908-911

Paulsrud JR, Pensler L, Whitten CF, Stewart S, Holman RT (1972) Essential Fatty Acid Deficiency in Infants Induced by Fat-free Intravenous Feeding. Am J Clin Nutr 25:897-904

Rahm JJ, Holman (1964). Effect of Linoleic Acid upon the Metabolism of Linolenic Acid. J Nutr 84:15-19

Rieckehoff I, Holman RT, Burr GO (1949) Polyethenoid Fatty Acid Metabolism. Effect of Dietary Fat on Polyethenoid Fatty Acids of Rat Tissues. Arch Biochem 20:331-340

Schlenk H (1971) Odd Numbered Polyunsaturated Fatty Acids. Prog Chem Fats Other Lipids 9:587-606

III. Effects of Dietary Fat on Carcinogenesis in Laboratory Animals

Dietary Fat and Cancer, pages 231–248
© 1986 Alan R. Liss, Inc.

EXPERIMENTAL STUDIES ON DIETARY FAT AND CANCER IN RELATION
TO EPIDEMIOLOGICAL DATA

Kenneth K. Carroll[1]

Department of Biochemistry, University of Western
Ontario, London, Ontario, Canada, N6A 5C1

INTRODUCTION

From evidence collected over the past 50 years, it is
clear that animals fed high-fat diets develop some kinds
of tumors more readily than those fed low-fat diets. This
has been demonstrated most clearly for tumors of the skin,
mammary gland, intestine and pancreas (Tannenbaum and
Silverstone, 1953; Carroll and Khor, 1975; Reddy et al,
1980; Longnecker et al, 1984). Interest in these
observations has been greatly stimulated by analyses of
epidemiological data on human populations showing strong
positive correlations between dietary fat and cancer,
particularly cancer of the breast and colon (Armstrong and
Doll, 1975; Carroll and Khor, 1975; Reddy et al, 1980).

In studying effects of dietary fat on tumorigenesis
and the mechanisms by which these effects are produced,
there are a number of different dietary variables to be
considered. These include the level of fat in the diet,
the nature of the dietary fat, the timing and duration of
feeding of the high-fat diet, and the composition of the
diet as a whole. These variables can be investigated most
easily in experiments on animals, but the results of
animal studies are not necessarily applicable to humans.
As far as possible, it is therefore desirable to relate
the results of animal experimentation to epidemiological
data for human populations.

[1]Career Investigator of the Medical Research Council of
Canada

The literature relating dietary fat to cancer has been reviewed at numerous symposia and workshops in recent years, and various aspects of the subject are discussed in detail in other chapters of this volume. The aim of this chapter is to provide an overview of experimental studies in relation to epidemiological data and to discuss possible mechanisms of action of dietary fat in these terms.

EFFECTS OF AMOUNT AND TYPE OF DIETARY FAT ON TUMORIGENESIS IN ANIMALS

In early studies on dietary fat and tumorigenesis reviewed by Carroll and Khor (1975), effects of high- and low-fat diets were compared without much attention being given to the type of fat. In such experiments, animals fed high-fat diets containing from 12 to 30% by weight of fat nearly always showed a higher incidence of skin tumors and mammary tumors than those fed low-fat diets containing 0.5 to 3% fat.

A number of different dietary fats and oils were compared in our studies on mammary carcinogenesis induced by 7,12-dimethylbenz(a)anthracene (DMBA), and the results showed clearly that polyunsaturated fats caused a marked increase in tumor yields while saturated fats had little or no effect (Gammal et al, 1967; Carroll and Khor 1971). Similar observations have been made for pancreatic cancer (Birt and Roebuck, 1986). The situation for intestinal cancer is less clear, but there is some evidence that polyunsaturated fats are more effective than saturated fats in this case as well (Reddy et al, 1980; Reddy, 1986).

Further studies on mammary carcinogenesis in our laboratory indicated that saturated fats were ineffective because of their low content of essential fatty acids. When fed with a small amount of polyunsaturated fat or with pure ethyl linoleate, saturated fats were found to increase the tumor yield as effectively as polyunsaturated fats at comparable levels of intake (Hopkins et al. 1981). These experiments indicated that a certain amount of essential fatty acid was required in addition to a high-fat diet for enhancement of the tumor yield. In our original experiments, it appeared that the maximum effect could be obtained by feeding linoleate at a level of 2 to 3% by weight, but recent studies by Ip et al (1985) have indicated that this should be revised upward to about 4% by weight, or more than 8% of total calories. The requirement for essential fatty acid in promotion of pancreatic cancer has been estimated to be even higher, in the range of 4 to 8% (Roebuck et al. 1985).

The polyunsaturated fats that have been investigated in studies on dietary fat and cancer are mostly vegetable oils that contain linoleic acid as the main essential fatty acid (Carroll and Khor, 1971). Fish oils also contain substantial amounts of polyunsaturated fatty acids, but they have an additional double bond at the 3-position relative to the methyl end of the chain, whereas in linoleic acid the double bond nearest to the methyl end is at the 6-position. The n-3 fatty acids are also considered to be essential fatty acids. Like the n-6 fatty acids, they cannot be synthesized de novo by animals, but their biological properties are different from those of the n-6 fatty acids (Holman, 1986). It is thus of interest to consider the effects of dietary fish oils on tumorigenesis (Ip et al. 1986).

Comparative studies on a polyunsaturated vegetable oil (corn oil) and a polyunsaturated fish oil (menhaden oil) at different levels of intake showed that rats treated with DMBA and fed corn oil at levels of 10 or 20% by weight of the diet developed many more tumors than rats fed menhaden oil at these levels. The tumor yields were relatively low in rats fed these oils at 3% by weight, but in this case the rats fed menhaden oil showed a higher tumor yield (Braden and Carroll, 1986). Similar results were obtained by Jurkowski and Cave (1985) using rats treated with N-nitrosomethylurea to induce mammary tumors. Dietary fish oils also failed to exert a stimulatory effect in other models of mammary cancer (Karmali et al, 1984; Gabor and Abraham, 1985) or pancreatic cancer (O'Connor et al, 1985; Birt and Roebuck, 1986).

In their studies on mammary tumors induced by N-nitrosomethylurea (NMU), Chan et al. (1983) reported that the total dietary intake of oleic acid and linoleic acid was positively correlated with tumor incidence. Oleic acid is the most abundant monounsaturated fatty acid in dietary fats and is the major fatty acid in olive oil. Studies in our laboratory showed that olive oil has a promoting effect on DMBA-induced mammary tumorigenesis, but this was not attributed to any specific effect of oleic acid since olive oil also contains a substantial amount of linoleic acid (Carroll and Khor, 1971). Cohen (1986) reported that olive oil failed to show promoting activity on mammary tumors induced by N-nitrosomethylurea (NMU) and a similar lack of promoting activity on colon carcinogenesis was reported by Reddy and Maeura (1984), (see also Reddy, 1986).

The presence of relatively large amounts of trans fatty acids in the American diet has led to concern about their effects on carcinogenesis (Enig et al. 1978). However, experiments on animal models of mammary cancer or colon cancer have failed to provide evidence of tumor promotion by trans fatty acids (Ip et al. 1986; Reddy 1986).

Medium-chain fatty acids (MCT) are major components of coconut oil and are present in small amounts in butterfat, but these fats showed no promoting effect on DMBA-induced mammary tumors (Carroll and Khor 1971). Cohen et al. (1984) also failed to observe any promotion of NMU-induced mammary tumors in rats fed MCT. There is likewise no evidence that thermally oxidized fats have tumor-enhancing effects in experimental animal models (Cohen, 1986).

AMOUNT AND TYPE OF DIETARY FAT IN RELATION TO CANCER INCIDENCE AND MORTALITY IN HUMAN POPULATIONS

As indicated in the Introduction, dietary fat shows strong positive correlations with cancer at sites such as breast and colon, and this applies to both incidence and mortality. The values for dietary fat used to demonstrate these correlations are usually based on disappearance data and are commonly expressed as grams of fat per capita available for consumption in different countries (Armstrong and Doll, 1975; Carroll and Khor, 1975). Such values do not allow for fat discarded during the preparation and consumption of food and are typically substantially higher than actual consumption in most

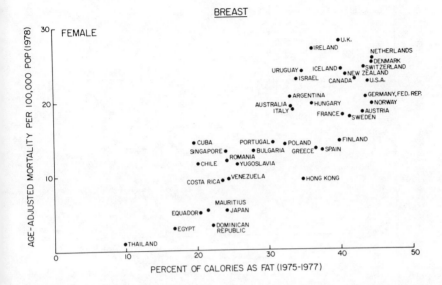

Fig. 1 Positive correlation between age—adjusted mortality
from breast cancer (Segi Institute of Cancer
Epidemiology, 1984) and percentage of dietary
calories as fat calculated from data provided by
FAO (1980).

countries. It is assumed, however, that the values are
overestimated to a similar degree in different countries,
so that the observed correlations may still be valid.

Dietary guidelines with respect to fat and cancer are
usually expressed in terms of percent of total calories
derived from fat (Committee on Diet, Nutrition, and
Cancer, 1982; Disogra and Disogra, 1985). It is thus more
pertinent to compare cancer incidence and mortality to fat
consumption expressed in these terms. As illustrated for
breast cancer in Fig. 1, mortality shows a strong positive
correlation similar to that seen when dietary fat is
expressed as amount per capita available for consumption.
However, the values for percent of calories as fat are
much more in line with accepted values based on other

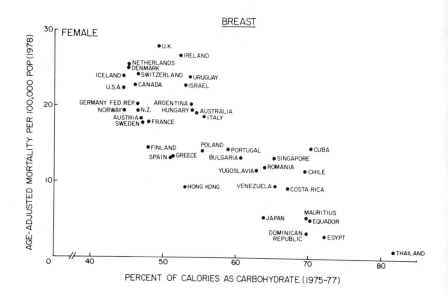

Fig. 2 Negative correlation between age-adjusted mortality from breast cancer and percentage of calories as carbohydrate. Sources of data as for Fig. 1.

measurements. For example, the results in Fig. 1 show that fat comprises about 40% of total calories in the diets of many of the Western industrialized countries.

As calories derived from fat increase, those from carbohydrate tend to decrease, since protein, the other major source of dietary calories, varies over a narrower range from country to country than either fat or carbohydrate. It is therefore not surprising that the percentage of calories from carbohydrate shows a strong negative correlation with mortality from breast cancer (Fig. 2).

As discussed above, studies on experimental cancer models have shown that polyunsaturated fats increase tumor yields more effectively than saturated fats. It was therefore disconcerting to find that mortality from cancers of the breast and colon correlated strongly with total dietary fat and with fat available for consumption

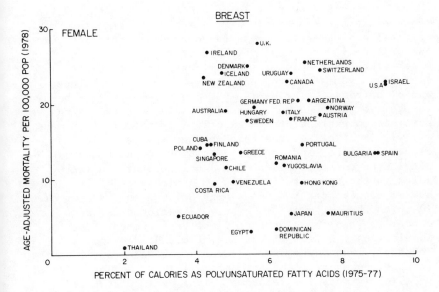

Fig. 3 Lack of correlation between age-adjusted mortality from breast cancer and percentage of calories as polyunsaturated fatty acids. Mortality data as for Fig. 1. Data on polyunsaturated fatty acids from FAO (1982).

from animal sources, but showed little or no correlation with vegetal fat (Carroll, 1975, 1983). This seemed at odds with the experimental data since vegetal fats derived from plant sources are in general more polyunsaturated than fats from animals.

This was explained on the basis that most human diets contain enough polyunsaturated fatty acids to satisfy the relatively small amount of essential acid required for maximum enhancement of tumor yields in experimental animal models. Thus, if this requirement were satisfied by the diet of every country, one might not expect to see any correlation with polyunsaturated fat, and the strong positive correlations observed in epidemiological data could then be attributed to the other, less specific requirement for a high level of dietary fat (Carroll et al, 1981).

The recent report of Ip et al (1985) that the requirement for essential fatty acid is higher than our original estimate has necessitated a reevaluation of our explanation for the apparent discrepancy between the experimental and epidemiological data. As illustrated in Fig. 3, polyunsaturated fatty acids account for between 4 and 8% of total calories in most countries. This is below the threshold found by Ip et al. (1985), but it may not be possible to extrapolate so exactly from animals to humans.

It is likewise uncertain whether any variations in cancer incidence and mortality in human populations can be attributed to consumption of n-3 polyunsaturated fatty acids in the form of fish oils or other marine oils. Some Eskimo populations consume a high polyunsaturated fat diet in which the fat consists mainly of marine oils, and cancer is less frequent than might be expected in Eskimo populations (Neilson and Hansen, 1980; Hildes and Schaefer, 1984). The low incidence of breast cancer may be related, however, to other factors such as the practice of suckling infants for relatively long periods of time.

EFFECTS OF TIMING AND DURATION OF FEEDING OF HIGH-FAT DIET IN CARCINOGENESIS

One of our early studies on effects of dietary fat on DMBA-induced mammary carcinogenesis was designed to provide information on the stage of carcinogenesis at which fat had the greatest influence on tumor yield (Carroll and Khor, 1970). The results showed that feeding a high-fat diet after treatment with DMBA gave the maximum effect, whereas feeding it only before the carcinogen was given had little or no influence on tumor incidence. This suggested that dietary fat was acting primarily at the promotional stage of carcinogenesis (Carroll and Khor, 1975), and in subsequent studies it has been our practice to wait until about a week after treatment with the carcinogen to initiate the high-fat diet (Hopkins et al, 1981).

Other workers have also studied the effect on mammary tumorigenesis of the timing and duration of the feeding of dietary fat. Such studies have indicated that the effect of dietary fat is enhanced by prolonging the time of feeding a high-fat diet (Dao and Chan, 1983). There is also evidence that dietary fat can influence the initiation stage of carcinogenesis (Rogers, 1986; Sylvester et al, 1986). However, the fact that the stimulatory effect of dietary fat on carcinogenesis can be demonstrated with tumors induced by a wide variety of carcinogenic agents helps to support our suggestion that it acts primarily as a promoting agent (Carroll, 1980).

This concept is important in considering the possibility of influencing cancer risk in humans by altering fat intake. Initiation is considered to occur rapidly and to be essentially irreversible, whereas the subsequent proliferation of transformed cells occurs over a much longer time span and appears to be more reversible, particularly during the early stages when the number of transformed cells is still relatively small. Tumor promotion is thought to require more or less continuous exposure to the promoting agent over a prolonged period of time, and this means that withdrawal of the promoting stimulus at any time could help to reduce cancer risk.

Experiments have shown that reducing the level and degree of unsaturation of dietary fat after a period of promoting with a high, polyunsaturated fat diet, can reduce the yield of mammary tumors induced by DMBA (Kalamegham and Carroll, 1984). It is less certain that an achievable decrease in the level of dietary fat with no change in degree of unsaturation will be effective (Carroll et al, 1986).

If the positive correlation between dietary fat and breast cancer mortality in human populations is causative, a reduction in dietary fat would be expected to decrease cancer risk. An important question, however, is how long it would be necessary to remain on a low-fat diet in order to achieve a significant effect. There are, at present, no data to answer this question, although there is some evidence with respect to increasing risk in people whose fat intake has increased. This can be seen in populations migrating from areas of low fat intake to areas of high fat intake (Gori, 1978). There is also evidence that breast cancer and colon cancer are increasing in countries such as Japan, where fat intake has increased in recent years (Hirayama, 1979).

Recurrence of disease due to metastatic growth constitutes the major problem in cancer and is responsible for most cancer deaths. Since dietary fat appears to affect the proliferation of cancer cells, a reduction in dietary fat should theoretically delay or even prevent the development of metastases. There is evidence that recurrence of breast cancer is less frequent in Japanese than in American women (Wynder and Cohen, 1982), and this offers some hope that a reduction in dietary fat might reduce the risk of recurrence in cancer patients. It may only be possible to assess this by controlled clinical trials (Greenwald, 1986; Rose and Boyar, 1986).

EFFECTS OF DIETARY COMPONENTS OTHER THAN FAT

Experiments in our laboratory have shown that rats fed semipurified diet develop DMBA-induced mammary tumors more readily than animals on commercial feed at comparable levels of fat intake (Carroll, 1975). This finding has recently been confirmed and extended by Ip (1986). It is thus evident that experimental mammary carcinogenesis can be influenced by dietary components other than fat (Hopkins and Carroll, 1985). Experiments in our laboratory have provided evidence that rats fed diets containing simple sugars develop mammary tumors more readily than those fed starches at comparable levels of fat intake. There is also some indication of a positive correlation between dietary sucrose and breast mortality in human populations (Hoehn and Carroll, 1979). Effects of dietary carbohydrate have recently been reinvestigated by Klurfeld et al (1984).

Interactions between dietary fat and protein and between dietary fat and fiber are considered by other authors in this volume (Hawrylesicz, 1986; Visek, 1986; Kritchevsky, 1986). It is well-known that retinoids (Moon et al, 1983) and selenium (Ip, 1985) can markedly inhibit tumorigenesis in experimental animals, and the process may also be influenced by other vitamins and trace elements (Committee on Diet, Nutrition, and Cancer, 1982; Newberne and Conner, 1986). It is less certain, however, whether human cancer is significantly influenced by such dietary components within the normal range of intake. Recently, there has been an upsurge of interest in dietary calcium, which may have an important modifying influence on effects of dietary fat (Lipkin and Newmark, 1985; Bruce, 1986).

MECHANISM OF ACTION OF DIETARY FAT

Since it appears that dietary fat exerts its main effects at the promotional stage of carcinogenesis, this discussion will be confined to mechanisms by which dietary fat may act as a promoter. A hormonal mechanism was suggested by Chan and Cohen (1975) in the case of mammary cancer. The original idea that dietary fat alters circulating hormone levels seems improbable in the light of subsequent studies, but dietary fat may influence tumorigenesis by increasing the responsiveness of the target tissue to hormones and/or growth factors (Welsch, 1986).

Some of the proposed mechanisms of action of dietary fat apply to effects that are primarily related to a need for polyunsaturated fatty acids. These include effects of changes in the fatty acid composition of membrane lipids (Hopkins and West, 1976). Such changes would probably occur mainly as a result of alterations in the intake of polyunsaturated fatty acids that cannot be synthesized in the animal body. The fatty acid composition of membrane lipids could be a factor in the proposed mechanism involving junctionally-mediated intercellular communication (Aylsworth, 1986).

Polyunsaturated fatty acids are likely to be involved in promoting effects mediated by the immune system (Vitale and Broitman, 1981; Erickson, 1986). Intake of polyunsaturated fatty acids will also influence tumor promotion by eicosanoids, since eicosanoids are derived from polyunsaturated fatty acids (Karmali, 1986). The mechanism proposed by Kidwell (1986) was developed from observations on stimulation of the growth of cultured cells by polyunsaturated fatty acids, and Abraham and Hillyard (1983) have described marked stimulatory effects of polyunsaturated fatty acids on transplantable mammary tumors.

Although polyunsaturated fatty acids are clearly required for promotion of mammary cancer, pancreatic cancer and possibly other types of cancer in experimental animals, the positive correlations between dietary fat and cancer in human populations are related more to the amount than to the type of fat in the diet (Figs. 1,3). Animal tumor models also show an increase in tumor yields with increasing amounts of fat in the diet, and this seems to be relatively independent of the type of fat after the requirement for polyunsaturated fatty acids has been met (Carroll et al, 1981; Ip, 1986). From a practical standpoint, therefore, it is of particular interest to understand the mechanisms involved in this non-specific promoting effect of dietary fat.

High-fat diets have a high caloric density and cancer mortality is positively correlated with caloric intake as well as with dietary fat in human populations (Carroll and Khor, 1975). It is well-known that caloric restriction can inhibit tumorigenesis in animals (Tannenbaum and Silverstone, 1953; Kritchevsky, 1986; Sylvester, 1986), and the promoting effect of high-fat diets may be due at least in part to increased caloric intake. High-fat diets have been postulated to promote colon tumors by increasing the concentration of bile acids and fatty acids in the intestinal lumen (Reddy et al, 1980; Bruce, 1986). This effect may also be related more to the amount than to the type of fat in the diet. High levels of dietary fat can undoubtedly have other effects on cellular metabolism that serve to promote tumorigenesis. Knowledge of such mechanisms could help to maximize the effectiveness of dietary approaches to reduction of cancer risk.

CONCLUSIONS

Studies on experimental animals and analysis of epidemiological data for human populations have indicated that high-fat diets stimulate the development and growth of tumors at sites such as the mammary gland, colon and pancreas. In animals, the effect is only observed if the dietary fat contains an adequate amount of linoleic acid, an n-6 polyunsaturated fatty acid. Fish oils containing n-3 polyunsaturated fatty acids derived from linolenic acid are ineffective. In human populations, cancer mortality correlates best with total dietary fat and shows no correlation with dietary polyunsaturated fatty acids, possibly because most human diets contain substantial amounts of linoleic acid.

Dietary components other than fat can also influence tumorigenesis in experimental animals, and effects of dietary fat may be modified by components such as carbohydrate, protein or fiber. In human populations, breast cancer mortality is positively correlated with the percentage of calories derived from dietary fat and negatively correlated with the percentage derived from carbohydrate.

Dietary fat appears to act primarily as a promoter of tumorigenesis in experimental animals but may also affect initiation of tumors. The mechanisms of action are still unclear, but various possibilities have been suggested. Some of these are related mainly to the requirement for polyunsaturated fatty acids and others to the less specific requirement for a high-fat diet. The latter is of particular interest from a practical point of view, since cancer mortality in humans correlates better with total dietary fat than with any particular dietary fatty acids.

Promotion of carcinogenesis normally depends on continuing exposure to the promoting agent over a prolonged period of time. If dietary fat is a promoter, reducing fat intake might help to delay or prevent recurrence of disease in cancer patients as well as helping to reduce the overall risk of cancer. This can perhaps best be assessed by controlled clinical trials.

REFERENCES

Abraham S, Hillyard LA (1983). Lipids, lipogenesis, and the effects of dietary fat on growth in mammary tumor model systems. In Perkins EG, Visek WJ "Dietary Fats and Health" Champaign IL: American Oil Chemists' Society, pp 817-853.
Armstrong B, Doll R (1975). Environmental factors and cancer incidence and mortality in different countries, with special reference to dietary practices. Int J Cancer 15:617-631.

Aylsworth CF (1986). Effects of lipids on gap junctionally-mediated intercellular communication: possible role in the promotion of tumorigenesis by dietary fat. This volume.

Birt D, Roebuck BD (1986). Pancreatic cancer. This volume.

Braden LM, Carroll KK (1986). Dietary polyunsaturated fat in relation to mammary carcinogenesis in rats. Lipids (in press).

Bruce WR (1986). Induction of colon toxicity by bile acids, fatty acids, fiber, cholesterol; calcium effects in colon. This volume.

Carroll KK (1975). Experimental evidence of dietary factors and hormone-dependent cancers. Cancer Res 35:3374-3383.

Carroll KK (1980). Lipids and carcinogenesis. J Environ Pathol Toxicol 3(4):253-271.

Carroll KK (1983). Diet and carcinogenesis. In Schettler G, Gotto AM, Middelhoff G, Habenicht AJR, Jurutka KR (eds): "Atherosclerosis VI," Berlin: Springer-Verlag, pp 223-227.

Carroll KK, Braden LM, Bell JA, Kalamegham R (1986). Fat and cancer. Cancer (in press).

Carroll KK, Hopkins GJ, Kennedy TG, Davidson MB (1981). Essential fatty acids in relation to mammary carcinogenesis. Prog Lipid Res 20:685-690.

Carroll KK, Khor HT (1970). Effects of dietary fat and dose level of 7,12-dimethylbenz(α)anthracene on mammary tumor incidence in rats. Cancer Res 30:2260-2264.

Carroll KK, Khor HT (1971). Effects of level and type of dietary fat on incidence of mammary tumors induced in female Sprague-Dawley rats by 7,12-dimethylbenz(α)anthracene. Lipids 6:415-420.

Carroll KK, Khor HT (1975). Dietary fat in relation to tumorigenesis. Prog Biochem Pharmacol 10:308-353.

Chan P-C, Cohen LA (1975). Dietary fat and growth promotion of rat mammary tumors. Cancer Res 35:3384-3386.

Chan P-C, Ferguson KA, Dao TL (1983). Effects of different dietary fats on mammary carcinogenesis. Cancer Res 43:1079-1083.

Cohen LA (1986). Dietary fat and mammary cancer. In Reddy BS, Cohen LA (eds): "Diet, Nutrition, and Cancer: A Critical Evaluation," Boca Raton FL: CRC Press, Inc, pp 77-100.

Cohen LA, Thompson DO, Maeura Y, Weisburger JH (1984). Influence of dietary medium-chain triglycerides on the development of N-methylnitrosourea-induced mammary tumors. Cancer Res 44:5023-5028.

Committee on Diet, Nutrition, and Cancer, Assembly of Life Sciences, National Research Council (1982). "Diet, Nutrition, and Cancer." Washington DC: National Academy Press.

Dao TL, Chan P-C (1983). Effect of duration of high fat intake on enhancement of mammary carcinogenesis in rats. JNCI 71:201-205.

Disogra CA, Disogra LK (1985). Nutrition and cancer prevention. A perspective on dietary recommendations. In Weininger J, Briggs GM (eds): "Nutrition Update, Vol. 2," New York: John Wiley & Sons, pp 3-27.

Enig MJ, Mann RJ, Keeney M (1978). Dietary fat and cancer trends - a critique. Fed Proc 37:2215-2220.

Erickson KL, (1986). Mechanisms of dietary fat modulation of tumorigenesis: changes in immune response. This volume.

FAO (1980). "Food Balance Sheets 1975-77 Average and Per Caput Food Supplies 1961-65 Average, 1967 to 1977." Rome: Food and Agriculture Organization of the United Nations.

FAO (1982). FAO Monthly Bull Statist 5(2):17-18.

Gabor H, Abraham S (1985). Effect of dietary menhaden oil on growth and cell loss of transplantable mammary adenocarcinoma in mice. Proc Am Assoc Cancer Res 26:126.

Gammal EB, Carroll KK, Plunkett ER (1967). Effects of dietary fat on mammary carcinogenesis by 7,12-dimethylbenz(α)anthracene in rats. Cancer Res 27:1737-1742.

Gori GB (1978). Diet and nutrition in cancer causation. Nutr Cancer 1:5-8.

Greenwald, P (1986). Intervention trials. In "Proc of Symp on Calories and Energy Expenditure in Carcinogenesis," Washington DC, Feb 24-25, 1986 (in press).

Hawrylewicz EJ (1986). Fat-protein interaction, defined 2-generation studies. This volume.

Hildes JA, Schaefer O (1984). The changing picture of neoplastic disease in the western and central Canadian Arctic (1950-1980). Can Med Assoc J 130:25-32.

Hirayama T (1979). Diet and cancer. Nutr Cancer 1(3):67-81.

Hoehn SK, Carroll KK (1979). Effects of dietary carbohydrate on the incidence of mammary tumors induced in rats by 7,12-dimethylbenz(a)anthracene. Nutr Cancer 1(3):27-30.

Holman RT (1986). Nutritional and functional requirements for essential fatty acids. This volume.

Hopkins GJ, Carroll KK (1985). Role of diet in cancer prevention. J Envir Pathol Toxicol Oncol 5(6):279-298.

Hopkins GJ, Kennedy TG, Carroll KK (1981). Polyunsaturated fatty acids as promoters of mammary carcinogenesis induced in Sprague-Dawley rats by 7,12-dimethylbenz(a)anthracene. JNCI 66:517-522.

Hopkins GJ, West CE (1976). Possible roles of dietary fats in carcinogenesis. Life Sci 19:1103-1116.

Ip C (1985). Selenium inhibition of chemical carcinogenesis. Fed Proc 44:2573-2578.

Ip C (1986). Fat and essential fatty acid in mammary carcinogenesis. In "Proc of Symp on Calories and Energy Expenditure in Carcinogenesis," Washington DC, Feb 24-25, 1986. (in press).

Ip C, Carter CA, Ip MM (1985). Requirement of essential fatty acid for mammary tumorigenesis in the rat. Cancer Res 45:1997-2001.

Ip C, Ip MM, Sylvester P (1986). Relevance of trans fatty acids and fish oil in animal tumorigenesis studies. This volume.

Jurkowski JJ, Cave WT Jr (1985). Dietary effects of menhaden oil on the growth and membrane lipid composition of rat mammary tumors. JNCI 74:1145-1150.

Kalamegham R, Carroll KK (1984). Reversal of the promotional effect of high-fat diet on mammary tumorigenesis by subsequent lowering of dietary fat. Nutr Cancer 6:22-31.

Karmali RA (1986). Eicosanoids and cancer. This volume.

Karmali RA, Marsh J, Fuchs C (1984). Effect of omega-3 fatty acids on growth of a rat mammary tumor. JNCI 73:451-461.

Kidwell WR (1986). Fatty acid growth requirements of normal and neoplastic mammary epithelium. This volume.

Klurfeld DM, Weber MM, Kritchevsky D (1984). Comparison of dietary carbohydrates for promotion of DMBA-induced mammary tumorigenesis in rats. Carcinogenesis (London) 5:423-425.

Kritchevsky D (1986). Fat, calories, fiber. This volume.

Lipkin M, Newmark H (1985). Effect of added dietary calcium on colonic epithelial-cell proliferation in subjects at high risk for familial colonic cancer. N Engl J Med 313:1381-1384.

Longnecker, DS, Wiebkin P, Schaeffer BK, Roebuck BD (1984). Experimental carcinogenesis in the pancreas. Int Rev Exp Pathol 26:177-229.

Moon RC, McCormick DL, Mehta RG (1983). Inhibition of carcinogenesis by retinoids. Cancer Res (Suppl) 43:2469s-2475s.

Newberne PM, Conner MW (1986). Nutrient influences on toxicity and carcinogenecity. Fed Proc 45:149-154.

Nielsen NH, Hansen JPH (1980). Breast cancer in Greenland-selected epidemiological, clinical, and histological features. J Cancer Res Clin Oncol 98:287-299.

O'Connor TP, Roebuck BD, Peterson F, Campbell TC (1985). Effect of dietary intake of fish oil and fish protein on the development of L-azaserine-induced preneoplastic lesions in the rat pancreas. JNCI 75:959-962.

Reddy BS (1986). Amount and type of dietary fat and colon cancer: animal model studies. This volume.

Reddy BS, Cohen LA, McCoy GD, Hill P, Weisburger JH, Wynder EL (1980). Nutrition and its relationship to cancer. Adv Cancer Res 32:237-345.

Reddy BS, Maeura Y (1984). Tumor promotion by dietary fat in azozymethane-induced colon carcinogenesis in female F344 rats: influence of amount and source of dietay fat. JNCI 72:745-750.

Roebuck BD, Longnecker DS, Baumgartner KJ, Thron CD (1985). Carcinogen-induced lesions of the rat pancreas: effects of varying levels of essential fatty acid. Cancer Res 45:5252-5256.

Roebuck BD, Yager JD Jr, Longnecker DS (1981). Dietary modulation of azaserine-induced pancreatic carcinogenesis in the rat. Cancer Res 41: 888-893.

Rogers AE (1986). Chemically-induced mammary tumors. This volume.

Rose DP, Boyar AP (1986). Dietary fat and cancer risk: the rationale for intervention. In Reddy BS, Cohen LA (eds): "Diet, Nutrition, and Cancer: A Critical Evaluation," Boca Raton FL: CRC Press, Inc., pp 151-166.

Segi Institute of Cancer Epidemiology (1984). "Age-Adjusted Death Rates for Cancer for Selected Sites (A-Classification) in 46 Countries in 1978." Nagoya, Japan: Segi Institute of Cancer Epidemiology.

Sylvester PW (1986). Role of acute caloric-restriction in murine tumorigenesis. This volume.

Sylvester PW, Russell M, Ip MM, Ip C (1986). Comparative effects of different animal and vegetable fats fed before and during carcinogen administration on mammary tumorigenesis, sexual maturation, and endocrine function in rats. Cancer Res 46:757-762.

Tannenbaum A, Silverstone H (1953). Nutrition in relation to cancer. Adv Cancer Res 1:451-501.

Visek WJ (1986). Fat-protein interaction on mammary, colon and pancreas cancers. This volume.

Vitale JJ, Broitman SA (1981). Lipids and immune function. Cancer Res 41: 3706-3710.

Welsch CW (1986). Interrelationship between dietary fat and endocrine processes in mammary gland tumorigenesis. This volume.

Wynder EL, Cohen LA (1982). A rationale for dietary intervention in the treatment of postmenopausal breast cancer patients. Nutr Cancer 3:195-199.

Dietary Fat and Cancer, pages 249–253
© 1986 Alan R. Liss, Inc.

INTRODUCTION TO THE EFFECTS OF NEUTRAL FATS AND FATTY
ACIDS ON CARCINOGENESIS IN EXPERIMENTAL ANIMALS

Diane F. Birt

Eppley Institute for Research in Cancer,
University of Nebraska Medical Center, Omaha,
Nebraska 68105

INTRODUCTION

Dietary fat effects on carcinogenesis have been
assessed at a wide variety of sites with a number of different cancer models. Separate chapters in this book will
review dietary fat effects on carcinogenesis in the mammary gland (Chapter by Adrianne Rogers), colon (Chapters
by Bandaru Reddy and by Paul Newberne), liver (Chapter by
Hisashi Shinozuka) and the pancreas (Chapters by Diane
Birt and Bill Roebuck and by Robert Landers). Cancer at
several other sites, which have been studied for effects
of dietary fat, will be briefly summarized in this chapter. In addition, this introductory chapter will discuss
changing methodologies applied to assessing dietary fat
effects on carcinogenesis.

DIETARY FAT EFFECTS ON CARCINOGENESIS AT SITES OTHER THAN THE MAMMARY GLAND, COLON, LIVER OR PANCREAS

Early studies on the influence of dietary fat on carcinogenesis were reviewed in 1975 by Carroll and Kohr and
more recent work was summarized by Birt (1986). Dietary
fat effects on skin carcinogenesis were evaluated extensively in work by Dr. Albert Tannenbaum and other investigators of that time, as reviewed (Tannenbaum and
Silverstone, 1953). These studies usually employed benzo-
(a)pyrene (BP) or ultraviolet light as the carcinogen and
commercial dog or rodent food as the diet. Consistent
enhancement of skin carcinogenesis was observed in mice

fed increasing fat levels and the effects were greatest when the high fat diets were fed following carcinogen treatment (Tannenbaum and Silverstone, 1953). Recent studies with ultraviolet light-induced skin cancer demonstrated an increased probability of tumors in mice fed 4% or 12% corn oil diets, in comparison with those given 12% hydrogenated corn oil (Black et al., 1983).

In early studies on spontaneous lung tumors in ABC mice, high fat diet had no influence on cancer yield (Tannenbaum, 1942). Spontaneous lung cancer in TM mice was, however, elevated in those fed diet supplemented with ether or alcohol extracts of egg in comparison with mice fed unsupplemented diet or diets supplemented with the extracted egg powder (Szepsenwol, 1964). Studies with Syrian hamsters demonstrated enhanced carcinogenesis by BP in the lungs, when 20% beef tallow was added to diets, and further enhancement, when 20% sunflower oil was added (Beems and van Beek, 1984). These diets were fed before, during and after BP treatment. Separate hamster studies indicated that feeding 20.4% corn oil either before or after treatment with N-nitrosobis(2-oxopropyl)amine (BOP) elevated lung adenoma yields (Birt and Pour, 1983). In both hamster studies the animals fed high fat diets gained 15-30% more weight (Beems and van Beek, 1984; Birt and Pour, 1983).

Other sites at which effects of dietary fat on carcinogenesis were assessed are the brain, earduct, kidneys, prostate and muscle. Brain nerve cell tumors were observed in mice fed diets supplemented with various combinations of lipids and lipid fractions for several generations (Szepsenwol, 1969). Renal cancer was observed only in hamsters fed 9 or 20.4% corn oil, in comparison with 4.2% corn oil, before and after treatment with BOP (Birt and Pour, 1983). However renal cancer induced by 1,2-dimethylhydrazine (DMH) or methylazoxymethanol acetate (MAM) was not influenced by dietary fat (Reddy et al., 1977). Spontaneous prostatic cancer in Lobund strain Wistar rats treated with testosterone was found in a preliminary report (Pollard and Luckert, 1985) to be elevated in rats fed diets supplemented with 20% corn oil. However, prostatic carcinogenesis induced by cyproterone acetate and testosterone was not influenced by the level or type of dietary fat in a separate study (Kroes et al., 1986). Earduct cancer induced by DMH or MAM was not influenced by

dietary fat (Reddy et al., 1977) and early reports indicated no effect of dietary fat on sarcoma incidence
(reviewed in Carroll and Khor, 1975).

METHODS FOR ASSESSING DIETARY FAT EFFECTS ON CARCINO-
GENESIS

Several general changes in experimental approach have
occurred, since effects of dietary fat on chemical carcinogenesis were first observed. In particular:

1) Early studies often added crude dietary fat to complete diets, which were generally natural ingredient diets
that are noted for variability (Greenman et al., 1980).
More refined fats, sometimes purified essential fatty
acids (EFA), and purified diets are generally used now.
This change avoids the undesirable contaminants present in
natural ingredient diets, in addition to allowing the
investigator improved control in diet formulation.

2) Concern for the types of fatty acids fed has
increased with a growing understanding of the importance
of differences in fatty acids.

3) As the use of semipurified diets increased, experiments often compared excessively low dietary fat levels
(<0.5%) to excessively high levels (20-30%), without
including an intermediate level (4-8%). A basis for inclusion of intermediate levels was provided by the National
Research Council Subcommittee on Laboratory Animal Nutrition (National Research Council, 1978). Recent studies
compare adequate dietary fat with excessive levels and
include adequate controls when diets insufficient in fat
are studied.

4) As information developed on stages in the carcinogenesis process, e.g., via initiation/promotion models,
researchers on dietary fat have shown more concern for the
period of time experimental dietary fat levels are fed
relative to the time of carcinogenic treatment. In addition carcinogenesis models have been developed for more
human cancers and more single or limited treatment models
are available to study stages of carcinogenesis.

5) Investigators are adjusting their diets for the nutrient dilution observed when fat is added to diets (Newberne et al., 1978; Visek and Clinton, 1983). In the past fat was often supplementary to a complete diet, with considerable caloric dilution of the other nutrients in the diet, or it was substituted for an equal number of grams of carbohydrate with a more modest, but significant, dilution of nutrient density. The method of substituting fat for an equivalent number of calories from carbohydrate has now been recognized as an appropriate correction for this nutrient dilution. However, there is some dispute regarding the values for nutrient density, which should be used in formulating diets, since numerous factors can influence the caloric value of fat, protein and carbohydrate. It should be recognized that the recommended adjustment results in much lower carbohydrate intakes in the high fat diets.

ACKNOWLEDGEMENTS

Research conducted in this laboratory was supported by a Public Health Service grant R01 CA31655-02 from the National Cancer Institute and preparation of this chapter was aided by a Laboratory Cancer Research Center grant P30 CA36727-02 from the National Cancer Institute.

REFERENCES

Beems RB, van Beek L (1984). Modifying effect of dietary fat on benzo(a)pyrene-induced respiratory tract tumors in hamsters. Carcinogenesis 5:413-417.

Birt DF (1986). Dietary fat and experimental carcinogenesis: A summary of recent in vivo studies. In Poirier LA, Pariza M, Newberne PM (eds): "Essential Nutrients in Carcinogenesis", New York, NY: Plenum Press, in press, 1986.

Birt DF, Pour PM (1983). Increased tumorigenesis induced by N-nitrosobis(2-oxopropyl)amine in Syrian golden hamsters fed high-fat diets. J Natl Cancer Inst 70:1135-1138.

Black HS, Lenger W, Phelps AW, Thornby JI (1983). Influence of dietary lipid upon ultraviolet-light carcinogenesis. Nutr Cancer 5:59-68.

Carroll KK, Khor HT (1975). Dietary fat in relation to tumorigenesis. Prog Biochem Pharmacol 10:303-353.

Greenman DL, Oller WL, Littlefield NA, Nelson CJ (1980). Commercial laboratory animal diets: Toxicant and nutrient variability. J Toxicol Env Health 6:235-246.

Kroes R, Beems RB, Bosland MC, Bunnik GSJ, Sinkeldam EJ (1986). Nutritional factors in lung, colon, and prostate carcinogenesis in animal models. Federation Proc 45:136-141.

National Research Council (1978). "Nutrient Requirements of Laboratory Animals." Washington, D.C.: National Academy Press, Third Revised Edition.

Newberne PM, Bieri JG, Briggs GM, Nesheim MC (1978). Control of diets in laboratory animal experimentation. Inst Lab Animal Res News 21:A1-A12.

Pollard M, Luckert PH (1985). Promotional effects of testosterone and dietary fat on prostate carcinogenesis in genetically susceptible rats. Prostate 6:1-5.

Reddy BS, Watanabe K, Weisburger JH (1977). Effect of high fat diet on colon carcinogenesis in F344 rats treated with 1,2-dimethylhydrazine, methylazoxymethanol acetate or methylnitrosourea. Cancer Res 37:4156-4159.

Szepsenwol J (1969). Brain nerve cell tumors in mice on diets supplemented with various lipids. Pathol Microbiol 34:1-9.

Szepsenwol J (1964). Carcinogenic effect of ether extract of whole egg, alcohol extract of egg yolk and powdered egg free of the ether extractable part in mice. Proc Soc Exp Biol Med 116:1136-1139.

Tannenbaum A (1942). The genesis and growth of tumors. III. Effects of a high fat diet. Cancer Res 2:468-475.

Tannenbaum A, Silverstone H (1953). Nutrition in relation to cancer. Adv Cancer Res I:451-501.

Tucker MJ (1979). The effect of long term food restriction on tumors in rodents. Int J Cancer 23:803-807.

Visek WJ, Clinton SK (1983). Dietary fat and breast cancer. In Perkins EG, Visek WJ (eds): "Dietary Fats and Health", Champaign, Illinois: American Oil Chemists Society, pp 721-740.

Dietary Fat and Cancer, pages 255–282

CHEMICALLY-INDUCED MAMMARY GLAND TUMORS IN RATS: MODULATION BY DIETARY FAT

Adrianne E. Rogers and Soon Y. Lee

Department of Pathology
Boston University School of Medicine
Boston, MA 02118 (AER) and Department of Applied
Biological Sciences, Massachusetts Institute of
Technology,
Cambridge, MA 02139 (SYL)

Introduction

Dietary fat content has highly significant, reproducible and consistent effects on chemically induced mammary gland tumorigenesis in female rats. The fats that are effective reduce tumor latency and may increase final tumor incidence and number. The enhancement of tumorigenesis by fat can be reduced by addition of selenium to the diet, by treatment with indomethacin and by hormonal manipulations. The mechanism of the fat effect is not known. It may be due in part to enhanced growth from highly efficient utilization of calories from fat, oxidative damage to cell constituents, subtle endocrine alterations or abnormal metabolism of carcinogens and promoting agents. These and other potential factors have been reviewed recently (Welsch, 1985) and are the subjects of other chapters in this volume. The effect of fat can be demonstrated if it is fed throughout the rat's lifetime or if it is fed only before or only after carcinogen exposure. This suggests that fat influences mammary tumorigenesis by more than one mechanism.

Chemically-Induced Mammary Gland Tumors in Rats

The rat models for breast cancer are reasonably well standardized and widely used and have produced a large body of useful information. The tumors induced are, however, often benign or of borderline malignancy, particularly when the carcinogens are given in low doses to detect subtle dietary effects. Further development and analysis of the models are needed to resolve conflicts in the experimental data and increase correspondence between the rat mammary gland tumors and human breast cancer.

DMBA

With Huggins' description of induction of mammary gland tumors in rats by a single dose of 7, 12-dimethylbenzanthracene (DMBA) in 1961 there began a period of intense and productive investigation of mammary gland tumorigenesis. Earlier models, the development of the single dose model and the major results derived from the model have been reviewed (Welsch, 1985). The single dose model has permitted elucidation of factors that act at initiation of neoplasia in the gland and at the subsequent steps in tumor development and has provided a large amount of information on mammary gland tumors. Review of papers published in the last 10 years from several laboratories shows good agreement on tumorigenesis induced in female Sprague-Dawley (S-D) rats by DMBA with only the minor variations that can be expected on the basis of biological variation or differences in protocols in different laboratories. Characteristic results are summarized in Tables 1 & 2. Other rat strains respond to DMBA, but S-D rats are the most widely used and are the basis of discussion in this chapter.

Factors in the experimental protocol that have the greatest influence on tumor latency, incidence and number are age of the rat at DMBA exposure, her reproductive history and endocrine status and composition of the diet fed; dose and route of administration of DMBA have variable effects. Rats show maximum sensitivity to DMBA tumorigenesis in the period beginning shortly after vaginal opening and ending after establishment of regular estrous cycles. This is a period of rapid growth of the gland and occurs between approximately 35 and 60 days of age. Increasing age, completed pregnancy and lactation all decrease susceptibility of the gland to chemical carcinogenesis and increase the proportion of tumors that are benign. The relatively resistant epithelium is characterized by a low growth fraction and a lengthened G_1 phase in the cell cycle (Russo et al., 1983). Induction of tumors by DMBA is dependent upon a normal hormonal environment. Hormone dependence demonstrated by ovariectomy, occurs in about 80% of DMBA-induced tumors. The hormone-dependent tumors regress if circulating estrogen and prolactin are reduced or withdrawn or if tissue hormone receptors are blocked. The small number of tumors induced in rats treated at the time of DMBA administration with tamoxifen and bromocryptine to block estrogen effects and prolactin release, respectively, are much less likely to be hormone-dependent than tumors induced in normal rats. (Sylvester et al., 1986a).

There are several nutrients and other components of diet that influence tumorigenesis; they will be discussed below. In general, rats fed natural ingredient diets are somewhat less susceptible to chemical carcinogens than rats fed purified diets. This effect is not prominent in the mammary tumor models. Comparison of results in rats fed purified or natural ingredient diets, such as the data summarized in Tables 1 and 2, does not indicate major differences between the 2 types of diet. In a direct comparison of tumorigenesis induced by intravenous (iv) injection of 5 mg DMBA in rats fed natural product or purified diets, rats fed the purified diet had a slightly but not significantly shorter latent period and a higher incidence and multiplicity of tumors than rats fed a natural product diet. (Aylsworth et al., 1984).

Dose responses are detectable in reduced latency (time to first palpable tumor or, in some reports, to all palpable tumors) with increasing dose and, less consistently, in increased tumor incidence and number. Because new tumors continue to appear with time after exposure, final tumor incidence and number may not show a clear dose response. Complete reporting of data including latency, cumulative tumor incidence and number and time between treatment with DMBA and necropsy is required for full evaluation of experimental results in the model. Review of results summarized in Tables 1 & 2 shows that a wide range of doses of DMBA has been used to induce tumors, and that parenteral (iv or subcutaneous, sc) administration as well as administration by gastric gavage (ig) is effective. Latency to first palpable tumor induced by a given dose of DMBA following the same protocol in the same laboratory can vary by many weeks; tumor incidence and number also vary between experiments (Tables 1 and 2; Ip et al. 1985). It is important to recognize the variability of results and take it into consideration when evaluating potential tumorigenesis-modulating factors. Enteral and intravenous administration of DMBA give similar results (Tables 1 & 2). The choice depends upon convenience and the importance of including or avoiding effects due to gastrointestinal absorption and first pass hepatic metabolism of DMBA. Direct application of DMBA to the surgically exposed gland or injection of carcinogen into the gland can be used and are useful in examining local factors in tumorigenesis. Preliminary experiments suggest that it may be possible to alter the histologic spectrum of tumors induced and increase the fraction of malignant tumors by using local injection since large local doses can be given without causing systemic toxicity. (Rogers, unpublished).

TABLE 1

MAMMARY TUMORS INDUCED BY DMBA IN 50-60 DAY OLD, FEMALE SPRAGUE-DAWLEY RATS FED NATURAL INGREDIENT DIETS

DMBA Dose(mg)	Route	Weeks DMBA-Necropsy	Mammary Tumors			Reference
			Latency[a] (wks)	Incidence	No/Rat at Risk	
20	ig	32	12	91	5.4	McCormick, et. al., 1982
20	ig	28	20	60	0.7	Minton et al., 1983
20	ig	17	7	85	2.6	Thompson, et al., 1982
15	ig	40	16	89	1.0	
20	ig	11	--	100	3.9	Welsch & Dehoog, 1983
10	ig	12	--	90	4.5	
5	ig	26	--	85	2.0	
15	ig	30	--	75	1.6	Moon et. al., 1976
5	ig	30	--	46	0.6	
2.5	ig	30	--	8	0.1	
8	ig	30	14	88	8.6	McCormick et al., 1984
5	ig	28	22	63	2.4	Welsch et al., 1981
3/100g	iv	--	11	80	1.5	Sinho & Dao, 1980
5	iv	21	15	81	2.6	Sylvester et al., 1982
5	iv	16	11	72	2.7	Sylvester et al., 1983
5	iv	26	12	97	2.6	Nagasawa et al., 1976
1	sc[b]	--	9	100	1.0	Sinho & Dao, 1980
0.5	sc[b]	19	12	63	0.63	Jabara & Anderson, 1982
0.1	sc[b]	19	17	30	0.30	
0.03	sc[b]	19	11	5	0.05	

[a] DMBA to first palpable tumor; value read from graphs if not stated in text in reference cited.

[b] applied locally to the surgically exposed gland.

TABLE 2

MAMMARY TUMORS INDUCED BY DMBA GIVEN TO 50-55 DAY OLD FEMALE
SPRAGUE-DAWLEY RATS FED PURIFIED, CONTROL DIETS CONTAINING 3-5% FAT[a]

DMBA Dose(mg)	Route	Weeks DMBA-Necropsy	Latency	%Incidence	No/Rat At Risk	Reference
5	ig	17	--	70	2.3	Hopkins & Carroll, 1979
		19	--	70	2.1	Hopkins et al., 1981
		17	11	77	2.3	Carroll & Khor, 1971
5	ig	20-22	--	46	1.3	Ip & Ip, 1981
		22	13	40	0.9	Ip & Sinha, 1981
		22	17	44	1.0	Carter et al., 1983
2.5	ig	35	16	68	1.4	Rogers et al., 1986
		35	22	83	1.7	Lee & Rogers, 1983
		10-12	9	78	2.9	Rogers, et al., 1986
		32	16	52	1.4	Rogers et al., 1985
5	iv	16	10	88	5.4	Aylsworth et al., 1984a
		16	11	75	3.0	Aylsworth et al., 1984b
2.5	iv	19	13	83	1.7	Rogers et al., 1986
1	sc	19	6	84	1.8	
0.5	sc	25	15	79	1.3	
0.25	sc	17	11.	80	1.3	

a   In some experiments rats were fed natural ingredient diets up to
    DMBA administration and then fed purified diets. The types of
    fat included polyunsaturated vegetable oils and mixed or largely
    saturated animal fats.

b   DMBA to 1st palpable tumor; value read from graphs if not stated
    in text in reference cited.

The mammary gland tumors induced in rats by a single dose of DMBA comprise a spectrum of morphology from benign, typical fibroadenomas and adenomas to papillomas with hyperplastic, atypical or dysplastic epithelium and significant stromal and myoepithelial components, to tumors that are architecturally and cytologically malignant and invade adjacent normal tissue. Metastases from even the most anaplastic tumors are rare. The pathogenesis of DMBA-induced mammary tumors has been thoroughly and elegantly described (Russo et al., 1983). Morphologic characterization of normally developing mammary glands in female S-D rats has been made using whole mounts, autoradiographs to detect DNA synthesis and histologic and histochemical methods to characterize stem cells and their progeny differentiating into epithelial and myoepithelial, alveolar and ductal elements (Dulbecco et al., 1982, 1983; Russo et al., 1983; Warburton et al. 1982).

Carcinogenesis is thought to occur primarily in the epithelium of the terminal end buds (TEB's) while they are developing into alveolar buds and terminal ducts; these structures make up the terminal duct lobular units (TDLU's). Excessive epithelial proliferation and development of progressive cytologic abnormality result from carcinogen exposure and ultimately produce tumors. Several classifications of rat mammary tumors have been presented (Young & Hallowes, 1973; Greaves & Faccini, 1984; Van Zwieten, 1984). The most highly malignant tumors (histologically) are similar in appearance to intraductal and infiltrating ductal carcinomas in humans. They are, however, a minority of the tumors induced in rats by the commonly used regimens. Similarly, benign fibroadenomas and adenomas that occur in rats resemble closely the human benign tumors but compose only a few percent of tumors induced in most studies. The majority of induced tumors are papillomatous with hyperplastic epithelium that may contain 2 cell types (epithelial and myoepithelial) and appear cytologically benign or that may be composed of epithelial cells with varying degrees of cytological atypia, growing in solid, papillary or adenomatous patterns. The abnormal epithelium tends to remain rigidly confined by the adjacent stroma, show no clear evidence of invasion and vary considerably within and between tumors. All of these features contribute to the difficulty of making clear distinctions between benign and malignant lesions and raise questions about the validity of all but the most malignant tumors as models for human breast cancer.

Factors and pathways that result in the different histologic types of tumors are largely unknown. High single doses of DMBA generally induce a greater fraction of histologically malignant tumors than the low doses often used to evaluate dietary and other tumorigenesis-modulating effects. In an examination of relationships between DMBA dose and number of histologically malignant tumors induced, Isaacs (1985) reported that a single 5 mg dose of DMBA induced a low yield of carcinomas in rats treated at age 36, 43, 50 or 57 days and examined 200 days later. Final results were similar in the 4 age groups. He reported markedly lower malignant tumor incidences than McCormick et al., 1985, using similar protocols (Table 3). The number and percent of malignant tumors was increased synergistically by repeated doses of carcinogen with yields of 1.2, 2.4 and 4 malignant tumors per rat induced by, respectively, 2, 3 or 4 doses of DMBA, 5 mg each; with a single dose he obtained only 0.2 tumors per rat at risk. In studies using a single low dose of DMBA, the fraction of mammary tumors that was malignant and the incidence of malignant tumors were increased if a high fat diet was fed (Rogers et al., 1986; Clinton et al., 1984). Examples of tumor histologic classification in the DMBA or N-nitrosomethylurea (MNU) (to be discussed below) models are given in Table 3.

The single-dose models have been extraordinarily useful in the development of theories of the carcinogenic process in the mammary gland. They have produced many of the data that make up our knowledge of the events and modulating factors in initiation, promotion and progression of tumors. However, the predominance of benign tumors or mixed tumors of questionable malignancy may be a disadvantage when one extrapolates data form them to predict behavior of malignant tumors. Dietary and other factors significant in development of malignant mammary gland tumors might be defined more clearly if data are reported separately for malignant tumors and for borderline and benign lesions. For example, in a recent examination of indomethacin suppression of DMBA mammary tumorigenesis, induction of malignant tumors by a high dose of DMBA (16 mg) showed less evidence of an effect of indomethacin than induction of the (largely) benign tumor population by 8 mg DMBA (McCormick et al., 1985). Sensitivity of the model for detection of dietary effects is enhanced when histologic classification of tumors is taken into consideration (Rogers et al., 1986). Use of multidose models may be indicated in studies of dietary and other tumorigenesis modulating factors in which timing of specific events in the process is not critical.

DMBA is activated in the liver, mammary gland and other tissues. Binding of labeled DMBA or its metabolites to mammary gland nuclei and DNA after in vivo or in vitro

TABLE 3
MAMMARY GLAND TUMOR HISTOLOGY IN RATS GIVEN A SINGLE
DOSE OF DMBA OR MNU
AT 50-60 DAYS AND FED DIETS CONTAINING 4-5% FAT

Carcinogen	Dose[a]	Weeks Carcinogen To Necropsy	Malignant No/Rat	% All Tumors Malignant	Reference
DMBA	20	32	3.8	81	McCormick, et al., 1982
DMBA	16	21	6.4	74	McCormick, et al., 1985
DMBA	8	30	3.2	34	
DMBA	8	30	2.2	26	McCormick, et al., 1984
DMBA	20	28	2.5	b	Isaacs, 1985
	15	28	1.5		
	10	28	0.7		
	5	28	0.2		
	2.5	28	0.04		
DMBA	7.5	19	1.2	100	Sylvester, et al., 1986
DMBA	2.5	10-12	0.5	17[c]	Rogers, et al., 1986
MNU	50	3.0	3.2	82	Grubbs, et al., 1983a
MNU	50	26	3.5	78	Grubbs, et al., 1983b
MNU	35	--	2.3	79	McCormick et al., 1983
MNU	50(7.5)[d]	28	5.3	b	Isaacs, 1985
	40(6.0)	28	2.5		
	30(4.5)	28	1.6		
	20(3.0)	28	0.5		
	10(1.5)	28	0.2		

a   DMBA mg/rat given by gastric gavage; MNU: mg/kg given by intravenous injection.

b   In this study only malignant tumors were reported.

c   An additional 48% was classified as borderline, giving a total of 1.9 malignant or borderline malignant tumors composing 65% of all tumors. (see Table 8).

d   The dose per rat was reported and is given in parenthesis; the mg/kg dose was calculated assuming an average rat weight of 150 grams.

exposure has been demonstrated by autoradiographic and chromatographic procedures. (Russo et al., 1983; Vigny et al., 1985). The mammary gland DNA adducts detected 24 hours after exposure to a 20 mg, ig dose of DMBA were consistent with activation by formation of vicinal diol-expoxides in the 1,2,3,4-ring and agreed with results of activation studies in other tissues (Vigny et al., 1985).

Toxicokinetic studies of DMBA after ig or ip administration have been reported, and the information has been expanded recently to include rats fed high fat diets. (Lee et al., 1986) Absorption from the GI tract is rapid with peak blood levels at 1-3 hours. Clearance curves are biphasic (Levine 1974, Lee et al. 1986). Blood radioactivity declines rapidly for about 6 hours; decay then slows, and label is still detectable at 30 hours. The peak concentration in the gland occurs at 3-6 hours. There is about 100 times more total radioactivity in mammary fat pad cells than in mammary parenchymal cells (Gammal et al., 1965; Janss and Moon, 1970, Lee et al., 1986). A high lard diet, fed as in the carcinogenesis protocol up to 48 hours before administration of DMBA, had no effect on absorption or clearance, but polar metabolites persisted in the blood and liver at a higher level in rats fed high fat than in controls. (Lee et al, 1986).

MNU

MNU (N-nitrosomethylurea) has been used increasingly in the last ten years to induce mammary tumors. It is administered parenterally, usually by iv injection but also by sc injection into the back (Thompson and Meeker, 1983) or into the mammary fat pad (Rogers, unpublished). It was reported to induce significantly more malignant tumors than were induced by DMBA (Gullino et al, 1975; McCormick et al. 1982). The differences are not large, however, and are not consistently found (Williams et al., 1981; Isaacs, 1985). The percent malignant tumors increases, and the histologic patterns may alter, with increasing number of doses of MNU (Rose et al., 1980; Isaacs, 1985). MNU is effective in Fischer 344, Buffalo and 3-D rats (Chan et al., 1977; Chan & Dao, 1981). As with DMBA, tumors arise more often in the upper (cervicothoracic) than in the lower glands (Thompson & Meeker, 1983). Characteristic results are given in Tables 6 and 7. Purified and natural ingredient diets appear to support similar tumorigenesis, but in a direct comparison of the 2 types of diet in 3 strains of rat, Chan and Dao (1981) found reduced latency and increased tumor numbers in rats fed the purified diet. The sample of results of MNU tumorigenesis in Sprague-Dawley rats given in Tables 4

TABLE 4

MAMMARY TUMORS INDUCED BY INTRAVENOUS ADMINISTRATION OF MNU
TO 50-60 DAY OLD SPRAGUE DAWLEY RATS FED NATURAL INGREDIENT DIETS

MNU mg/kg b.w.	Weeks MNU to Necropsy	Latency (wks)	% Incidence	No/Rat[a]	Reference
50	26	15	70	3.3	Chan & Dao, 1981
50	32	8	100	4.8	McCormick et al., 1982
50	26	11	90	4.5	Grubbs, et al., 1983b
50[b]	21	10-12	70-89	1.4-2.0	Ratko & Beattie, 1985
50	30	14	90	3.9	Grubbs et al., 1983a
50	26	10	90	4.3	Thompson & Meeker, 1983
50	14-68	9	100	7.5	McCormick et al., 1981
25	14-80	34	70	2.7	
10	37-86	--	45	2.6	
50x2	25	15	41	1.1	Rose et al., 1980
50x2	26	9	94	6.8	Grubbs et al., 1983c
25x2	31	--	73	2.7	Welsch et al., 1980
12.5x2	25	--	27	0.5	

a   No. per rat at risk; recalculated from published data if given as
    no per tumor-bearing rat.

b   Lower latency and higher incidence and multiplicity values are
    for rats treated at proestrus or estrus, others for rats treated
    at diestrus.

TABLE 5

MAMMORY TUMORS INDUCED BY PARENTERAL ADMINISTRATION OF MNU
TO 50-60 DAY OLD, SPRAGUE-DAWLEY RATS FED PURIFIED CONTROL
DIETS CONTAINING 3-5% FAT

| MNU mg/kg b.w. | Weeks MNU To Necropsy | Mammary Tumors | | | Reference |
		Latency (wks)	%Incidence	No/Rat[a]	
50 (iv)	26	14	88	6.4	Chan & Dao, 1981
50 (iv)	18	11	91	2.4	Silverman et al., 1980
50 (iv)	18	14	50	1.0	Wei et al., 1985
	28	16	90	1.8	
50 (sc)	26	7	100	7.6	Thompson et al., 1984
35 (sc)	26	11	96	4.1	Thompson et al., 1985

a No per rat at risk (recalculated from published data if
   expressed as no. per tumor-bearing rat).

and 5 shows that average latency can be expected to be 8-16 weeks if one uses the most frequently used protocol, a single iv injection of 50 mg/kg. A tumor incidence of nearly 100% can be expected at 6 months with 2-7 tumors per rat. In an early characterization of the model, McCormick et al., (1981) reported that malignant tumors appeared earlier than benign tumors and that the percent of tumors that were benign tended to increase as dose decreased; this observation was due in part to the appearance with increasing age of spontaneous tumors. At the highest MNU doses (35-50 mg/kg) 86-94% of tumors were malignant; at lower doses, the percent malignant tumors was 42-70%.

Susceptibility to tumorigenesis by MNU is strongly age-dependent. Grubbs et al. (1983b) found a marked decrease in tumor incidence and multiplicity with age at first dose in Sprague-Dawley rats given 2 doses of MNU, 50 mg/kg each, 1 week apart, as age increased from 35 to 200 days. Chan and Dao (1983) reported similar results in Fischer rats given a single dose of MNU at 35, 50, 90 or 130 days; results were not different in rats treated at 35 or 50 days. There is an influence of stage of the estrous cycle at the time of carcinogen exposure. Tumor response is higher and latency shorter in rats given MNU at proestrus or estrus than at diestrus (Lindsey et al., 1981; Ratko & Beattie, 1985). Tumor induction is reduced by prior pregnancy and lactation (Grubbs et al., 1983c) and by treatment with pharmacological doses of 17-B-estradiol or oophorectomy after carcinogen administration. Progesterone also has some inhibitory effect. The inhibitory endocrine treatments reduced slightly, but not significantly, the proportion of malignant tumors (Grubbs et al., 1983a). The tumors are hormone-dependent and responsive (Gandilhon et al., 1983); hormone receptors have been identified and measured (Lindsey et al., 1981). MNU-induced tumors may be somewhat more responsive to estrogen and less to prolactin than DMBA-induced tumors, but the responses are similar in direction. (Welsch, 1985).

The cellular Ha-ras-1 oncogene locus is activated in 83% of MNU-induced tumors tested from 3 rat strains. An identical G --> A transition in the 2nd nucleotide of the 12th codon was found in all cases. Activation of the same oncogene by DMBA was observed in 21% of tumors examined; the activating mutation occurred in the 2 deoxyadenosine residues in codon 61. The authors conclude that the MNU-induced activation is concomitant with initiation by MNU, but the significance of the DMBA activation is not clear (Zarbl et al., 1985).

Dietary Fat and Mammary Tumorigenesis

In both rat models described, tumor development is markedly influenced by dietary fat. In experiments based on epidemiological evidence that breast cancer is associated with dietary fat intake, Carroll and his colleagues, (Carroll and Khor, 1975) and subsequently many other investigators have shown that feeding rats diets high in certain fats increases the tumorigenic effect of DMBA and MNU on the mammary gland. The influence of high dietary fat has been shown primarily by demonstration of decreased tumor latency. Increased tumor incidence and number may be found at termination of experiments if termination is relatively early. (Tables 6 and 7)

The dietary fat contents compared have been generally 3-5% by wt. for control and 20-25% for high fat, values that will be so designated in this chapter. Investigators have used lower, and rarely higher, fat content. Diets lower than 3% in fat are often not fully supportive of growth and may be deficient in essential fatty acids (EFA). They may not permit normal hormone synthesis and secretion or growth and differentiation of the mammary gland . They are, therefore, not suitable controls for high fat diets, although they may provide useful information about basic fat requirements of the gland. Polyunsaturated fats and their constituent fatty acids (PUFA) from vegetable sources are more effective in enhancing tumorigenesis than fats from animal sources. Saturated and monounsaturated fats have little or no effect. Polyunsaturated w-3 fats have recently been reported to be inhibitory. These polyunsaturated fats derived from fish oils and some plants contain largely C_{20} and C_{22} w-3 fatty acids rather than the C_{18} w-6 fatty acids (Jurkowsky and Cave, 1985).

The enhancing effect of fat shows a dose response to linoleic acid content with added effects of other constituents. Carroll and Khor (1975) reported that enhancement occurred after some minimum level of PUFA had been provided and that the remaining fat content could be composed of saturated fats. They demonstrated enhancement by feeding 3% oil (about 2% linoleate) and 17% saturated fat. The minimum level of PUFA required for tumorigenesis enhancement was greater than the dietary requirement of rats since rats fed 1% corn oil and 19%-23% of beef tallow or rapeseed oil showed no enhancement of tumorigenesis (Lee & Rogers, 1983). Rats fed 1% corn oil and 19-23% lard, providing a total of about 2.7% linoleate, did show tumorigenesis enhancement. (Rogers et al. 1985, Wetsel et al 1981). Ip et al. (1985) demonstrated a dose responsive effect of DMBA-induced

TABLE 6

DMBA-INDUCED MAMMARY TUMORIGENESIS IN SPRAGUE-DAWLEY RATS

FED HIGH CORN OIL DIETS

Dietary Corn Oil		Mammary Gland Tumors			DMBA		DMBA-	Reference
%	Wks Fed[a]	Latency (wks)	Incidence (%)	No.	mg/ rat	route	Necropsy (wks)	
5	0-16	11	77	2.3	5	ig	16	Carroll & Khor, 1971
10	0-16	10	93	4.0				
20	0-16	10	90	3.6				
5	0-22	13	33	0.5	5	ig	22	Ip & Sinha, 1981
25	0-22	12	60	1.6				
5	-5-36	16	68	2.0	2.5	ig	36	Wetsel et al., 1981
20	-5-36	14	83	2.0				
5	0-24	13	44	1.1	5	ig	24	Selenskas et al. 1984
20	0-24	10	80	2.9				
4.5	0-16	11	75	3.6	5	iv	16	Aylsworth et al. 1984
20	0-16	9	78	6.5				
	4-7	11	96	5.0				

[a] Zero = DMBA administration at 50-60d of age

TABLE 7

MNU INDUCED MAMMARY TUMORIGENESIS IN FISCHER 344 RATS FED HIGH

FAT DIETS

Dietary Corn Oil		Mammary Gland Tumors[a]		No.	Reference
%	Wks Fed[b]	Latency (wks)	Incidence (%)		
5	-4-24	11	36	0.6	Chan & Dao, 1983
25	-4-24	8	79	1.7	
5	0-24	--	39	0.6	Dao & Chan, 1983
25	1-24	--	70	1.7	
25	8-24	--	62	1.5	
5	0-22	17	66	--	Cohen et al, 1984
23	0-22	12	87	--	

[a] Time from MNU to necropsy was 22-24 weeks in all experiments.

[b] Zero = MNU administration at 50-60 days of age.

tumorigenesis to dietary linoleic acid provided by corn oil with a plateau at 8% corn oil, which corresponded to 4.8% lineolate. The total fat content was 20% with the balance provided saturated fatty acids in by palm oil or coconut oil. However in a study in Fischer rats using MNU rather than DMBA, Cohen et al, (1984) found no enhancing effect of a diet containing 6% corn oil and 17.6% medium chain triglycerides, the major component of coconut oil. Chan et al. (1983) reported data indicating that several fatty acids contributed to the effect of fat. The variable results obtained in different studies examining the relative importance of amounts of unsaturated and saturated fatty acids fed and the interactions between type and amount of fat indicate a need for further studies. The results may be clarified by consideration of tumor histology.

In a series of experiments in rats examining the effect on DMBA mammary tumorigenesis of feeding a high lard diet, tumor latency and growth rate were measured, and the tumors were classified histologically into benign (fibroadenoma, adenoma, papilloma), borderline malignant and malignant categories. All were single dose experiments; DMBA, 2.5 mg, was given by gastric intubation (Rogers et al., 1986). Rats fed high fat regimens that supported increased tumorigenesis, manifested by decreased tumor latency or increased tumor number or incidence, had a significantly increased fraction of tumors that were malignant compared to control rats (Table 8). There was a greater number of tumors per rat at risk in the high-fat groups; the increase was composed of an approximately 2.8 times increase in malignant tumors and a smaller increase in borderline and benign tumors (Table 8). The average growth rate, using geometric mean diameter, of all malignant tumors was 0.32 cm/wk $^+_-$ 0.22 (SD.); for borderline and benign tumors the rate was 0.20 cm/wk $^+_-$ 0.22; the difference was highly significant, P < 0.0001. There was no effect of dietary fat content on growth rate within the histological categories. Clinton et al. (1984, 1986) reported a higher incidence of malignant tumors in DMBA-treated rats fed a high corn oil diet. It may be necessary to use a relatively small dose of DMBA to demonstrate the effect of high fat diets on tumor histology since it has not been reported in earlier studies.

Aylsworth et al., (1986) reported that a diet high in corn oil that decreased latency of DMBA-induced tumors did not increase tumor growth rate. This agrees with our result in rats fed a high lard diet. It appears that the effective high fat diets do not influence growth of malignant or benign tumors after they become palpable and

TABLE 8
DMBA-INDUCED TUMORS IN RATS FED CONTROL OR HIGH-LARD DIETS

Diet	No of Rats	Incidence (%)	Total	Malignant[b]	Borderline	Benign
				Number per rat at risk[a]		
Control	99	78	2.9	0.5(28)	1.4	1.0
High Lard	100	85	4.3	1.4(41)	1.7	1.2

a   Rats were killed and necropsied 10-12 weeks after DMBA.
b   Percent of rats bearing malignant tumors shown in parenthesis.

TABLE 9

MAMMARY TUMORS INDUCED BY PARENTERAL DMBA IN RATS FED
CONTROL PURIFIED DIET CONTAINING 5% FAT

DMBA Route	Dose (mg/rat)	Total	Malignant	Borderline	Benign
			No. Mammary Tumors[a]		
sc	1	1.8	0.4	0.7	0.7
	0.5	1.2	0.2	0.6	0.4
	0.25	1.4	0.4	0.8	0.2
iv	2.5	1.6	0.3	0.6	0.7

a   Per rat at risk; 18-20 rats per group. Rats were killed
and necropsied when they bore a 2 cm tumor or at termination of the experiments 4-6 months after DMBA administration. Tumor incidence was 68-95% in different groups.

measurable but exert their effect on the stages from initiation to appearance of palpable tumor. Studies using local injection of carcinogen may be useful in studying dietary fat effects on tumor histology and growth. Histology of tumors induced by DMBA injection in rats fed a control fat diet was similar to histology of tumors induced by ig DMBA. (Tables 8,9)

In mouse models it has been clearly demonstrated that EFA are required for growth of transplanted mammary tumors. If mice are fed fat-free diets or diets that contain hydrogenated coconut oil or oleic acid, and therefore do not supply EFA, tumor growth is reduced compared to growth in mice fed corn oil or linoleic acids. Linolenic acid also did not support tumor growth despite its ability to meet EFA requirements. (Abraham and Hillyard, 1983); Abraham et al., 1984; Gabor et al, 1985) Menhaden oil, a source of w3 fatty acids found to reduce rather than enhance DMBA tumorigenesis in rats, reduced tumor growth in mice fed corn oil if the menhaden oil was fed at a ratio of 9:1 corn oil. (Gabor and Abraham, 1985; Abraham, et al., 1986)

Dietary fat effects on MNU-induced tumorigenesis have been reported primarily in Fisher 344 rather than S-D Dawley rats. Characteristics of the fat effects are similar to findings using DMBA in S-D rats insofar as they have been studied. Corn oil is highly effective when fed after administration of a single dose of MNU. It enhances tumorigenesis over a wide age range (Chan & Dao, 1983) and range of doses of MNU (Dao & Chan, 1983). Lard fed at 25% of the diet gave an enhancement similar to but somewhat less than corn oil and beef tallow had little if any effect (Chan & Dao, 1983).

The mechanisms of the high fat effect are not known. Hypotheses proposed and tested fall into 2 groups; mechanisms specific for the mammary gland and mechanisms that may be generally applicable to the several organs in which high fat diets enhance carcinogenesis. Many of these are discussed in detail elsewhere in this volume. Specific mechanisms examined in the mammary gland include effects of high fat diets on circulating hormones, mammary gland tissue hormone receptors, mammary gland growth and differentiation and mammary gland metabolism and binding of DMBA. More generalized hypotheses include effects of the high fat diets on caloric balance, carcinogen kinetics, tissue peroxide content, cellular immunological responses, prostaglandin secretion, balance and distribution and cell membrane composition and response to growth factors. Examination of proposed mechanisms has provided a large amount of useful information about interactions of dietary fat and mammary tumorigenesis even if the mechanisms of the interactions have not been identified.

Because of the availability of single dose models for mammary tumorigenesis, it has been possible to investigate extensively the timing and duration of the enhancing effect of high dietary fat. The predominant effect is exerted after carcinogen exposure, is directly correlated to duration of feeding of the high fat diet and inversely correlated to the time between carcinogen exposure and introduction of the high fat diet. The polyunsaturated vegetable oils appear to act primarily during the post-exposure period although data have been reported that show that this is partially due to the longer feeding period (Dao and Chan, 1983). Recent reports using a low dose of DMBA show an inhancing effect of corn oil fed only before DMBA exposure (Clinton et al, 1986). Lard, which is a mixed, predominantly monounsaturated fat, enhances tumorigenesis when fed only before carcinogen exposure (Rogers et al., 1982; Rogers et al, 1986; Sylvester et al., 1986), and beef tallow, which is highly saturated, may have an effect at or before exposure. The determinants of the effect at initiation are not known. Contributions of fatty acid composition, the antioxidants butylated hydroxyanisole (BHA) and -- toluene (BHT) to the effect of lard, which is somewhat variable, or evidence of contaminating estrogenic or toxic or carcinogenic compounds were not found in an extensive series of experiments examining timing of the activity of lard. (Rogers et al, 1986).

The importance of active DNA synthesis in the TDLU in governing age-related susceptibility of the gland to carcinogenesis, led to examination of DNA synthesis in mammary glands of rats fed high lard or control diets prior to DMBA administration. Increased DNA synthesis could contribute to the enhancing effect of fat at initiation or at later stages. DNA synthesis was evaluated by isolation and counting of DNA from TDLU and counting labeled cells in autoradiographs. It was not different in the 2 diet groups at the time of DMBA administration (55 days) or at later times examined until the period at which tumors began to appear, about 10 weeks after DMBA was given. At that time counts of ^{3}H-thymidine incorporation were higher in nontumorous glands from rats fed high lard than from control rats. Autoradiographic examination of the glands showed increased small ducts with heavily labeled epithelium. (Lee et al., 1986) Flow cytometric measurements of cells isolated from the glands showed no abnormalities of cell cycle patterns or of ploidy.

The search for hormonal mechanisms to explain the effect of fat has yielded essentially negative results and is discussed in a separate chapter (Welsch). A recent study (Sylvester et al., 1986a) indicated that a high corn oil diet stimulated development of both hormone-dependent and hormone independent tumors induced by DMBA, but did not influence the hormone responsiveness of the tumors.

The question of the relative importance of fat and the calories it provides was raised by Kritchevsky (1984) in his studies of mammary tumorigensis by DMBA. The question is relevant to all tissues in which tumorigenesis is enhanced by high fat diets and has been a subject of discussion for about 40 years. The marked effect of specific fats, such as corn oil and lard, on mammary tumorigenesis and the absent or reduced effects of other, equally well-utilized fats, such as supplemented beef tallow or olive oil indicates that the effective fats have an activity aside from their caloric contributions.

Interaction of dietary protein (casein) and fat (corn oil) content has been studied in the DMBA model. (Clinton et al., 1984) S-D rats fed purified diets that provided 8,16 or 32% calories from casein and 12,24 or 48% calories from corn oil were given DMBA, 2 mg/g body wt at 50 days of age. Tumor latency was inversely proportional to dietary corn oil content in all 3 dietary protein groups except the lowest in which only the highest corn oil content reduced latency. Tumor incidence and multiplicity increased with dietary fat content. Dietary protein content had no detectable effect on tumorigenesis. Effects of dietary protein alone in the DMBA model are considered in a seperate chapter in this volume. (Hawrylewicz)

Effect of Other Nutrients and Selected Chemicals on Mammary Tumorigenesis

Dietary supplementation by selenium at levels in the toxic or near-toxic range partially inhibits tumorigenesis, particularly in rats fed diets high in polyunsaturated fat The inhibiting effect is detectable at initiation and during promotion of tumorigenesis, is maximized by continuous administration of selenium, and is enhanced by additional supplementation with vitamin E, a nutrient that does not by itself inhibit DMBA tumorigenesis. (Ip, 1985). Selenium supplementation (5mg/kg) of a nutritionally complete, natural product diet significantly reduced tumor multiplicity but not incidence in MNU-treated rats and caused a significant decrease in weight gain which may have contributed to the decrease in tumor numbers. Selenium- deficient rats given MNU had increased tumor multiplicity but no change in incidence (Thompson & Becci, 1980). Vanadyl (IV) sulfate (Thompson et al., 1984) and molybdenum supplementation (Wei et al., 1985) both reduced MNU tumorigenesis without reducing weight gain.

Reduction of tumorigenesis by feeding high levels of retinyl acetate or less toxic synthetic retinoids has been demonstrated repeatedly in several laboratories. As with selenium, long-term administration is most effective, but inhibition can be demonstrated by short periods of feeding at the time of initiation or during promotion. Tumors may appear rapidly after retinoid administration is stopped. The retinoids retard growth and development of the normal mammary gland when fed at tumor-inhibiting doses. (Welsch, 1985; Moon et al, 1983).

Pharmacological and dietary non-nutrient modulating factors have been described also. Among these, coffee and caffeine are of particular interest because associations between coffee intake and benign or malignant breast disease has been reported, although inconsistently, in epidemiological studies. (Reviewed in Petrek et al. 1985, and Welsch et al., 1983). In a two-year study in which S-D female rats were fed brewed coffee and given no known carcinogen, the incidence of mammary tumors was unchanged compared to controls, but the mammary tumors appeared somewhat earlier in coffee-fed rats. (Palm et al., 1984). In DMBA-treated rats, consumption of caffeine in a 20% fat, purified diet decreased latency to tumor and increased tumor multiplicity but did not influence final tumor incidence; when given with a natural product diet, however, caffeine had the opposite effect; it increased tumor latency and reduced incidence. (Minton et al., 1983). Food intake and body weight are not discussed, and the basis for the inconsistent results can not be determined. Welsch et al. (1983), using a larger amount of caffeine, found consistent evidence that caffeine increased the incidence and number of tumors induced by DMBA in S-D rats. In contrast, similar doses of caffeine inhibited mammary tumorigenesis by diethylstilbestrol (DES) in ACI rats. (Petrek et al., 1985). The differences in strain and carcinogen may be responsible for the different results; specific information on tumor histology is not given in the reports and may also be of interest in view of the variable results.

Several food antioxidants, including BHA and BHT, other chemicals such as B-naphthoflavone and cysteamine, cruciferous vegetables and green coffee beans reduce DMBA tumorigenesis. (Welsch, 1985). BHA and BHT must be fed at high doses (0.3 - 0.6%) to inhibit tumorigenesis; when BHA was fed at the maximum level permitted in foods (0.02%), it had no detectable effect. (Rogers et al, 1986).

REFERENCES

Abraham S, Faulkin LJ, Hillyard LA (1984). Effect of dietary fat on tumorigenesis in the mouse mammary gland. J Natl Cancer Inst 72:1421-1429.

Abraham S, Faulkin LA, Hillyard LA, Mitchell DJ (1986). Effect of dietary fat on various states of mammary gland development and tumorigenesis in mice. Proc AACR 27.

Abraham S, Hillyard LA (1983). Effect of dietary 18-carbon fatty acids on growth of transplantable mammary adenocarcinomas in mice. J Natl Cancer Inst 71:601-605.

Aylsworth CF, Cullum ME, Zile MH, Welsch CW (1986). Influence of dietary retinyl acetate on normal rat mammary gland development and on the enhancement of 7,12-dimethylbenz[a]antracene-induced rat mammary tumorigenesis by high levels of dietary fat. J Natl Cancer Inst 76:339-345.

Aylsworth CF, Jones C, Trosko JE, Meites J, Welsch CW (1984). Promotion of 7,12-dimethylbenz[a]anthracene-induced mammary tumorigenesis by high dietary fat in the rat: Possible role of intercellular communication. JNatl Cancer Inst., 72:637-645.

Alysworth CF, Van Vugt DA, Sylvester W, Meites J, (1984a) Role of estrogen and prolactin in stimulation of carcinogen-induced mammary tumor development by a high-fat diet. Cancer Res 44: 2835-2840.

Carroll KK, Khor HT (1975). Dietary fat in relation to tumorigenesis. Prog. Biochem Pharmacol 10:308-322.

Carroll KK, Khor HT, ((1971) Effects of level and type of dietary fat on incidence of mammary tumors induced in female Sprague-Dawley rats by 7,12-dimethylbenz(a)Anthracene. Lipids 6:415-420.

Carter CA, Milholland RJ, Shea W, Ip MM (1983). Effect of the prostaglandin synthetase inhibitor indomethacin on 7,12-dimethylbenz(a)anthracene-induced mammary tumorigenesis in rats fed different levels of fat. Cancer Res 43:3559-3562.

Chan P-C, Dao TL (1981). Enhancement of mammary carcinogenesis by a high-fat diet in Fischer, Long-Evans, and Sprague-Dawley rats. Cancer Res 41:164-167.

Chan P-C, Dao TL (1983). Effects of dietary fat on age-dependent sensitivity to mammary carcinogenesis. Cancer Letters 18:245-249.

Chan P-C, Ferguson KA, Dao TL (1983). Effects of different dietary fats on mammary carcinogenesis. Cancer Res 43:1079-1083.

Chan P-C, Head JF, Cohen LA, Wynder EL (1977). Influence

of dietary fat on the induction of mammary tumors by N-nitrosomethylurea: Associated hormone changes and differences between Sprague-Dawley and F344 rats. J Natl Cancer Inst 59:1279-1283.

Clinton SK, Alster JM, Imrey PB, Nandkumar S, Truex R, Visek W, (1986) Dietary protein, fat and caloric intake during an initiation phase study of 7,12-dimethylbenz(a)anthracene-induced breast cancer in rats. J Nutr in press.

Clinton SK, Imrey PB, Alster JM, Simon J, Truex CR, Visek WJ (1984). The combined effects of dietary protein and fat on 7,12-dimethylbenz(a)anthracene-induced breast cancer in rats. J Nutr 114:1213-1223.

Cohen LA, Thompson DO, Maeura Y, Weisburger JH (1984). Influence of dietary medium-chain triglycerides on the development of N-methylnitrosourea-induced mammary tumors. Cancer Res 44:5023-5026.

Dao TL, Chan P-C (1983). Effect of duration of high fat intake on enhancement of mammary carcinogenesis in rats. J Natl Cancer Inst 71:201-205.

Dulbecco R, Henahan M, Armstrong B (1982). Cell types and morphogenesis in the mammary gland. Proc Natl Acad Sci 79:7346-7350.

Dulbecco R, Unger M, Armstrong B, Bowman M, Syka P (1983). Epithelial cell types and their evolution in the rat mammary gland determined by immunological markers. Proc Natl Acad Sci 80:1033-1037

Gabor H, Abraham S (1985). Effect of dietary menhaden oil on growth and cell loss of transplantable mammary adenocarcinoma in mice. Proc. AACR 26:126.

Gabor H, Hillyard LA, Abraham S (1985). Effect of dietary fat on growth kinetics of transplantable mammary adenocarcinoma in BALB/c mice. J Natl Cancer Inst 74:1299-1305.

Gammal EB, Carroll KK, Muhlstock BH, Plunkett ER (1965). Quantitative estimation of 7,12-dimethylbenzanthracene in rat mammary tissue by gas liquid chromatography. Proc Soc Exp Bio Med 119:1086-1089.

Gandilhon P, Melancon R, Djiane J, Kelly P (1983). N-nitroso-N-methylurea-induced mammary tumors in the rat: Role of prolactin and a prolactin-lowering drug. J Natl Cancer Inst 70:105-109.

Greaves P, Faccini JM, (1984). Tumors of the mammary gland. In "Rat Histopathology", Amsterdam: Elsevier, 10-14.

Grubbs CJ, Peckham JC, McDonough KD (1983a). Effect of ovarian hormones on the induction of 1-methyl-1-nitrosourea-induced mammary cancer. Carcinogenesis 4:495-497.

Grubbs CJ, Peckham JC, Cato KD (1983b). Mammary carcinogenesis in rats in relation to age at time of N-nitroso-N-methylurea administration. J Natl Cancer Inst

70:209-212.

Grubbs CJ, Hill DL, McDonough KC, Peckham JC (1983c). N-Nitroso-N-methylurea-induced mammary carcinogenesis: Effect of pregnancy on preneoplastic cells. J Natl Cancer Inst 71:625-628.

Gullino PM, Pettigrew HM, Grantham FH (1975). N-Nitrosomethylurea as mammary gland carcinogen in rats. J Natl Cancer Inst 54:401-414.

Hopkins GJ, Carroll KK, (1979). Relationship between amount and type of dietary fat in promotion of mammary carcinogenesis induced by 7,12-dimethylbenzanthracene. J Natl Cancer Inst 62:1009-1012.

Hopkins GJ, Kennedy TG, Carroll KK, (1981). Polyunsaturated fatty acids as promoters of mammary carcinogenesis induced in Sprague-Dawley rats by 7,12-dimethylbenzanthracene. J Natl Cancer Inst 66:517-522.

Ip C, Ip M, (1981) Serum estrogens and estrogen responsiveness in 7,12-dimethylbenz(a)anthracene-induced mammary tumors as influenced by dietary fat. J Natl Cancer Inst 66:291-295.

Ip C (1985). Selenium inhibition of chemical carcinogenesis. Fed Proc 44:2573-2578.

Ip C, Carter CA, Ip M (1985). Requirement of essential fatty acid for mammary tumorigenesis in the rat. Cancer Res 45:1997-2001.

Ip C, Sinha DK (1981). Enhancement of mammary tumorigenesis by dietary selenium deficiency in rats with a high polyunsaturated fat intake. Cancer Res 41:31-34.

Isaacs JT (1985). Determination of the number of events required for mammary carcinogenesis in the Sprague-Dawley female rat. Cancer Res 45:4827-4832.

Jabara AG, Anderson PS, (1982) Effects of progesterone on mammary carcinogenesis when various doses of DMBA were applied directly to rat mammae. Pathology 14:313-316.

Janss DH, Moon RC (1970). Uptake and clearance of 9,10-dimethyl-1,2-benzathrancene-9-^{14}C by mammary parenchymal cells of the rat. Cancer Res 30:473-479.

Jurkowski JJ, Cave WT (1985). Dietary effects of menhaden oil on the growth and membrane lipid composition of rat mammary tumors. J Natl Cancer Inst 74:1145-1150.

Kritchevsky D, Weber MM, Klurfeld DM, (1984). Dietary fat versus caloric content in initiation and promotion of 7,12-dimethylbenzanthracen-induced mammary tumorigenesis in rats. Cancer Res 44:3174-3177.

Lee S-Y, Rogers AE (1983). Dimethylbenzanthracene mammary tumorigenesis in Sprague-Dawley rats fed diets differing in content of beef tallow or rapeseed oil. Nutr Res 3:361-371.

Lee S-Y, Walsh CT, Ng SF, Rogers AE (1986). Toxicokinetics of 7,12-dimethylbenz(a)anthracene (DMBA) in rats fed high lard or control diet (submitted for publication).

Levine, WG (1974). Hepatic uptake, metabolism, and biliary excretion of 7,12-dimethylbenzanthracene in the rat, Drug Metab Dispos 2: 169-177.

Lindsey WF, Das Gupta TK, Beattie CW (1981). Influence of the Estrous cycle during carcinogen exposure on nitrosomethylurea-induced rat mammary carcinoma. Cancer Res 41:3857-3862.

McCormick DL, Adamowski CB, Fiks A, Moon RC, (1981) Lifetime dose-response relationships for mammary tumor induction by a single administration of N-Methyl-N-nitrosourea. Cancer Res 41:1690-1694.

McCormick DL, Madigan MJ, Moon RC (1985). Modulation of rat mammary carcinogenesis by indomethacin. Cancer Res 45:1803-1808.

McCormick DL, Major N, Moon RC (1984). Inhibition of 7,12-dimethylbenz(a)anthracene-induced rat mammary carcinogenesis by concomitant or postcarcinogen antioxidant exposure. Cancer Research 44:2858-2863.

McCormick DL, Mehta RG, Thompson CA, Dinger N, Caldwell JA, Moon RC (1982). Enhanced inhibition of mammary carcinogenesis by combined treatment with N-(4-hydroxyphenyl) retinamide and ovariectomy. Cancer Res 42:508-512.

McCormick DL, Sowell ZL, Thompson CA, Moon RC (1983). Inhibition by retinoid and ovariectomy of additional primary malignancies in rats following surgical removal of the first mammary cancer. Cancer 51:594-599.

Minton JP, Abou-Issa H, Foecking MK, Sriram MG (1983). Caffeine and unsaturated fat diet significantly promotes DMBA-induced breast cancer in rats. Cancer 51:1249-1253.

Moon RC, Grubbs CJ, Sporn MB, (1976) Inhibition of 7,12-dimethylbenz(a)anthracene-induced mammary carcinogenesis by retinyl acetate. Cancer Res 36:2626-2630.

Moon RC, McCormick DL, Mehta RG (1983). Inhibition of carcinogenesis by retinoids. Cancer Res 43:2469s-2475s.

Nagasawa H, Yanai R, Taniguchi H, (1976) Importance of mammary gland DNA synthesis on carcinogen-tumorigenesis in rats. Cancer Res 36:2223-2226.

Palm PE, Arnold EP, Nick MS, Valentine JR, Doerfler TE (1984). Two-year toxicity/carcinogenicity study of fresh-brewed coffee in rats initially exposed in Utero. Toxicol Appl Pharm 74:364-382.

Petrek JA, Sandberg WA, Cole MN, Silberman MS, Collins DC (1985). The inhibitory effect of caffeine on hormone-induced rat breast cancer. Cancer 56:1977-1981.

Ratko TA, Beatie CW (1985). Estrous cycle modification of rat mammary tumor induction by a single dose of N-methyl-N-nitrosourea. Cancer Res 45:3042-3047.

Rogers AE, Conner BH, Boulanger CL, Lee SY, Carr FA, Dumouchel WH (1985). Enhancement of 7,12-dimethylbenz(a)anthracene mammary carcinogenesis by a high lard diet. In Vahouny GV, Kritchevsky D (eds):

"Dietary Fiber," New York, Plenum, pp 444-455.
Rogers AE, Fernstrom JD, GE K, McConnell RG, Leavitt WW, Wetsel WC, Yang SO, Camelio EA (1982). Endocrine interactions in the nutritional modulation of mammary carcinogenesis in rats. In Arnott, MS, Van Eys J., Wang YM (eds): "Molecular Interrelations of Nutrition and Cancer," New York: Raven. pp 381-399.
Rogers AE, Connor B, Boulanger C, Lee S (1986). Mammary tumorigenesis in rats fed diets high in lard. Lipids (in press)
Rose DP, Pruitt B, Stauber P, Erturk E, Bryan GT (1980). Influence of dosage schedule on the biological characteristics of N-nitrosomethylurea-induced rat mammary tumors. Cancer Res 40:235-239.
Russo J, Tay LK, Ciocca DR, Russo IH (1983). Molecular and cellular basis of the mammary gland susceptibility to carcinogenesis. Environmental Health Perspectives 49:185-199.10
Selenskas SL, Ip MM, Ip C (1984). Similarity between trans fat and saturated fat in the modification of rat mammary carcinogenesis. Cancer Res. 44:1321-1326.
Silverman J, Shellabarger CJ, Holtzman S, Stone JP, Weisburger JH, (1980) Effect of dietary fat on x-ray-induced mammary cancer in Sprague-Dawley rats. J Natl Cancer Inst 64: 631-634.
Sinha DK, Dao TL, Induction of mammary tumors in aging rats by 7,12-dimethylbenz(a)anthracene: role of DNA synthesis during carcinogenesis. J Natl Cancer Inst 64:519-521.
Sylvester PW, Aylsworth CF, Van Vugt DA, Meites J, (1982) Influence of underfeeding during the "critical period"or thereafter on carcinogen-induced mammary tumors in rats. Cancer Res 42:4943-4947.
Sylvester PW, Aylsworth CF, Van Vugt DA, Meites J, (1983) Effects of alterations in early hormonal environment on development and hormone dependency of carcinogen-induced mammary tumors in rats. Cancer Res 43:5342-5346.
Sylvester PW, Ip C, Ip M (1986a). Effects of high dietary fat on the growth and development of ovarian-independent carcinogen-induced mammary tumors in rats. Cancer Res 46:763-769.
Sylvester PW, Russell M, Ip MM, Ip C (1986a). Comparative effects of different animal and vegetable fats fed before and during carcinogen administration on mammary tumorigenesis, sexual maturation and endocrine function in rats. Cancer Res 45:757-762.
Thompson HJ, Becci PJ (1980). Selenium inhibition of N-methyl-N-nitrosourea-induced mammary carcinogenesis in the rat. J Natl Cancer Inst 65:1299-1301.
Thompson HJ, Chasteen ND, Meeker LD (1984). Dietary vanadyl(IV) sulfate inhibits chemically-induced mammary carcinogenesis. Carcinogenesis 5:849-851.

Thompson HJ, Meeker DL (1983). Induction of mammary gland carcinomas by the subcutaneous injection of 1-Methyl-1-nitrosourea. Cancer Research 43:1628-1629.

Thompson HJ, Meeker LD, Herbst EJ, Ronan AM, Minocha R (1985). Effect of concentration of D,L-2-difluoromethylornithine on murine mammary carcinogenesis. Cancer Res 45:1170-1173.

Thompson HJ, Meeker LD, Tagliaferro AR, Becci PJ, (1982) Effect of retinyl acetate on the occurrence of ovarian hormone-responsive and nonresponsive mammary cancers in the rat. Cancer Res 42:903-905.

VanZwieten, MJ (1984). The Rat as Animal Model in Breast Cancer Research, The Hague: Martinus Nijhoff.

Vigny P, Brunissen A, Phillips DH, Cooper CS, Hewer A, Grover PL, Sims P (1985). Metabolic activation of 7,12-dimethylbenz(a)anthracene in rat mammary tissue: Fluorescence spectral characteristics of hydrocarbon-DNA adducts. Cancer Letters 26:51-59.

Warburton MJ, Mitchell D, Ormerod EJ, Rudland P (1982). Distribution of myoeptihelial cells and basement membrane proteins in the resting, pregnant, lactating, and involuting rat mammary gland. J Histochem Cystochem 30:667-676.

Wei J, Luo X-M, Yang SP (1985). Effects of molybdenum and tungsten on mammary carcinogensis in SD rats. J Natl Cancer Inst 74:469-473.

Welsch CW (1985). Host factors affecting the growth of carcinogen-induced rat mammary carcinomas: A review and tribute to Charles Brenton Huggins. Cancer Res 45:3415-3443.

Welsch CW, Brown CK, Goodrich-Smith M, Chiusano J, Moon RC (1980). Synergistic effect of chronic prolactin suppression and retinoid treatment in the prophylaxis of N-methyl-N-nitrosourea-induced mammary tumorigenesis in female Sprague-Dawley rats. Cancer Res 40:3095-3098.

Welsch CW, DeHoog JV (1983). Retinoid feeding, hormone inhibition, and/or immune stimulation and the genesis of carcinogen-induced rat mammary carcinomas. Cancer Res 43:585-591.

Welsch CW, Goodrich-Smith M, Brown CK, Greene HD, Hamel E, (1981) Selenium and the genesis of murine mammary tumors. Carcinogenesis 2:519-522.

Welsch CW, Scieszka KM, Senn ER, DeHoog JV (1983). Caffeine (1,3,7-trimethylxanthine), a temperate promoter of DMBA-induced rat mammary gland carcinogenesis. Int J Cancer 32:479-484.

Wetsel WC, Rogers AE, Newberne PM, (1981) Dietary fat and DMBA mammary carcinogenesis in rats. Cancer Detection Prevention 4:535-543.

Williams, JC, Gusterson B, Humphreys J, Monaghan P, Coombes RC, Rudland P, Neville AM (1981). N-methyl-N-nitrosourea-induced rat mammary tumors. Hormone

responsiveness but lack of spontaneous metastasis.   J.
Natl Cancer Inst 66:147-155.
Young S, Hallowes RC: (1973).   Tumors of the Mammary Gland
   In Turosov VS (ed); "Pathology of Tumors in Laboratory
   Animals" Vol. 1 Lyons: IARC, pp 31-74.
Zarbl H, Sukumar S, Arthur AV, Martin-Zanca D, Barbacid M
   (1985).   Direct mutagenesis of Ha-ras-1 oncogenes by N-
   nitroso-N-methylurea during initiation of mammary
   carcinogenesis in rats. Nature 315:382-385.

Dietary Fat and Cancer, pages 283–294
© 1986 Alan R. Liss, Inc.

RELEVANCE OF TRANS FATTY ACIDS AND FISH OIL IN ANIMAL
TUMORIGENESIS STUDIES

Clement Ip, Margot M. Ip and Paul Sylvester
Department of Breast Surgery (C.I.), and
Grace Cancer Drug Center (M.M.I., P.S.),
Roswell Park Memorial Institute, Buffalo,
New York 14263

INTRODUCTION

Throughout this book, there are many chapters
comparing the effects of animal versus vegetable fats on
experimental tumorigenesis. In recent years, investigators
are beginning to show an interest in two other types of
dietary lipid, namely trans fatty acids and fish oil. The
purpose of this article is to summarize the existing,
although limited, literature regarding the modification of
tumor development as a result of feeding animals diets
containing either trans fat or fish oil.

Nature and Occurrence of Trans Fatty Acids

Since the turn of this century, there has been a trend
towards an increasing per capita consumption of fat in the
United States (Rizek, 1981). Virtually all of the increase
can be accounted for by vegetable fats, most of which are
subjected to a series of processing steps to convert them
from seed oils to various food products. After extraction
and refining, it is estimated that about 70% of vegetable
fats are partially hydrogenated for marketing. Partial
hydrogenation is important for imparting desirable stability
and physical properties to many edible oil products such as
salad and cooking oils, mayonnaise, shortenings and
margarines.

Hydrogenated fats differ in many ways from natural
vegetable fats; the most significant change is the
introduction of trans fatty acids. In addition to a

reduction in the number of double bonds through hydrogenation, some double bonds rearrange from the cis to the trans configuration and some double bonds migrate to new positions in the fatty acid chain. Industrial hydrogenation is thus known to produce positional and geometric isomers of the natural unsaturated fatty acids, resulting in a product that is high in trans-monoenes. The orientation of a trans double bond results in straightening of the hydrocarbon chain, forming a structure resembling more closely a saturated fatty acid chain molecule. Since most of the polyunsaturated fatty acids in vegetable oils contain a high proportion of linoleic acid, the majority of trans acids generated during hydrogenation have a chain length of 18 carbon atoms. Smaller amounts of geometric and/or positional isomers of dienoic acids are also formed; these are mainly cis-trans, trans-cis and trans-trans isomers of octadecadienoic acid. The levels and types of cis and trans isomers present depend on the hydrogenation conditions such as temperature, time and the kind of catalyst used.

Data available to the Institute of Shortenings and Edible Oils indicate that most liquid or solid cooking fats contain 5 to 25% trans isomers, while most stick margarines contain 20 to 35% trans isomers. There is currently no reliable information on the consumption of trans fat in the United States, although it has been estimated that hydrogenated fats may constitute about 44% of the "visible fat" in American diets (Emken, 1980). It should be noted that small amounts of isomeric fatty acids occur naturally in foods such as milk, butter and tallow as a result of microbial biohydrogenation in ruminants (Parodi, 1976).

Design of Trans Fat and its Appropriate Control in the Study of DMBA-Induced Mammary Carcinogenesis

The first study examining the relationship between trans fat intake and tumor growth in an animal model was published only a few years ago. Awad (1981) reported that ingestion of elaidic acid (9-trans-C18:1) reduced the survival time of mice bearing the Ehrlich ascites tumor. The control animals in this study were fed a similar amount by weight of olive oil, which is high in oleic acid (9-cis-C18:1). Results of this study are difficult to interpret because it is inappropriate to compare the feeding of a triglyceride (olive oil) with the feeding of a free fatty acid (elaidic acid). Elaidic acid has a melting point of

$45^{\circ}C$ and is therefore very poorly digested. Moreover, the two lipids differ substantially in fatty acid composition, thus invalidating the conclusion that the shortened survival time of tumor-bearing mice was due to elaidic acid exclusively.

Food products contain trans fatty acids as triglycerides. In order to properly evaluate the effect of trans fat intake, a lipid in triglyceride form of similar fatty acid composition and in the cis configuration should be used as a control. The use of the parent fat source (from which the hydrogenated fat is derived) as control would be misleading, since the two lipids would have different fatty acid profiles. We have investigated the effect of feeding a fat which contained approximately 38% trans fatty acids (designated as trans fat) on the induction of mammary tumors by dimethylbenz(a)anthracene (DMBA) in rats (Selenskas et al, 1984). The corresponding control fat (designated cis fat) was specially blended to have a fatty acid composition similar to that of the trans fat, but consisted only of cis isomers. Since both the cis and trans fats were rather saturated in nature, a comparison was made between these two types of fats and corn oil, which contains about 60% linoleic acid (9-cis, 12-cis, C18:2).

The fatty acid composition of these three fats, as determined by gas chromatograhy, is shown in Table 1. The trans fat was a partially hydrogenated mixture of 50% soybean oil and 50% cottonseed oil. It was high in monoenes and low in dienes and other polyenes. The cis fat consisted of 58% olive oil, 40% cocoa butter, and 2% coconut oil. Animals were fed purified diets containing either 5% or 20% fat by weight. Considering the virtual absence of linoleic acid in the trans fat (as indicated by the cis, cis-lipoxygenase value), 1% of corn oil was added to the trans fat diet to prevent essential fatty acid deficiency. The same amount of corn oil was also added to the cis fat diets to minimize differences in fatty acid composition between the cis fat and trans fat diets. Therefore, the low fat diets contained 4% trans or cis fat plus 1% corn oil, and the high fat diets contained 19% trans or cis fat plus 1% corn oil. As a matter of convenience, the low fat and high fat trans or cis diets will be referred to as 5% and 20% trans or cis diets, respectively. The concentrations of linoleic acid and trans acids in each diet are shown in Table 2.

Table 1   Fatty acid composition of dietary fats[a]

Fatty Acid	Trans Fat	Cis Fat	Corn Oil
10:0	–	0.1	–
12:0	1.3	0.8	–
14:0	1.0	0.4	–
16:0	17.6	17.1	10.4
16:1	–	–	0.1
17:0	–	–	–
18:0	15.9	15.7	1.9
18:1	57.5	54.7	24.9
18:2	6.1	8.5	60.8
18:3	0.2	0.6	1.3
20:0	0.3	0.8	0.6
22:0	–	0.3	–
% Trans	38.3[b]	ND[c]	ND
cis, cis-lipoxygenase	ND	8.4	61.9
Iodine Value	59	65	130

[a] Expressed as percent of total fatty acids.

[b] Capillary GC and IR spectroscopy gave comparable results for total trans levels. Capillary GC indicated that the trans fat consisted of about 92% trans monoenes.

[c] Not detectable.

Table 2   Levels of linoleic acid and trans acids in
various diets

Dietary Fat	5% Dietary Fat		20% Dietary Fat	
	Linoleic Acid	Trans Acids	Linoleic Acid	Trans Acids
		(g/100 g of diet)		
Trans fat[a]	0.61	1.5	0.61	7.2
Cis fat[a]	0.95	–	2.2	–
Corn oil	3.0	–	12.2	–

[a] Includes the contribution of 1% corn oil added to the
diet.

Results of this study are illustrated in Fig. 1.
Although rats fed the 20% trans fat or cis fat diets had a
slightly higher tumor incidence and yield than those on the
corresponding 5% fat control diets, the difference was not
statistically significant. In contrast, rats fed the 20%
corn oil diet developed a much greater number of tumors than
did rats fed a diet containing only 5% corn oil. Further
analysis of the data showed that diets containing either
trans fat or cis fat were much less effective than the corn
oil diets in promoting the development of mammary neoplasia
at either the 5% or 20% level. Since the cis fat was the
appropriate control for the trans fat in this experiment, it
can be concluded that trans versus cis isomerization of
fatty acids has no detectable effect in the modification of
mammary carcinogenesis.

Trans Fat and Other Tumor Models

Following the publication of our work in 1984, several
papers have appeared in the literature examining the effect
of trans fat intake on other tumor models. Hogan and
Shamsuddin (1984) have compared the effect of a high trans
fatty acid diet (25% elaidic acid) with a high cis fatty
acid diet (25% oleic acid) on the development of
azoxymethane-induced colon tumors in rats. Although they
found that the incidence of large intestinal carcinoma was
higher in the trans fatty acid group (37%) than in the cis

fatty acid group (23%), the difference was not statistically significant. Using the _trans_ and _cis_ fats similar to those in our study described above, Erickson et al (1984) observed that there was no difference in tumor growth rate or final tumor size in mice carrying a subcutaneous mammary tumor implant and fed these diets. Moreover, when tumor cells were injected intravenously to the animals, _trans_ fatty acids were found to be less effective in promoting distant metastasis. Further studies examining the effect of _trans_ fat on colon carcinogenesis induced by either dimethylhydrazine or azoxymethane have recently been reported (Watanabe et al, 1985; Reddy et al, 1985). These studies differed in the levels of _trans_ fatty acids given to the animals. However, they nonetheless suggest that the _trans_ monoene behaves like _cis_ monoene in modifying cancer risk and that it is less effective than the _cis_-polyunsaturated fatty acid in stimulating the development of colon tumors.

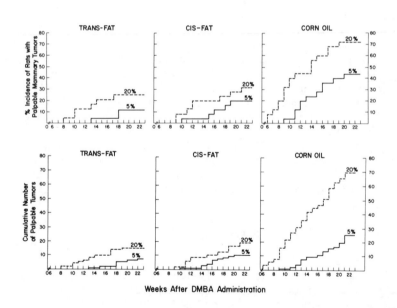

Fig. 1. Incidence and cumulative number of palpable mammary tumors in rats fed either _trans_ fat, _cis_ fat or corn oil at a level of 5 or 20% in the diet. There were 25 rats/group. (Selenskas et al, 1984, with permission).

Biological Significance of Trans Fatty Acids

It is established that trans fatty acids are readily absorbed and are incorporated mainly into the neutral triglyceride fraction (Beare-Rogers, 1983). Several workers have reported that the trans fatty acids are oxidized at rates equivalent to the corresponding cis isomers (Coots, 1964; Lawson and Kummerow, 1979; Stearns et al, 1967). On the other hand, in vitro studies have shown that mitochondria from rats fed trans fatty acids were more susceptible to swelling and have a lower rate of oxidation (Hsu and Kummerow, 1977), although it should be pointed out that the rats in this study were apparently deficient in essential fatty acid. Kinsella and coworkers (1981) have recently reported that high levels of dietary trans, trans-C18:2 impair   6-desaturase activity and decrease prostaglandin synthesis. Although there is legitimate concern as to the biochemical consequence of this metabolic perturbation, suffice it to note that trans, trans-dienes are present in only trace amounts in hydrogenated fats (Marchand and Beare-Rogers, 1982). In general, several carefully controlled long-term animal studies have shown that feeding high levels of trans monoenes, in the presence of adequate linoleic acid, did not result in any overall deleterious effects (Aaes-Jorgensen et al, 1956; Alfin-Slater et al, 1957; Mattson, 1960). Watanabe et al (1985) showed that fecal neutral steroid excretion was higher in rats given trans fat, but there was no change in the excretion and composition of fecal bile acids. Since increased levels of bile acids have been associated with enhanced colon carcinogenesis (Cohen and Reicht, 1981), the lack of stimulation by trans fat of bile acid production would suggest that trans fat is no more likely than cis fat to promote the development of colon tumors.

Fish Oil and Experimental Tumorigenesis

Fish oils are generally high in eicosapentaenoic and docosahexaenoic acids. These are long chain omega-3 polyunsaturated fatty acids with 5 and 6 double bonds, respectively. In contrast, linoleic and arachidonic acids belong to the family of omega-6 polyunsaturated fatty acids. When omega-3 fatty acids are ingested, they are incorporated into tissue lipids in place of omega-6 fatty acids. The omega-3 fatty acids may exert their effects by competing with arachidonic acid for the cyclooxygenase and lipoxygenase enzymes which regulate the synthesis of a host of active metabolites including thromboxanes, prostaglandins, prostacyclin, hydroxyeicosatetraenoic acids and leukotrienes. Thus, perturbation of the arachidonic acid metabolic cascade could form the biochemical basis by which fish oil influences cellular functions and the disease processes.

Research on the relationship of fish oil and cancer risk is still in its infancy, with only a handful of publications appearing in the literature in the last two years. Karmali et al (1984) showed that supplementation of the diet with fish oil significantly reduced the size of the transplantable R3230AC mammary tumor in rats after four weeks of treatment. Both tumor content and in vitro synthesis of prostaglandins of the two series were inhibited in the fish oil-treated group. Using the mammary tumor model induced by N-methyl-N-nitrosourea, Jurkowski and Cave (1985) reported that a diet containing 20% menhaden oil actually produced a reduction in tumor incidence and yield when compared to diets containing lower levels of menhaden oil (3% or 0.5%). Similar findings were also observed by Carroll and Braden (1985) with the DMBA-induced mammary tumor model. This is the only type of dietary fat known to produce an inverse relationship between intake and tumorigenesis. The effect of fish oil on the development of pancreatic preneoplastic lesions induced by L-azaserine in rats was examined by O'Connor and coworkers (1985). They found that a 20% menhaden oil diet produced a significant decrease in the size and number of atypical acinar cell nodules when compared to a 20% corn oil diet.

We have previously shown that the essential fatty acid requirement (linoleic acid) for maximal expression of mammary tumorigenesis is approximately 4% (Ip et al, 1985). Corn oil contains high levels of linoleic acid (about 60%) and has been demonstrated consistently by many investigators to be very effective in stimulating tumor development if present in large quantities in the diet. Menhaden oil contains about 2% linoleic acid and may not be enough to support optimal neoplastic growth even at a dietary level of 20%. Consequently, we have decided to examine whether menhaden oil could modulate the effect of corn oil on DMBA-induced mammary carcinogenesis. Results of this experiment are shown in Table 3. Compared to a 20% corn oil diet, 20% fat diets containing either 12% or 19% menhaden oil significantly reduced mammary carcinogenesis, based on decreases in tumor incidence and tumor number. This decrease in tumorigenesis is not due to insufficient essential fatty acid levels, which could be argued for the results of the above studies, since we observed the lowest tumor incidence and number in rats receiving 12% menhaden oil plus 8% corn oil. Interestingly, there were also a much larger number of tumor regressions noted in the menhaden oil groups.

Table 3   Effect of dietary menhaden oil on DMBA-induced mammary carcinogenesis

Diet Group	Tumor Incidence (%)	Tumors per rat	No. of regressing tumors
20% corn oil	87	3.22	1
12% menhaden oil + 8% corn oil	47	1.96	8
19% menhaden oil + 1% corn oil	70	2.46	6

Conclusion

Widespread usage of partially hydrogenated vegetable oil in the U.S. during the past 60 to 70 years has raised some concern about possible adverse consequences of consuming isomeric fatty acids present in these products. Previous studies on nutritional and biological effects of isomeric fatty acids have focused primarily on whether or not trans fatty acids may play a role in the development of atherosclerosis. In general, these studies have shown that diets high in trans monoene, but adequate in essential fatty acid, are not uniquely atherogenic (Applewhite, 1981; Kritchevsky, 1982). Recent reports on the relationship between trans fat intake and cancer risk have been in agreement suggesting that trans fatty acids behave like saturated fatty acids and are no more tumor promoting than the cis isomers. These findings should be comforting in view of the variety of food products containing <u>trans</u> fatty acids that are in the typical American diet.

The verdict on the potential protective effect of fish oil against neoplastic growth is still in the hands of the jury. However, preliminary studies from several laboratories using different animal models have been consistent and encouraging. The question that needs to be settled is whether fish oil can modulate the influence of other dietary fats on tumor development, and if so, what is the critical level that has to be present in the diet. Mechanistic studies are important, but they should go hand in hand with animal experiments so that the significance of the problem can be put in the proper perspective. Research in nutrition and cancer is rewarding because of the potential of translating what we learn in the laboratory into preventive measures and intelligent recommendations.

REFERENCES

Aaes-Jorgensen E, Funch JP, Dam JH (1956). The role of fat in the diet of rats. 8. Influence on growth of shortening products, emulsifiers and polymerized linseed oil. Brit J Nutr 10: 317-324.

Alfin-Slater RB, Wells AF, Aftergood L, Deuel HJ (1957). Nutritive value and safety of hydrogenated vegetable fats as evaluated by long-term feeding experiments with rats. J Nutrition 63: 241-261.

Applewhite TH (1981). Nutritional effects of hydrogenated soya oil. J Am Oil Chem Soc 58:260-269.

Awad AB (1981). Trans fatty acids in tumor development and the host survival. J Natl Cancer Inst 67: 189-192.

Beare-Rogers JL (1983). Trans and positional isomers of common fatty acids. Adv Nutr Res 5: 171-200.

Carroll KK, Braden LM (1985). Dietary fat and mammary carcinogenesis. Nutrition and Cancer 6: 254-259.

Cohen BI and Raicht RF (1981). Effects of bile acids on colon carcinogenesis in rats treated with carcinogens. Cancer Res 41: 3759-3760.

Coots RH (1964). A comparison of the metabolism of cis, cis-linoleic, trans, trans-linoleic and a mixture of cis, trans- and trans, cis-linoleic acids in the rat. J Lipid Res 5: 473-476.

Emken EA (1980). Nutritional aspects of soybean oil utilization. In: World Soybean Research Conference II -

Proceedings, Corbin FT (ed.), Boulder, CO, Westview Press, p. 667-679.

Erickson KL, Schlanger DS, Adams DA, Fregeau DR, Stern JS (1984). Influence of dietary fatty acid concentration and geometric configuration on murine mammary tumorigenesis and experimental metastasis. J Nutrition 114: 1834-1842.

Hogan ML, Shamsuddin AM (1984). Large intestinal carcinogenesis. I. Promotional effect of dietary fatty acid isomers in the rat model. J Natl Cancer Inst 73:1293-1296.

Hsu CML, Kummerow FA (1977). Influence of edaidate and erucate on heart mitochondria. Lipids 12: 486-494.

Ip C, Carter CA, Ip MM (1985). Requirement of essential fatty acid for mammary tumorigenesis in the rat. Cancer Res. 45: 1997-2001.

Jurkowski JJ, Cave WT (1985). Dietary effects of menhaden oil on the growth and membrane lipid composition of rat mammary tumors. J Natl Cancer Inst 74: 1145-1150.

Karmali RA, Marsh J, Fuchs C (1984). Effect of omega-3 fatty acids on growth of a rat mammary tumor. J Natl Cancer Inst 73: 457-461.

Kinsella JE, Bruckner G, Mai J, Shimp J (1981). Metabolism of trans fatty acids with emphasis on the effects of trans, trans-octadecadienoate on lipid composition, essential fatty acid, and prostaglandins: an overview. Am J Clin Nutr 34: 2307-2318.

Kritchevsky D (1982). Trans fatty acid effects in experimental atherosclerosis. Fed Proc 41: 2813-2817.

Lawson L, Kummerow F (1979). B-Oxidation of the coenzyme A esters of vaccenic, elaidic, and petroselaidic acids of rat heart mitochondria. Lipids 14: 501-503.

Mattson FH (1960). An investigation of the essential fatty acid activity of some of the geometrical isomers of unsaturated fatty acids. J Nutrition 71: 366-370.

O'Connor TP, Roebuck BD, Peterson F, Campbell TC (1985). Effect of dietary intake of fish oil and fish protein on the development of L-azaserine-induced preneoplastic lesions in the rat pancreas. J Natl Cancer Inst 75: 959-962.

Parodi PW (1976). Distribution of isomeric octadecenoic fatty acids in milk fat. J Dairy Sci 59: 1870-1873.

Reddy BS, Tanaka T, Simi B (1985). Effect of different levels of dietary trans fat or corn oil on azoxymethane-induced colon carcinogenesis in F344 rats. J Natl Cancer Inst 75: 791-798.

Rizek RL (1981). Food supply studies and consumption survey statistics on fat in United States diets. Can Res 41: 3729-3730.

Selenskas SL, Ip MM, Ip C (1984). Similarity between trans fat and saturated fat in the modification of rat mammary carcinogenesis. Cancer Res 44: 1321-1326.

Stearns EM, Rysavy JA, Privette OS (1967). Metabolism of cis-11, cis-14, and trans-11, trans-14 eicosadienoic acids in the rat. J Nutrition 93: 485-490.

Watanabe M, Koga T, Sugano M (1985). Influence of dietary cis- and trans-fat on 1,2-dimethylhydrazine-induced colon tumors and fecal steroid excretion in Fischer 344 rats. Am J Clin Nutrition 42: 475-484.

Dietary Fat and Cancer, pages 295–309
© 1986 Alan R. Liss, Inc.

AMOUNT AND TYPE OF DIETARY FAT AND COLON CANCER: ANIMAL MODEL STUDIES

Bandaru S. Reddy

Division of Nutrition and Endocrinology
Naylor Dana Institute for Disease Prevention
Valhalla, NY 10595

INTRODUCTION

Since Wynder et al. (1969) and Burkitt (1978)first suggested that dietary fat and fiber might play a role in enhancing or inhibiting colon cancer in man, there have been numerous human epidemiologic and animal model studies to test this hypothesis. Since then, a substantial amount of progress has been made in understanding the relationship between dietary factors and colon cancer, but the conduct and interpretation of some epidemiologic studies have been complicated by inherent problems in testing dietary hypothesis for their reliability, validity and sensitivity to reveal narrow but biologically significant differences and to achieve some degree of dose stratification. For example, the major difficulty with most studies has been the lack of measurement of types of saturated and types of polyunsaturated fat content of food in the population being studied. The importance of types of fat with different fatty acid composition rather than total fat cannot be discounted since animal model studies provided evidence that colon tumor promoting effect depends on the type of fat (Reddy, 1986[b]). Several other studies in humans did not take into consideration other confounding factors, such as consumption of cruciferous vegetables and dietary fiber, that have been shown to reduce the risk of colon cancer. Therefore, the lack of consistent findings does not necessarily mediate against a dietary

etiology of colon cancer since the discrepancies may
have arisen atleast in part from methodological limitations of the studies (McKeown-Eyssen, 1985). However,
when another line of evidence based on biochemical
(metabolic epidemiology) and laboratory animal model
studies supports the hypothesis, the relationship between fat and colon cancer deserves a great deal of
attention (Reddy, 1986b).

ANIMAL MODELS FOR COLON CANCER

A number of distinct animal models of colon cancer
induced by chemicals and operating by different metabolic mechanisms are available for studying the pathogenesis of colon cancer and comparing similar stages of
the disease seen in man (Weisburger and Fiala, 1983).
Of all the model systems tested, use of rats and azoxymethane (AOM) as carcinogen seems to be the best
(Shamsuddin, 1983). In that regard, rats, particularly
F344 rat colons, have light and electron microscopic
morphology as well as histochemical properties that are
quite similar to that of the humans (Shamsuddin, 1983).
Besides, AOM-induced colon carcinomas readily metasta-
size to regional lymph nodes and liver, and these carcinomas are easily transplantable. Thus, the biological behaviors of AOM-induced rat colon carcinomas have
close similarity with that of human colon carcinomas.
Other chemicals that are routinely used to induce colon
tumors are (1) aromatic amines such as 3,2'-dimethyl-
4-aminobiphenyl (DMAB), (2) 1,2-dimethylhydrazine (DMH)
and methylazoxymethanol (MAM) acetate; and (3) intrarectal administration of direct-acting carcinogens such
as methylnitrosourea (MNU) or N-methyl-N'-nitro-N-
nitrosoguanidine (MNNG). The spectrum of lesions obtained in rats is similar to the various types of neoplastic diseases observed in the colon and rectum of
humans.

DIETARY FAT AND COLON CARCINOGENESIS

In several earlier studies on dietary fat and
colon cancer, interpretation of results between high-
and low-fat diets was confounded by different intakes
of total calories, protein, vitamins, minerals and non-
nutritive fiber between high- and low-fat fed animals.
In addition, the animals were challenged with multiple

high doses of carcinogen. However, recent studies in which the intake of all nutrients and total calories was controlled between the low-fat and high-fat groups, indicated that not only the amount but the type of fat are determining factors in colon carcinogenesis.

Many carcinogens require metabolic activation in order to exert their carcinogenic effects and the liver is the major site of this process (Fiala et al., 1985). Moreover, even for many carcinogens that affect other target organs including the colon, a first step of hepatic metabolism is required in addition to metabolism by target organs (Fiala et al. 1985). The hepatic and extrahepatic (such as colon) metabolism of several carcinogens has been shown to be affected by dietary fat. The possibility thus exists that the effect of dietary fat on colon carcinogenesis can be demonstrated during the stage of initiation as well as at the stage of promotion.

Effect and Type and Amount of Dietary Fat on Colon Carcinogenesis

Early studies conducted in our laboratory and elsewhere on the effect of dietary fat in colon carcinogenesis did not distinguish whether the effect of fat is at the initiation and post-initiation (promotion) stage of carcinogenesis. In these studies, animals were fed the experimental high-fat diets before, during and after carcinogen treatment, making it difficult to separate the effect of diet between the initiation and promotion stages of colon carcinogenesis. Our early experiments on the effect of type and amount of dietary fat fed before, during and after carcinogen treatment are discussed in this section.

Inasmuch as men in various population groups usually eat comparable regimens over generations, we designed our experiments in a manner so that animals are exposed to a given regimen for 2 generations prior to treatment with a carcinogen (Reddy et al., 1976). Virgin female F344 rats fed semipurified diets containing 5% corn oil, 20% corn oil, 5% lard or 20% lard were bred, and the litters were weaned to the same diets consumed by the mothers. The fat content in high fat

diets was adjusted at the expense of sucrose. At 7
weeks of age, all second generation female rats fed the
experimental diets containing 5% corn oil, 20% corn
oil, 5% lard or 20% lard were given 20 weekly s.c.in-
jections of DMH (10 mg/kg body wt/wk) and necropsied 10
weeks after the last injection. Animals fed 20% lard
or 20% corn oil diets were more susceptible to DMH-induced colon tumors compared to those fed 5% lard or 5%
corn oil diets (Table 1, Experiment 1). The type of
fat appears to be immaterial at the 20% level, however,
at the 5% fat level, unsaturated fat (corn oil) induced
more colon tumors than saturated fat (lard).

Table 1.

Colon Tumor Incidence in F344 Rats Fed Diets High in
Fat Before, During and After Carcinogen Treatment

Dietary fat(%)	Carcinogen	Rats with colon tumors(%)
Experiment 1		
Lard		
5	DMH	17 [a]
20	DMH	67
Corn Oil		
5	DMH	36 [a]
25	DMH	64
Experiment 2		
Beef fat		
5	DMH	27 [a]
20	DMH	60
5	MNU	33[a]
20	MNU	73
5	MAM acetate	45 [a]
20	MAM acetate	80
5	DMAB	26 [a]
20	DMAB	74

[a] Significantly different from high-fat diet

Investigations were also carried out to test the effect of high dietary beef fat on colon carcinogenesis by a variety of carcinogens, DMH, MAM acetate, DMAB, or MNU which differ in metabolic activation (Reddy et al., 1977; Reddy and Ohmori, 1981). In these studies, semi-purified diets containing high and low fat were fed to animals before, during and after carcinogen treatment to study the effect during initiation and promotion stages of colon carcinogenesis (Table 1, Experiment 2). Male F344 weanling rats were fed semipurified diets containing 20% or 5% beef fat. At 7 weeks of age, animals fed the high and low fat diets were given DMH (150 mg/kg body wt, s.c. once), MAM acetate (35 mg/kg body wt, i.p., once), or MNU (2.5 mg/rat/wk, intrarectally, 2 doses). All animals were fed the experimental diets until termination of the experiment which was 30 weeks after the last carcinogen injection. In another study, male F344 weanling rats were fed the semipurified diets (AIN Standard Reference Diet) containing 5% and 23.3% beef tallow and at 7 weeks of age, they were given DMAB (50 mg/kg body wt/wk, s.c., weekly for 20 weeks) and necropsied 20 weeks later. The percent composition of high-fat and low-fat diets was adjusted so that all dietary groups consumed the same amount of total calories, protein, vitamins, minerals and nonnutritive fiber, except for the number of calories from fat. Combined results of these 2 studies (Reddy et al., 1977; Reddy and Ohmori, 1981) indicate that, irrespective of colon carcinogens which differ in metabolic activation, animals fed the diet containing high beef fat had a greater incidence of colon tumors than did rats fed a low beef fat diet. This study also provides evidence that the amount of fat in the diet rather than the number of total calories is one of the determining factors in colon cancer.

Effect of Type and Amount of Dietary Fat Fed During the Stage of Initiation

A pioneering study of Bull et al. (1979) indicates that ingestion of high beef fat increased the intestinal tumor incidence when fed after AOM treatment but not during or before the carcinogen administration, suggesting that excess of dietary beef fat acts at the promotion (post-initiation) stage of colon carcinogenesis but not at the initiation stage of carcinogenesis. Since the activity of enzyme system which metabolizes procarcinogens into active metabolites has been shown to be influenced by dietary fats, particularly unsaturated fat, it is possible that different types of fat may have an effect during the stage of initiation. To answer this question, we investigated the effect of various levels of polyunsaturated (corn oil) and saturated (lard) fats fed during the initiation phase of colon carcinogenesis (Reddy, 1986a). Male F344 rats (5 weeks of age) were fed the semipurified diets containing 5%, 13.6% and 23.5% corn oil or lard. At 7 weeks of age, animals received 2 weekly injections of AOM (15 mg/kg body wt/wk). One week after AOM treatment, groups of animals receiving the 13.5% and 23.5% corn oil or lard diets were transferred to 5% corn oil or lard diets and the groups receiving 5% corn oil or lard diet were continued on same diets. This experimental design will study the effect of high fat diets during the stage of initiation. Additional groups receiving 5% corn oil or lard diets were transferred to 23.5% corn oil or lard diets to study the effect of high corn oil or lard during the stage of promotion. These experimental diets were fed until termination of the experiment. Body weights and the intakes of total calories, protein, vitamins, minerals and nonnutritive fiber were comparable among the dietary groups. The results of this study are of interest in several respects. When the animals were fed the diets containing 13.6% and 23.5% corn oil during the stage of initiation, there was no increase in the incidence of colon tumors compared to animals on a 5% corn oil diet. When the 23.5% corn oil diet was fed during the promotion (post-initiation) stage of carcinogenesis, there was a significant increase in colon tumor incidence compared to animals fed the 5% corn oil diet during the stage of promotion and to those fed the 23.5% corn oil diet during the initiation stage. These results thus suggest that the effect of high corn oil diet in colon carcinogenesis is mainly observed during the promotion stage rather than at the initiation stage of carcinogenesis. In contrast, animals fed the 23.5% and 13.6% lard diet during the stage of initiation had a significant increase of colon tumors in a dose-response manner compared to those fed the 5% lard diet. In addition, animals fed the 23.5% lard diet during the promotion period also had a higher colon tumor inci-

dence than did those fed the 23.5% lard diet during initiation as well as those fed the 5% lard diet during
the promotion stage, suggesting the importance of dietary fat during the promotion stage of colon carcinogenesis.

The results presented above from our laboratory
(Reddy, 1986a) and those of others (Bull et al., 1979)
demonstrate that the role of dietary fat during the initiation stage of colon carcinogenesis depends on the
type of fat.

Effect of Type and Amount of Dietary Fat Fed During the Stage of Promotion (Post-initiation)

Effect of dietary corn oil, safflower oil, coconut oil
and olive oil. The role of type and amount of dietary
fat during the promotional phase of colon carcinogenesis has been studied in our laboratory (Reddy and
Maeura, 1984). At 5 weeks of age, groups of female
F344 rats were fed the semipurified diets (AIN-76) containing 5% corn oil, 5% safflower oil or 5% olive oil
and continued on these diets during and until 1 week
after carcinogen treatment. At 7 weeks of age, groups
of animals were treated subcutaneously with AOM (20
mg/kg body wt, once). One week after AOM treatment,
groups of animals receiving the diets containing 5%
corn oil, safflower oil or olive oil were transferred
to their respective high-fat (23.5%) diets, whereas
additional groups consuming 5% corn oil diet was transferred to high coconut oil diet. Additional groups
were continued on low corn oil, safflower oil and olive
oil diets. All animals were fed these diets until termination of the experiment. Body weights and consumption of total calories, protein, micronutrients and
fiber except the amount of calories from fat were comparable between high- and low-fat fed animals. The
animals fed the high corn oil or high safflower oil
diets had a higher incidence of colon tumors than those
fed the diets low in fat (Table 2). In contrast, diets
high in coconut oil or olive oil had no colon tumor
promoting effect compared to diets high in corn oil or
safflower oil. The varied effects of different types
of fat on colon carcinogenesis suggest that the fatty
acid composition is one of the determining factors in
colon tumor promotion. Thus, the colon tumor induction

effects differ in diets high in saturated fats of vegetable origin (coconut oil) or monounsaturated fat of
vegetable origin (olive oil) and polyunsaturated fats
of vegetable origin (corn oil or safflower oil).

Table 2.

Colon Tumor Incidence in F344 Rats Fed High Fat Diets
During Promotional Phase of Carcinogenesis

Type and amount of fat	% animals with colon tumors[a]	Type and amount of fat	% animals with colon tumors
5% corn oil	17[b]	5% olive oil	10
23.5% corn oil	46	23.5% olive oil	13
5% safflower oil	13[b]	23.5% coconut oil	13
23.5% safflower oil	36		

[a] Female F344 rats were given a single s.c. injection of AOM at a dose level of 20 mg/kg body wt.

[b] Significantly different from 23.5% fat diet.

Effect of dietary trans fat and Menhaden fish oil.
There was an increase in per capita consumption of fat
for the last 50 years in the United States and this increase can be partly accounted for by a trend toward
greater use of vegetable oils which include partially
hydrogenated fats and processed vegetable oils that
contain trans fatty acids. The most common isomers
which occur in processed fats are 9-trans-18:1 (elaidic
acid) and cis-trans-octadecadienoic acid. Fish oils
which contain highly polyunsaturated fatty acids, eico-
sopentaenoic acid and docosahexaenoic acid are unique
fats that have not been studied in colon cancer. Two
separate experiments were conducted in our laboratory
in which one study tested the effect of high fat
(23.5%) diets containing different levels of trans fat
(Reddy et al., 1985b) and the second study tested the
effect of high and low levels of Menhaden fish oil
(Reddy, 1986a) on the promotion phase of AOM-induced
carcinogenesis in F344 rats.

In the trans fat study, high fat diets (23.5%) containing low trans fat (5.8% corn oil + 5.9% trans fat + 11.8% oleinate), intermediate trans fat (5.8% corn oil + 11.8% trans fat + 5.9% oleinate) and high trans fat (5.8% corn oil + 17.6% trans fat) and high corn oil (23.5%) were tested for colon tumor promoting effect. Animals fed the high fat diets containing different levels of trans fat developed significantly fewer colon tumors than did the rats fed the high corn oil diet (Reddy et al., 1985b; Table 3). There was no difference between low corn oil diet and high fat diets containing different levels of trans fat. Thus, high trans fat had little or no promoting effect in colon carcinogenesis when used in a diet that contained about 5.9% corn oil.

In the Menhaden fish oil study, high fat diets containing 23.5% corn oil or 1% corn oil + 22.5% Menhaden oil and low fat diets containing 5% corn oil or 1% corn oil + 4% Menhaden oil were compared for AOM-induced colon tumor promoting activity in male F344 rats. Colon tumor incidence was significantly inhibited in animals fed the high Menhaden oil diet as compared to those fed the high corn oil diet (Reddy, 1986a). It is possible that lack of colon tumor promoting effect by Menhaden oil might be due to its inhibitory effect on prostaglandin synthesis. However, additional studies are warranted in this aspect.

The above studies conducted in our laboratory demonstrate that the effect of dietary fat during the promotion stage of carcinogenesis depends on the type and amount of fat. In these studies, the body weights of animals fed the high and low fat diets were comparable. The intakes of total calories, protein, micronutrients and fiber, with the exception of fat calories, were similar in all dietary groups. Thus, the observed differences in colon tumor incidences in animals fed various levels and types of fat cannot be ascribed to total calories consumed but can be related to total fat calories and to the fatty acid composition of dietary fat.

Table 3.

Colon Tumor Incidence in F344 Rats Fed High Corn Oil or High Trans Fat Diets During Promotional Phase of Carcinogenesis

Type and amount of fat	% animals with colon tumors[a]	No. colon tumors/ animal	
		Adenomas	Adenocarc.
5% corn oil	67[b]	0.57[b]	0.50[b]
23.5% corn oil	93	0.90	0.87
23.5% high-fat diet containing			
low trans fat	63[b]	0.73	0.37[b]
intermed. trans fat	67[b]	0.90	0.43[b]
high trans fat	57[b]	0.57[b]	0.53[b]

[a] Male F344 rats were given s.c. injections of AOM at a dose rate of 15 mg/kg body wt/week for 3 weeks

[b] Significantly different from the groups fed 23.5% corn oil diet.

MECHANISMS OF DIETARY FAT IN COLON CANCER

The biological plausibility of dietary fat in the etiology of colon cancer is reflected in a number of hypotheses for the mechanism of action (Reddy, 1983; Hill et al., 1971). Currently, much of our knowledge on the mechanism of dietary fat on colon carcinogenesis is based on experiments conducted in humans and animal models.

The search for genotoxic carcinogens associated with the etiology of colon cancer has been initiated by several laboratories including our laboratory (Ehrich et al., 1979; Reddy et al., 1985a; Bruce et al., 1977). These studies demonstrate that the populations who are at high-risk for colon cancer and consuming a high-fat diet excrete increased levels of fecal mutagens (or presumptive carcinogens) compared to low-risk populations who consume a low-fat diet. However, the carcinogenic activity of these mutagens is yet to be determined.

The role of dietary fat as a promoting stimuli in colon cancer has been based on the hypothesis that the amount of dietary fat modulates the concentration of colonic secondary bile acids which have been shown to act as colon tumor promoters but do not have the properties of genotoxic carcinogens (Reddy, 1983). This is important since current views on properties of promoters note that the effect of such agents is highly dependent on dose and on length of exposure, and thus provides an opportunity of reducing the risk of colon cancer development by lowering the concentration of bile acids by dietary means. It has been demonstrated in humans that the concentration of fecal deoxycholic acid and lithocholic acid is much lower in low-risk populations consuming a low-fat diet when compared to high-risk populations consuming a high-fat diet (Reddy, 1986b). The concentration of secondary bile acids can be reduced by lowering the amount of dietary fat in high-risk populations (Reddy, 1986b). In animal model experiments, the excretion of secondary bile acids is positively correlated with colon tumor promotion by various types of dietary fat (Reddy and Maeura, 1984; Reddy et al., 1985b). For example, the concentrations of fecal deoxycholic acid and lithocholic acid were unaffected in animals fed the diets containing high coconut oil, olive oil, trans fat or Menhaden fish oil, whereas the diets containing high levels of corn oil, safflower oil, lard or beef tallow increased the concentration of fecal secondary bile acids. Although the molecular mechanisms to tumor promoting effect of dietary fat via the action of bile acids are incompletely understood, recent studies of Takano et al. (1981) and Rozhin et al. (1984) indicate that the induction of colonic epithelial ornithine decarboxylase activity by the bile acids may play a role in these mechanisms. Deschner et al. (1981) demonstrated that bile acids enhance epithelial cell proliferation in the colon. Our recent study also provided additional evidence to indicate a relationship between dietary fat fed during promotion stage of colon carcinogenesis, colonic mucosal ornithine decarboxylase activity, secondary bile acids and colon tumor promotion (Reddy, 1986a).

CONCLUSION

During the last 15 years, human and animal model experiments conducted in our laboratory indicate that dietary fat plays an important role in colon carcinogenesis. The effect of dietary fat during the initiation as well as promotion stage of colon carcinogenesis depends on the type of fat and its fatty acid composition. The mechanisms by which various types of fat increase the colon carcinogenesis is not fully understood; however, in most instances, the high fat diet appears to enhance colon carcinogenesis through its elevation of agents that act as promoters of tumor development. In certain instances, liver and extrahepatic tissue (colon) enzymes responsible for the metabolism of a variety of carcinogens and cocarcinogens may be mediating factors in the relationship between dietary fat and colon cancer.

ACKNOWLEDGMENTS

This research was supported in part from grants and contracts CP-33208, CA-16382, CA-17613, CA-29602, CA-36892, and CA-37663 from the National Cancer Institute. Expert editorial assistance of Ms. Arlene Banow is gratefully appreciated.

REFERENCES

Bruce WR, Varghese AJ, Furrer R, Land PC (1977). A mutagen in the feces of normal human. In: Hiatt HH, Watson JP, Winston JA, (eds). "Origins of Human Cancer", Cold Spring Harbor Conf. Cell Proliferation, Cold Spring Harbor, New York 4:1641-1645.

Bull AW, Soullier BK, Wilson PS, Haydon MT, Nigro ND (1979). Promotion of azoxymethane-induced intestinal cancer by high-fat diets in rats. Cancer Res 39:4956-4959.

Burkitt DP (1978). Colonic-rectal cancer: fiber and other dietary factors. Am J Clin Nutr 31:S58-S64.

Deschner EE, Cohen BI, Raicht RF (1981). Acute and chronic effect of dietary cholic acid on colonic epithelial cell proliferation. Digestion 21:290-296.

Ehrich M, Ashell JE, Van Tassell RL, Wilkins TD, Walker ARP, Richardson NJ (1979). Mutagens in the feces of 3 South African populations at different levels of risk for colon cancer. Mut Res 64:231-240.

Fiala ES, Reddy BS, Weisburger JH (1985). Naturally occurring anticarcinogenic substances in foodstuffs. Ann Rev Nutr 5:295-321.

Hill MJ, Drasar BS, Aries VC, Crowther JS, Hawksworth GB, Williams REO (1971). Bacteria and etiology of cancer of large bowel. Lancet 1:95-100.

Manousos O, Day NE, Trichopoulous D, Gervassilis E, Tzonow A, Polychronopoulous A (1983). Diet and colorectal cancer: A case-control study in Greece. Int J Cancer 32:1-5.

McKeown-Eyssen G. Dietary approaches to the prevention of large bowel cancer. In: Ingall JRF, Mastromarino AJ (eds). "Carcinoma of the Large Bowel and its Precursors. Progress in Clinical and Biological Research". New York:Alan R. Liss 4:277-284.

Reddy BS (1983). Tumor promotion in colonic carcinogenesis. In: Slaga TJ (ed). "Mechanisms of Tumor Promotion", Boca Raton:CRC Press, 1:107-129.

Reddy BS (1986a). Unpublished observation.

Reddy BS (1986b). Diet and colon cancer: Evidence from human and animal model studies. In: Reddy BS, Cohen LA (eds). "Diet, Nutrition and Cancer: A Critical Evaluation, Macronutrients and Cancer", Boca Raton:CRC Press 1:47-76.

Reddy BS, Maeura Y (1984). Tumor promotion by dietary fat in azoxymethane-induced colon carcinogenesis in female F344 rats: Influence of amount and source of dietary fat. J Natl Cancer Inst 72:745-750.

Reddy BS, Narisawa T, Vukusich D, Weisburger JH, Wynder, EL (1976). Effect of quality and quantity of dietary fat and dimethylhydrazine in colon carcinogenesis in rats. Proc Soc Exp Biol Med 151:237-239.

Reddy BS, Ohmori T (1981). Effect of intestinal microflora and dietary fat on 3,2'-dimethyl-4-aminobiphenyl-induced colon carcinogenesis in F344 rats. Cancer Res 451:1363-1367.

Reddy BS, Sharma C, Mathews L, Engle A, Laakso K, Choi K, Puska P, Korpella R (1985a). Metabolic epidemiology of colon cancer: Fecal mutagens in healthy subjects from rural Kuopio and urban Helsinki, Finland. Mutation Res 152:97-105.

Reddy BS, Tanaka T, Simi B (1985b). Effect of different levels of dietary trans fat or corn oil on azoxymethane -induced colon carcinogenesis in F344 rats. J Natl Cancer Inst 75:791-798.

Reddy BS, Watanabe K, Weisburger JH (1977). Effect of high fat diet on colon carcinogenesis in F344 rats treated with 1,2-dimethylhydrazine, methylazoxymethanol acetate or methylnitrosourea. Cancer Res. 37:4156-4159.

Rozhin J, Wilson PS, Bull AW, Nigro ND (1984). Ornithine decarboxylase activity in the rat and human colon. Cancer Res 44:3226-3230.

Shamsuddin AKM (1983). In vivo induction of colon cancer dose and animal species. In: Autrup H, Williams GM (eds). "Experimental colon carcinogenesis", Boca Raton:CRC Press, pp 51-62.

Stemmermann GN, Nomura AMY, Heilbrun L (1984). Dietary fat and risk of colorectal cancer. Cancer Res 44: 4633-4677.

Takano S, Matsushima M, Erturk E, Bryan GT (1981). Early induction of rat colonic epithelial ornithine and S-adenyl-L-methionine decarboxylase activities by N-methyl-N'-nitro-N-nitrosoguanidine or bile salts. Cancer Res 41:624-628.

Weisburger JH, Fiala ES (1983). Experimental colon carcinogens and their mode of action. In: Autrup H, Williams GM (eds). "Experimental Colon Carcinogenesis", Boca Raton:CRC Press, pp 27-50.

Wynder EL, Kajitani T, Ishikawa S, Dodo H, Takano A (1969). Environmental factors of the colon and rectum. II. Japanese epidemiological data. Cancer 23:1210-1220.

Dietary Fat and Cancer, pages 311–330
© 1986 Alan R. Liss, Inc.

DIETARY FAT AND COLON CANCER: VARIABLE RESULTS IN ANIMAL MODELS

Paul M. Newberne[1,2] and Kathleen M. Nauss[1]
Department of Applied Biological Sciences,[1]
Massachusetts Institute of Technology, Cambridge,
MA 02139; and Department of Pathology,[2] Boston
University School of Medicine, Boston, MA 02118

INTRODUCTION

Cancer of the large bowel appears to be increasing in some segments of the populations of the industrialized world. It is these same societies which, with the exception of Japan, consume diets high in fat. The rate of colon cancer is also low in Japan, but high in North America and Europe, but relatively low in Africa, Asia and South America (Armstrong and Doll, 1975; Doll and Peto, 1981).

Observations from epidemiological studies and from experiments in animal models have, in some instances, linked dietary fat to colon cancer. A general observation is that industrialized societies eat diets which are high in fat, compared to non-industrialized societies, and this correlates with the colon cancer incidence rate in those societies. It is essential however, to bear in mind that the epidemiological data which support a linkage between fat and colon cancer are tenuous and controversial (Byers and Graham, 1984; Marshall, 1986). Moreover, total food intake has sometimes been used to show an effect of one dietary component (fat) as the culprit when other factors (protein) may be equally significant (Enstrom, 1975).

Hill et al. (1979) found that high socioeconomic status (SES) groups in Hong Kong experienced over twice the colon cancer rates as low SES groups. Dietary surveys showed that the high SES group ate more meat, but also more of almost

every other type of food as well, than the low SES group.
Ecological studies also suggest meat to be a risk factor
(Enstrom, 1975). Colorectal cancer is much lower in
Seventh-Day Adventists, who are often lacto-ovo-vegetarian,
as compared to nonadventists (Phillips, 1975). Similarly,
Mormons also have relatively low rates, yet a special
dietary survey in Southern Utah which is almost entirely
Mormon, showed meat consumption levels to be virtually iden-
tical to the remainder of the United States suggesting that
factors other than low meat consumption may be important in
explaining the low colon cancer rates in this area (Lyon and
Sorenson, 1978).

A comparative study by Kinlen (1982) of strict religious
orders in Britain showed that colon cancer mortality was not
lower in an order which ate no meat as compared to one which
did. In addition, there are some ecological patterns which
are not entirely consistent with the fats hypothesis.
Dietary fat intake is very high in Finland, yet colon cancer
rates are relatively low, and within the United States there
is no correlation between regional beef fat consumption and
colorectal cancer rates (Enstrom, 1975).

Case-control studies have not always confirmed the
suspicion generated from experimental and ecological studies
that fat is a risk factor for colon cancer. This fits particularly well with the recent observations from our laboratory (Nauss et al., 1983; 1984; Locniskar et al., 1985;
Newberne et al., 1985) and from the observations in Hawaiian
studies (Stemmerman et al., 1984).

Higginson (1966) reported no case-control differences in
dietary fat. In a study conducted in Minnesota (Bjelke,
1973) there was no association between dietary fat and colon
cancer. Dales et al. (1978), however, reported higher risk
for those who ate diets that were both high in fat and low
in fiber, and Jain et al. (1980) reported a study in Canada
in which cases reported eating more fat than controls.

These reports represent a cross-section of a large
number of epidemiologic and case-control studies, pointing
out the difficulties in assessing data on human dietary fat
and colon cancer.

When critically evaluated, the data from studies using
animal models to demonstrate an effect of dietary fat on

colon carcinogenesis, as a single variable, are less than exact; enthusiasm seems to have run ahead of the available data. The literature has provided numerous reports from proponents of the hypothesis that increased dietary fat is associated with increased susceptibility to the induction of colon cancer (Reddy et al., 1974; 1976; 1977; 1981; 1984; Broitman et al., 1977; Nigro et al., 1975; Bull et al., 1979). However other investigators have been unable to demonstrate an effect of fat on chemically induced colon cancer (Nutter et al., 1983; Nauss et al., 1983; 1984; Locniskar et al., 1985; Schmähl et al., 1983; Bansal et al., 1978; Glauert et al., 1983).

Table 1

Effect of High Levels of Dietary Fat on
Experimental Colon Carcinogenesis

Type of Fat	Number of Studies	Increased Frequency	Increased Incidence	No Change
Polyunsaturated Vegetable Fat	12	2	5	5
Saturated Vegetable Fat	3	1	0	2
Saturated Animal Fat	13	5	4	5
TOTAL	28	8	9	12

To date, there have been approximately 28 different trials published by nine laboratories examining the influence of dietary fat on chemically-induced colon cancer in rodents. These trials have been described in more detail in an earlier review (Rogers and Nauss, 1985) and are sum-marized in Table 1. It is apparent that in half of these studies, high levels of dietary fat resulted in either an increased incidence or frequency of colon tumors but in 42% of the studies no effect of high levels of dietary fat was observed.

Table 2

Two Studies Demonstrating an Enhancing Effect of

Dietary Fat on Colon Cancer in Rats[1]

Basal Diet	Fat Level	Carcinogen	Colon Tumor Incidence	Tumors/Tumor Bearing Rat				
				Total	Colon	Small Intestine	Adenocarcinoma	Adenoma
	(%)		(%)					
Study 1 Chow	5	AOM	100	5.9	3.1	2.8	ND	ND
Chow[2]	35	AOM	100	10.5	4.6	6.0	ND	ND
p value			NS	<0.01	<0.05	<0.025		
Study 2 Semi-purified	5	DMH	23	1.14	ND	ND	0.57	0.57
Semi-purified[3]	20	DMH	60	1.33	ND	ND	0.28	1.06
p value			<0.05	NS	-	-	NS	NS

[1] Abbreviations used; AOM = azoxymethane, DMH = 1,2-dimethylhydrazine, ND = not determined, NS = not significant.

[2] Fat added to chow.

[3] Fat substituted for carbohydrate.

Study 1 (Nigro et al., 1975)

Study 2 (Reddy et al., 1977)

The divergent effects of dietary fat on experimental colon carcinogenesis are probably a reflection of differences in diet and experimental protocol as well as a lack of consistency in assessing colon tumorigenesis. Two examples of studies which have demonstrated an enhancing effect of dietary fat on chemically-induced colon carcinogenesis illustrate these points (Table 2).

Nigro et al. (1975) demonstrated that if beef tallow were added to laboratory animal chow the frequency of azoxymethane (AOM)-induced intestinal tumors in rats was increased (Table 2, Study 1). Since the total dose of carcinogen was high, all treated rats developed intestinal tumors and incidence rates could not be analyzed. Multiple tumors (5-10/rat) were produced and animals fed the high fat diet had a 114% increase in small intestinal tumors and a 48% increase in colon tumors. Histopathologic examination of representative tumors indicated that they were all carcinomas.

Reddy and co-workers (1977) induced intestinal tumors using 1,2-dimethylhydrazine (DMH) which is a precursor of AOM (Table 2, Study 2). Since the total dose of carcinogen was lower than that used in Study 1, not all animals developed intestinal tumors and overall incidence data could be evaluated. Colon tumor incidence was significantly ($p < 0.05$) higher in animals fed 20% beef tallow compared to those fed 5% tallow. However there were no significant differences in tumor frequency. The histopathology data indicated that adenomas rather than adenocarcinomas accounted for the increased tumors in animals fed the high fat diets. No data were presented regarding the incidence of adenocarcinomas. These two studies demonstrate that more attention must be directed to developing a uniform system of assessing experimental tumorigenesis which would include histopathologic classification of all masses as well as analysis of tumor incidence and frequency.

The results from several studies in our laboratory have failed to support the hypothesis that dietary fat, quality or quantity, alone influence experimental colon cancer (Nauss et al., 1983; Nauss et al., 1984; Locniskar et al., 1985). There are suggestions, however, that other factors, interacting with dietary fat, may participate in the potential for susceptibility to colon cancer (Nauss et al. submitted for publication). A summary of these results is presented in this paper.

MATERIALS AND METHODS

Animals

Male weanling rats of the Sprague-Dawley, (Crl:CD®(SD)BR)(SD) and Fischer (CDF-F344/Crl BR) (F-344) strains were obtained from the Charles River Breeding Laboratories, Inc., Wilmington, MA, systematically randomized and assigned to experimental groups of the various studies. They were housed individually in stainless steel wire-mesh suspended cages in climate controlled quarters (72°+4°F) with a 12-hour light/dark cycle. They were given distilled water and one of several diets described in the various tables of the results section or as noted below.

Diets

We have used diets, defined in every detail, utilizing a number of fats with respect to quality and quantity (Table 3). Generally, the diets have used five percent as the low level and either 20% or 24% as the high level. In all cases, the diets were isocaloric and balanced with respect to nutrient to calorie ratio. The levels of fat are shown in the various tables. The carcinogens have been used at different levels and according to different protocols.

Tumor incidences and differences in weight gain or food consumption were compared by X^2 test or by analysis of variance (Helwig and Couacil, 1979).

Routine necropsy procedures were used except that all tumors or suspicious lesions were carefully identified as to location in the colon and measurements were made of those of a millimeter or more.

RESULTS

The results of three different trials using an indirect carcinogen (DMH) or the direct acting N-methylnitrosourea (NMU) are shown in Table 4. A comparison is also shown of intragastric and subcutaneous administration of DMH. There were no significant differences in colon tumor incidences, frequency, or cumulative probability of death between rats fed 5% fat or those which received 24% fat diets.

Table 3

Isocalorically Balanced High Fat Diets[a]

	5% Mixed Fat (g)	24% Beef Tallow (g)	24% Corn Oil (g)	24% Crisco® (g)
Casein[b]	20	24	24	24
Sucrose[c]	21	12	12	12
Dextrose[c]	21	12	12	12
Dextrin[c]	21	12	12	12
Vitamin Mix	2	2.4	2.4	2.4
Salts	5	6	6	6
Cellulose	4	5	5	5
Beef Tallow[b]	1.6	22	--	--
Corn Oil[b]	1.6	2	24	--
Crisco®[b]	1.6	--	--	24
Total	100	100	100	100

a All diets were mixed in a 1:1 ratio into a 5% agar solution; the 5% fat control diet contains 5% Rogers-Harpers salts and 2% vitamin mix. The vitamin content of the 5% fat diet is vitamin A, 10 mg/kg; vitamin D_2, 3000 IU; vitamin E, 169 IU; menadione, 1 mg/kg; niacin, 50 mg/kg; calcium pantothenate, 20 mg/kg; riboflavin, 4 mg/kg; thiamin HCl, 8 mg/kg; pyridoxine HCl, 8 mg/kg; folic acid, 10 mg/kg; choline, 3.0 g/kg; inositol, 250 mg/kg; vitamin B_{12}, 0.05 mg/kg. The salt and vitamin content of the 24% fat diets is increased to 6% and 2.4% respectively to allow for decreased food consumption in animals consuming diets of higher caloric density.

b Vitamin-free casein was purchased from Teklad Test Diets, Madison, WI; Newell Beef Tallow, Mazola® corn oil and Crisco® vegetable shortening were purchased from McKinnon and McKenzie, Brighton, MA.

c The carbohydrate is mixed from 3 sources: dextrose (CPC International, Engelwood Cliffs, NJ); dextrin (American Maize Products, Hammond, IN); and sucrose (Savage Co., Waltham, MA).

In view of these negative results we considered the possibility that an enhancing effect of dietary fat might be

Table 4

Three Studies Demonstrating No Effect of Dietary Fat on
Chemically-Induced Colon Cancer in Rats[1]

Dietary Fat(%)	Study 1[2] DMH (i.g.)[5]		Study 2[3] NMU(i.r.)		Study 3[4] DMH (i.g. vs. s.c.) i.g.		s.c.	
	Incidence(%)[5]	Frequency[6]	Incidence(%)	Frequency	Incidence(%)	Frequency	Incidence(%)	Frequency
Mixed Fat (5)	77	1.6	55	1.6	--	--	--	--
Corn Oil (5)	--	--	--	--	63	1.4	58	1.3
Beef Tallow (24)	68	1.5	63	1.4	--	--	--	--
Corn Oil (24)	63	1.4	55	1.2	68	1.3	48	1.6
Crisco® (24)	55	1.5	38	1.1	--	--	--	--

1 Abbreviations: DMH = 1,2-dimethylhydrazine, NMU = N-methylnitrosourea, i.g. = intragastric, s.c. = subcutaneous, i.r. = intrarectal.
2 Nauss et al., 1983, total dose = 75 mg DMH·2HCl/kg body wt.
3 Nauss et al., 1984, total dose NMU = 6 mg/rat.
4 Locniskar et al., 1985, total dose = 150 mg DMH·2HCl/kg body wt.
5 Incidence = % of animals in a group bearing colon tumors (N = 40).
6 Frequency = number of tumors per tumor bearing rat.

restricted to special aspects of experimental conditions
including the strain of rat. We examined this possibility
by using two different strains of rats, the Fischer-344
(F-344) and Sprague-Dawley (SD). Diets of different
nutrient composition were also used and the differences in
fat were 5% or 20% beef fat with or without added corn oil.

There are three methods of adding fat to an experimental
diet,the choice of which can have a profound effect on animal nutrient consumption. If extra fat is added to a chow
or natural product diet there is an overall dilution of
nutrients. The substitution of fat for carbohydrate in
semipurified diets increases the caloric density and unless
the concentration of other nutrients is increased accordingly, the animals fed the high fat diets will consume less
protein, fiber, vitamins and minerals.

We prepared two semipurified diets which differed in the
method of fat addition as well as in the concentration of
certain micronutrients. The first diet, which was isocalorically balanced,was identical to the diet used in our
earlier studies (Table 4). It contained levels of certain
vitamins and minerals in excess of the recommended requirements for normal growth (Report on the American Institute of
Nutrition ad hoc Committee on Standards for Animal Studies,
1977). With the exception of the addition of agar, the composition of the second diet was the same as that used in
studies where an enhancing effect of dietary fat on
DMH-induced colon tumors was reported (Table 2, Study 2).
It was not isocalorically balanced.

The salient features of this study are shown in Table 5.
Although the dose of DMH was adjusted on a body weight
basis, the response of an animal to the toxic effects of the
carcinogen was dependent on strain and diet composition.
F-344 rats were more sensitive to the toxic effects of DMH
and the deficit in weight gain was greatest for animals fed
the non-isocalorically balanced diet with the lowest concentration of certain vitamins and minerals. This same
trend was evident in S.D. rats.

The effect of the four different diets on colon tumorigenesis is presented in Table 5. In the SD group, colon
tumor incidence was 57% in rats fed Diet 1 which contained
20% fat compared to 27-33% in the other three groups. When

Table 5

Effect of DMH on Colon Tumor Induction:
Strain and Body Weight Differences[1,2]

Dietary Fat(%)	Nutrient to Calorie Ratio	Vitamins and Minerals	Final Body Wt ($\overline{X}$+SD)	Tumor Incidence(%)	Tumors/ TBR
		Sprague-Dawley			
5%	Balanced	Supplemented	495 ± 38	27	1.5
20%	Balanced	Supplemented	580 ± 27	57	1.5
5%	Not Balanced	Not Supplemented	412 ± 30	30	1.1
20%	Not Balanced	Not Supplemented	467 ± 35	33	1.2
Significance (p)			< 0.01	< 0.07	NS
		Fischer-344			
5%	Balanced	Supplemented	342 ± 20	27	1.6
20%	Balanced	Supplemented	373 ± 23	37	1.1
5%	Not Balanced	Not Supplemented	221 ± 12	27	1.4
20%	Not Balanced	Not Supplemented	236 ± 14	33	1.0
Significance (p)			< 0.01	NS	0.06

[1] DMH (200 mg DMH·2HCl/kg) administered subcutaneously (10 mg/kg·wk·20). Animals killed 10 weeks after the last dose of carcinogen.

[2] Abbreviations: TBR = tumor bearing rat. NS = not significant.

the four groups were compared by a chi-squared test, the effect was not significant (p = 0.07 level). When the Diet 1-5% group was compared to the Diet 1-20% group, the p value was 0.02. If multiple comparisons are made, it is generally recommended that the value for significance be lowered, making the effect of marginal significance. There were no significant effects on tumor frequency (number of tumors per tumor bearing rat). Dietary treatment had no significant effect on colon tumor incidence or frequency in F-344 rats. In neither strain were differences observed in tumor size, degree of differentiation or extent of invasion through the colon wall.

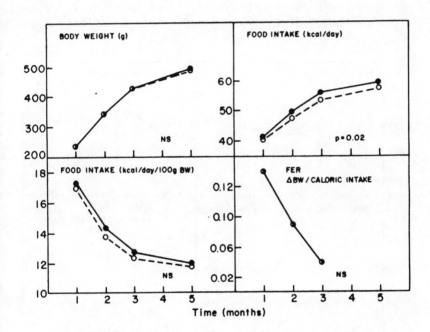

Figure 1. Food intake and body weight gain in tumor-bearing (•-•) and tumor-free (o--o) Sprague-Dawley rats.

Since Sprague-Dawley and Fischer rats differ significantly in rate of weight gain and final body mass, it was of interest to examine the relationship between food consumption and colon tumorigenesis in these two strains. One way of looking at the data is to determine mean food consumption and energy intake in tumor-bearing and tumor-free animals. We carried out such calculations for rats in each strain at four time periods: 1. Prior to DMH treatment, 2. During treatment (two and three months) and immediately prior to the terminal sacrifice. For SD rats (Fig. 1) there were no significant differences in mean body weight of tumor-bearing and tumor-free animals. Food intake expressed as kcal/day was higher in animals with colon tumors. This effect was not significant when the data were expressed as kcal/day/100 g body weight. If one calculated the food efficiency ratio, no differences were seen. For the leaner F-344 animals, no differences were seen in body weight, caloric intake or food efficiency ratio between tumor-bearing and tumor-free rats (Fig. 2).

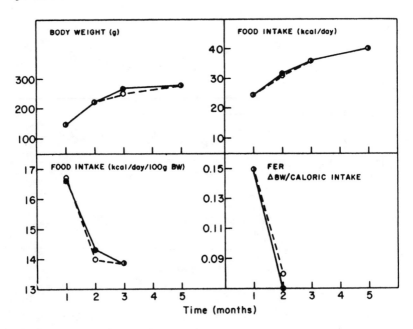

Figure 2. Food intake and body weight gain in tumor bearing (•-•) and tumor free (o--o) F-344 rats.

We then decided to look at the data in a slightly different way. Visek and co-workers (1983) had observed that if animals were ranked according to their caloric intake, breast tumor incidence and frequency were higher in SD rats

ranked in the upper two thirds according to calories consumed. We did a similar analysis of the data from our most
recent study. Colon tumor incidence and frequency in SD
rats increased as one moved from the lower to the upper
levels of food intake (Fig. 3). A significant and
interesting aspect of these data were the one month intake
data, prior to carcinogen treatment; these data showed that
SD rats which were eating more prior to DMH treatment, were
more likely to develop tumors. Similar results were
obtained for the three and five month intake data (data not
shown).

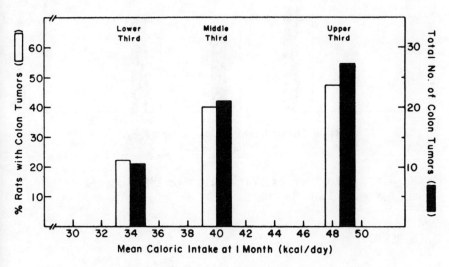

Figure 3. Effect of caloric intake on DMH-induced colon
tumorigenesis in Sprague-Dawley rats.

When we carried out the same calculations for Fischer
animals (Fig. 4) no association was observed between level
of caloric intake and colon tumorigenesis. It may be that
the effect of calories is more pronounced in a rapidly
growing strain than in slower growing, leaner animals.

Results from three separate long term trials in our own
laboratory with SD rats showed no effect of dietary fat on
DMH or NMU induced colon tumorigenesis. In our most recent
trial using a longer carcinogen treatment procedure, 20%
beef fat did not increase colon tumorigenesis in Fischer
rats. The effect of dietary fat in SD rats was mixed.

Animals fed a diet which promoted optimal growth had a barely significant increase in colon tumor incidence but not in frequency or size. This effect was not observed using a second diet which resulted in slower growth.

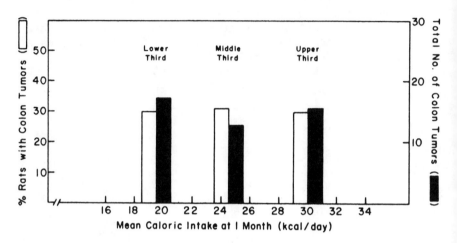

Figure 4. Effect of caloric intake on DMH-induced colon tumorigenesis in F-344 rats.

DISCUSSION

These studies have shown that dietary variables, other than fat level have an effect on animals' response to a colon carcinogen. When diets are not isocalorically balanced the levels of protein, fiber, vitamins and minerals consumed by animals in a high fat group may be inadequate under stressful conditions, such as periods of long-term carcinogen administration We observed this effect to be more pronounced in F-344 rats than in SD animals. Failure to recognize the importance of marginal nutriture and the variable responses of different rodent strains to carcinogen administration may explain, in part, the inconsistencies in the literature regarding the effect of dietary fat on experimentally induced colon tumorigenesis.

The hypothesis that high dietary fat intake enhances colon tumorigenesis receives support from international studies demonstrating a correlation between per capita fat intake and mortality from colon cancer (Armstrong and Doll, 1975), but findings from case-control studies have been contradictory (Byers and Graham, 1984). In a fifteen year prospective study, Stemmerman and co-workers (1984) actually found a negative association between colon cancer and saturated fat intake. In a more recent prospective study involving 8006 Hawaiian Japanese men, these investigators found no association between total fat intake and colon cancer, confirming their earlier findings (personal communication, in press).

Animal studies from a number of laboratories have produced equivocal results regarding the influence of dietary fat on experimentally-induced colon carcinogenesis. No two investigators have used the exact same diet formulation or carcinogen treatment protocol,making comparisons among studies difficult or impossible as implied by the results reported here. An enhancing effect of dietary fat on experimentally-induced colon tumors in rodents is generally observed in models where additional fat was added to chow or natural product diets, a procedure which results in an overall dilution of nutrients with consequent imprecise interpretation of results. An improved formulation was provided by semipurified diets where excess fat was substituted for carbohydrate on a weight basis, although such diets do not take into account the increased caloric density of the high-fat diets and the reduction in nutrient intake by animals consuming such diets. Isocaloric formulations increase the levels of protein, fiber, vitamins and minerals in the high fat diets to maintain a constant nutrient to calorie ratio. Even these designs are subject to criticism because the values used for available energy of fat may have been underestimated (Donato and Hegsted, 1985).

Since caloric intake appears to have a significant bearing on risk for tumors, diets which differ in calories and which modify food intake must be taken into consideration. Human and animal studies have shown that consumption of high fiber diets is associated with increased fecal loss of fat and nitrogen and therefore a reduced availability of calories (Nyman and Asp, 1982; Cummings et al., 1976; Isaksson et al., 1984). Much remains to be done to clarify this issue but more evidence is accumulating in animal and human studies to suggest a complex phenomenon is

operating and that a number of factors may interact to produce increased risk.

The fat-fiber relationship in colon carcinogenesis has
been examined by a number of investigators with conflicting
results. Its complexity is illustrated by some preliminary
data from Kroes' laboratory (Table 6). Nine different fat-
fiber combinations were tested in Wistar rats which received
either the direct acting colon carcinogen
(N-methyl-N'-nitro-N-nitrosoguanidine) (MNNG) or the
indirect carcinogen DMH (Kroes et al., 1986). No relationship between tumor incidence and fat was seen for
either carcinogen at the medium or high fiber levels. Tumor
frequency was enhanced by high fat diets containing low or
medium levels of fiber. MNNG-treated animals in the low
fiber group demonstrated a fat associated increased incidence and frequency of colon tumors, while frequency, but not
incidence, was increased in DMH-treated rats.

Table 6

Fiber and Fat Influence on
Colon Tumorigenesis*

Fiber Level	Fat Level	MNNG Incidence %	MNNG Tumors/ TBR	DMH Incidence %	DMH Tumors/ TBR
Low	Low	40	1.4	78	2.0
Low	Medium	60	1.4	78	2.0
Low	High	73	2.9	81	3.7
Medium	Low	60	1.8	60	1.8
Medium	Medium	80	1.8	73	1.7
Medium	High	53	3.1	65	2.6
High	Low	43	1.7	48	2.0
High	Medium	37	1.8	38	1.8
High	High	52	1.8	61	1.9

*Adapted from Kroes et al., Fed. Proc. 45:136 (1986).

All components of the diet must be carefully evaluated
and their input to overall energy consumption and utiliza-

tion taken into consideration. It is now clear, for example, that not only fat, but fiber may contribute significantly to available energy and influence the human digestive tract or colon tumorigenesis in the rat (Cummings, 1983; Kritchevsky, 1983; Jacobs, 1983a, 1983b). Moreover, fat and fiber influences the availability of calories, under some conditions (Kaur et al., 1985) and thus result in additional confounding variables.

CONCLUSIONS

Dietary total fat (quality and quantity)has been associated with increased risk for colon cancer in humans and experimental animals. Results from various laboratories and between investigators are highly variable and subject to differences in interpretation. It seems likely that effects attributed to fat are a result of much more complex interactions of other dietary factors and nutrients. We must begin to dissect the complexity by addressing interactions and other factors which affect overall growth and development and the progress of initiated cells to neoplasia.

This is not to infer that dietary fat is not important as a risk factor in human colon cancer. We believe that it is a significant factor but, most likely, acting in concert with other dietary variables. We also believe that there is sufficient evidence to suggest to populations at high risk for colon cancer to reduce their fat intake, even though we do not know now the exact nature of fat effects and the interactions of fat and other variables. Fundamental research in experimental animals and carefully designed and conducted human studies should provide some of these answers.

REFERENCES

Armstrong B, Doll R (1975). Environmental factors and cancer incidence and mortality in different countries with special reference to dietary practices. Int J Cancer 15:617.
Bansal BR, Rhoads JE, Bansal SC (1978). Effects of diet on colon carcinogenesis and the immune system in rats treated with 1,2-dimethylhydrazine. Cancer Res 38:3293.
Bjelke E (1973). Ph.D. thesis, U of Minnesota, University Microfilms, Ann Arbor, Michigan.

Broitman SA, Vitale JJ, Jakuba EV, Gottlieb LS (1977).
  Polyunsaturated fat, cholesterol and large bowel tumorige-
  nesis. Cancer 40:2455.
Bull AW, Soullier BK, Wilson PS, Hayden MT, Nigro ND (1979).
  Promotion of azoxymethane-induced intestinal cancer by
  high fat diet in rats. Cancer Res 39:4956.
Byers T, Graham S (1984). The epidemiology of diet and
  cancer. In Klein G, Weinhouse S (eds): "Advances in
  Cancer Research." Orlando: Academic Press, pp 1.
Cummings JH, Hill MJ, Jenkins DJA, Pearson JR, Wiggins HS
  (1976). Changes in fecal composition and colonic function
  due to cereal fiber. Am J Clin Nutr 29:1468.
Cummings JH (1983). Fermentation in the human large
  intestine: evidence and implications for health. Lancet
  1:1206.
Dales LG, Friedman GD, Ury HK, Grossman S, Williams SR
  (1978). A case control study of relationships of diet and
  other traits to colorectal cancer in American Blacks. Am
  J Epidemiol 109:132-144.
Doll R, Peto R (1981). The causes of cancer: quantitative
  estimates of avoidable risks of cancer in the United
  States today. J Natl Cancer Inst 66:1191.
Donato K, Hegsted DM (1985). Efficiency of utilization of
  various sources of energy for growth. Proc Natl Acad Sci
  USA 82:4866-4870.
Enstrom JE (1975). Colorectal cancer and consumption of
  beef and fat. Brit J Cancer 32:432-439.
Glauert HP, Bennink MR, Sander CH (1981). Enhancement of
  1,2-dimethylhydrazine induced colon carcinogenesis in mice
  by dietary agar. Fd Cosmet Toxicol 19:281.
Higginson J (1966). Etiological factors in gastrointestinal
  cancer in man. JNCI 37:527-545.
Hill M, MacLennan R, Newcombe K (1979). Diet and large
  bowel cancer in three socio-economic groups in Hong Kong.
  Lancet 1:436 (Letter to Editor).
Isaksson G, Lundquist I, Akesson B, Ihse I (1984). Effect
  of pectin and wheat bran on intraluminal pancreatic enzyme
  activities and on fat absorption as examined with the
  triolein breath test in patients with pancreatic insufficiency. Scand J Gastroenterol 19:467.
Jacobs LR (1983a). Effects of dietary fiber on mucosal
  growth and cell proliferation in the small intestine of
  the rat: a comparison of oat bran, pectin and guar with
  total fiber deprivation. Am J Clin Nutr 37:954.
Jacobs LR (1983b). Enhancement of rat colon carcinogenesis

by wheat bran consumption during the stage of
1,2-dimethylhydrazine administration. Cancer Res 43:4057.
Jain M, Cook GM, Davis FG, Grace M, Howe GR, Miller AB
(1980). A case control study of diet and colorectal
cancer. Internat J Cancer 26:757-768.
Kaur AP, Bhat CM, Grewal RB (1985). Effect of cellulose
incorporation in a low fiberdiet on fecal excretion and
digestibility of nutrients in adolescent girls. Nutr Rep
Int 32:383.
Kinlin LJ (1982). Meat and fat consumption and cancer
mortality: A study of strict religious orders in Britain.
Lancet 1:946-949.
Kritchevsky D (1983). Fiber, steroids and cancer. Cancer
Res 43:2491s.
Kroes R, Beems RB, Bosland MC, Bunnik GSJ, Sinkeldam EJ
(1986). Nutritional factors in lung, colon, and prostate
carcinogenesis in animal models. Federation Proc
45:136-141.
Locniskar M, Nauss KM, Kaufmann P, Newberne PM (1985).
Interaction of dietary fat and route of carcinogen admi-
nistration on 1,2-dimethylhydrazine-induced colon tumori-
genesis in rats. Carcinogenesis 6:349-354.
Lyon JL, Sorenson AW (1978). Colon cancer in a low-risk
population. Am J Clin Nutr 31:5227-5230.
Marshall E (1986). Diet advice with a grain of salt and a
larger helping of pepper. Science 231:537-539.
Nauss KM, Bueche D, Newberne PM. Effect of beef fat on
DMH-induced colon tumorigenesis: Influence of rat strain
and nutrient composition. (submitted for publication).
Nauss KM, Locniskar M, Newberne PM (1983). Effects of
alterations in the quality and quantity of dietary fat
on 1,2-dimethylhydrazine-induced colon tumorigenesis in
rats. Cancer Res 43:4083-4090.
Nauss KM, Locniskar M, Sondergaard D, Newberne PM (1984).
Lack of effect of dietary fat on N-nitrosomethylurea
(NMU)-induced colon tumorigenesis in rats. Carcinogenesis
5:225-260.
Newberne PM, Schrager TF, Conner MW (1985). Nutrients and
other risk factors associated with cancer. In Meyskens
FL, Prasad KN (eds): "Vitamins and Cancer- Human Cancer
Prevention by Vitamins and Micronutrients." Clifton, NJ:
Humana Press, Inc., pp 113-138.
Nigro ND, Singh DV, Campbell RL, Pak MS (1975). Effect of
dietary fat on intestinal tumor formation by azoxymethane
in rats. J Natl Cancer Inst 54:439.

Nutter RL, Gridley DS, Kettering JD, Goude AG, Slater JM (1983). BALB/c mice fed milk or beef protein: Differences in response to 1,2-dimethylhydrazine carcinogenesis. J Natl Cancer Inst 71:867.

Nyman M, Asp N-G (1982). Fermentation of dietary fiber components in the rat intestinal tract. Br J Nutr 47:357.

Phillips RL (1975). Role of lifestyles and dietary habits in risk of cancer among 7th Day Adventists. Cancer Res 35:3513-3522.

Reddy BS, Maeura Y (1984). Tumor promotion by dietary fat on azoxymethane-induced colon carcinogenesis in female F-344 rats: Influence of amount and source of fat. JNCI 72:745-750.

Reddy BS, Narisawa T, Weisburger JH (1976). Effect of a diet with high levels of protein and fat on colon carcinogenesis in F344 rats treated with 1,2-dimethylhydrazine. J Natl Cancer Inst 57:56-569.

Reddy BS, Ohmori T (1981). Effect of intestinal microflora and dietary fat on 3,2'-dimethyl-4-aminobiphenyl-induced colon carcinogenesis in F344 rats. Cancer Res 41:1363-1367.

Reddy BS, Watanabe K, Weisburger JH (1977). Effect of high fat diet on colon carcinogenesis in F344 rats treated with 1,2-dimethylhydrazine, methylazoxymethanol acetate or methylnitrosourea. Cancer Res 37:4156-4159.

Reddy BS, Weisburger JH, Wynder EL (1974). Effects of dietary fat level and dimethylhydrazine on fecal acid and neutral sterol excretion and colon carcinogenesis in rats. J Natl Cancer Inst 52:507-511.

Report of the American Institute of Nutrition ad hoc Committee on Standards for Animal Studies (1977). J Nutr 107:1340.

Rogers AE, Nauss KM (1985). Contributions of laboratory animal studies of colon carcinogenesis. In Mastromarino AJ, Brattain MG (eds): "Large Bowel Cancer: Clinical and Basic Science Research." New York: Praeger, p 1.

Schmähl D, Habs M, Habs H (1983). Influence of a non-synthetic diet with a high fat content on the local occurrence of colonic carcinomas induced by N-nitroso-acetoxymethylmethylamine (AMM) in Sprague Dawley rats. Hepato-gastroenterol 30:30.

Stemmerman GN, Nomura AMY, Heilbrun LK (1984). Dietary fat and the risk of colorectal cancer. Cancer Res 44:4633-4637.

Visek WJ, Clinton SK (1983). Dietary fat and breast cancer. In Perkins EG, Visek WJ (eds): "Dietary Fats and Health," Champaign, IL: American Oil Chemists Society, p 721.

Dietary Fat and Cancer, pages 331–355
© 1986 Alan R. Liss, Inc.

ENHANCEMENT OF PANCREATIC CARCINOGENESIS BY DIETARY FAT IN
THE HAMSTER AND RAT MODELS

D.F. Birt and B.D. Roebuck

The Eppley Institute for Research in Cancer,
University of Nebraska Medical Center, 42nd and
Dewey Avenue, Omaha, NE 68105, U.S.A. (D.F.B.) and
Department of Pharmacology and Toxicology, Dartmouth
Medical School, Hanover, NH 03756 U.S.A. (B.D.R.)

INTRODUCTION

Fpidemiological investigations of dietary fat and
pancreatic cancer have largely consisted of ecological
correlations of incidence and/or death rates and the intake
of nutrients (Wynder et al., 1973; Wynder, 1975; Lea, 1967;
Meyer, 1977; Zaldivar et al., 1981; Armstrong and Doll,
1975; Miller, 1980). Such studies have suggested increased
pancreatic cancer rates in groups consuming diets high in
fat (Wynder et al., 1973; Wynder, 1975; Lea, 1967; Meyer,
1977; Zaldivar et al., 1981) and/or protein (Meyer, 1977;
Zaldivar et al., 1981). However, other reports have failed
to show these associations (Mack and Paganini-Hill, 1981).
One of the difficulties in studying the etiology of
pancreatic cancer has been diagnosing the disease (Zaldivar
et al., 1981; Armstrong and Doll, 1975; Mack and Paganini-
Hill, 1981; Cubilla and Fitzgerald, 1978). Thus, the actual
strength of association between dietary fat intake and
pancreatic cancer cannot readily be derived from available
data. For this reason, data in which an elevated rate of
pancreatic cancer has been found in hamsters and rats fed
high fat diets are particularly noteworthy.

Two models for experimental pancreatic cancer have been
used to assess the relationship between dietary fat and the
disease. Experimental pancreatic ductal/ductular cell
cancer induced by N-nitrosobis(2-oxopropyl)nitrosamine (BOP)
in the Syrian hamster is a particularly useful model,

because of the morphological resemblance between the induced tumors and the most common forms of the comparable human disease (Cubilla and Fitzgerald, 1978). The hamster model also has the advantage of being induced by a single carcinogen injection (Pour et al., 1978). Thus the time of cancer initiation can be more closely defined than in models requiring multiple exposures to the carcinogen. This characteristic is most appropriate for dietary studies, because the influence of nutrient intake on initiation and/or development of tumors can be examined separately.

Experimental pancreatic cancer in the rat has been induced by a variety of chemicals (Roebuck et al., 1983), including one of the same nitrosamines which induces ductal/ductular cell cancer in the hamster model (Longnecker et al., 1985). The most extensive series of studies in the rat have utilized the carcinogen azaserine (Roebuck et al., 1983; Longnecker et al., 1984). Studies have shown a positive relationship between pancreatic DNA damage by azaserine and its ability to induce pancreatic tumors (Zurlo et al., 1984). These studies strongly suggest that azaserine is activated by a pyridoxal-dependent enzyme. Within a few weeks following injection of azaserine, foci of atypical acinar cells appear in the pancreas. These lesions are hyperplastic, apparently irreversible, and a fraction of them appear to give rise to adenomas and adenocarcinomas (Longnecker et al., 1981). The carcinomas predominately retain a degree of acinar cell character, although a few cancers possess duct-like characteristics. With this rat model, quantitation of the number of foci, focal size, and focal growth has proven to be particularly easy (Roebuck et al., 1984; Roebuck 1986b; Roebuck, 1986c). Another advantage of the rat model is the extensive literature available concerning the nutritional requirements and physiology of the rat. The considerable use of the rat in biochemical studies, as well as the lengthy history of its application in cancer research, are important considerations for the use of the rat as a model for the study of pancreatic cancer.

There is currently considerable dispute regarding the cell of origin of pancreatic cancer in humans and in the hamster model (Flaks et al., 1982; Moore et al., 1983; Parsa et al., 1985). The authors believe that both the hamster and the rat models for pancreatic carcinogenesis are extremely valuable. In some cases in which both models have been used, the conclusions drawn from one model have been confirmed in the other. As with all experimental cancer models, results in one model must be carefully considered in relation to similar manipulations in other organ specific models.

STUDIES WITH HAMSTERS

In the initial studies, dietary fat effects on pancreatic carcinogenesis were evaluated with each of three levels of dietary protein. Such a design was used because human diets that are low in protein are also often low in fat, and those high in protein are generally high in fat. Using epidemiological studies, it is difficult to assess which of these two dietary components influences pancreatic cancer development. We addressed this important issue by investigating the interaction between dietary fat and protein on pancreatic carcinogenesis in hamsters. Diets were formulated to contain three levels of dietary corn oil (low fat, 4.5 g/385 Kcal; medium fat, 9.0 g/385 Kcal; high fat, 18 g/385 Kcal) with each of three levels of casein (low protein, 9 g/385 Kcal; medium protein, 18 g/385 Kcal; high protein, 36 g/385 Kcal). These diets were fed either before treatment with a single BOP injection (10 mg/kg body weight, s.c.) at eight weeks of age to determine the effects on initiation, or beginning two days after BOP treatment to measure effects on pancreatic tumor development. Diets were formulated on a nutrient/Kcal basis to avoid dilution of dietary protein, fiber, vitamins and minerals with calories, as the caloric density of the diets was elevated with each increment of dietary fat. As such, carbohydrate was added or reduced to account for the calories (not the grams) of fat removed or added to the diet in the low or high fat diets, respectively. The control level of dietary fat was formulated at 100 g diet/385 Kcal. Similar diets were used in studies of mammary carcinogenesis (Visek and Clinton, 1983) and are recommended for investigations of dietary fat and cancer, because they generally confound fat effects with carbohydrate only, not with all the other nutrients in the diet.

Among the nine dietary groups, the lowest rate of pancreatic cancer resulted when the low fat/low protein diet was fed preceding BOP treatment of the hamsters (Figure 1) (Birt et al., 1983). There were no observed differences

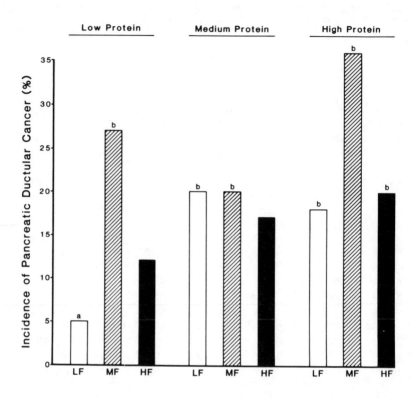

Figure 1. Effect of dietary fat and protein levels fed before carcinogen treatment on pancreatic ductular cancer incidence in hamster. IF, low fat level, 4.5 g/385 Kcal; MF, medium fat level, 9 g/385 Kcal; HF, high fat level, 18 g/385 Kcal. Letters above the bars indicate significant differences by Chi square comparisons, a<b (P<0.05).

between male and female hamsters, and no independent effects of protein (at the medium fat level) or fat (at the medium protein level) were seen (Birt et al., 1981; Pour and Birt, 1983).

Further studies in this laboratory determined the influence of prefeeding with low fat/low protein diet or higher fat and protein levels on single strand breaks in pancreatic ductular DNA. The single strand breaks were measured by alkaline elution. The resultant elution constants are a measure of the elution rate of DNA from a cellulose acetate filter. Higher elution constants denote a more rapid elution and thus more single strand breaks (Kohn, 1979). As shown in Table 1 for BOP-treated hamsters, fewer single strand breaks (as indicated by lower elution constants) were found in pancreatic ductular DNA from hamsters fed the low fat/low protein diet, than were observed in hamsters fed higher levels of fat and/or protein. The lowest elution constant was consistently seen in DNA from hamsters fed low fat/low protein diet and the highest value was observed in the high fat/medium protein group at 6 and 24 hours and 1 week. Elution constants did

Table 1. Elution constants of DNA from pancreatic ductular cells in hamsters prefed levels of dietary fat and protein and treated with BOP (10 mg/kg body weight)[1]

Time after BOP	Low fat/ low protein	Low fat/ medium protein	High fat/ low protein	High fat/ medium protein
0	0.001	0.001	0.001	0.001
6 h	0.032^c	0.049^d	0.040^d	0.051^e
24 h	0.034^c	0.044^d	0.043^d	0.061^f
1 wk	0.028^b	0.040^d	$0.038^{c,d}$	0.045^d
4 wk	0.019^a	0.041^d	0.025^b	$0.028^{b,c}$

[1]Each value represents the mean of 2 sets of observations at 0 and 6 h and at 4 weeks and of 3 observations at 24 h and 1 week; SEM = 0.002. Superscripts indicate the results of multiple comparison tests. Numbers in the BOP treatment groups not sharing a common superscript are significantly different (P <0.005).

not differ between dietary groups in non-BOP-treated
hamsters. These results suggest that the feeding of low
protein diet may have decreased damage to pancreatic
ductular DNA and thus offered some protection against BOP
carcinogenicity. Repair in acinar cells was generally
reduced by prefeeding higher protein levels, and was not
consistently influenced by dietary fat level (Birt and
White, unpublished data).

High fat diet, when given with both medium and high
protein levels following BOP treatment, resulted in elevated
incidences and numbers of ductal/ductular cell carcinomas
(Birt et al., 1983; Birt, et al., 1981). High fat levels,
when administered at a low protein level, however, did not
influence pancreatic carcinogenesis (Figure 2) (Birt et al.,
1983). There were no sex differences observed with these
diets. However, dietary protein effects with the medium fat
level differed according to the sex of the animals, and
therefore these results were not included in Figure 2. The
low protein-medium fat diet inhibited pancreatic cancer
development in females, but not in male hamsters (Pour and
Birt, 1983).

Dietary fat and protein levels also influenced
induction of atypical acinar cell nodules (AACN) in
hamsters. Such nodules have not occurred spontaneously in
hamsters fed natural ingredient diets (Takahashi and Pour,
1978), nor have they been induced by BOP treatment in
hamsters fed natural ingredient diets (Pour et al., 1981).
However, AACN were previously reported in hamsters treated
with azaserine (Roebuck and Longnecker, 1977) and with a
nitrosourea amino acid (Longnecker et al., 1979). In the
studies on the effect of fat and protein on pancreatic
carcinogenesis, AACN developed in a few non-BOP-treated
hamsters; however their incidence was not clearly associated
with diet in these groups. AACN developed in higher yields
in BOP-treated hamsters and were responsive to diet in these
groups. The high fat-low protein experimental diets, when
given prior to BOP treatment, caused the greatest yield of
AACN in female hamsters (52 AACN/28 hamsters, or 1.9
AACN/hamster) in comparison with the high protein level (17
AACN/85 hamsters, or 0.2 AACN/hamster) or with the low fat
level (8 AACN/86 hamsters, 0.1 AACN/hamster) (Birt et al.,
1983; Birt et al., 1981; Pour and Birt, 1983). Male values
were lower and not significantly related to dietary fat and
protein.

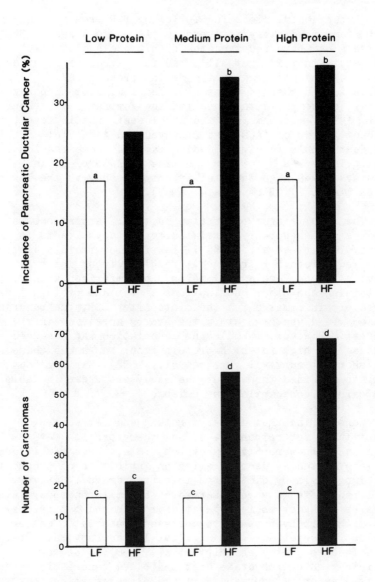

Figure 2. Effect of dietary fat and protein levels fed after carcinogen treatment on pancreatic ductular carcinogenesis in hamsters. LF, low fat level, 4.5 g/385 Kcal; HF, high fat level, 18 g/385 Kcal. Letters above the bars indicate significant differences by Chi square comparisons, a<b (P<0.05) and c<d (P<0.05).

Experimental diets fed following BOP treatment had the most dramatic dietary influence on AACN, as shown in Table 2. When hamsters received the high protein diet, AACN were completely inhibited at all three fat levels (Birt et al., 1983). In hamsters given the medium protein level, AACN yields were higher in those also fed medium or high levels of fat, as compared to those fed the low fat level (Pour and Birt, 1983). In hamsters fed the lowest protein level, the highest yields of AACN were observed and AACN yield doubled between animals receiving medium fat and those fed low fat diet. There was a further doubling of AACN yield in hamsters given high fat diet in comparison with the low fat level (Table 2) (Birt et al., 1983).

The results from pancreatic ductular carcinogenesis studies were generally unrelated to dietary effects on survival (Birt et al., 1982). Low fat-low protein diet, when fed before BOP treatment, resulted in an intermediate survival among females and males, in comparison with diets containing the other combinations of fat and protein levels. Moreover, in females fed the diets after BOP, the pancreatic cancer yield was highest in the groups surviving the longest. However, in males no association was observed, because the high fat-high protein group was among those with the shortest survival (Birt et al., 1982). Maximal body weights attained throughout the study are shown in Table 3 and calorie consumption is in Table 4.

Considering that dietary protein and fat were substituted for carbohydrate, and therefore low fat-low protein diets were high in carbohydrate, these results could be interpreted as demonstrating an inhibition of pancreatic carcinogenesis by diets high in carbohydrate. However, different effects were observed with similar carbohydrate intakes in hamsters fed elevated protein and fat levels. Low fat-high carbohydrate diets decreased pancreatic cancer yields in comparison with high fat-low carbohydrate diets in both females and males (Birt et al., 1981), but low protein-high carbohydrate diet inhibited pancreatic cancer in females only (Pour and Birt, 1983), suggesting that the observed results were not simply due to an influence of dietary carbohydrate. In addition, a differing fat-to-protein ratio cannot explain the results, since diets with similar ratios resulted in different effects on pancreatic carcinogenesis (Birt et al., 1983).

Table 2. Pancreatic atypical acinar cell nodule yield in BOP-treated hamsters fed experimental diets after 8 weeks of age[1]

Sex	Dietary fat (g/385 Kcal)	Dietary protein (g/385 Kcal)					
		9		18		36	
		EFA[2]	Ave. No. AACN/EFA	EFA	Ave. No. AACN/EFA	EFA	Ave. No. AACN/EFA
Female	4.5	27	3.4[d]	29	0.1[a]	27	0.0[a]
	9.0	28	1.2[c]	43	1.4[c]	27	0.0[a]
	18.0	28	7.3[e]	29	1.6[c]	26	0.0[a]
Male	4.5	27	2.5[d]	29	0.1[a]	26	0.0[a]
	9.0	29	1.0[c]	42	0.4[b]	24	0.0[a]
	18.0	29	7.1[e]	27	0.6[b]	29	0.0[a]

[1]Results of chi-square tests indicated as superscripts a<b<c<d<e (p < 0.05).

[2]EFA = effective number of hamsters.

Table 3. Maximal body weight (g) for hamsters fed the experimental diets from 8 weeks of age until death[1]

Dietary fat (g/385 Kcal)	Dietary protein (g/385 Kcal)		
	9.0	18.0	36.0
	Females		
4.5	154[a]	160[a]	177[b]
9.0	172[b]	177[b]	189[c]
18.0	200[c]	229[d]	219[d]
	Males		
4.5	154[f]	155[f]	143[e]
9.0	153[f]	161[f]	156[f]
18.0	172[g]	176[g]	179[g]

[1]Data did not differ with BOP treatment. These values are for the non-BOP treated groups. Each number represents the mean of 26-30 animals (SEM=5) except for the control diet groups (9 g fat and 18 g protein/385 Kcal) in which 48-49 animals are represented (SEM=4). T-test comparisons: ($P<0.05$) a<b<c<d<e<f<g.

Diets high in corn oil enhanced BOP-induced carcinogenesis not only in the pancreas, but also in the lungs, liver and kidneys (Birt and Pour, 1983). These observations agree with results from high-fat diet studies from other laboratories using different cancer models (Carroll et al., 1975; Hopkins and West, 1976; Newberne et al., 1979; Hopkins et al., 1978; Reddy et al., 1977; Tannenbaum, 1942; Beems and Van Beek, 1984). High fat diets generally enhance carcinogenesis when given following carcinogen treatment (Carroll et al., 1975; Hopkins and West, 1976; Newberne et al., 1979; Hopkins et al., 1978;

Table 4. Daily caloric consumption of male hamsters fed three fat levels.

Experimental diet feeding period	Dietary fat (g/385 Kcal)	Calories consumed during weeks of age[3]			
		mean Kcal/day/animal			
		3-7	8-27	28-52	53-92
3-7 weeks[1]	4.5	25[a]	27	25	21
	9.0	30[b]	28	25	22
	18.0	34[c]	28	25	22
8 weeks-death[2]	4.5	28	26[d]	24[f]	20[h]
	9.0	29	27[d]	25[f]	21[h]
	18.0	29	33[e]	20[g]	28[i]

[1] Pooled across protein.

[2] Consumption at 18.0 g/385 Kcal level of protein.

[3] t-test comparisons a<b<c, d<e, f<g, h<i (P<0.005). Week during which calories were consumed and week by sex interaction significant for both feeding periods (P<0.001).

Reddy et al., 1977; Tannenbaum, 1942 and Beems and Van Beek, 1984).

Interactions between dietary fat and protein were previously studied in experimental mammary (Clinton et al., 1984), liver and urinary bladder (Frith et al., 1980) cancer models. Mammary cancer induced by 7,12-dimethylbenz-[a]anthracene (DMBA) was elevated by high fat diet at low, medium, and high protein levels when diets were consumed either before or after DMBA treatment (Clinton et al., 1984). Interactions between dietary fat and protein were not observed (Clinton et al., 1984). Liver and urinary bladder cancer incidences, induced by repeated N-2-fluorenylacetamide treatment, were reduced by feeding low fat-low protein diets and increased by elevations in fat at low and high protein levels during carcinogen treatment (Frith et al., 1980). In our studies on pancreatic carcinogenesis, BOP-induced lung adenomas were also influenced by the interaction between dietary fat and protein, with the highest yields observed in hamsters fed high fat-high protein diets (Birt and Pour, 1985). Nutrient interactions have received little attention in the evaluation of human data; however, an interaction between dietary fat and fiber was suggested as an important factor in human colon cancer (Reddy et al., 1980).

STUDIES WITH RATS

Initial studies in the rat, to evaluate the role of dietary fat on pancreatic carcinogenesis, simultaneously treated rats with the pancreatic carcinogen, azaserine, while feeding test diets with various fats (Roebuck et al., 1981). The unsaturated fat was corn oil and the saturated fat was hydrogenated coconut oil with 2% corn oil added to supply the essential fatty acid. These two high fat diets were fed at 20% total fat. Two other groups were fed diets with only 2% fat and 5% fat (both corn oil). All diets were modifications of the purified AIN-76 diet (Bieri, 1976; 1981). This initial experiment was of one year's duration. The differential diagnosis of pancreatic adenomas and well-differentiated adenocarcinomas in situ is difficult; therefore, these neoplasms were combined and are summarized in Table 5. The 20% unsaturated fat-fed group had a significantly higher incidence of neoplasms and more neoplasms per pancreas, and included three rats with locally

Table 5. Pancreatic neoplasms: concurrent azaserine treatment and dietary fats[1,2]

Dietary treatments	Total dietary fat (%)	Number of rats per group	Pancreatic adenomas and adenocarcinomas	
			Incidence (%)	Neoplasms per pancreas (mean)
AIN (saline)	5	16	0 (0)	0
AIN	5	17	12 (71)	2.4
Low fat	2	13	11 (85)	2.2
Saturated fat	20	20	15 (75)	2.4
Unsaturated fat	20	18	18 (100)[3]	>10

[1] From Roebuck et al. 1981a.

[2] Rats received intermittent azaserine injections (total azaserine dose of 160 mg/kg body weight) and the test diets concurrently during this experiment of 12 months duration. One group received only the solvent, saline, and served as a control.

[3] Three locally invasive pancreatic adenocarcinomas.

invasive pancreatic adenocarcinomas. The azaserine-treated
rats fed the lower levels of fats exhibited neoplastic
response similar to that in rats fed the 20% saturated fat
diet. These results could not be explained by differences
in growth of the rats or caloric intakes. For example, the
saturated fat group consumed more calories and attained a
greater body weight than did the unsaturated fat group,
although the neoplastic response was most similar to that in
the AIN and low fat groups.

The experiment described above does not indicate the
stage (initiation or postinitiation) of carcinogenesis in
which unsaturated fats preferentially enhance pancreatic
carcinogenesis. Experiments to evaluate this were undertaken
(Roebuck et al., 1981b). Ideally, experiments designed to
demonstrate promotion utilize a single, sub-carcinogenic
dose of carcinogen. With azaserine this dose was not known;
therefore, we utilized multiple injections over a relatively
short initiation phase. During an initiation phase of 7
weeks, rats received 6 consecutive weekly i.p. injections of
10 mg azaserine per kg body weight. During the
postinitiation phase, no further exposure to azaserine
occurred. The various test diets were fed either during the
initiation phase or during the postinitation phase. When
fed at 20% in the diet during the initiation phase, the
saturated and unsaturated fats had no effect on the
incidence or number of neoplasms as compared to rats fed the
5% AIN diet (for details see Roebuck et al., 1981b). When
fed during the postinitiation phase, the unsaturated fat
increased the incidence and multiplicity of pancreatic
neoplasms; whereas the saturated fat at the same high level
showed no enhancement. The results of the postinitiational
enhancement are summarized in Table 6. Also summarized in
Table 6 is an entirely separate replicate experiment of this
postinitiational effect due to 20% unsaturated fat. In
addition to corn oil, the unsaturated fat safflower oil was
also evaluated. Again when compared to either the AIN diet
(5% corn oil) or the 20% saturated fat diet, the unsaturated
diets at 20% fat enhanced pancreatic carcinogenesis. This
phenomenon has been termed promotion; however, until the
mechanism responsible for the enhancement is better
understood this term should probably be avoided in favor of
enhancement (Hicks, 1983).

Experiments similar to those described above require at
least one year to complete. To study the effects of dietary

Table 6. Effects of diet on initiation and postinitiation phases of azaserine-induced carcinogenesis in the rat[1]

Initiation phase		Postinitiation phase	Duration of experiment (month)	Pancreatic adenomas and adenocarcinomas	
Dietary treatment	Total azaserine dose (mg/kg)	Dietary treatment		Incidence[2] (%)	Neoplasia per pancreas (mean)
AIN	60	AIN	9	24	0.47
Saturated	60	AIN	9	11	0.11
Unsaturated	60	AIN	9	21	0.21
AIN	60	Saturated	9	15	0.20
AIN	60	Unsaturated	9	55	1.45
AIN	80	AIN	12	56	0.9
AIN	80	Saturated	12	69	1.3
AIN	80	Unsaturated	12	94	4.7
AIN	80	Safflower	12	94[3]	5.9

[1] For details see Roebuck et al., 1983.
[2] The effective number of rats ranged between 16 and 20 per group.
[3] Two locally invasive pancreatic adenocarcinomas.

fats on pancreatic carcinogenesis, we have developed a
short-term, quantitative model based upon the early
appearance of putative preneoplastic atypical acinar cell
nodules, AACN (for review see Roebuck, 1986b). In the
earliest experiments (Roebuck et al., 1977), the
susceptibility by species and strain of rodents to azaserine
was determined by the number of AACN found in histological
sections of the pancreases. Subsequently, the number of
AACN in tissue sections of pancreas has been related to the
dose of azaserine, the age at dosing, and the time to
autopsy (Yager et al., 1981). Success with these early
experiments has led to rigorous quantitation of the rat
model, which includes measurement of the size of the AACN
(Roebuck et al., 1984). AACN are three-dimensional
structures, but in the histological section we can identify,
count and measure only the two-dimensional transections of
these lesions. The techniques of quantitative stereology
have been applied to our two-dimensional observations of the
pancreatic lesions (Roebuck et al., 1984) in a manner
similar to their application to the study of
hepatocarcinogenesis (Pugh et al.,1983). The utilization of
these techniques to the study of the enhancement of
pancreatic carcinogenesis by dietary fats is discussed
below, but first, the model as it currently exists, will be
described.

The short term model is of approximately 4 months
duration. Male rat pups (usually of the Lewis strain) are
injected i.p. at 14 days of age with azaserine (30 mg/kg)
and weaned at 21 days of age to the test diets. Alternatively, weaned rats may be injected with the carcinogen and
then transferred to test diets. With no further azaserine
exposure, the young rats are usually fed the test diets for
4 months. At autopsy the entire pancreas is embedded and
routine histological sections are prepared, to allow the
maximum amount of pancreatic tissue to be examined without
encountering the same AACN more than once. Details of the
tissue preparation are covered elsewhere (Roebuck, 1986b).
Carcinogens, including azaserine, induce two phenotypically
different populations of AACN (Rao et al. 1983; Roebuck et
al. 1984; and Chiu, 1985). Identified AACN are counted and
measured with a computer-aided microscope system, and
quantitative stereological equations are applied. The
resulting data from experiments include the observed
two-dimensional counts and sizes of the foci, and the
computed mean number of foci per volume of tissue, the mean

size of the AACN, and the volume of pancreas occupied by the AACN.

The effects of the dietary unsaturated fat on the growth of azaserine-induced AACN are presented in Table 7. In this short-term experiment, dietary fat had differential effects on the two phenotypically different populations of AACN. Both unsaturated fat and saturated fats were fed at 20% in the diet. The pancreases of the group fed the unsaturated fat had significantly more, but not larger, acidophilic AACN than did the pancreases of those rats fed the saturated fat diet. Neither fat had an effect on the basophilic population of AACN. The volume of pancreas occupied by the acidophilic AACN was three times larger in the rats fed the unsaturated fat. This volume expression can be thought of as the "tumor" burden within the pancreas. In other experiments, the basophilic population of AACN generally shows little growth potential (Rao et al., 1983; Roebuck et al., 1985). Although the basophilic foci are carcinogen-induced, and at 2.5 months following initiation have a similarly high rate of growth as possessed by the acidophilic AACN, their rate of growth is not sustained. By 4 months postinitiation, both the nuclear labelling index and the mean size of the basophilic AACN are less than for the acidophilic population (Roebuck, 1986a). By an as yet unknown mechanism, the high level of dietary unsaturated fat enhances and sustains the growth of the acidophilic foci for a longer time than the basophilic population. The growth rate of the acidophilic AACN, but not the basophilic AACN, increases with increasing essential fatty acid (linoleic acid) content of the standard 20% by weight fat diet. This increase is especially large and obvious for the essential fatty acid range of 4 to 8% (Roebuck et al., 1985). Experiments similar to ours, with the DMBA-induced mammary tumorigenesis model, indicate that for diets of 20% fat, the minimum requirement of essential fatty acid is 4% (Ip et al., 1985).

Perturbation of the pancreatic tumor-enhancing effects of dietary unsaturated fat has been shown with this short-term model. At two months into the usual 4 month postinitiation phase, if the 20% unsaturated fat diet is switched to a 5% unsaturated fat diet, the resulting number and size of the AACN at 4 months resemble that seen in the group fed 5% fat throughout the 4 months of the postinitiation phase. This implies that the stimulus

Table 7. The effects of dietary modification of the postinitiation phase[1]

Focal phenotype and dietary fat treatment	Observed transectional data of foci		Calculated volumetric data of foci		
	No. per sq cm	Mean area (sq mm X 100)	No. per cu cm	Mean Diameter (μm)	Volume as % of pancreas
ACIDOPHILIC					
Saturated	1.3 ± 0.5	5.72 ± 1.81	52 ± 19	265 ± 17	0.136 ± 0.103
Unsaturated	5.2 ± 0.6	7.46 ± 0.85	171 ± 20	306 ± 27	0.397 ± 0.061
BASOPHILIC					
Saturated	1.8 ± 0.4	2.98 ± 0.52	86 ± 19	223 ± 16	0.053 ± 0.014
Unsaturated	1.0 ± 0.3	3.84 ± 0.84	52 ± 14	210 ± 21	0.040 ± 0.012

[1]Results are means ± standard errors of the mean with 10 rats per group. The duration of the postinitiation phase was 4 months during which the postinitiation diets were fed. See Roebuck et al., 1984 for details of the diet composition. All rats were fed the AIN control diet when initiated. The rats fed the high fat diets during the postinitiation phase were initiated at 7 weeks of age with a single (30 mg/kg) dose of azaserine.

produced by the high fat diet has to be continually present. However, a switch at two months from the low fat diet to the high fat diet resulted in the pattern of AACN being similar to that seen in the rats fed the high fat throughout the 4 months of postinitiation (O'Connor et al., 1985a). A tentative assumption is that the "fat effect" is reversible and maximum stimulation of AACN growth occurs over a short period (i.e., approximately 2 months). These dietary intervention studies clearly indicate that intervention by the modulation of the level of fat in the diet could have public health significance. In other experiments in which fats were fed at 20% in the diet, the feeding of menhaden oil (rich in omega-3, long-chain fatty acids) significantly inhibited the growth of AACN (O'Connor et al., 1985b). Others have reported similar findings in different tumor systems (Karmali et al., 1984). While the mechanisms involved in the enhancement of pancreatic carcinogenesis by unsaturated fat are at present unknown, experimental modulations as described above should aid in determining the underlying mechanisms leading to enhancement or promotion.

GENERAL DISCUSSION

Comparisons between pancreatic ductular carcinogenesis in the hamster and acinar cell carcinogenesis in the rat have generally led to similar conclusions concerning the action of dietary fat. From the above presentations, it is obvious that a high intake of unsaturated fat enhances pancreatic carcinogenesis. The use of these two models has not always lead to the same result; for example, various retinoids have been shown to inhibit carcinogenesis in the rat model but enhance carcinogenesis in the hamster model (Birt et al., 1983a). In spite of the general use of different initiator carcinogens and the apparently different target cell population, the intake of high levels of unsaturated fat enhanced tumorigenesis in both models of pancreatic cancer. This implies that the enhancement must be operating through a common mechanism. These critical mechanistic studies are currently lacking.

With respect to the models and their characterization, several issues are as yet unresolved. Interactions between dietary fat and protein have not been evaluated in the rat-acinar cell carcinogenesis model and the results of studies with fats other than corn oil have not been reported for the hamster model, although research comparing beef tallow with corn oil is currently under way in both rodent models. In contrast with observations of enhanced pancreatic ductal/ductular cell carcinogenesis in hamsters fed high protein diet, carcinogenesis in the acinar cell rat model was inhibited in rats fed diets containing 50% casein. However, the results from studies of acinar cell carcinogenesis agreed with the effects of dietary fat and protein on AACN in hamsters.

Although the individual attributes of each model are many, the demonstration that both models behave similarly with respect to the modulation of carcinogenesis by dietary fat cannot be overstated. This is certainly the case for the enhancement of pancreatic cancer by feeding high levels of unsaturated fat during the postinitiation phase of carcinogenesis. The development of critical studies to investigate the mechanisms is now the next step to understanding and perhaps controlling pancreatic cancer.

ACKNOWLEDGEMENTS

Research on the hamster model (D.F.B.) was supported by Public Health Service Contract NDICP-33278 from the Division of Cancer Cause and Prevention, NCI, Grant 1RO1CA31655 from NCI and funds from the Nebraska Department of Health. Preparation of this chapter was aided by NIH Research Grant CA36727 from NCI. Research on the rat model (B.D.R.) was supported by several grants including CA-20948 and CA-26594 from the Diet, Nutrition, and Cancer Program from NCI. We thank Karen J. Baumgartner and Linda V. Conrad for assistance in preparation of this chapter.

REFERENCES

Armstrong B, Doll R (1975). Environmental factors and cancer incidence and mortality in different countries, with special reference to dietary practices. Int J Cancer 15:617-631.
Beems RB, Van Beek L (1984). Modifying effect of dietary fat on benzo[a]pyrene-induced respiratory tract tumors in hamsters. Carcinogenesis 5:413-417.
Bieri G (1977). Report of the American Institute of Nutrition Ad Hoc Committee on standards of nutritional studies. J Nutr 107:1340-1348.

Bieri G (1980). Second report of the ad hoc committee on standards for nutritional studies. J Nutr 110:1726.

Birt DF, Davies MH, Pour PM, Salmasi S (1983). Lack of inhibition by retinoids of bis(2-oxopropyl)nitrosamine induced carcinogenesis in Syrian hamsters. Carcinogenesis 4:1215-1220.

Birt DF, Higginbotham SM, Patil K, Pour P (1982). Nutritional effects on the lifespan of Syrian hamsters. Age 5:11-19.

Birt DF, Pour PM (1983) Increased tumorigenesis induced by N-nitrosobis(2-oxopropyl)amine in Syrian golden hamsters fed high-fat diets. J Natl Cancer Inst 70:1135-1138.

Birt DF, Pour PM (1985) Effects of the interaction of dietary fat and protein on N-nitrosobis(2-oxopropyl)amine-induced carcinogenesis and spontaneous lesions in Syrian golden hamsters. 74:1121-1127.

Birt DF, Salmasi S, Pour PM (1981). The enhancement of experimental pancreatic cancer in Syrian golden hamsters by dietary fat. J Natl Cancer Inst 67:1327-1332.

Birt DF, Stepan KR, Pour PM (1983). Interaction of dietary fat and protein on pancreatic carcinogenesis in Syrian golden hamsters. J Natl Cancer Inst 71:355-360.

Carroll KK, Khor HT (1975). Dietary fat in relation to tumorigenesis. Prog Biochem Pharmacol 10:308-353.

Chiu T (1985). Hypertrophic foci of pancreatic acinar cells in rats. CRC Critical Rev. Toxicol. 14:133-157.

Clinton SK, Imrey PB, Alster JM, Simon J, Truex R, Visek WJ (1984). The combined effects of dietary protein and fat on 7,12-dimethylbenz(a)anthracene-induced breast cancer in rats. J Nutr 114:1213-1223.

Cubilla AL, Fitzgerald PJ (1978). Pancreas cancer (non-endocrine): A review, Part 1. Clin Bull 8:91-99.

Cubilla AL, Fitzgerald PJ (1978). Pancreas cancer (non-endocrine): A review, Part II. Clin Bull 8:143-155.

Flaks B, Moore MA, Flaks B (1982). Ultrastructural analysis of pancreatic carcinogenesis. 5. Changes in differentiation of acinar cells during chronic treatment with N-nitrosobis(2-hydroxypropyl)amine. Carcinogenesis 3:485-498.

Frith CH, Norvell MJ, Umholtz R, Knapka JJ (1980). Effect of dietary protein and fat levels on liver and urinary bladder neoplasia in mice fed 2-acetylaminofluorene. J Food Safety 2:183-198.

Hicks RM (1983). Pathological and biochemical aspects of tumor promotion. Carcinogenesis 4:1209.

Hopkins GJ, Hard GC, West CE (1978). Carcinogenesis induced

by 7,12-dimethylbenz(a)anthracene in C3H-A or fB mice: Influence of different fats. J Natl Cancer Inst 60:849-853.

Hopkins GJ, West CE (1976). Possible roles of dietary fats in carcinogenesis. Life Sci 19:1103-1116.

Ip C, Carter CA, Ip MM (1985). Requirement of essential fatty acid for mammary tumorigenesis in the rat. Cancer Res 45:1997-2001.

Karmali RA, Marsh J, Fuchs C (1984). Effect of omega-3 fatty acids on growth of a rat mammary tumor. J Natl Cancer Inst 73:457-461.

Kohn KW (1979). DNA as a target in cancer chemotherapy: Measurement of macromolecular DNA damage produced in mammalian cells by anticancer agents and carcinogens. Methods in Cancer Research 16:291-345.

Lea AJ (1967). Neoplasms and environmental factors. Ann R Coll Surg Engl 41:432-438.

Longnecker DS, Curphey TJ, French JI, Lilja HS (1979). Response of the Syrian golden hamster to a nitrosourea amino acid carcinogen. Cancer Lett 8:163-168.

Longnecker DS, Roebuck BD, Kuhlmann ET, Curphey TJ (1985). Induction of pancreatic carcinomas in rats with N-nitroso(2-hydroxypropyl)(2-oxopropyl)amine: histopathology. J Natl Cancer Inst 74:209-217.

Longnecker DS, Roebuck BD, Yager JD, Lilja HS, Siegmund B (1981). Pancreatic carcinoma in azaserine-treated rats: induction, classification and dietary modulation of incidence. Cancer 47:1562-1572.

Longnecker DS, Wiebkin P, Schaffer BK, Roebuck BD (1984). Experimental carcinogenesis in the pancreas. Int Rev Exp Pathol 26:177-229.

Mack TM, Paganini-Hill D (1981). Epidemiology of pancreas cancer in Los Angeles. Cancer 47:1474-1483.

Meyer F (1977). Relationship between diet and carcinoma of stomach, colon, rectum and pancreas in France. Gastroenterol Clin Biol 1:971-982.

Miller AB (1980). Nutrition and cancer. Prev Med 9:189-196.

Moore MA, Takahashi M, Iton BP (1983). Early lesions during pancreatic carcinogenesis induced in the Syrian hamster by DHPN and DOPN. II Ultrastructural findings. Carcinogenesis 4:439-448.

Newberne PM, Weigert J, Kula N (1979). Effects of dietary fat on hepatic mixed-function oxidases and hepatocellular carcinoma induced by aflatoxin B in rats. Cancer Res 39:3986-3991.

O'Connor TP, Roebuck BD, Campbell TC (1985). Dietary

intervention during the postdosing phase of L-azaserine-induced preneoplastic lesions. J Natl Cancer Inst 75:955-957.

O'Connor TP, Roebuck BD, Peterson F, Campbell TC (1985). Effect of dietary intake of fish oil and fish protein on the development of L-azaserine-induced preneoplastic lesions in the rat pancreas. J Natl Cancer Inst 75:959-962.

Parsa I, Longnecker DS, Scarpelli DG, Pour P, Reddy JK, Lefkowitz M (1985). Ductal metaplasia of human exocrine pancreas and its association with carcinoma. Cancer Res 45:1285-1290.

Pour PM, Birt DF (1983). Modifying factors in pancreatic carcinogenesis in the hamster model. IV. Effects of dietary protein. J Natl Cancer Inst 71:347-353.

Pour P, Runge R, Birt D, Gingell R, Lawson T, Nagel D, Wallcave L, Salmasi SZ (1981). Current knowledge of pancreatic carcinogenesis in the hamster and its relevance to the human disease. Cancer 47:1573-1587.

Pour PM, Salmasi SZ, Runge RG (1978). Selective induction of pancreatic ductular tumors by single doses of N-nitroso(2-oxopropyl)amine in Syrian golden hamsters. Cancer Lett 4:317-323.

Pugh TD, King JH, Koen H, Nychka D, Chover J, Wahba G, He Y, Goldfarb S (1983) Reliable stereological method for estimating the number of microscopic hepatocellular foci from their transections. Cancer Res 43:1261-1268.

Rao MS, Upton MP, Subbarao DG, Scarpelli DG (1982). Two populations of cells with differing proliferative capacities in atypical acinar cell foci induced by 4-hydroxyaminoquinoline-1-oxide in the rat pancreas. Lab Invest 46:527-534.

Reddy BS, Cohen LA, McCoy GD, Hill P, Weisburger JH, Wynder EL (1980). Nutrition and its relationship to cancer. Adv Cancer Res 32:237-345.

Reddy BS, Watanabe K, Weisburger JH (1977). Effect of high-fat diet on colon carcinogenesis in F344 rats treated with 1,2-dimethylhydrazine, methylazoxymethanol acetate or methylnitrosourea. Cancer Res 37:4156-4159.

Roebuck BD (1986a). Effects of high levels of dietary fats on the growth of azaserine-induced foci in the rat pancreas. Lipids (in press).

Roebuck BD (1986b). Enhancement of pancreatic carcinogenesis by raw soy protein isolate: Quantitative rat model and nutritional considerations. In Friedman M (ed): "Nutritional and Toxicological Significance of

Enzyme Inhibitors in Foods." Boston: Plenum Publishing
Corp. (in press).
Roebuck BD (1986c). Enhancement of pancreatic carcinogenesis
in the rat by dietary fats. In Scarpelli DG, Reddy J,
Longnecker DS (eds): "Experimental Pancreatic
Carcinogenesis." Boca Raton, Florida: CRC Press (in
press).
Roebuck BD, Baumgartner KJ, Thron CD (1984).
Characterization of two populations of pancreatic atypical
acinar cell foci induced by azaserine in the rat. Lab
Invest 50:141-146.
Roebuck BD, Longnecker DS (1977). Species and rat strain
variation in pancreatic nodule induction by azaserine.
J Natl Cancer Inst. 59:1273-1277.
Roebuck BD, Longnecker DS, Baumgartner KJ, Thron CD (1985).
Carcinogen-induced lesions in the rat pancreas: Effects of
varying levels of essential fatty acid. Cancer Res
45:5252-5256.
Roebuck BD, Longnecker DS, Yager JD (1983). Initiation and
promotion in pancreatic carcinogenesis. In Slaga TJ (ed)
"Mechanisms of tumor promotion, Volume 1: Tumor promotion
in internal organs." Boca Raton Florida: CRC Press, pp
151-171.
Roebuck BD, Yager JD, Longnecker DS (1981a). Dietary
modulation of azaserine-induced pancreatic carcinogenesis
in the rat. Cancer Res 41:888-893.
Roebuck BD, Yager JD, Longnecker DS, Wilpone SA (1981b).
Promotion by unsaturated fat of azaserine-induced
pancreatic carcinogenesis in the rat. Cancer Res
41:3961-3966.
Takahashi M, Pour P (1978). Spontaneous alterations in the
pancreas of the aging Syrian golden hamster. J Natl Cancer
Inst 60:355-364.
Tannenbaum A (1942). The genesis and growth of tumors. III.
Effects of a high fat diet. Cancer Res 2:468-475.
Visek WJ, Clinton SK (1983). Dietary fat and breast cancer.
In Perkins EG, Visek WJ (eds) "Dietary Fats and Health."
American Oil Chemists Society, Champaign, IL, pp 721-740.
Wyder EL (1975). An epidemiological evaluation of the
causes of cancer of the pancreas. Cancer Res
35:2228-2233.
Wynder EL, Mabuchi K, Maruchi N, Fortner JG (1973).
Epidemiology of cancer of pancreas. J Natl Cancer Inst
50:645-667.
Yager JD, Roebuck BD, Zurlo J, Longnecker DS, Weselcouch EO,
Wilpone SA (1981). Rationale for a single-dose azaserine

protocol for initiation of pancreatic carcinogenesis in the rat. Int J Cancer 28:601-606.

Zaldivar R, Wetterstrand WH, Ghai GL (1981). Relative frequency of mammary, colonic, rectal, and pancreatic cancer in a large autopsy series. Statistical association between mortality rates from these cancers: Dietary fat intake as a common etiological variable. Zentralbl Bakteriol [Naturwiss] 169:474-481.

Zurlo J, Roebuck BD, Rutkowski JV, Curphey TJ, Longnecker DS (1984). Effect of pyridoxal deficiency on pancreatic DNA damage and nodule induction by azaserine. Carcinogenesis 5:555-558.

Dietary Fat and Cancer, pages 357–374
© 1986 Alan R. Liss, Inc.

OIL GAVAGE TEST-COMPOUND ADMINISTRATION EFFECTS IN NTP CARCINOGENESIS-TOXICITY TESTING

Robert E. Landers, Michael J. Norvell and
Mark A. Bieber

Best Foods Research and Engineering Center, A
Division of CPC International, Inc., Union,
New Jersey 07083

INTRODUCTION

Interest in safety testing has grown rapidly in the chemical and food industries as carcinogenesis and toxicity methods have been developed and pressed into use. The National Cancer Institute's (NCI) Toxicology and Carcinogenesis Studies Program, to detect potential human carcinogens, was converted into the National Toxicology Program (NTP) and transferred to the National Institute of Environmental Health Sciences (NIEHS) in 1978. In an effort to enhance assurance that rodents were exposed to known amounts of the test compound, the NTP chemical managers increased use of oil gavage administration from about 10 to 28 percent.

Two widely used compounds administered by oil gavage, benzyl acetate (flavor/fragrance) and methylene chloride (degreaser/solvent) appeared to show carcinogenic responses in NTP carcinogenesis bioassays in 1982. The oil gavage technique soon caught the attention of consulting toxicologists who began to question its involvement in the unexpected carcinogenic responses. Ironically, the technique for oil gavage administration of test compounds to rodents has been widely used without prior validation. In this chapter the effects of oil gavage on the outcome of NTP carcinogenesis bioassays are examined for consistency with carcinogen animal model data, implications for data extrapolation and potential associations with overnutrition; related NTP research is summarized.

PRECHRONIC STUDIES

The prechronic studies include single acute dose, 14-day repeated dose, chemical disposition, fertility and reproduction, urinalysis, clinical chemistry, hematology and other compound specific tests (U.S. DHHS, 1985).

Maximum Tolerated Dose. Current testing protocols require use of maximum tolerated dose (MTD) and two intermediate doses to assure adequate exposure to the test compound (U.S. DHHS, 1985). Oil gavage could increase or decrease the MTD depending on the properties of the test compound as well as the nature, volume and frequency of the gavage vehicle. Data are very limited on most of the variables; complexity is increased by the frequently observed tumor depression in the two highest dose groups in long-term NTP studies.

Prioritization of the interactive oil gavage variables suggests that the properties of the test compound could have the largest effect on MTD. Withey et al., (1983) observed that the oil-water partition coefficient had a large effect on apparent absorption of a series of halogenated solvents, at pharmacokinetic dose levels. Eschenbrenner et al., (1943) observed that a four day interval between carbon tetrachloride dosing gave maximum mouse hepatoma response. The effects of the NTP five day oil gavage schedule with two days off on weekends need to be investigated.

Prediction of oil gavage effects in the MTD range is a real challenge. Modeling studies have extrapolated pharmacokinetic data into the MTD range to predict metabolism (Angelo and Pritchard, 1984); however, in this high dose range which is above the saturation kinetics state it appears virtually impossible to describe the actual metabolism of a specific test compound. An alternate acute oral LD_{50} bioassay approach (Lorke, 1983), to predict potential vehicle type and gavage volume effects, has been tested (Landers, original data 1986). Chloroform and carbon tetrachloride were selected for the LD_{50} evaluation because they were well tested compounds with a 10-fold difference in water solubility (1.0 ml per 200 and 2,000 mls of water respectively; Anon, 1976). Range finding LD_{50} studies in 5 ml/kg of corn oil indicated ml/kg doses of 0.1, 0.2, 0.3, 0.4, 0.8 and 0.2, 0.4, 0.8, 1.2, 1.6 for chloroform and carbon tetrachloride respectively.

Chloroform and carbon tetrachloride were administered, after an 18-hour fast, neat, and in 2.5, 5.0, 10 ml corn oil/Kg body wt/compound, 5.0 ml tricaprylin-compound/Kg or 5 ml toothpaste base-chloroform mixture/Kg (Roe et al., 1979) to 5 male and 5 female Fischer 344 rats (136-190 grams) per group. Rats were individually caged, fed Purina rat chow and observed for mortality or other signs of gross toxicity for 14 days. Gross necropsies were performed on all mortalities and on all survivors at terminal sacrifices. The defined oral LD_{50} values were calculated by probit analyses (Litchfield and Wilcoxon, 1949). Preliminary oral LD_{50} data suggest that in comparison to neat administration, corn oil gavage could increase the toxicity of chloroform and carbon tetrachloride thus reducing the apparent MTD, Figure 1. Tricaprylin may increase the toxicity even

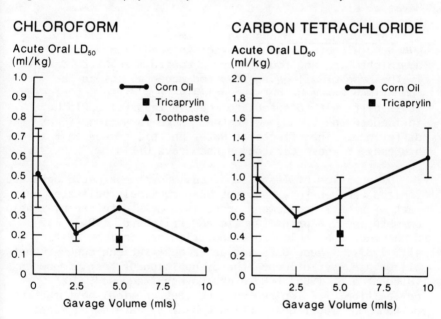

Figure 1. Acute oral LD_{50} (ml/kg) for chloroform and carbon tetrachloride administered neat, and in 2.5, 5.0, 10 ml corn oil/Kg body wt/compound or 5 ml/tricaprylin-compound/Kg or 5 ml toothpaste base-chloroform mixture/Kg to 5 male and 5 female Fischer 344 rats (136-190 grams) per group. The 95 percent confidence ranges are shown for means except for 3 chloroform points where variation of individual values prevented the calculation.

further due to its preferential absorption via the portal vein. Oil gavage may enhance the absorption of chloroform and carbon tetrachloride at lower gavage volumes but have opposite effects at higher volumes for some compounds.

An LD_{50} comparison for gavage administration of chloroform to mice in aqueous Emulphor (95/5) or corn oil (10 ml/kg) showed no differences in the 14 day study; however, in a 90 day gavage study there were some elevations in serum LDH enzyme activity in the corn oil gavage-treated rats (Hayes, JR, personal communication, 1985). Preliminary studies to evaluate aqueous versus oil-gavage vehicles in 90 day studies have shown that different compounds produce unpredictable effects based on LD_{50} results and known properties of the compounds (Condie, 1986; Hayes, 1984; Hayes et al., 1986).

Teratogenicity Bioassays. Kimmel et al., (1985) compared effects of water gavage versus oil gavage administration and found a trend toward more birth defects in the pups of oil gavage treated rodents. Since the comparison was made between animals from different studies it is difficult to speculate what variable(s) could have influenced the trend and whether there is a significant difference. The effects of water and oil gavage in the same bioassay of known teratogens needs evaluation.

Disposition of Test Compounds. Pharmacokinetic data are limited because they have not been routinely collected as part of safety assessment programs. Some data are available on methylene chloride (Angelo and Pritchard, 1984), 1,2-dichloroethane, chloroform and trichloroethylene (Withey et al., 1983). These data and other observations suggest that oil gavage may influence the disposition of test compounds (Bird et al., 1985). However, gavage frequency, diet composition, feeding regimen and test chemical perturbation of food and water consumption appear to have a far more consequential effect on lesion incidence than the oil vehicle per se (Eschenbrenner et al., 1943; Ross, 1961; Ross et al., 1982; Leveille, 1972; Jorgenson et al., 1985).

CHRONIC BIOASSAYS

The purpose of the NTP chronic carcinogenesis bioassays is to determine the carcinogenic potential of nominated chemicals (U.S. DHHS, 1985).

Protocol. A chronic two-year study uses two rodent species (usually Fischer 344/N rats and B6C3F$_1$ mice of both sexes). Animals are placed in the bioassay protocol after weaning and studied for two years. The current diet is the National Institute of Health 07 (NIH-07) cereal-based diet; however, the data discussed in this chapter were obtained from bioassays using both least-cost-formulated commercial chow and NIH-07 diets. Untreated control, vehicle control, low, intermediate, and high dose groups of animals (50 per group) are carried through the two-year bioassay. All tissues are submitted for pathology workup. The chemical is given by the feed, oil gavage, dermal, inhalation, drinking water or intraperitoneal injection route. Gavage oil volume is usually 5 ml/kg for the rat and 10 ml/kg for the mouse but it has varied from 1-10 ml/kg for the rat. The gavage frequency is 5 days/week for 2 years. The majority of the chemicals have been given by feed (about 55%) and oil gavage (about 28%; Haseman et al., 1984a).

Untreated (UC) Versus Vehicle Control (VC) Tumors. Oil gavage effects were analyzed for the large NTP data base on rats (3499 UC and 2200 VC) and mice (3582 UC and 2193 VC; Haseman et al., 1985). Gavaging errors, potential gavage stress and oil bolus effects have not been included in this analysis since available data are so limited. Untreated control rats and mice have a relatively high incidence of neoplasms (Haseman et al., 1984b; Haseman et al., 1985; Haseman, 1985) so one would expect the three-fold increase in fat intake from oil gavage would enhance the development of tumors (Welsch, 1985). Only two oil gavage related responses were found (Haseman et al., 1985). First, a sporadic weakly positive association between oil gavage use and background pancreatic acinar cell proliferative lesion incidence was observed in male Fischer 344/N rats only, Table 1.

The sporadic occurrence of the pancreatic proliferative lesions was not correlated with (1) the brand or lot of corn oil, (2) the brand or lot of rat chow or (3) the contract laboratory (Haseman et al., 1985). Hyperplasia incidence varied from 0-24 percent and was higher in heavier rats. The increased incidence of acinar cell hyperplasia remained significant (P <.05) after adjustment for body weight differences. The background incidence of pancreatic

TABLE 1. Percent Exocrine Pancreatic Acinar Cell Proliferative Lesions in Untreated (UC) and Vehicle Control (VC) Male Fischer 344/N Rats

Treatment	Hyperplasia	Adenomas	Adenocarcinomas
1041 UC	2.6	0.9	0
992 VC	12.6	4.9	0.2

adenomas is also increased; however, this has not increased the number of chemicals judged carcinogenic for the pancreas. Increased incidences of acinar cell adenomas observed in corn oil gavage controls were also correlated ($P < .05$) with increased body weight, Table 2 (Eustis and Boorman, 1985).

TABLE 2. Incidences of Acinar Cell Adenomas in Untreated and Corn Oil Gavage Treated Male Fischer 344/N Rats

Maximum body weight during study	Untreated			Oil gavage		
	No. studies	Adenomas	(%)	No. studies	Adenomas	(%)
400–455	15	3/656	0.5	8	6/393	1.5
456–487	7	5/287	1.7	6	12/299	4.0
488–499	2	1/48	1.0	4	12/200	6.0
500–525	0	–	–	2	25/100	25.0

In contrast to the pancreatic hyperplasia, there was no statistically significant corn oil gavage effect on acinar cell Adenomas above and beyond what was associated with increased body weight. The two corn oil gavage studies with the greatest mean body weights (511 and 520 g) also had the two highest rates of pancreatic acinar cell adenomas (11/50 and 14/50). The association between maximum mean body weight (ranged from 430 to 497 g) and incidence of pancreatic acinar cell adenomas is no longer significant when the two highest body weight studies are omitted.

Kociba et al., (1979) reported a 30 percent incidence of pancreatic adenomas in only untreated male rat controls (86) for a feed toxicology study of 2,4,5-trichlorophenoxyacetic acid. NTP pathologists have also observed pancreatic proliferative lesions in only male rats on chow diets with no treatment for 34 months; the pancreatic lesion incidence was comparable to that for the corn oil vehicle controls (McConnell, 1983). Therefore pancreatic adenomas are not limited to oil gavage vehicle control male rats. Oil gavage may be interacting with other factors (e.g., increased body weight) to shorten time to pancreas lesion.

The second oil gavage effect is a strong negative association with background incidence of leukemia in male Fischer 344/N rats, Table 3 (Haseman et al., 1985).

TABLE 3. Incidences of Leukemia in Untreated (UC) and Corn Oil Gavage-Treated Control (VC) Male Fischer 344/N Rats

Treatment	Rate	%	S.D.	Range
UC	458/1727	26	9.2	10-46
VC	152/1100	14	4.4	2-28

An 8 percent improvement in survival of male oil gavage-treated rats was observed. This is remarkable and consistent with the observations of Ross (personal communication, 1983) who noted that overnutrition was associated with an increase in hormone related neoplasms and a decrease in blood neoplasms. Oil gavage-treated male Fischer 344/N rats were significantly heavier than the untreated controls, Table 4 (Haseman et al., 1985).

The increased body weight in recent NTP studies which have used the NIH-07 diet also reflect an increase in some background lesions, Table 5 (Haseman et al., 1984b; Haseman et al., 1985; Haseman, 1985). The percent background lesion incidence for vehicle control rats is lower than untreated control values for (1) leukemia in male rats (15.9 versus 43.6), (2) adrenal pheochromocytoma in the male rat (25.0 versus 36.6) and (3) mammary fibroadenomas in the female rat (25.1 versus 38.5). Based on both statistical strength of

TABLE 4. Untreated and Corn Oil Gavage-Treated Fischer 344/N Rat and B6C3F$_1$ Mouse Body Weight Comparisons

Animal	Maximum mean body weight (g $\pm$ SD)	
	Untreated controls	Oil gavage-treated controls
Male rats	449 $\pm$ 23	480 $\pm$ 21[a]
Female rats	322 $\pm$ 23	302 $\pm$ 18[a]
Male mice	42.4 $\pm$ 2.8	45.6 $\pm$ 3.5[a]
Female mice	41.7 $\pm$ 6.1	41.2 $\pm$ 4.2

[a]P <.01 relative to untreated controls after adjusting for interlaboratory differences, time related trends, and supplier effects.

TABLE 5. Increased Background Lesion Incidence (%) Associated with Heavier Body Weight, Use of NIH-07 Diet and Improved Animal Care

Site	Untreated rats		Untreated mice	
	Male	Female	Male	Female
Leukemia	12 → 44	10 → 24	–	–
Pituitary adenomas	11 → 25	29 → 43	0.1 → 2	3 → 16
Adrenal pheochromocytomas	9 → 37	4 → 8	–	–
Liver neoplasms	3 → 7	–	21 → 31	4 → 11
Mammary fibroadenomas	–	24 → 38	–	–

the effects and survival data, one can conclude that oil gavage is much more protective than harmful.

The incidence of lesions in all other tissues was examined for potential oil vehicle related effects; no statistically significant effects were found as demonstrated by the mammary gland data, Table 6 (Haseman et al., 1985).

TABLE 6. Mammary Gland Tumor Incidence in Untreated and Vehicle Control Fischer 344/N Rats and B6C3F$_1$ Mice

	Fibroadenomas		Adenocarcinomas	
Rodent	Untreated controls (%)	Vehicle controls (%)	Untreated controls (%)	Vehicle controls (%)
Male rats	3.0	4.5	0.2	0.2
Female rats	27.8	25.5	2.5	1.5
Male mice	0.0	0.0	0.0	0.0
Female mice	0.3	0.4	1.7	1.3
Average Total	7.7 (549/7081)	7.6 (333/4394)	1.1 (79/7081)	0.8 (33/4394)

Several special analyses of the data add further support for the concluded absence of tumor promoting oil vehicle effects. Landers and Appleton (1984) determined that positive oil gavage and feed carcinogenesis bioassays show the same incidence of liver tumors (68 and 69 percent). Perera (personal communication, 1985) examined data on compounds listed in the Third Annual Report on Carcinogens, and found that out of 22 compounds which were positive in an oil gavage carcinogenesis bioassay, 20 were also positive when administered by another route (U.S. DHHS, 1983).

Extrapolation of Carcinogenesis Data. The absence of tumor growth enhancement in rodents receiving oil gavage is remarkable since fat intake was increased up to three-fold. Welsch (1985) reviewed the vast literature on carcinogen-induced rat mammary carcinomas which shows increased fat intake consistently enhances mammary tumorigenesis. There are a number of differences (duration, diet, fat intake, tumor type and dosage) between the typical rodent tumor models and the NTP carcinogenesis bioassay which may help to explain the lack of enhanced tumor growth in rodents receiving oil gavage, Table 7 (U.S. DHHS, 1985; Welsch, 1985). However, it is clear that one cannot extrapolate the tumor growth enhancing effect of a high fat diet from induced rodent tumor models to the NTP carcinogenesis bioassay (Appleton and Landers, 1985). This unexpected observation raises serious questions about extrapolating from animal tumor model studies to the human situation.

OVERNUTRITION CONCERNS

The bolus of gavage oil could exaggerate overnutrition effects observed in untreated controls (Haseman et al., 1985; Haseman, 1985). Members of a 1981 workshop on animal nutrition concluded that overnutrition is responsible for many nutritional problems in long-term carcinogenicity and toxicity testing (Coates, 1982).

Diet Composition. Rodent diets have not been specifically designed for long-term studies of carcinogenesis and toxicity. It has been assumed that maximum animal performance is ideal so diets have been formulated to achieve this goal; however, high consumption of nutrients and most rapid growth often do not correlate with longest life span and freedom from disease (Berg and Simms, 1960; Ross and Bras, 1965, 1973, 1975).

Comparison of rodent nutrient requirements with current diet composition reveals that 20-25 percent protein is 2 to 5 times too high and 5-6 percent fat is very low (NRC, 1978; U.S. DHHS, 1985). High protein diets are associated with increased food consumption, maximum tumor development and reduced life span (Ross, 1961; Ross et al., 1982). In contrast, several observations suggest that 5 percent fat may be too low and may be creating experimental artifacts. Temporary food intake depression and appetite loss lasts up to 21 days in rats when dietary fat is reduced from 20 to 5 percent (Ramirez, 1986). Increased leukemia occurs in male Fischer 344/N rats on 5 percent fat diets compared to vehicle controls consuming the equivalent of 16 percent fat diets (Haseman et al., 1985). Depressed DMBA-induced rat mammary tumors could be observed since linoleic acid intake would be about 1.5 percent lower than the required level of 4.5 percent observed for 20 percent fat diets (Ip et al.,

TABLE 7. Parameter Comparison for Rodent Tumor Models and the NTP Carcinogenesis Bioassay

Parameter	Tumor model	NTP carcinogenesis bioassay
Rat species	Sprague-Dawley, Wistar, Lewis, Fischer 344	Fischer 344/N
Mouse species	$B6C3F_1$, C3H	$B6C3F_1$
Rodents per group	10-30	50
Duration	Post puberty to 6 months	Weanling to 2 years
Diet	Purified	Natural ingredient (NIH-07)
Fat intake (%)	5-20 (in diet)	5-15 (in diet or diet & oil gavage)
Tumor type	Induced by potent and specific carcinogen	Induced by test chemical
Carcinogen administration routes and frequency	IG, IM or IP with limited doses (1-7)	Feed, oil gavage, dermal, inhalation, drinking water, or IP 5 days per week for 24 months
Dosage	Carcinogenic	1/4, 1/2 MTD & MTD
Pathology	Target organ	All tissues

1985); Carroll (1986) observed mammary tumor depression when he reduced dietary fat from 20 to 5 percent but no depression at 10 percent. Incomplete saturation of rat blood cholesterol esters with linoleic acid would occur and reduced rat prostaglandin synthesis would be observed since 9 percent of the calories must come from linoleic acid

(Dupont et al., 1980). Finally, loss of immune function occurs in owl monkeys on 5 percent fat chow diets for long time periods but this can be prevented and/or reversed by soaking the chow in a polyunsaturated vegetable oil (Meydani et al., 1983).

Ad Libitum Feeding. Ad libitum feeding could make customary rodent control groups unacceptable (Schneider and Reed, 1985). Restricting rats to 80 percent of the ad libitum intake quickly results in a shift in eating pattern to consumption of the allotted food within a 2-hour period (Schnakenberg et al., 1971). Meal-eating (access to food two hours per day) has three prominent effects: (1) meal-eating decreases food intake by 20-25 percent (rats were two months old, weighed 270 grams at the beginning of the experiment and declined in weight for about three weeks before resuming growth), (2) meal-eating reduces body weight by 25 percent and (3) meal-eating increases life span by 17 percent and presumably lowers tumor incidence (Leveille, 1972). Meal-eating or limiting food access time is a viable way of controlling food consumption and minimizing overnutrition modulated development of both naturally occurring and chemically induced tumors.

Lack of Exercise. Exercise is another means of helping rodents cope with the overnutrition associated with ad libitum feeding of low fat, high fat and high protein diets. Rusch and Kline (1944) studied the effect of forced exercise on male ABC mice and concluded that all procedures that have a significant effect on the energy requirements of animals will also influence tumor growth. Stern (1984) observed that genetically obese-prone yellow mice do not become obese when an exercise wheel is added to the end of the cage. Osborne-Mendel rats exercised on a treadmill and fed ad libitum maintain a lower body weight (Applegate et al., 1984).

Tumor Growth Modulation Mechanism. Roe (1981) proposed that caloric restriction has a widespread and profound effect on hormonal status of the animal. His thesis is that laboratory rodents maintained on ad libitum feeding regimens manifest numerous abnormalities in endocrine status from the age of six months onwards and are hardly suitable for investigating the chronic pharmacological or toxicological effects of exogenous substances. Since caloric restriction alone did not totally abolish background lesion incidence,

Roe concluded that other aspects of animal maintenance and handling are not satisfactory for long-term studies. For example, he suggests that pseudo-pregnancy and pathological changes in the gonads and genital tracts of both male and female rodents may be due to housing males and females sufficiently close to smell each other but not able to make contact. Calorie restriction reduces the level of serum hormones like prolactin (Roe, 1981; Sarkar et al., 1982). Exercise disrupts the estrous cycle in female Sprague-Dawley rats (Carlberg and Fregly, 1985). Caloric restriction, meal-eating, low protein diets and exercise all achieve about a 25 percent reduction in body weight and may be reducing tumor incidence through a common hormone-related mechanism.

NTP OIL GAVAGE RELATED RESEARCH

Oil Gavage Alternatives. Oil gavage use needs to be validated but this is even more true for suggested alternatives like microencapsulation. Preliminary data from the NTP microencapsulation research indicate that considerable research will be needed to perfect and validate this approach (Melnick et al., 1984; Melnick et al., 1985). Tricaprylin, high oleic acid safflower oil, peanut oil, and sunflower oil are being compared with corn oil as gavage oil vehicles (Rall, 1984).

Teratogenicity. Effects of corn oil versus water gavage of known teratogenic compounds will be compared in Fiscal 1986 to determine if corn oil gavage is influencing the outcome of teratogenicity bioassays (Schwett BN, personal communication, 1985).

Pancreas Effects. Three cooperative agreement research projects have been awarded for study of dietary oil effects on the pancreas (RFA number NIEHS 84-3; Anon., 1984). A contract has been awarded to EG&G Mason Research Institute to (1) assess the effect of various levels of corn oil in gavage studies, (2) evaluate several other vehicles for water insoluble chemicals, (3) study the restriction of the pancreatic lesions to the male Fischer 344/N rat, (4) investigate the interaction of the oil vehicle with benzyl acetate and methylene chloride proliferative exocrine pancreas lesions and (5) determine the biological nature of the induced pancreatic lesions (Rall, 1984).

Diet Optimization. A 1985 "NIEHS, TRTP/NTP Workshop to Optimize Diet for Rodents in Chemical Carcinogenicity Studies" explored imbalances and ways to correct them. The 1986 NTP program includes diet studies (Rao GN, personal communication, 1985) and the National Center for Toxicological Research (NCTR) is comparing effects of caloric restriction, and natural ingredient versus purified diets (Anon., 1985).

Food Restriction. Food intake restriction will be studied since this appears to occur in some high dose groups and is associated with depressed tumor response (Abdo, KM, personal communication, 1985).

SUMMARY

Consulting toxicologists began in 1982 to question the use and potential involvement of oil gavage test-compound administration in unexpected NTP carcinogenesis responses. Investigations have focused on corn oil gavage alternatives, vehicle type and volume, alteration of MTD, teratogenic effects, disposition of test compounds, and target tissues. Micoencapsulation will require considerable development research to make it a suitable alternative. Vehicle type and volume appear to have different effects on the apparent MTD, teratogenicity and disposition of very similar compounds. Only two tissue effects have been observed in the NTP oil gavage bioassay data. First, there is a sporadic and weak association with exocrine pancreatic acinar cell proliferative lesions; these lesions are highly correlated with overweight male Fischer 344/N rats. Second, leukemia is reduced about 50 percent in the male Fischer 344/N rats; this is a strong association which results in an 8-10 percent increase in survival. The protective effect of corn oil gavage is remarkable and there is no significant enhancement of tumor development. Corn oil gavage under the conditions of the NTP carcinogenesis bioassay does contribute to overnutrition and undesirable increased body weight, especially in male Fischer 344/N rats. The NTP and NCTR research programs include research plans to address critical oil gavage, diet composition feeding regimen, exercise and hormonal status questions. Results of these studies will point the way to improving long-term carcinogenesis and toxicity testing.

ACKNOWLEDGEMENTS

The authors thank J. K. Haseman for providing NTP data and statistical analyses, B. S. Appleton and P. L. Kraft for data analyses, T. DeGisi-Heinaman and E. J. Turick for assistance in preparation of the manuscript.

REFERENCES

Angelo MJ, Pritchard AB (1984). Simulations of methylene chloride pharmacokinetics using a physiologically based model. Reg Toxicol Pharmacol 4:329-339.

Anon (1976). In Windholz M, Budavari S, Stroumtsos LY, Fertig MN (eds): "The Merck Index, 9th Edition," Rahway, NJ: Merck & Company, Inc, monographs 1821, 2120.

Anon (1984). NTP expects to award corn oil gavage contract early next year. Food Chem News 26(34):52-53.

Anon (1985). Hart estimates 70% of NCTR budget will be used for basic research. Food Chem News 27(37):51-52.

Applegate EA, Upton DE, Stern JS (1984). Exercise and detraining: Effect on food intake, adiposity and lipogenesis in Osborne-Mendel rats made obese by a high fat diet. J Nutr 114:447-459.

Appleton BS, Landers RE (1986). Oil gavage effects on tumor incidence in the National Toxicology Program's two-year carcinogenesis bioassay. In Poirier LA, Newberne P, Pariza MW (eds): "Role of Nutrients in Carcinogenesis." New York: Plenum Publishing Corp.

Berg BN, Simms HS (1960). Nutrition and longevity in the rat. II. Longevity and onset of disease with different levels of food intake. J Nutr 71:255-263.

Bird RP, Medline A, Furrer R, Bruce WR (1985). Toxicity of orally administered fat to the colonic epithelium of mice. Carcinogenesis 6:1063-1066.

Carlberg KA, Fregly MJ (1985). Disruption of estrous cycles in exercise-trained rats. Proc Soc Exp Biol Med 179:21-24.

Carroll KK (1986). Fat and cancer. In "Second National Conference on Diet, Nutrition and Cancer," Cancer (Suppl), In Press.

Coates ME (1982). Workshop on laboratory animal nutrition (letter to the editor). Food Chem Toxicol 20:149.

Condie LW, Laurie RD, Mills T, Robinson M, Bercz JP (1986). Effect of gavage vehicle on hepatoxicity of carbon tetrachloride in CD-1 mice: Corn oil versus Tween-60 aqueous emulsion. Toxicol Appl Pharmacol, In press.

Dupont J, Mathias MM, Connally PT (1980). Effects of
dietary essential fatty acid concentration upon prostanoid
synthesis in rats. J Nutr 110:1695-1702.
Eschenbrenner AB, Miller E (1943/44). Studies on hepatomas.
1. Size and spacing of multiple doses in the induction of
carbon tetrachloride hepatomas. J Natl Cancer Inst
4:385-388.
Eustis SL, Boorman GA (1985). Proliferative lesions of the
exocrine pancreas: Relationship to corn oil gavage in the
National Toxicology Program. J Natl Cancer Inst
75:1067-1071.
Haseman JK (1985). Growth, body weight, survival and tumor
incidences of F344/N rats and B6C3F$_1$ mice on NIH-07 diet.
In "NIEHS, TRTP/NTP Workshop to Optimize Diet for Rodents
in Chemical Carcinogenicity Studies," Research Triangle
Park, NC: NIEHS.
Haseman JK, Crawford DD, Huff JE, Boorman GA, McConnell EE
(1984a). Results from 86 two-year carcinogenicity studies
conducted by the National Toxicology Program. J Toxicol
Environ Health 14:621-639.
Haseman JK, Huff JE, Boorman GA (1984b). Use of historical
control data in carcinogenicity studies in rodents.
Toxicol Pathol 12:126-135.
Haseman JK, Huff JE, Rao GN, Arnold JE, Boorman GA,
McConnell EE (1985). Neoplasms observed in untreated and
corn oil gavage control groups of F344/N rats and
(C57BL/6NXC3H/HeN)F$_1$ (B6C3F$_1$) mice. J Natl Cancer Inst
75:975-984.
Hayes JR, Condie LW, Borzelleca JF (1984). Subchronic
toxicity of carbon tetrachloride (CT) administered by oral
gavage to CD-1 mice. Toxicologist 4:183.
Hayes, JR, Condie LW, Borzelleca JF (1986). Acute, 14-day
repeated dosing and 90-day subchronic toxicity studies of
carbon tetrachloride in CD-1 mice. Fundam Appl Toxicol,
In press.
Ip C, Carter CA, Ip MM (1985). Requirement of essential
fatty acid for mammary tumorigenesis in the rat. Cancer
Res 45:1997-2001.
Jorgenson TA, Meierhenry EF, Rushbrook CJ, Bull RJ, Robinson
M (1985). Carcinogenicity of chloroform in drinking water
to male Osborne-Mendel rats and female B6C3F$_1$ mice. Fundam
Appl Toxicol 5:760-769.
Kimmel CA, Price CJ, Sadler BM, Tyl RW, Gerling FS (1985).
Comparison of distilled water (DW) and corn oil (CO)
vehicle controls from historical teratology study data.
Toxicologist 5:185.

Kociba RJ, Keyes DG, Lisowe RW, Kalnins RP, Dittenber DD, Wade CE, Gorzinski SJ, Mahle NH, Schwetz BA (1979). Results of two-year chronic toxicity and oncogenic study of rats ingesting diets containing 2,4,5-trichlorophenoxy-acetic acid (2,4,5-T). Food Cosmet Toxicol 17:205-221.

Landers RE, Appleton BS (1984). Oil gavage testing procedures. In "Proceedings of the European Toxicology Forum Meeting," Washington, DC: Toxicology Forum Inc, 1:172-195.

Leveille GA (1972). The long-term effects of meal-eating on lipogenesis, enzyme activity, and longevity in the rat. J Nutr 102:549-556.

Litchfield JJ, Wilcoxon F (1949). A simplified method of evaluating dose-effect experiments. J Pharmacol Exp Therap 96:99-115.

Lorke D (1983). A new approach to practical acute toxicity testing. Arch Toxicol 54:275-287.

McConnell E (1983). National Toxicology Program view. In "Proceedings of the Toxicology Forum Winter Meeting," Washington DC: Toxicology Forum Inc, pp 351-358.

Melnick RL, Goehl T, Collins B, Jameson CW, Maronpot R, Greenwell A, Harrington F, Wilson R, Tomaszewski K, Agarwal D (1985). Toxicity of microencapsulated trichloroethylene (TCE) in rats. Toxicologist 5:228.

Melnick RL, Jameson CW, Goehl T, Kuhn G (1984). Microencapsulation of chemicals for toxicologic studies. Toxicologist 4:49.

Meydani SN, Nicolosi RJ, Sehgal PK, Hayes KC (1983). Altered lipoprotein metabolism in spontaneous vitamin E deficiency of owl monkeys. Am J Clin Nutr 38:888-894.

National Research Council (1978). Nutrient requirements of the laboratory rat. In "Nutrient Requirements of Laboratory Animals, No. 10, 3rd Edition," Washington, DC: National Academy Press, pp 7-37.

Rall DP (1984). National Toxicology Program: Proposal to sponsor studies on the significance of increased acinar cell lesions of the pancreas in rats given oil gavage and their relevance in the interpretation of these studies; request for comments. Fed Reg 49:38366-38367.

Ramirez I (1986). Recovery from dietary obesity. Physiol Behav, In press.

Roe FJC, Palmer AK, Worden AN Van Abbé NJ (1979). Safety evaluation of toothpaste containing chloroform. 1. Long-term studies in mice. J Environ Pathol Toxicol 2:799-819.

Roe FJC (1981). Are nutritionists worried about the epidemic of tumours in laboratory animals? Proc Nutr Soc 40:57-65.

Ross MH (1961). Length of life and nutrition in the rat. J Nutr 75:197-210.

Ross MH, Bras G (1965). Tumor incidence patterns and nutrition in the rat. J Nutr 87:245-260.

Ross MH, Bras G (1973). Influence of protein under- and overnutrition on spontaneous tumor prevalence in the rat. J Nutr 103:944-963.

Ross MH, Bras G (1975). Food preference and length of life. Science 190:165-167.

Ross MH, Lustbader ED, Bras G (1982). Dietary practices of early life and spontaneous tumors of the rat. Nutr Cancer 3:150-167.

Rusch HP, Kline BE (1944). The effect of exercise on the growth of a mouse tumor. Cancer Res 4:116-118.

Sarkar NH, Fernandes G, Telang NT, Kourides IA, Good RA (1982). Low-calorie diet prevents the development of mammary tumors in C3H mice and reduces circulating prolactin level, murine mammary tumor virus expression and proliferation of mammary alveolar cells. Proc Natl Acad Sci 79:7758-7762.

Schnakenberg DD, Krabil LF, Weiser PC (1971). The anorexic effect of high altitude on weight gain, nitrogen retention and body composition of rats. J Nutr 101:787-796.

Schneider EL, Reed JD, Jr (1985). Life extension. N Engl J Med 312:1159-1168.

Stern JS (1984). Is obesity a disease of inactivity? In Stunkard AJ (ed): "Eating Disorders," New York: Raven Press.

U.S. Department of Health and Human Services (1983). "Third Annual Report on Carcinogens - Summary," Research Triangle Park, NC, NTP-82-330.

U.S. Department of Health and Human Services (1985). "National Toxicology Annual Plan for Fiscal Year 1985," Research Triangle Park, NC, NTP-85-055.

Welsch CW (1985). Host factors affecting the growth of carcinogen-induced rat mammary carcinomas: a review and tribute to Charles Brenton Huggins. Cancer Res 45:3415-3443.

Withey JR, Collins BT, Collins PG (1983). Effect of vehicle on the pharmacokinetics and uptake of four halogenated hydrocarbons from the gastrointestinal tract of the rat. J Appl Toxicol 3:249-253.

IV. Studies of Interaction of Fat With Other Nutritional Factors in Experimental Carcinogenesis

Dietary Fat and Cancer, pages 377–401
© 1986 Alan R. Liss, Inc.

THE MACRONUTRIENTS IN EXPERIMENTAL CARCINOGENESIS OF THE BREAST, COLON, AND PANCREAS

Steven K. Clinton
University of Chicago
Department of Medicine
5841 South Maryland Avenue
Chicago, IL 60637

Willard J. Visek
University of Illinois College of Medicine
506 South Mathews Avenue
Urbana, IL 61801

INTRODUCTION

Malignant cells, like their normal counterparts, depend upon nutrients for energy and the synthesis of biochemical catalysts and structural components. The evidence that the nutritional status of the host can modify the development and growth of neoplasms was obtained early in experimental oncology. Pioneering studies near the turn of the century by Rous (1914) and others (Moreschi, 1909) showed depression of tumor incidence in laboratory animals by underfeeding. During subsequent decades there were infrequent studies describing effects of nutrients on carcinogenesis, however few met current nutritional standards. Since the early 1940s, there has been an acceleration in the accumulation of knowledge concerning diet and cancer brought about by the availability of numerous organ-specific carcinogenic agents, multiple strains of transplantable tumors, spontaneous tumor models in inbred rodents, purified dietary components, and more precise knowledge of nutrient requirements for laboratory animals. The present chapter is intended to review selected studies describing the individual effects and interactions of caloric intake, dietary fat, and protein in experimental carcinogenesis of the breast, colon, and pancreas.

Experimental Methodology

Investigators need to be aware of many factors which influence the quality of information obtained from studies of nutrition and carcinogenesis in laboratory experiments. These include the selection of appropriate experimental models, use of an adequate number of experimental animals, careful histopathologic evaluation of the tissues, and applications of appropriate experimental designs and statistical analyses. The formulation of experimental and control diets is of special importance for reliably determining the effects of specific nutritional variables. The use of more chemically defined dietary ingredients has eliminated many of the variables characteristic of unrefined diets containing natural ingredients of unknown composition.

Although purified diets offer significant advantages in defining dietary conditions, they also fail to meet nutritional requirements unless properly formulated. Greenfield and Briggs (1971) compared a large number of the mineral mixtures that have been used, and found serious imbalances or deficiencies of nutrients recognized as essential. Such errors or omissions can now be readily avoided because dietary requirements of laboratory animals are periodically reassessed by expert committees whose recommendations incorporate recent information (NAS-NRC-1978). Guidelines for diets of satisfactory compostion for long-term studies in rats and mice have also been developed by a committee of the American Institute of Nutrition (AIN, 1977). The original recommendations of this group have been slightly modified in accord with subsequent experience (AIN, 1980) and are a reliable guide for scientists from diverse fields who may have limited experience in nutritional studies. Wider application of the information in these reports would make it possible to obtain more definitive data in diet and cancer research and greatly facilitate comparisons between laboratories. The AIN-76A diet (AIN, 1977) modified as to carbohydrate source, vitamin K, and antioxidant content (AIN, 1980) lends itself readily to changes in single nutrients.

Experimental variables can have significant influence on food intake. A change in nutrient content or addition of a chemical agent can reduce food consumption. Under these conditions, it is difficult to differentiate between a response due to test conditions from one secondary to a reduction in food intake. To assess the effects of reduced food intake in experimental animals it may be necessary to utilize pair-feeding techniques. Regardless, it is highly desirable and sometimes critical to document feed intake. Reports of diet and cancer studies would have their usefulness significantly enhanced for comparisons between laboratories if they contained detailed descriptions of the diets fed and the source of the dietary ingredients used.

Dietary Fat and Breast Cancer

Numerous experimental models have been used to investigate the relationship between dietary lipids and breast cancer. Increasing the proportion of fat in the diet increased the incidence of spontaneous mammary tumors in both mice (Tannenbaum, 1942) and rats (Benson et al., 1956). Similar results have been obtained with representatives of different classes of carcinogens including diethylstilbesterol, (Dunning et al., 1949), 2-acetylaminofluorene, (Engle and Copeland, 1951), 7,12-dimethylbenz(a)anthracene (DMBA) (Gammal et al., 1967) and methylnitrosourea (MNU) (Chan et al., 1977). Silverman et al. (1980) found that rats fed a high fat diet developed slightly more x-irradiation induced mammary tumors than rats fed low fat diets. The growth rates of several strains of transplantable breast tumors were also increased in animals fed high fat diets (Giovarelli et al., 1980; Hillyard and Abraham, 1979; Hopkins and West, 1977; Rao and Abraham, 1976).

Several studies have employed graded levels of dietary fat to characterize the dose-response relationship between fat intake and breast tumorigenesis. Silverstone and Tannenbaum (1950) found that the incidence of spontaneous mammary tumors in mice increased in proportion to the content of a partially hydrogenated mixture of cottonseed and soybean oil ranging from 2 to 16% of the diet. Further increments in dietary fat had no effect. Carroll and Khor (1971) fed 0.5, 5.0, 10.0, and 20.0% corn oil and found the increase in DMBA-induced tumorigenesis to be the largest when fat was increased from 5 to 10%. In contrast, Ip and Ip

(1981) using a similar model found successive increases in the number of rats with mammary tumors and the total tumor number as dietary corn oil was increased from 0.5 to 5.0 and 20%. In our laboratory the effects of dietary corn oil on DMBA-induced breast cancer were best described as linear between 12 and 48% of calories (approximately 6 to 24% by weight). Each doubling of dietary fat approximately doubled the odds of tumor development (Clinton et al., 1984).

Although it is increasingly evident that tumor development is a complex multistep process, the original two-stage, initiation and promotion model of carcinogenesis has proven useful in studies with laboratory animals to determine mechanisms whereby dietary fat influences experimental mammary carcinogenesis. Carroll and Khor (1970) concluded that high fat diets exert their effects on the promotion phase of DMBA-induced breast cancer. This has been confirmed in other studies utilizing carcinogen-treated mammary gland explants (Ip and Sinha, 1981) and transplantable tumors (Giovarelli et al., 1980; Hillyard and Abraham, 1979). However, recent studies show that high-fat diets may also influence initiation. Dao and Chan (1983) reported that fat acts during both the initiation and promotion phases of MNU-induced breast carcinogenesis (Dao and Chan, 1983). Our laboratory has also obtained evidence that increasing dietary corn oil increases DMBA-induced tumor incidence in the initiation phase (Clinton et al., 1981; Clinton and Visek, 1985). Other reports using diets high in lard (Rogers, 1983), or coconut oil (Kritchevsky et al., 1984) also suggest a role for fat during the initiation of DMBA-induced mammary cancer.

The mechanism whereby fats influence cancer initiation is unclear. The effects of fat on hepatic enzymes involved in polycyclic aromatic hydrocarbon metabolism appear to be minimal (Visek and Clinton, 1983). Gammel et al. (1968) found no differences in the uptake or clearance of DMBA by mammary tissue of rats fed 0.5 or 20.0% corn oil. The observation that high corn oil diets enhance the tumorigenic response to NMU, a direct acting water-soluble carcinogen, suggests that the mechanism is independent of carcinogen distribution or metabolism (Dao and Chan, 1983).

A number of studies have shown that fat concentration also acts during the promotion phase (Visek and Clinton, 1983). Mechanisms proposed (Welsch and Aylsworth, 1983; Visek and Clinton, 1983) whereby fat concentration may influence promotion include: (a) alterations in the endocrine environment or hormone responsiveness, (b) modifications of cell membrane lipids, (c) changes in the immune system, (d) changes in the metabolism and biological activity of prostaglandins, (e) direct effects on tumor cell metabolism or genetic regulation, and (f) production of tumor-promoting oxidized products from unsaturated fatty acids.

Ovarian hormones clearly play a role in human and experimental breast cancer (Welsch and Aylsworth, 1983). The evidence that dietary fat level influences steroid hormone concentrations in rats has been inconsistent. Some studies suggest elevations of serum estrogens (Chan et al., 1975; Ip and Ip, 1981) while others (Wetzel et al., 1984; Clinton et al., 1982) show no effect of dietary fat. An additional study (Table 1), with ovariectomized rats treated with a constant level of estrogen, also showed that increasing corn oil enhanced the promotion of mammary cancer similarly to control animals fed identical diets (Clinton et al., 1982). The data provide clear evidence that dietary fat exerted its effects on breast cancer independently of estrogen homeostasis.

Table 1

The Effects of Dietary Corn Oil on the Promotion Phase of DMBA-Induced Breast Carcinogenesis in Control, Ovariectomized, and Ovariectomized-Estrogen Treated Rats.

Treatment Group	Tumor Incidence (%)		Tumor Number	
	4% Fat	20% Fat	4% Fat	20% Fat
Controls	59	84	53	117
Ovariectomy	12	22	6	10
Ovariectomy and Estrogen	47	81	61	95

Rats were treated with DMBA between 50-55 days of age. Hormonal treatments were initiated 48 hrs thereafter. Each group contained 30 to 34 rats.

Prolactin has been extensively studied as a mediator in the dietary fat-breast cancer relationship. Chan et al. (1975) observed two- to three-fold higher serum prolactin concentrations during proestrus and estrous in ether-anesthetized rats fed 20% lard compared to groups fed 0.5%. They subsequently observed higher serum prolactin concentrations during metestrus and diestrus in F344 rats fed 20% lard compared to those fed 0.5% (Chan et al., 1977). Ip et al. (1980) observed higher serum prolactin concentrations during proestrus in rats fed 20% corn oil than in those fed 0.5%. In contrast, our results (Clinton et al., 1984) agree with those of Wetzel et al. (1984) showing no effect of fat on serum prolactin levels throughout the estrous cycle. Likewise, we have observed no effect of fat on pituitary prolactin secretion, the metabolic clearance rate of prolactin (Clinton and Visek, 1985), or its peripheral metabolism (Clinton et al., 1984). These results fail to support the theory that fat increases breast cancer incidence by changes in prolactin homeostasis.

Our laboratory has recently been investigating the hypothesis that dietary fat may mediate its effect in mammary carcinogenesis via changes in the immune system. Olson et al. (1983) observed that 20% soybean oil (SBO) in a purified diet caused more frequent and larger spontaneous mammary tumors in C3H/OUJ mice compared to those fed 5% SBO. A subsequent experiment with identical diets showed that splenocytes from the same strain of mice fed the 20% SBO diet exhibited a decreased mitogenic response to the T-cell mitogens concanavalin-A and phytohemagglutin. However, fat intake showed no effect on B-cell mitogenesis. The next study examined the effects of fat intake on the kinetics of T-cell cytotoxicity. Mice fed 5 or 20% SBO by weight were immunized with allogeneic P815 mastocytoma cells (mast cell tumor line) 10 days prior to harvest of splenocytes. A constant number of splenocytes was then incubated with varying concentrations of chromium-51 labeled P815 cells for varying periods. The rate of tumor cell lysis (target cells killed per hour) showed that T-cytotoxic cells from mice fed 20% SBO had a lower killing capacity (V_{max}) without changes in the apparent affinity ($K_{\frac{1}{2}}$) for their targets (Figure 1).   Dietary fat concentration did not influence the fatty acid composition of the two major lymphocyte phospholipids: phosphatidylethanolamine and phosphatidylcholine.   Thus, the decline in killing capacity was unrelated to splenocyte membrane fatty acid composition.   These studies suggest that the decline in killing capacity may be due to fewer active T-cytotoxic cells or a reduced lytic efficiency.   Further investigations should define the reasons for the immunosuppressive effects of high fat diets and their influence on tumor immuno-surveillance.

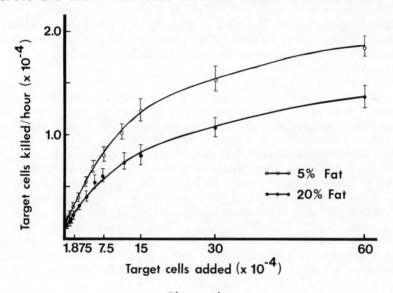

Figure 1:

The effect of soybean oil concentration on the kinetics of splenocyte T-cell cytotoxicity.   Initial velocities (target cells killed/hour) were plotted against initial substrate concentrations for splenocytes from female C3H/OUJ mice fed either 5 or 20% soybean oil for 12 weeks.   There was no effect of soybean oil concentration on the $K_{\frac{1}{2}}$ of the reaction.   The calculated V_{max} was significantly lower ($p<0.05$) for mice fed 20% soybean oil than for mice fed 5% soybean oil (1.4 ± 0.2 x 10^4 vs 2.3 ± 0.4 x 10^4 target cells killed/hour, respectively).   Values represent means $\pm$ SEM, for 18 fed each diet.

The type of fat also influences the genesis of mammary tumors. Polyunsaturated fats like corn, sunflower seed, olive, soybean, and cottonseed oil lead to more mammary tumors than saturated fats like beef tallow, lard, coconut, or hydrogenated vegetable oil (Carroll and Khor, 1971; Chan et al., 1983). However, Carroll and coworkers (Hopkins and Carroll, 1979; Carroll and Hopkins, 1978) found that saturated fats could be as effective as unsaturated fat in promoting tumorigenesis if a small quantity of polyunsaturated fat (i.e., 3% of the diet) was fed with the saturated fat (17% of the diet). Ip et al. (1985), using diets containing 20% coconut oil found that raising the linoleate content from 0.5 to 4.4% by the substitution of palm oil for coconut oil increased DMBA-induced tumors. Further increases in linoleate had no significant effect. This has been interpreted to mean that once the requirements for unsaturated fatty acids are fulfilled, a further increase in tumor incidence is related to the level of total fat, and not its source. However, other studies provide evidence that the enhancement of mammary carcinogenesis is directly related to the percentage of polyunsaturated fat (Clinton et al., 1984; Rogers and Wetzel, 1981). More studies are needed to characterize the effects of fat source or essential fatty acid intake.

Dietary Protein and Breast Cancer

The effects of dietary protein on mammary carcinogenesis are much less consistent than those noted for dietary fat or caloric intake. Several investigators found no effect on breast cancer from increasing dietary protein (Tannenbaum and Silverstone, 1949; Ross and Bras, 1973), whereas others have noted an enhancement (Shay et al., 1964; Hawrylewicz et al., 1982), or a reduction (Engle and Copeland, 1952; Clinton et al., 1979). We have recently completed three studies with over 1,000 rats to evaluate the interactions of protein, fat, and caloric intake in DMBA induced mammary carcinogenesis (Clinton and Visek, 1985). There was no effect of protein in the combined or promotion phases. However, increasing dietary protein from 8 to 16% of calories during the initiation phase was associated with a significant reduction in tumor incidence. These results are similar to those reported earlier (Table 2) on the effect of protein on breast cancer (Clinton et al., 1979).

The mechanisms underlying the influence of protein in DMBA-induced carcinogenesis during the initiation phase are not known. We have observed that hepatic enzymes involved in carcinogen metabolism are elevated with increased protein intake (Clinton et al., 1979). Our data support the hypothesis that dietary protein modifies the carcinogenic response by enhancing DMBA metabolism to more water soluble and readily excretable products. This agrees with other studies where pretreatment with inducers of hepatic carcinogen metabolizing enzymes prior to DMBA administration reduced the number of tumors subsequently produced. (Wattenberg et al., 1976). Human studies also show that the metabolism and clearance of various pharmacologic agents is enhanced by diets higher in protein (Kappas et al., 1976).

Our results showing no effect of protein on the promotion of DMBA-induced breast cancer agree with others. (Tannenbaum and Silverstone, 1949; and Ross and Bras, 1973) showing no effect of protein on spontaneous breast tumorigenesis. In contrast, Shay et al. (1964) reported increased 3-methylcholanthrene-induced breast cancer as rats were fed greater concentrations of protein. Significant differences were reported, but their interpretation is questionable because the control diet was standard laboratory chow and the experimental diets containing the higher levels of protein were composed of purified ingredients. Recently Hawrylewicz et al. (1982) also reported more DMBA-induced breast tumors in rats fed increasing amounts of protein as casein. In their studies the experimental diets were fed throughout the initiation and promotion phases to offspring of dams fed the same diets during mating, gestation, and lactation.

The published data on the influence of dietary protein in experimental mammary carcinogenesis are limited. Most studies of protein and cancer have employed a variety of experimental models and protocols, and in some instances the dietary controls have been inappropriate. The formulation of a unifying hypothesis

Table 2

The Effects of Dietary Protein on the Initiation and Promotion of DMBA-induced Breast Carcinogenesis in Rats[1]

Dietary Protein (% of Kcal)	Initiation		Promotion	
	Incidence (%)	Tumors per rat	Incidence (%)	Tumor per rat
7.5%	85	2.2 ± 0.4	55	1.4 ± 0.1
15.0%	52	1.4 ± 0.2	55	1.4 ± 0.1
45.0%	30	1.1 ± 0.1	40	1.1 ± 0.1

[1]Weanling female Sprague-Dawley rats were utilized in each study and DMBA was administered after 4 weeks of feeding. For the initiation-phase study, diets varied in protein only for the 4 weeks prior to DMBA administration. Diets varying in protein were fed only following carcinogen administration in the promotion-phase study.

concerning the effects of dietary protein on experimental mammary cancer would be premature.

Energy Intake and Breast Cancer

Energy-supplying components (carbohydrate, lipid, and protein) are essential for normal growth, reproduction, and lactation. The overall requirement depends upon factors such as the animal strain or species, age, sex, method of housing, physical exercise, and ambient temperature. Standards for optimum body weight and caloric intake have not been defined. Some investigators have expressed the opinion that laboratory animals in confined quarters fed ad libitum on semi-purified diets consume excessive calories and became overweight.

Of all the nutritional factors evaluated, caloric intake has had the most consistent influence on the development of malignant neoplasms in experimental animals. Numerous investigations, many completed in the 1940s and 1950s, clearly established that caloric restriction inhibits the incidence of leukemia, sarcomas, and tumors of the breast, lung, liver, and skin. These early studies were reviewed by Tannenbaum (1959). Experiments for evaluating calories have employed several techniques. Underfeeding involves withholding feed without any change in diet composition. All dietary components are therefore restricted proportionately with feed intake. In contrast, caloric restriction restricts the energy content of the diet. Usually carbohydrate is limited while the amount of fat, protein, fiber, vitamins, and minerals is the same as consumed by control groups. However, the attempt to control these variables while limiting calories may not give a reliable reflection of metabolic and biochemical aberrations which may ensue. When calories are decreased significantly, protein is utilized for energy and diverted from the synthesis of cellular or regulating proteins and other processes. Secondly, some vitamins and minerals are utilized in proportion to energy consumption and their supply may therefore exceed requirements when calories alone are restricted. Most studies utilizing caloric restriction or underfeeding have been designed to reduce caloric intake by 20 to 50% below ad libitum which is associated with significant decreases in growth and final body weight.

A number of breast cancer studies have utilized underfeeding or caloric-restriction to inhibit tumor formation. A classic study by Tannenbaum (1947) showed that caloric-restriction decreased breast tumor incidence and prolonged the latency period. The restricted mice were also smaller, lived longer, and had fewer non-neoplastic lesions. A subsequent study showed that successive decreases in caloric restriction resulted in a proportional decrease in tumor incidence (Tannenbaum, 1959). Caloric-restriction was most effective during the longer promotion stage of mammary tumorigenesis (Tannenbaum, 1959). Twice-weekly fasts lasting 24 hours with ad libitum feeding between fasts had no effect on mammary tumor development (Tannenbaum, 1959). Over the entire experiment the total caloric intake and average final body weights of both groups were equal. Tannenbaum also completed a series of studies to evaluate the interrelationships between tumor incidence, caloric intake, body weight, and metabolic rate (Tannenbaum and Silverstone, 1949). Incorporating sodium fluoride or dinitrophenol into the diet or placing the mice in a cooler environment with a caloric intake equal to control mice dramatically decreased spontaneous mammary tumor incidence. Sodium fluoride reduced food intake while dinitrophenol and a cooler environmental temperature increased metabolism. Since compensatory increases in food intake were prevented, there was a restriction in food intake relative to need with a decrease in body weight and tumor incidence.

Our laboratory has investigated other methods for evaluating the influence of caloric intake in carcinogenesis (Clinton et al., 1984). In recent experiments involving large numbers of rats, we observed a variation in ad libitum intake which approached a normal distribution. Using established statistical techniques involving multiple logistic regression, we assessed the effects of caloric intake in breast tumorigenesis based on the observed variation in voluntary intake. The data (Table 3) derived from our studies on the interactions of fat and protein, on DMBA-induced breast cancer in rats (Clinton et al., 1984) showed a highly significant effect of ad libitum caloric intake on tumorigenesis. The effects of caloric intake were best illustrated by dividing the 351 rats into three groups according to ad libitum caloric intake

(Table 3). Based on statistical analysis, the odds of developing an adenocarcinoma, adenoma, or tumor of any type were increased by a factor of 1.10, 1.14, and 1.09 respectively, for each additional one kilocalorie consumed. Conversely, a drop in caloric consumption by 12-13% was associated with about a 25% reduction in the prevalence of any type of breast tumor. The interrelationships between caloric intake, body weight, metabolic rate, carcinogenesis, and longevity are complex and deserve further investigation.

Dietary Fat and Colon Cancer

Studies of colon carcinogenesis in laboratory animals gained impetus in the late 1960s and early 1970s, when experimental models were developed which mimic human colon cancer. These utilize chemicals representing different classes of carcinogens including: cycasin and its derivatives 1,2-dimethylhydrazine (DMH), methylazoxymethanol (MAM), and azoxymethane (AOM); an aromatic amine 3,2'-dimethyl-4-aminobiphenyl (DMAB); and the direct acting nitrosoureas methylnitrosourea (MNU) and N-methyl-N'-nitrosoguanidine (MNNG). Nigro et al. (1975) initially reported the enhancement of AOM-induced colon cancer in rats fed high fat diets. A chow diet containing 5% fat was compared with chow diluted with beef tallow to a final fat concentration by weight of 35%. Unfortunately, this diluted the other nutrients resulting in reduced intake of protein, vitamins, minerals, and fiber by the rats fed the high fat diet. A number of subsequent experiments, reviewed by Reddy (1983), utilized semi-purified diets with fat varied by substitution for carbohydrate on a weight basis. Studies with a number of different carcinogens (DMAB, DMH, AOM, MAM, and MNU) showed an increase in colon tumorigenesis with high fat diets. Although the diets were an improvement over previous studies, they failed to control for increased caloric density and decreased nutrient to calorie ratios, characteristic of high fat diets formulated by the substitution method. A recent study by Reddy and Maema (1984), equalized the nutrient to calorie ratios between the low and high fat diets. They again observed that diets high in corn oil or safflower oil increased the incidence of AOM-induced colon tumors. In contrast, Nauss et al. (1983, 1984) using rigidly controlled dietary regimens combined with detailed histopathologic techniques found no effect of high fat on DMH- or NMU-induced colon carcinogenesis. Thus, compared to the data concerning dietary fat concentration and breast cancer, recent studies in experimental colon carcinogenesis are inconsistent. Further study will be needed to determine how specific details of experimental design, such as diet composition, type of carcinogen, method of administration, sacrifice scheduling, and histopathologic techniques interact to produce the divergent results between laboratories.

The effects of fat source on colon cancer have not been extensively evaluated, however, it appears that at higher levels of fat intake, the source of dietary lipid has little influence on colon tumorigenesis (Reddy, 1983; Nauss et al., 1983, 1984). Some studies suggest that at lower levels of total fat, unsaturated fats are more effective promotors than saturated fats (Sakaguchi, 1984).

Evidence that high fat diets may act primarily during the promotion phase of colon carcinogenesis is based on a study which showed that intestinal tumor incidence was increased by a high-fat diet following but not before or during AOM treatment (Reddy, 1983). A popular hypothesis (Reddy, 1983) suggests that high-fat diets alter the gut microflora and increase the concentrations of bile acids or their metabolites which reach the colon. These changes are believed to enhance bacterial production of tumor-promoting substances from bile acids. As with breast cancer, it may be that fat inhibits tumoricidal immuno-surveillance. Dietary fat may also influence enzyme systems within the colonic mucosa which activate or detoxify xenobiotics such as mutagens or tumor promotors. Others suggest that dietary fat, fatty acids, prostaglandins, or other metabolites may influence DNA metabolism or genomic regulation to favor tumorigenesis (Bull et al., 1984; Rozhin et al., 1984). At this stage it is not known how fat or its saturation influence colon cancer incidence in laboratory animals.

Table 3

DMBA-induced mammary tumors in rats divided into three groups based upon ad libitim caloric consumption.

	Lower third	Middle third	Upper third
Number of rats	117	117	117
Range of Kcal intake, Kcal/day	29.96-46.06	46.13-48.53	48.53-55.32
Mean Kcal intake, Kcal/day	42.77	47.31	50.84
Weight at 4 wks	150±2	156±1	154±2
Weight at 30 wks	250±3	265±2	269±3
Percentage of rats with tumors (number of tumors)			
Any tumor	40(88)	58(103)	57(137)
Adenocarcinoma	27(62)	42(66)	45(84)
Adenoma	8(12)	12(15)	19(25)
Fibroadenoma	8(13)	17(22)	14(27)

Data from Clinton et al. (1984).

Dietary Protein and Colon Cancer

Few studies have been conducted on the relationship of dietary protein to colon carcinogenesis. Topping and Visek (1976) examained DMH-induced carcinogenesis in male rats ad libitum fed one of three purified diets containing 7.5, 15.0, or 22.5% casein as protein. Although the percentage of rats with tumors of the colon or small intestine was not influenced by diet, the total number of tumors per rat was greater with 15.0 or 22.5% protein (Table 4). In addition, DMH-induced tumors of the inner ear developed earlier and with a higher incidence as the percent of protein in the diet was increased. As with other nutrients the mechanism whereby dietary protein influences DMH-carcinogenesis is unknown. One factor which may enhance colon tumor growth is the higher lipid content in the feces as observed in mice when dietary protein was increased from 10 to 40% (Hevia et al., 1984; Anderson et al., 1985). The possible relationships between fecal lipids, bile acid metabolism, fecal steroid excretion, and colon cancer have been reviewed (Reddy, 1983).

Our laboratory has observed changes in DMH metabolism associated with increased dietary protein. Kari et al. (1983) found that the percentage of DMH metabolized to mutagenic end-products in protein-deficient mice was lowered apparently because the volatile metabolite, azomethane, was more readily expired and not further metabolized to the ultimate carcinogen. Further examination implicates a decrease in conversion of AOM to MAM in protein-deficient mice allowing for the build up of azomethane and its loss in the expired gases.

At the present time, no studies have documented significant effects of protein source on incidence of colon cancer in laboratory animals. We observed (Clinton et al., 1979) no difference in DMH-induced tumor incidence in rats fed diets containing 20% protein derived from soybean meal, or raw or charcoal broiled beef. In summary, the concentration rather than source of protein appears to be more important in DMH-induced colon cancer. Studies also suggest that the effect of protein on DMH-induced colon carcinogenesis may be related to its effects on DMH metabolism.

Table 4

Incidence and total number of DMH-induced tumors in the small and large intestine, and the inner ear of rats fed different levels of protein.[1]

| | % of rats with tumors | | | Ave. no. of tumors/rats | |
	Small Intestine	Large Intestine	Inner Ear	Small Intestine	Large Intestine
Diet (n)					
7.5% Protein (32)	31	84	47	0.37	1.03
15.0% Protein (31)	65	87	58	0.74	1.68
22.5% Protein (33)	52	91	78	0.78	1.67

[1]Male rats were given DMH via intraperitoneal injection at 15 mg/Kg body weight each week for 24 weeks. Rats were necropsied between 28 and 32 weeks after the initiation of the experiment.

Caloric Intake and Colon Cancer

Although epidemiologic studies suggest that caloric intake may be associated with a higher risk of colon cancer, few laboratory studies have investigated this hypothesis. Pollard et al. (1984) recently completed a preliminary study evaluating the role of caloric intake in MAM-induced colon cancer in rats. Caloric intake was restricted to 67-75% of ad libitum fed controls beginning 10 days after carcinogen treatment. The incidence and frequency of colon tumors was reduced in restricted rats.

The Macronutrients and Pancreatic Cancer

Two animal models of pancreatic cancer have been well characterized and utilized to investigate the role of nutrients in pancreatic carcinogenesis. N-nitrosobis(2-oxopryl)amine, (BOP), induces a high yield of ductal pancreatic carcinomas in Syrian golden hamsters after a single injection (Birt et al., 1981). Pancreatic carcinomas can also be produced in rats by multiple injections of azaserine or its incorporation into the diet (Longnecker et al., 1981).

Several studies suggest that both dietary fat and protein influence experimental pancreatic carcinogenesis. Roebuck et al. (1981) reported that diets containing 20% corn oil or 20% safflower oil (% of weight) enhanced the promotion of azaserine induced pancreatic tumors compared to diets containing similar amounts of a saturated fat. In a recent study, Roebuck et al. (1985) fed diets containing 20% fat composed of various combinations of coconut oil and corn oil to provide a range of essential fatty acids (EFA). They found that the number of grossly visible azaserine-induced pancreatic nodules increased in approximate proportion to increases in EFA intake (0.5 to 11.5% of the diet). The incidence and size of microscopic premalignant acidophilic foci was increased most dramatically when the diet contained between 4.4 and 8.5% EFA, suggesting a minimum dietary EFA requirement for producing these lesions. Birt et al. (1981) showed that a greater total concentration of dietary fat enhanced BOP-induced pancreatic tumors in both male and female Syrian golden hamsters.

Pour et al. (1983) observed that a protein-free diet fed prior to or following BOP administration inhibited tumor incidence. Further studies showed that females fed 9% casein developed fewer BOP-induced cancers than those fed 18 or 36% casein. However, they observed no effect on the number of lesions in males (Pour and Birt, 1983). A study by Birt et al. (1983) suggests a significant interaction between dietary fat and protein on BOP-induced tumor incidence and multiplicity. Enhanced carcinogenesis by high-fat diets (42% of calories as corn oil vs 10%) occurred only in hamsters fed the high-protein diet. Conversely, the significant effects of protein were seen only with high-fat diets. These results suggest positive effects of both dietary protein and fat, and possible interactions which warrant further investigation.

REFERENCES

American Institute of Nutrition (1977). Report of the AIN ad hoc committee on standards for nutritional studies. J Nutr 107:1340-1348.

American Institute of Nutrition (1980). Second report of the ad hoc committee on standards for nutritional studies. J Nutr 110:1726.

Anderson P, Alster J, Clinton S, Imrey P, Mangian H, Truex C, Visek W (1985). Plasma amino acids and excretion of protein end products by mice fed 10 or 40% soybean protein diets with or without dietary benzo(a)pyrene or 1,2-dimethylhydrazine. J Nutr 115:1515-1527.

Benson J, Lev M, Grand C (1956). Enhancement of mammary fibroadenomas in the female rat by a high fat diet. Cancer Res 16:135-137.

Birt D, Salmasi S, Pour P (1981). Enhancement of experimental pancreatic cancer in Syrian golden hamsters by dietary fat. J Natl Cancer Inst 67:1327-1332.

Birt D, Stepan K, Pour P (1983). Interaction of dietary fat and protein on pancreatic carcinogenesis in Syrian golden hamsters. J Natl Cancer Inst 71:355-360.

Bull A, Nigro N, Golembeski W, Crissman J, Marnett L (1984). In vivo stimulation of DNA synthesis and induction of ornithine decarboxylase in rat colon by fatty acid hydroperoxides, autoxidation products of unsaturated fatty acids. Cancer Res 44:4924-4928.

Carroll K, Khor H (1971). Effects of level and type of dietary fat on incidence of mammary tumors induced in female Sprague-Dawley rats by 7,12-dimethylbenz(a)-anthracene. Lipids 6:415-420.

Carroll K, Hopkins G (1978). Dietary polyunsaturated fat versus saturated fat in relation to mammary carcinogenesis. Lipids 14:155-158.

Chan P, Didato F, Cohen L (1975). High dietary fat, elevation of rat serum prolactin, and mammary cancer. Proc Soc Exp Biol Med 149:133-135.

Chan P, Head J, Cohen L, Wynder E (1977). Influence of dietary fat on the induction of mammary tumors by N-nitrosomethylurea: associated hormone changes and differences between Sprague-Dawley and F344 rats. J Natl Cancer Inst 59:1279-1283.

Chan P, Ferguson K, Dao T (1983). Effects of different dietary fats on mammary carcinogenesis. Cancer Res 43:1079-1083.

Clinton S, Destree R, Anderson D, Truex C, Imrey P, Visek W (1979). 1,2-dimethylhydrazine-induced intestinal cancer in rats fed beef or soybean protein. Nutr Reports International 20:335-342.

Clinton S, Truex C, Visek W (1979). Dietary protein, aryl hydrocarbon hydroxylase and chemical carcinogenesis in rats. J Nutr 109:55-62.

Clinton S, Truex C, Nandkumar S, Imrey P, Visek W (1981). Dietary protein-fat interactions in the initiation and promotion of 7,12-dimethylbenz(a)-anthracene mammary cancer. Fed Proc 40:948 (Abs 4071).

Clinton S, Mulloy A, Visek W (1982). The effects of dietary fat on mammary carcinogenesis in intact, ovariectomized, and ovariectomized-estrogen treated rats. 13th International Cancer Congress, Seattle, WA.

Clinton S, Imrey P, Alster J, Simon J, Truex C, Visek W (1984). The combined effects of dietary protein and fat on 7,12-dimethylbenz(a)anthracene-induced breast cancer in rats. J Nutr 114:1213-1223.

Clinton S, Li P-H, Mulloy A, Visek W (1984). Dietary fat, size heterogeneity of circulating prolactin, and their role in breast cancer. Fed Proc 43:614 (Abs 1922).

Clinton S, Mulloy A, Visek W (1984). Effects of dietary lipid saturation on prolactin secretion carcinogen metabolism, and mammary carcinogenesis in rats. J Nutr 114:1630-1639.

Clinton S, Li P-H, Visek W (1985). The combined effects of dietary protein and fat on prolactin in female rats. J Nutr 115:311-318.

Clinton S, Visek W (1985). Nutrition and experimental breast cancer: the effects of dietary fat and protein. In Finley JW, Schwass DE (eds): "Xenobiotic Metabolism-Nutritional Effects," Chapter 24, pp. 309-325, American Chemical Society Symposium Series, 277.

Committee on Animal Nutrition (1978). Nutrient requirements of laboratory animals. 3rd Ed., National Academy of Sciences, Washington DC.

Dao T, Chan P (1983). Effect of duration of high fat intake on enhancement of mammary carcinogenesis in rats. J Natl Cancer Inst 71:201-205.

Dunning W, Curtis M, Maun M (1949). The effect of dietary fat and carbohydrate on diethylstilbesterol-induced mammary cancer in rats. Cancer Res 9:354-361.

Engel R, Copeland D (1951). Influence of diet on the relative incidence of eye, mammary, ear-duct, and liver tumors in rats fed 2-acetylaminofluorene. Cancer Res 11:180-183.

Engle R, Copeland D (1952). The influence of dietary casein level on tumor induction by 2-acetylaminofluorene. Cancer Res 12:905-908.

Gammal E, Carroll K, Plunkett E (1967). Effects of dietary fat on mammary carcinogenesis by 7,12-dimethylbenz(a)anthracene in rats. Cancer Res 27:1737-1742.

Gammal E, Carroll K, Plunkett E (1968). Effects of dietary fat on the uptake and clearance of 7,12-dimethylbenzanthracene in rats. Cancer Res 28:384-385.

Giovarelli M, Padula E, Ugazio G, Forni G, Cavallo G (1980). Strain and sex-linked effects of dietary poly-unsaturated fatty acids on tumor growth and immune functions in mice. Cancer Res 40:3745-3749.

Greenfield H, Briggs G (1971). Nutritional methodology in metabolic research with rats. Ann Rev Biochem 40:549-571.

Hawrylewicz E, Huang H, Kissane J, Drab E (1982). Enhancement of 7,12-dimethylbenz(a)anthracene (DMBA) mammary tumorigenesis by high dietary protein in rats. Nutr Rept Int 26:793-806.

Hevia P, Truex C, Imrey P, Clinton S, Mangian H, Visek W (1984). Plasma amino acids and excretion of protein end products by mice fed 10 to 40% soybean protein diets with or without dietary 2-acetylaminofluorene or N,N-dinitropiperazine. J Nutr 114:555-564.

Hillyard L, Abraham S (1979). Effect of dietary poly-unsaturated fatty acids on growth of mammary adenocarcinomas in mice and rats. Cancer Res 39:4430-4437.

Hopkins G, West C (1977). Effect of dietary polyunsaturated fat on the growth of a transplantable adenocarcinoma in C3HA ^{vy}fB mice. J Natl Cancer Inst 58:753-756.

Hopkins G, Carroll K (1979). Relationship between amount and type of dietary fat in promotion of mammary carcinogenesis induced by 7,12-dimethylbenz(a)-anthracene. J Natl Cancer Inst 62:1009-1012.

Ip C, Yip P, Bernardis L (1980). Role of prolactin in the promotion of dimethylbenz(a)anthracene-induced mammary tumors by dietary fat. Cancer Res 40:374-378.

Ip C, Ip M (1981). Serum estrogens and estrogen responsiveness in 7,12-dimethylbenz(a)antracene-induced mammary tumors as influenced by dietary fat. J Natl Cancer Inst 66:291-295.

Ip C, Sinha D (1981). Neoplastic growth of carcinogen-treated mammary transplants as influenced by fat intake of donor and host. Cancer Lett 11:277-283.

Ip C, Carter C, Ip M (1985). Requirement of essential fatty acid for mammary tumorigenesis in the rat. Cancer Res 45:1997-2001.

Kappas A, Anderson K, Conney A, Alvares A (1976). Influence of dietary protein and carbohydrate on anti-pyrine and theophylline metabolism in man. Clinical Pharm and Therapeutics 20:643-653.

Kari F, Johnson J, Truex C, Visek W (1984). Effect of dietary protein concentration on yield of mutagenic metabolites from 1,2-dimethylhydrazine in mice. Cancer Res 43:3674-3679.

Kritchevsky D, Weber M, Klurfeld D (1984). Dietary fat verses caloric content in initiation and promotion of 7,12-dimethylbenz(a)anthracene-induced mammary tumori-genesis in rats. Cancer Res 214:3174-3177.

Longnecker D, Roebuck B, Yager J, Lilja H, Siegmund B (1981). Pancreatic carcinoma in azaserine-treated rats: induction, classification, and dietary modulation of incidence. Cancer 47:1562-1572.

Moreschi C (1909). Beziehungen Zwischen Ernahrung und Tumorwachstein Z. Immunitaetsforsch Immunobiol 2:651-685.

Nauss K, Locniskar M, Newberne P (1983). Effects of alterations in the quality and quantity of dietary fat on 1,2-dimethylhydrazine-induced colon tumorigenesis in rats. Cancer Res 43:4083-4090.

Nauss K, Locniskar M, Sandergaard D, Newberne P (1984). Lack of effect of dietary fat on N-nitrosomethylurea (NMU)-induced colon tumorigenesis in rats. Carcinogenesis 5:255-260.

Newberne P, Bieri J, Briggs G, Nesheim M (1978). Control of diets in laboratory animal experimentation. Institute of Laboratory Animal Resources News 21:A1-A12.

Nigro N, Singh D, Campbell R, Pak M (1975). Effect of dietary beef fat on intestinal tumor formation by Azoxymethane in rats. J Natl Cancer Inst 54:439-442.

Olson L, Clinton S, and Visek W (1983). Soybean oil (SBO) and the immune response in C2H/OUJ mice. Fed Proc 42:1186 (Abs 5240).

Pollard M, Luckert P, Pan G-Y (1984). Inhibition of intestinal tumorigenesis in methylazoxymethanol treated rats by dietary restriction. Cancer Treat Rep 68:405-408.

Pour P, Birt D (1983). Modifying factors in pancreatic carcinogenesis in the hamster model. IV. Effects of dietary protein. J Natl Cancer Inst 71:347-353.

Pour P, Birt D, Salmasi S, Gotz U (1983). Modifying factors in pancreatic carcinogenesis in the hamster model. I. The effect of protein-free diet fed during early stages of carcinogenesis. J Natl Cancer Inst 70:141-146.

Rao G, Abraham S (1976). Enhanced growth rate of transplanted mammary adenocarcinoma induced in C3H mice by dietary linoleate. J Natl Cancer Inst 56:431-432.

Reddy B (1983). Experimental research on dietary lipids and colon cancer. In Perkins EG, Visek WJ (eds): "Dietary Fats and Health," pp. 741-760. Am Oil Chemists Society, Champaign, IL.

Reddy B, Maeura Y (1984). Tumor promotion by dietary fat in azoxymethane-induced colon carcinogenesis in female F344 rats: influence of amount and source of dietary fat. J Natl Cancer Inst 72:745-750.

Roebuck B, Yager J, Longnecker D (1981). Dietary modulation of azaserine-induced pancreatic carcinogenesis in rats. Cancer Res 41:888-893.

Roebuck B, Longnecker D, Baumgartner K, Thron C (1985). Carcinogen-induced lesions in the rat pancreas: Effects of varying levels of essential fatty acid. Cancer Res 45:5252-5256.

Rogers A (1983). Influence of dietary content of lipids and lipotropic nutrients on chemical carcinogenesis in rats. Cancer Res 43:2477-2484.

Rogers A, Wetsel W (1981). Mammary carcinogenesis in rats fed different amounts and types of fat. Cancer Res 41:3735-3737.

Ross M, Bras G (1973). Influence of protein under- and over-nutrition on spontaneous tumor prevalence in the rat. J Nutr 103:944-963.

Rous P (1914). The influence of diet on transplanted and spontaneous mouse tumors. J Exptl Med 20:433-451.

Rozhin J, Wilson P, Bull A, Nigro N (1984). Ornithine decarboxylase activity in the rat and human colon. Cancer Res 44:3226-3230.

Sakaguchi M, Hiramatsu Y, Takada H, Yamamura M, Hicki K, Saito K, Yamamoto M (1984). Effect of dietary unsaturated and saturated fats on azoxymethane-induced colon carcinogenesis in rats. Cancer Res 44:1472-1477.

Shay H, Gruenstein M, Shimkin M (1964). Effect of casein, lactalbumin, and ovalbumin on 3-methylcholanthrene-induced mammary carcinoma in rats. J Natl Cancer Inst 33:243-253.

Silverman J, Shallabarger C, Holtzman S, Stone J, Weisburger J (1980). Effect of dietary fat on x-ray-induced mammary cancer in Sprague-Dawley rats. J Natl Cancer Inst 64:631-634.

Silverstone H, Tannenbaum A (1950). The effect of the proportion of dietary fat on the rate of formation of mammary carcinoma in mice. Cancer Res 10:448-453.

Tannenbaum A (1942). The genesis and growth of tumors. III. Effect of high fat diet. Cancer Res 2:468-475.

Tannenbaum A (1947). The role of nutrition in the origin and growth of tumors. In "Approaches to Tumor Chemotherapy," pp. 96-127. Lancaster, PA, Science Press.

Tannenbaum A, Silverstone H (1949). The genesis and growth of tumors. Effects of varying the proportion of protein (casein) in the diet. Cancer Res 9:162-173.

Tannenbaum A, Silverstone H (1949). Effect of low environmental temperature, dinitrophenol, or sodium fluoride on the formation of tumors in mice. Cancer Research 9:403-410.

Tannenbaum A (1959). Nutrition and cancer. In Homburger F (ed): "The Pathophysiology of Cancer," pp. 517-562, Holber-Harper.

Tinsley I, Schmitz J, Pierce D (1981). Influence of dietary fatty acids on the incidence of mammary tumors in the C_3H mouse. Cancer Res 41:1460-1465.

Topping D, Visek W (1976). Nitrogen intake and tumorigenesis in rats injected with 1,2-diemthylhydrazine. J Nutr 106:1583-1590.

Visek W, Clinton S (1983). Dietary fat and breast cancer. In Perkins E, Visek W (eds): "Dietary Fats and Health," pp. 721-740. Am Oil Chemists Society, Champaign, IL.

Wattenberg L, Loub W, Lam L, Speier J (1976). Dietary constituents altering the responses to chemical carcinogens. Fed Proc. 35:1327-1331.

Welsch C, Aylsworth C (1983). The interrelationship between dietary lipids, endocrine activity, and the development of mammary tumors in experimental animals. In Perkins E, Visek W (eds): "Dietary Fats and Health," pp. 790-816. Am Oil Chemists Society, Champaign, IL.

Wetsel W, Rogers A, Rutledge A, Leavitt W (1984). Absence of an effect of dietary corn oil content on plasma prolactin, progesterone, and 17β-estradiol in female Sprague-Dawley rats. Cancer Res 44:1420-1425.

Dietary Fat and Cancer, pages 403–433
© 1986 Alan R. Liss, Inc.

FAT-PROTEIN INTERACTION, DEFINED 2-GENERATION STUDIES

E.J. Hawrylewicz, Ph.D.

Director, Department of Research, Mercy Hospital
and Medical Center, Stevenson Exp. at King Drive,
Chicago, Illinois 60616

INTRODUCTION

Epidemiologic studies indicate that total dietary
protein and animal protein intake correlated positively
with the incidence and mortality from breast cancer (Armstrong et al., 1975). Drasar and Irving (1973) evaluated
the per capita consumption of total fat, and animal protein
in 37 countries as function of breast cancer incidence.
These studies showed a Pearson's correlation coefficient
for animal fat of 0.75; however the coefficient for animal
protein was also 0.75. Hems (1978) in a similar study
concluded that because the dietary factors correlated so
closely it was not possible to state which factor related
most closely with breast cancer.

Hems (1980) also studied the breast cancer rates in
England as a function of social class and concluded that
changes in breast cancer mortality was associated with
changes in consumption of fat, animal protein and sugar one
to two decades earlier.

Earlier studies by Tannenbaum and Silverstone (1947)
examined the relationship between dietary protein and the
incidence of spontaneous mammary tumors in C3H-female mice.
Dietary fat was constant at 2 percent, composed of equal
parts of cod liver oil and wheat germ oil, and protein
(casein) varied in 5 increments from 9 to 45 percent. Test
diets were initiated at a mature age of 14 weeks. Body
weights in the first year did not vary significantly
between dietary groups. Mammary tumor incidence was

between 92 and 98 percent for all groups except the 45 percent casein group which was 84 percent. Subsequently Tannenbaum and Silverstone (1953) reported that mice which were fed isocaloric diets and maintained at equal body weight, developed spontaneous mammary carcinomas which correlated positively to the level of dietary protein (10 to 46 percent).

Ross et al. (1982) developed a dietary model in which rats were permitted to select their own diets over an entire life-time. They determined that the combination of variables that maximized the probability of developing a neoplasm included a high absolute protein intake shortly after weaning and a high level of protein intake relative to body weight during the early adult period. Dietary fat (corn oil) was maintained at a constant level of 13.5 percent.

Reported studies with chemically induced tumors generally demonstrated a positive correlation between the level of dietary protein and the tumor incidence. Early studies by Madhaven et al. (1968) and Wells et al. (1976) demonstrated an increased incidence of aflatoxin induced hepatomas in rats fed higher levels of protein. Topping and Visek (1976) showed that induction of adenocarcinoma of the small and large intestines with 1,2-dimethylhydrazine was greater in rats fed 22 percent rather than 7.5 percent protein diet.

However the relationship between the level of dietary protein and chemically induced tumors in the mammary gland is not clearly established. Engel and Copeland (1952) reported that 2-acetylaminofluorene induced similar numbers of mammary tumors in rats fed diets with casein concentrations at 9, 20 and 27 percent and lard at 15 percent and cod liver oil at 1 percent. At 40 and 60 percent casein a significant decrease in body weight and tumor incidence occurred. However the mammary tumor incidence was equivalent in animals fed either 60 or 27 percent casein diet if the body weights were equal. Shay et al. (1964) fed rats semi-purified diets with casein concentrations of 27 or 64 percent, and vegetable oil level at 8 percent. The rats were individually housed and the diets initiated at 5 weeks of age. The carcinogen, 3-methylcholanthrene, was continuously administered six days per week. A similar mammary tumor incidence occurred in both casein groups. However in both diets the mammary tumor incidence was greater than in the control chow fed animals.

Clinton et al. (1979) reported on the effect of 7,12-dimethylbenz(a)anthracene (DMBA) induction of mammary tumors as a function of dietary protein fed during tumor initiation or promotion phases. The semi-purified diets contained corn oil at 10 percent and casein at 7.5, 15 or 45 percent. Rats were individually housed and the test diets initiated after weaning. These studies indicated that animals fed 7.5 and 45 percent casein diets for four weeks prior to DMBA treatment gained less body weight compared to those fed 15 percent casein diet. Following DMBA treatment all animals were fed a 15 percent casein diet; body weights were similar at termination. The mammary tumor incidence was inversely proportional to the dietary protein concentration fed prior to DMBA treatment. Rats fed a 15 percent casein diet prior to DMBA treatment followed with either a 7.5, 15 or 45 percent casein diet showed no differences in bodyweight at treatment or termination age. Tumor burden was similar in all groups. The authors concluded that high concentration of dietary protein inhibits tumor initiation but no protein effect was noted on tumor promotion.

Continuing these studies these authors (Clinton et al., 1984) reported on the interaction of dietary protein-fat on DMBA induced mammary tumor burden. They utilized a 3x3 factorial design with casein at 8, 16 or 32 percent and corn oil at 12, 24 or 48 percent of total dietary calories. The diets were initiated in weanling rats and continued for 30 weeks. The authors concluded that in-creasing dietary corn oil increased the incidence of palpable mammary tumors; however dietary protein did not affect tumor prevalence. Also no substantial interaction of protein and fat were observed on tumor incidence.

Our studies utilized a rat model in which the isocaloric, protein test diets are fed to mothers prior to conception. The neonates were continued on the test diet throughout their life and functioned as the test animal. These studies indicate a positive correlation between dietary protein concentration and chemically induced mammary tumor incidence. The data from these studies are summarized in this paper.

METHODOLOGY

Two diet models, moderate and high fat levels, with several concentrations of protein were evaluated in these studies. One protocol utilized diets composed of casein at 8, 19.5 and 31 percent and corn oil at a level of 10 percent (Table 1). Diets were isocaloric (4.07 Kcalories /g): sucrose provided the balance of calories. the pelletized diets were fed ad libitum and stored at $5^{\circ}C$. The animals had free access to water; group housed in plastic cages and the room maintained at $24 \pm 2^{\circ}C$ with 14 hours of illumination (Hawrylewicz et al., 1982).

Diets containing an increased level of corn oil enhance carcinogen-induced mammary tumor incidence (Carroll et al. 1970). To determine whether dietary protein could further enhance tumor growth a high protein-high fat diet was tested (Table 2, Hawrylewicz et al., 1986).

In order to assess the effect of the test diets on development of the breast gland and neuroendocrine function, the diets were fed to adult female rats prior to conception and continued through gestation and lactation. Female neonates were continued on their respective diets for the duration of the study and constituted the test groups.

Specifically adult virgin female Sprague-Dawley (Harlan Sprague-Dawley Farm) rats were upon receipt conditioned on laboratory chow (Ralston Purina Co.) for two weeks. The test diet replaced the chow diet and the conditioning continued for three weeks. Subsequently three females were housed with one male and the diet continued through gestation and lactation. At birth the pups were immediately sexed and the litter was adjusted to eight pups, females if possible. Weaning occurred at 21 days of age and the female neonates continued on the diet as the test group.

In one series of experiments dimethylbenz(a)anthracene (DMBA) was utilized as the carcinogen. DMBA in sesame oil was administered intragastrically (3mg/100g body weight) at seven weeks of age. It was established that the level of dietary protein influenced the age of sexual maturation and that animals fed a 8 percent protein diet were sexual

Table 1. Diet Composition (19.5% Casein)[a]

Ingredients	g/Kg
Casein (Protein 90%)	195.0
L-Methionine	3.0
Sucrose	455.0
Cornstarch	150.0
Corn Oil	100.0
Non-Nutritive Fiber	50.0
Mineral Mix (AIN-76)	35.0
Vitamin Mix (AIN-76)	10.0
Choline Bitartrate	2.0
K-Calories/Gram	4.10

[a]8% and 31% Isocaloric Casein Diets Blended with an Adjustment of Sucrose

(Hawrylewicz et al., 1982)

Table 2. Composition of Test Diets[a]

Ingredients	Normal Protein (NP, 19%) High Fat (HF, 15%)	High Protein (HP, 33%) High Fat (HF, 15%)
Casein (vitamin free)	19	33
Corn Oil	15	15
Corn Starch	25	25
Sucrose	31	17
Non-Nutritive Fiber	5	5
Mineral Mix (AIN)	3.5	3.5
Vitamin Mix (AIN)	1	1
Choline Bitartrate	0.2	0.2
DL Methionine	0.3	0.3

[a]4.35 Kcalories/g

(Hawrylewicz et al., 1986)

immature at 7 weeks of age. Therefore another group of
animals were treated three weeks after sexual maturation
(vaginal opening).

Estrous cycles were monitored for 3 cycles before DMBA
treatment and thereafter for 10 cycles. The pattern of
estrus was not changed. Before DMBA injection the average
length of estrous cycle was 4.91+0.15 days (N=23) and post
treatment 4.74+0.07 days in the NP-NF group. Level of
dietary protein had no significant effect on the length of
the estrous cycle.

To determine whether increased dietary protein could
enhance the effect of fat enriched diets, animals were
treated with N-nitrosomethylurea (NMU), a direct acting
carcinogen. At 7 and 8 weeks of age the sexual mature rat
was treated with NMU (50mg/kg, ICN Pharmaceutical, Inc.).
NMU was administered I.V. via the tail vein under light
ether anesthesia; controls were injected with saline. NMU
treatment or increased dietary protein had no effect on the
length of the estrous cycle (Hawrylewicz et al., 1986).

RESULTS

Effect of Diet on Food Consumption and Body Weight Gain

Compared to the control group, NP-NF, rats consuming
high protein-normal fat (HP-NF) diets consumed equivalent
amounts of food (Figure 1) and gained equivalent body
weight (Figure 2) in the post weaning period. These groups
of animals were essentially pair-fed. Conversely the low
protein diet (LP-NF) group consumed 35 percent more food
but gained significantly less weight (Figures 1 and 2).
Animals fed the high fat diets with either normal (NP-HF)
or high (HP-HF) protein levels consumed equivalent amount
of food and gained comparable weight over 32 weeks of life
(Hawrylewicz et al., 1986). Also irrespective of the level
of dietary fat, the normal and high protein diet groups in
the two experiments had similar food consumption and growth
curves.

In spite of the increased calories consumed, the
animals fed the low protein diets experienced a retarded
growth rate. No physical differences were noted in the

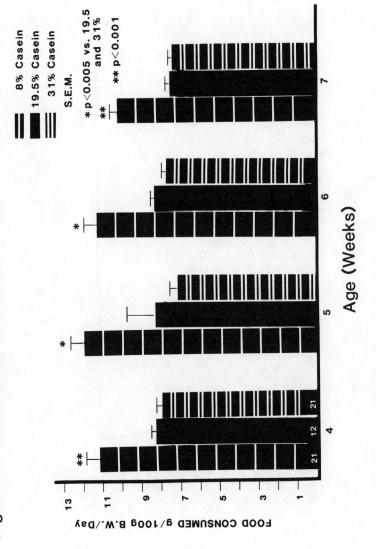

Figure 1. Protein Diet Consumed as Function of Body Weight

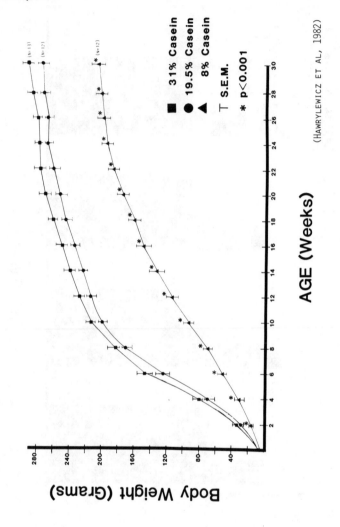

Figure 2. Effect of Protein Diet on Body Weight

(Hawrylewicz et al, 1982)

animals consuming adequate or enriched protein diets.

In addition to affecting body growth, the protein limiting diet (LP-NF) markedly delayed the age of sexual maturation as noted by vaginal opening (Table 3). Interestingly, repeated observations indicate that animals fed enriched protein diets (HP-NF) reach sexual maturation at a younger age (Table 3). Enriched protein diets do influence physiologic development inspite of a normal growth rate.

Effect of Diet on Hormone Regulation

Growth of mammary tumors is controlled in part by prolactin (Meites, 1972). Therefore the effect of the test diets on serum prolactin activity was determined. Serum was collected each day throughout the first estrous cycle following DMBA treatment at 7 weeks of age or 3 weeks after sexual maturation (SM+3). At 7 weeks of age, prolactin activity in the normal protein group (NP-NF) rose from a basel level of 47.0 ± 9.3 ng/ml (N=8) at 10.00 h at diestrus to surge values of 377.3 ± 67.5 (N=12) at proestrus (17:00 h) and subsequently fell to 82.2 ± 11.7 (N=10). Equivalent values were noted for animals fed the protein enriched diets. The low protein group was sexual immature and did not experience an estrous cycle (Huang et al., 1982).

Animals fed the normal and high protein diets and examined 3 weeks after sexual maturation showed a similar surge of prolactin activity on proestrus afternoon (Figure 3). As noted the animals were treated with DMBA 3 weeks after sexual maturation to insure the growth of hormone dependent tumors. However sexually mature animals (SM+3) fed low protein diets (LP-NF) experienced a marked repression of the prolactin surge (Figure 3). In the adult animal the prolactin activity normalized in the low protein group and was equivalent to the normal and enriched protein groups (Figure 4). The exact age for normalization of the prolactin surge has not been determined (Huang et al., 1982).

Release of prolactin from the anterior pituitary is under inhibitory control of dopamine released from the

Table 3. Effects of Protein Diet on Sexual Maturation and
Estrous Cycle

Dietary Group (% Protein)	Number of Rats	Age at Vaginal Opening	Estrous Cycles 2-3 Weeks After Vaginal Opening
8%	17	68.6 ± 3.6^a	Normal (4-5 day cycle)
19.5%	13	37.0 ± 0.45^b	Normal
31%	17	30.5 ± 0.3	Normal

$\pm$ S.E.M.
a: Significantly different from 31% and 19% ($p < 0.001$)
b: Significantly different from 31% ($p < 0.002$)

(Hawrylewicz et al., 1982)

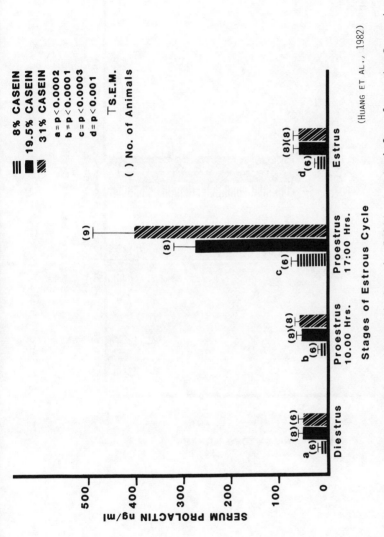

Figure 3. Serum prolactin activity in DMBA treated female rats 3 weeks after sexual maturity.

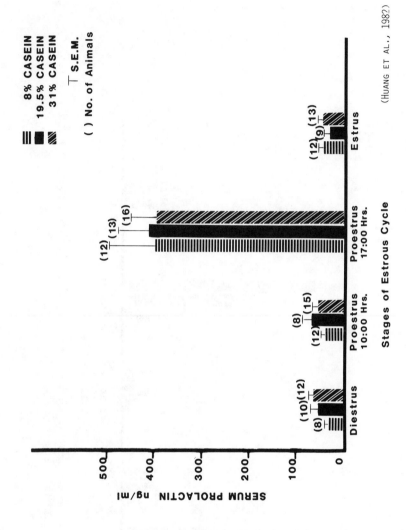

Figure 4. Serum prolactin activity 6 months after DMBA treatment.

(HUANG ET AL., 1982)

median eminence. The drug α-methylparatyrosine (α-MPT) inhibits the enzyme tyrosine hydroxylase and the synthesis of dopamine. Consequently the amount of dopamine released from the median eminence can be determined following injection of α-MPT. The data shown in Figure 5 indicates an increased release of dopamine from the median eminence in the low protein-normal fat (LP-NF) group compared to the normal or high protein groups. Serum prolactin activity consequently is depressed in the low protein group (Figure 6). Low protein-normal fat (LP-NF) diet fed during early development appears to alter neuroendocrine regulation. Animals fed normal or high protein-normal fat diets responded equivalently to α-MPT treatment and prolactin release.

Similarly rats fed high fat diets with either normal protein (NP-HF) or high protein (HP-HF) levels had at 7 weeks of age equivalent serum prolactin activities and an appropriate proestrus surge (Hawrylewicz et al., 1986, Figure 7). Following injection of NMU or saline at 7 and 8 weeks of age, the prolactin activity was equivalent in both dietary groups and both treatment procedures (Figure 8). The animals were further tested during the tumor growth phase at 28 and 33 weeks of age. The prolactin activity was equivalent throughout the estrous cycle in all diet and treatment groups.

With the exception of the low protein group (LP-NF), the diet did not affect neurohormone regulation and prolactin activity.

Growth of DMBA-induced mammary tumors are also enhanced by ovarian hormones, estrogen and progesterone (Leung, 1975). Serum estradiol and progesterone measured 3 weeks after sexual maturity showed a repressed surge during proestrus in the low protein-normal fat (LP-NF) group (Figure 9). The normal and high protein groups were equivalent and exhibited an appropriate hormone surge. These observations further support the premise that a low protein diet delays endocrine development.

Effect of Diet on Breast Development

The effect of dietary protein on the development of the breast gland was investigated. Wholemount preparations

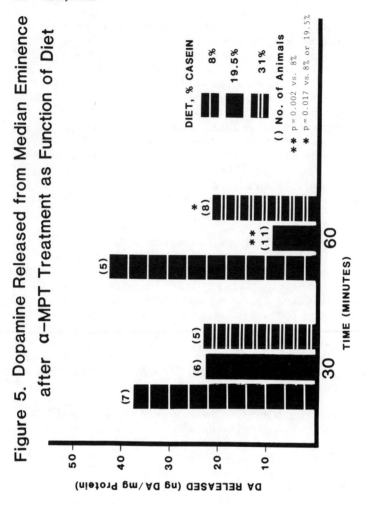

Figure 5. Dopamine Released from Median Eminence after α–MPT Treatment as Function of Diet

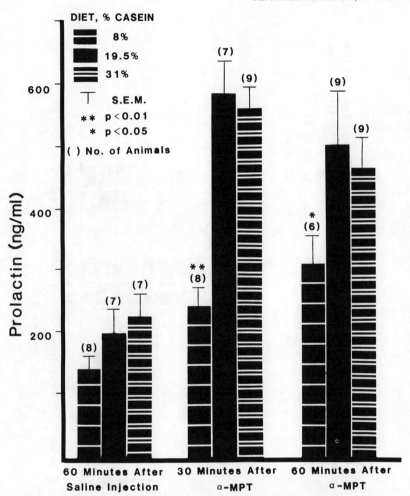

Figure 6. Serum Prolactin Concentration after α-MPT Treatment

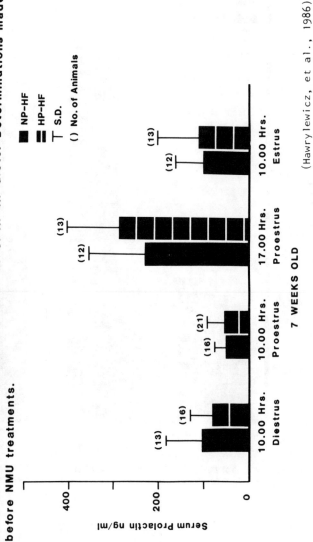

Figure 7. Serum prolactin concentration (ng/ml) measured at four stages of the estrous cycle in rats fed isocaloric NP-HF or HP-HF diets. Determinations made before NMU treatments.

(Hawrylewicz, et al., 1986)

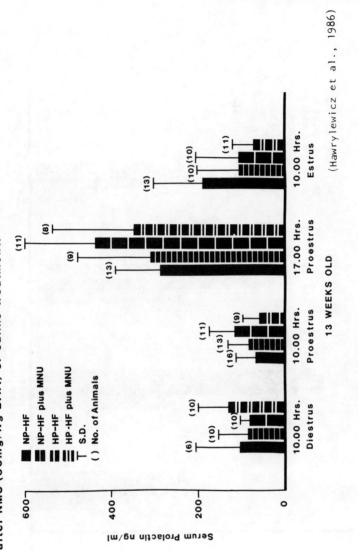

Figure 8. Serum prolactin (ng/ml) measured at four stages of the estrous cycle in rats fed isocaloric NP-HF or HP-HF diets. Determinations made five weeks after NMU (50mg/Kg B.W.) or saline treatment.

(Hawrylewicz et al., 1986)

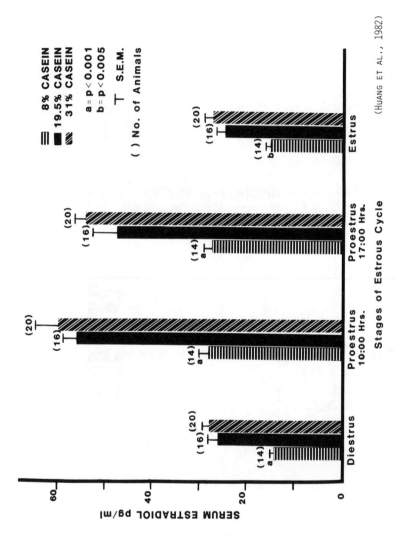

Figure 9. Serum estradiol activity in DMBA treated female rats 3 weeks after sexual maturity.

(HUANG ET AL., 1982)

showed that ductal development in the mammary gland is markedly reduced 3 weeks after sexual maturation in the low protein-normal fat (LP-NF) group compared to rats fed normal or high protein, normal fat diets (Sanz et al., 1986). Development of the mammary gland is dependent on estrogen and prolactin hormones. The depressed hormone activities observed in the low protein (LP-NF) group at this age contributed to the observed attenuated ductal growth. The extent of mammary ductal development in the normal and high protein diet groups 3 weeks after sexual maturity appeared equivalent.

Morphologic development of the mammary ducts were assessed by determining the number of terminal end buds (TEB), alveolar buds (AB), lobules (LOB) and terminal ducts (TD). At seven weeks of age the TEB structure dominated in the sexual immature low protein-normal fat (LP-NF) group. The TEB progressed to AB and LOB structures in the animals fed normal or high protein-normal fat diets and the number of these structures were significantly greater compared to the low protein group (Figure 10).

Three weeks after sexual maturity the number of TEB decreased and AB increased significantly in the low protein diet group (Figure 11). Inspite of this morphologic progression, the number of structures still remained significantly different than that observed for animals fed either normal or high protein-normal fat diets.

Effect of Diet on [^{3}H]-Thymidine Incorporation

The actively growing mammary gland, determined by [^{3}H-] thymidine incorporation into cellular DNA, is most sensitive to administered carcinogens (Russo et al., 1978). Therefore uptake of labeled thymidine into breast tissue fractions was determined as a function of diet. Three weeks after sexual maturation, the age of maximum sensitivity to carcinogens, [^{3}H]-thymidine was administered (50 Ci, I.P.) to animals fed normal fat diets (10%) with protein content at 3 (LP), 19.5 (NP) or 31 (HP) percent. Animals were sacrificed two hours later. The breast tissue from the abdominal and inguinal area was removed for analysis. Following collagenase digestion, the fat cells were removed and the ductal tissue processed for determination of DNA content and [^{3}H]-thymidine incorporation.

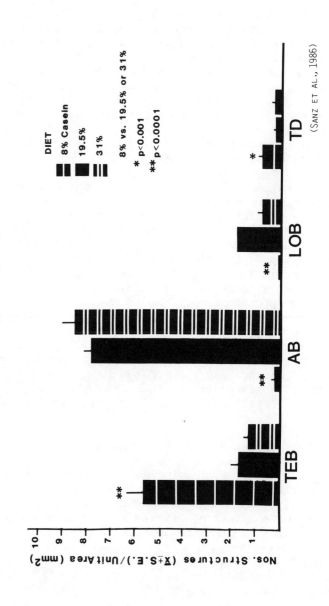

Figure 10. Morphologic Structures as Function of Dietary Protein

Age: 7 Weeks

(SANZ ET AL., 1986)

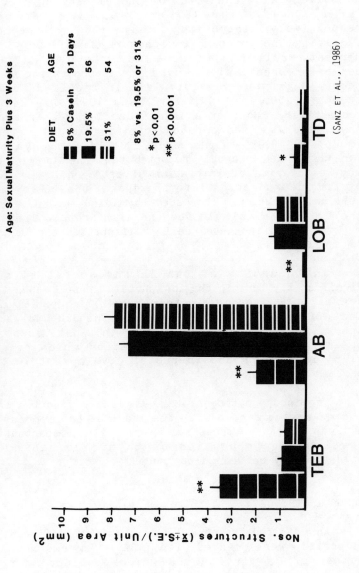

Figure 11. Morphologic Structures as Function of Dietary Protein

Age: Sexual Maturity Plus 3 Weeks

(SANZ ET AL., 1986)

The fat content in the breast tissue correlated negatively with the level of protein in the diet: 56.9 (LP-NF), 49.5 (NP-NF) and 40.5 (HP-NF) percent respectively. Increasing dietary fat to 15 percent and adjusting the protein to either 19 (NP-HF) or 33 (HP-HF) percent resulted in a tissue fat content of 45.1 and 45.4 percent respectively. Thymidine incorporation in the fat pad (DPM/g fat) was equivalent in the LP-NF and NP-NF groups (2100.09 $\pm$ 449, N=15, and 1997.36 $\pm$ 283, N=18, respectively. However a significantly greater amount of thymidine was incorporated into the fat pad in the HP-NF group (3419.92 $\pm$ 551, N=18, $p < 0.05$). Shyamala and Ferenczy (1984) recently reported that the mammary fat pad may be the site of initiation of estrogen action followed by its incorporation into the ductal tissue for mammary cell proliferation. Increased thymidine incorporation into the fat pad of animals fed the high protein diet (HP-NF) may relate to increased cell proliferation and sensitivity to carcinogens.

The quantity of DNA in the ductal tissue was significantly less in the low protein group compared to the normal (NP-NF) or high potein (HP-HF) groups (Figure 12). The amount of DNA in the ductal tissue did not vary with the stage in the estrous cycle. This data supports the breast tissue wholemont observation which revealed a significant decrease in ductal development in the low protein group (LP-NF).

The incorporation of $[^3H]$-thymidine into DNA from the ductal tissue varied with the stage of the estrous cycle, and was lowest at proestrus (Figure 13). Importantly, the level of incorporation of thymidine did not vary significantly between diet groups.

TUMOR INCIDENCE

Animals fed the normal fat diets with different levels of protein were treated with DMBA at 7 weeks of age. The number of mammary tumors which developed correlated positively with the level of dietary protein (Table 4). The tumor latency period and the number of tumors per tumor bearing rat were similar in all groups. The low protein (LP-NF) group developed tumors in approximately half the

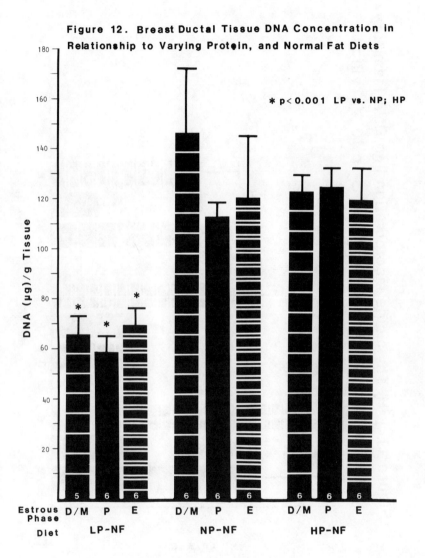

Figure 12. Breast Ductal Tissue DNA Concentration in Relationship to Varying Protein, and Normal Fat Diets

* p < 0.001 LP vs. NP; HP

Figure 13. [³H]–Thymidine Incorporation Into DNA Mammary Gland Ductal Tissue in Relationship to Varying Protein and Normal Fat Diets

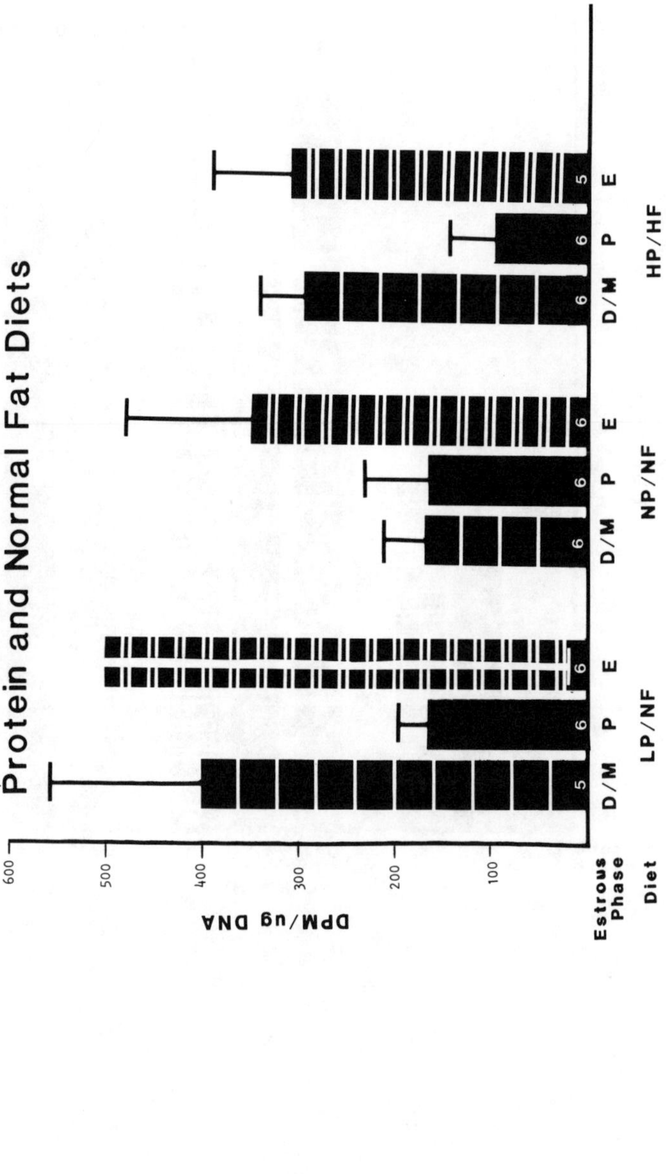

Table 4. Mammary tumor incidence following administration of DMBA to rats fed either an 8%, 19.5% or 31% protein and 10% fat diet. Rats were killed 25 weeks after administration of 5mg DMBA per rat at 7 weeks of age.

DIETARY GRP. (% PROTEIN)	NUMBER OF RATS	NO. OF RATS W/PALPABLE AND/OR NONPALPABLE TUMORS	NO. OF RATS W/PALPABLE TUMORS	NO. OF RATS W/NONPALPABLE TUMORS	TOTAL NO. OF TUMORS		TUMORS / TUMOR BEARING RAT	AV. LATENCY PERIOD (WEEKS)
					PALPABLE	NONPALPABLE		
8.	28	16 (58%)	12 (43%)	9 (32%)	17	14	1.94 ± 0.22	15.5 ± 1.70 (N=12)
19.5	25	19 (76%)	16 (64%)[b]	10 (46%)	28	13	2.16 ± 0.31	15.3 ± 1.27 (N=16)
31.	29	29 (100%)[a]	24 (83%)[c]	20 (70%)[c]	44	30	2.55 ± 0.23	15.6 ± 1.00 (N=24)

[a] SIGNIFICANTLY DIFFERENT FROM 8% and 19.5% (p < 0.005)
[b] SIGNIFICANTLY DIFFERENT FROM 8% (p < 0.05)
[c] SIGNIFICANTLY DIFFERENT FROM 8% and 19.5% (p < 0.025, p < 0.05 RESPECTIVELY)
± S.E.M.

(HAWRYLEWICZ ET AL., 1982)

animals inspite of their sexual immaturity and repressed mammary ductal development. The high protein group (HP-NF) was indistinguishable from the control normal protein (NP-NF) group with regard to mammary ductal development, hormone regulation and physical characteristics, nevertheless they experienced a significantly greater number of palpable and nonpalpable mammary tumors.

The experiment was repeated, DMBA was administered 3 weeks after sexual maturation: LP-NF at 90, NP-NF at 58 and HP-NF at 52 days of age. At 90 days of age the low protein group (LP-NF) was sexually mature however the cyclic hormone surges were repressed and morphologic development of the breast was delayed. Neither morphologic or hormonal differences were observed between the normal and high protein groups. As noted in the previous experiment the tumor incidence was directly related to the level of dietary protein (Table 5). In addition 41 percent of the mammary tumors in the low protein (LP-NF) group were classified as fibroadenomas as compared to fourteen percent in the high protein-normal fat (HP-NF) group. Sinha et al. (1983) reported that administration of DMBA prior to sexual maturation resulted in a higher incidence of fibroadenomas.

To determine whether dietary protein could augment the effect of a high fat diet on mammary carcinogenesis, rats were fed a high protein-high fat (HP-HF) diet. The animals were treated with the carcinogen N-methyl-N-nitro-sourea (NMU, 50mg/Kg B.W.) at 7 and 8 weeks of age. The average latency period for tumor appearance was similar and the tumor incidence was 100 percent in the two diet groups (Table 6). However the number of tumors per animal increased by 52.6% and the average tumor weight increased by 80.8% in animals fed the high protein-high fat (HP-HF) diet compared to the normal protein-high fat (NP-HF) group. Physical characteristics and hormone activities in these two groups of animals were similar; nevertheless increased dietary protein stimulated in the presence of high dietary fat an increased tumor burden.

SUMMARY

Mammary tumor burden, in rats fed either normal or high fat diets related positively to the level of protein in the diet. This relationship existed with either a

Table 5. Mammary tumor incidence following administration of DMBA to rats fed either an 8.1%, 19.5%, or 31% protein and 10% fat diet. Rats were killed 25 weeks after administration of 3mg DMBA per 100 gram body weight at 3 weeks after vaginal opening.

DIETARY GRP. (% PROTEIN)	NUMBER OF RATS	NO. OF RATS W/PALPABLE AND/OR NONPALPABLE TUMORS	NO. OF RATS W/PALPABLE TUMORS	NO. OF RATS W/NONPALPABLE TUMORS	TOTAL NO. OF TUMORS		TUMORS / TUMOR BEARING RAT	AV. LATENCY PERIOD (WEEKS)
					PALPABLE	NONPALPABLE		
8.0	30	10 (33%)	6 (20%)	6 (20%)	11	7	1.80 ± 0.38	15.2 ± 2.30 (N=6)
19.5	23	11 (48%)	10 (43%)[b]	6 (20%)	17	8	2.27 ± 0.51	15.0 ± 1.32 (N=10)
31	26	19 (73%)[a]	16 (62%)[c]	10 (40%)	23	11	1.79 ± 0.15	15.6 ± 0.91 (N=16)

[a] SIGNIFICANTLY DIFFERENT FROM 8% and 19.5% ($p < 0.005$, $p < 0.05$ RESPECTIVELY)
[b] SIGNIFICANTLY DIFFERENT FROM 8% ($p < 0.05$)
[c] SIGNIFICANTLY DIFFERENT FROM 8% and 19.5% ($p < 0.05$)
± S.E.M.

(HAWRYLEWICZ ET AL., 1982)

Table 6. Mammary Tumor Incidence 28 Weeks Following Administration of NMU. Rats Fed Either a High Protein-High Fat (HP-HF) or Normal Protein-High Fat (NP-HF) Isocaloric Diet.

Dietary Group	Treatment	Number of Rats	Number of Rat Bearing Tumors	Total Number of Tumor	Average No. of Tumor per Tumor Bearing Rat	Average Weight of Tumor per Tumor Bearing Rat (g)	Average Latency Period (Weeks)
HP-HF	Saline	24	0	0	0	0	0
	NMU	39	39 (100%)	171	$4.38 \pm 0.37^{a,b}$	17.97 ± 2.63^{b}	12.58 ± 0.77
NP-HF	Saline	25	0	0	0	0	0
	NMU	24	24 (100%)	69	2.87 ± 0.35	9.94 ± 2.92	14.0 ± 1.23

[a] Mean $\pm$ S.E.M.

[b] Significant difference ($p < 0.002$)

(HAWRYLEWICZ ET AL., 1986)

direct (NMU) or indirect carcinogen (DMBA).

Significant differences in body growth, sexual maturation, morphologic structures in the mammary duct, and hormone activities during the estrous cycle probably contributed to lower tumor burden in the low protein-normal fat (LP-NF) group. Animals fed a high protein-normal fat (HP-NF) diet throughout their entire life have, with the exception of early sexual maturation, no distinctive characteristics compared to the control group. Inspite of these physical and physiologic similarities, increased dietary protein enhanced the effect of administered carcinogens.

Animals fed a high protein-high fat (HP-HF) diet were compared to rats fed a normal protein-high fat (NP-HF) diet.

Increased dietary protein further enhanced the effect of the high fat diet resulting in an increased carcinogen-induced tumor burden.

These studies indicate that the design of the animal model, i.e. age of initiation of a test diet, appears to have a significant bearing on mammary tumor development.

The biologic mechanisms which respond to diet modifications and which may influence breast tumor growth have not been thoroughly elaborated and require additional study.

REFERENCES

Armstrong B, Doll R (1975). Environmental factors and cancer incidence and mortality in different countries, with special references to dietary practices. Int J Cancer 27:617-631.

Carroll KK, Khor HT (1970). Effect of dietary fat and dose level of 7,12-dimethylbenz(a)anthracene on mammary tumor incidence in rats. Cancer Res 30:2260-2264.

Clinton SK, Imrey PB, Alster JM, Simon J, Truex CR, Visek WJ (1984). The combined effects of dietary protein and fat on 7,12-dimethylbenz(a)anthracene-induced breast cancer in rats. J Nutr 114:1213-1223.

Clinton SK, Truex CR, Visek WJ (1979). Dietary protein, aryl hydrocarbon hydroxylase and chemical carcinogenesis in rats. J Nutr 109:55-62.

Drasar BS, Irving D (1973). Environmental factors and cancer of the colon and breast. Br J Cancer 27:167-172.

Engel RW, Copeland DH (1952). The influence of dietary casein level of tumor induction with 2-acetylamino-fluorene. Cancer Res 12:905-908.

Hawrylewicz EJ, Huang HH, Kissane JQ, Drab EA (1982). Enhancement of 7,12-dimethylbenz(a)anthracene (DMBA) mammary tumorigenesis by high dietary protein in rats. Nutr Rep Int 26:793-806.

Hawrylewicz EJ, Huang HH, Liu J.M (1986). Dietary protein, enhancement of N-nitrosomethylurea (NMU) induced mammary carcinogenesis and effect on hormone regulation. Cancer Res (Submitted).

Hems G (1973). The contributions of diet and child bearing to breast cancer rates. Br J Cancer 37:974-982.

Hems G (1980). Association between breast-cancer mortality rates, child-bearing and diet in the United Kingdom. Br J Cancer 41:429-437.

Huang HH, Hawrylewicz EJ, Kissane JQ, Drab EA (1982). Effect of protein diet on release of prolactin and ovarian steroids in female rats. Nutr Rep Int 26:807-820.

Leung BS, Sasaki GH, Leung JS (1975). Estrogen-prolactin dependency in 7,12-dimethylbenz(a)anthracene-induced tumors. Cancer Res 35:621-627.

Madhavan TV, Gopalan C (1968). The effect of dietary protein on carcinogenesis of aflatoxin. Arch. Pathol. 85:133-137.

Meites J (1972). Relation of prolactin and estrogen to mammary tumorigenesis in the rat. J Natl Cancer Inst 48:1217-1224.

Ross MH, Lustbader ED, Bras G (1982). Dietary practices of early life and spontaneous tumors of the rat. Nutr and Cancer 3:150-167.

Russo J, Russo IH (1978). DNA labeling index and structure of the rat mammary gland as determinants of its susceptiblity to carcinogenesis. J Natl Cancer Inst 61:1451-1459.

Sanz MCA, Liu JM, Huang HH, Hawrylewicz EJ (1986). Dietary protein, morphologic development of the rat mammary gland. J Natl Cancer Inst (Submitted).

Shay H, Gruenstein M, Shimkin MB (1964). Effect of casein,

lactalbumin and ovaltumin on 3-methylcholanthrene-induced mammary carcinoma in rats. J Natl Cancer Inst 33:243-253.

Shyamala G, Ferenczy A (1984). Mammary fat pad may be a potential site for initiation of estrogen action in normal mouse mammary glands. Endocrinology 115:1078-1081.

Sinha DK, Pazik JE, Dao TL (1983). Progression of rat mammary development with age and its relationship to carcinogenesis by a chemical carcinogen. Intl J Cancer 31:321-327.

Tannenbaum A, Silverstone H (1949). The genesis and growth of tumors IV. Effects of varying the proportion of protein (casein) in the diet. Cancer Res 9:162-173.

Tannenbaum A, Silverstone H (1953). Mammary carcinoma in the mouse. Proc Amer Assoc Cancer Res 1:56.

Topping DC, Visek WJ (1976). Nitrogen intake and tumorigenesis in rats injected with 1,2-dimethylhydrazine. J Nutr 106:1583-1590.

Wells P, Alftergood L, Alfin-Slater RB (1976). Effect of varying levels of dietary protein on tumor development and lipid metabolism in rats exposed to aflatoxin. J Amer Oil Chem Soc 53:559-562.

Dietary Fat and Cancer, pages 435–459
© 1986 Alan R. Liss, Inc.

CHOLESTEROL CONUNDRUMS: THE RELATIONSHIP BETWEEN DIETARY AND
SERUM CHOLESTEROL IN COLON CANCER

Selwyn A. Broitman

Department of Microbiology and Pathology
Boston University School of Medicine
Boston, MA 02118

Supported in part by Grants CA 16750 from the National Large
Bowel Cancer Project and T32-CA 09423, National Cancer
Institute, National Institutes of Health.

Abbreviations

AOM = azoxymethane
CHD = coronary heart disease
DMH = 1,2 dimethyl hydrazine
FAO = Food and Agriculture Organization
MNNG = N-methyl-N'-nitro-N-nitrosoguanidine
MNU = N-methyl-N-nitrosurea
WHO = World Health Organization
LRC-CPPT = Lipid Research Clinics Coronary Primary Preven-
tion Trial

INTRODUCTION

The etiology of cancer is generally considered to be
the result of a variety of elements, and as such, those
agents that result in carcinogenesis at one site may have
negligible effects in another region. Historic studies have
implied a number of relationships on the role of cholesterol
in tumorigenesis. Still controversial, current discussion
has revolved about the relationship between dietary
cholesterol and a variety of cancers, as well as the role of
serum/plasma cholesterol levels in oncogenesis. Diet would
appear to affect cancer at different sites. Additionally, it
may occur by specific carcinogenic tropism, altered latency,
and clinically display wide symptomatology and changeable

metabolism, resulting in a variety of clinical courses and outcomes. As a result, no clear correlation can be drawn regarding a given nutrient or its metabolism, or its resultant effect on cancers of various histologic types at a multiplicity of sites. With few exceptions this review is limited to the relationship of cholesterol and cancer at a single location, the colon, except in those cases where colorectal cancer is considered a single site. Further, animal studies are cited to examine if agreement exists in experimental and epidemiological studies. While many reports and reviews are available (Feinleib, 1981; Lilienfeld, 1981; Feinleib, 1982; Lowenfels, 1983; Sidney, 1983, McMichael, 1984), this inquiry will be restricted as follows: Is the risk of colon cancer increased in the presence of dietary cholesterol? Do individuals with hypocholesterolemic serum levels have greater risk for colon carcinogenesis? Does preclinical colonic cancer contribute or cause serum hypocholesterolemia? Does dietary restriction or pharmacochemical treatment for hypercholesterolemia alter risk factors for colon cancer? What is the relationship, if any, of these elements to each other?

DIETARY CHOLESTEROL AND COLON CANCER:

Epidemiologic Studies

Although a number of epidemiologic studies have assessed the relationship between dietary cholesterol and tumors at all sites, few have focused specifically on the relationship between dietary cholesterol and colon cancer.

The descriptive study of Liu and associates (1979) correlated food disappearance data between 1954 to 1965 in 20 industrialized countries (from the Food and Agriculture Organization (FAO)) with age-specific mortality rates (from the World Health Organization (WHO)) for the years 1967, 1969, 1971, and 1973. Mortality rates were studied from these specific years to account for the 10-year latency period for tumorigenesis. By simple correlation analysis, dietary intake of total saturated and monounsaturated fat, cholesterol, and fiber were shown to be highly correlated with the colon cancer mortality rate. Controlling for fat or fiber, the partial correlation of dietary cholesterol with colon cancer remained highly significant. However, controlling for cholesterol, the partial correlation of fat and fiber with colon cancer was not. In other words, a highly significant mean effect for cholesterol was demonstrated by cross classification but not fat or fiber. The authors suggested that there may be a causal relationship between dietary cholesterol and colon cancer mortality rates. Data from these studies are shown in Figure 1 (from Broitman 1986).

Kolonel and co-workers (1981) analyzed quantitative food consumption histories for 4,657 adults over the age of 45. The population was diverse, consisting of Caucasians, Chinese, Filipinos, and Hawaiians. The authors performed multiple regression analysis to assess the relationship of a variety of dietary variables with the corresponding population-based incidence of 15 selected cancer sites. No significant relationships were noted between dietary fat or cholesterol and colon or rectal cancers. Further, although the Hawaiians consumed high levels of dietary fat and the Japanese low levels, the incidence of colon cancer was paradoxically lower in the Hawaiians than in the Japanese.

A case control study of colorectal cancer conducted by Jain et al. (1980) compared 348 male and female patients with colon cancer and 194 male and female patients with rectal cancer to age-sex-matched community and in-hospital controls. On the basis of data from dietary questionnaires, the risk of colorectal cancer was increased for men and women who had high dietary cholesterol intake (relative risk for men, 1.8; relative risk for women, 1.6). Multivariate analysis revealed a dose responsive relationship between dietary cholesterol and colorectal cancer for each sex when other major nutrients were controlled.

Experimental Studies

Cruse et al. (1978) suggested a co-carcinogenic effect of dietary cholesterol when administered in conjunction with the colon carcinogen 1,2 dimethylhydrazine (DMH). They observed that female Wistar rats fed Vivonex (a commercial human food supplement) with 0.1% added cholesterol in conjunction with DMH had a greater incidence and increased number of bowel tumors per animal, as well as a higher frequency of metastases, in comparison with rats fed Vivonex alone. Although the validity of such a dietary regimen in experimental animals is subject to question, these studies

Figure 1. Prepared from data by Liu and associates (1979). Food disappearance information from FAO (1954-1965) and age-specific mortality rates of WHO (averaged for 1967, 1969, 1971 and 1973).

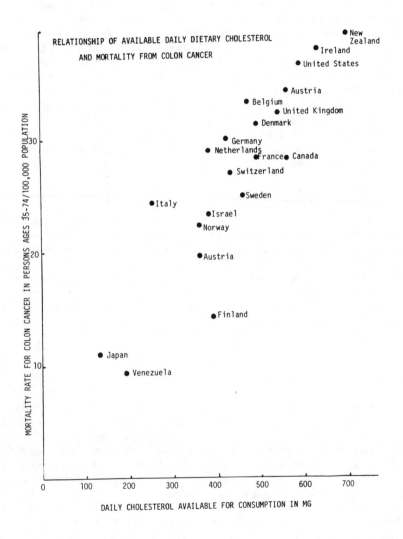

elicit concern about the relationship of dietary cholesterol to bowel tumorigenesis.

Hiramatsu and colleagues (1983) fed 1% cholesterol supplemented commercial chow to male Donryu rats injected with azoxymethane (AOM), a metabolite of DMH. Rats receiving the cholesterol supplemented diet had more tumors per animal and an increased number of distant metastases than rats not supplemented with cholesterol. In a similar study, Klurfeld et al. (1983) raised the serum cholesterol levels in male Fisher 344 rats with a semisynthetic diet containing 1.5% cholesterol, and then allowed serum cholesterol levels to decrease by removing cholesterol from the diet. The controls were given a diet devoid of cholesterol. DMH was used for bowel tumor induction and the authors found that rats fed a cholesterol supplemented diet had a significantly higher percentage of invasive tumors.

In serial studies of male Sprague Dawley rats fed semisynthetic diets with and without cholesterol, Broitman et al. (1986) used a direct acting carcinogen N-methyl N-nitrosourea (MNU) for bowel tumor induction. Rats consuming saturated or polyunsaturated fat diets with 1% supplemental cholesterol had augmented small and large bowel DMH-induced tumorigenesis in comparison with controls. For induction of large bowel tumors, MNU was administered rectally during either the initiation or promotional phase of carcinogenesis to rats fed cholesterol-supplemented diets. The results indicated that dietary cholesterol significantly enhanced bowel tumorigenesis in the late initiation or early promotional stage.

Contrasting results were reported by Cohen and associates (1982). These investigators used intrarectal MNU to induce colon tumors in Fischer F344 male rats who were fed a commercial lab chow (of undetermined cholesterol content) with and without 0.2% supplemental cholesterol. Using combined data from previous studies of rats given MNU but fed unsupplemented chow diets, the authors noted a decrease both in the incidence and multiplicity of bowel tumors.

Although the data are inconsistent, the bulk of the evidence points to a relationship between dietary cholesterol intake and colon tumor development. Moreover, the effect is apparent in diverse strains of rats receiving a variety of tumorigenic agents. It remains to be determined whether dietary cholesterol a) plays a role in the malignant potential of bowel tumors; b) controls bowel tumor multiplicity; c) diminishes the tumor latency period; d) affects absorption of carcinogenic agents; or e) influences the interaction of carcinogen with DNA and/or the DNA repair process. Nonetheless, results of experimental studies clearly echo epidemiologic observations that dietary cholesterol plays some as yet undefined role in large bowel carcinogenesis.

SERUM OR PLASMA CHOLESTEROL LEVELS IN RELATION TO COLON CANCER

Epidemiologic Studies

International surveys indicate that populations which consume diets high in animal fat and cholesterol (with a few notable exceptions) have higher colon cancer mortality rates than populations consuming less fat (Committee on Diet, Nutrition and Cancer, 1982). As one would expect, it also true that populations with high colon cancer mortality rates have high mortality rates for coronary heart disease (CHD). Rose et al. (1974), in fact, demonstrated a direct relationship (r = 0.775) between CHD and malignant intestinal growths using WHO national mortality rates. From these results the authors extrapolated that blood cholesterol would serve as a good predictor of colon cancer. In their "Six Countries" study (Table 1), Rose and associates followed 36,211 males (ages 35-64) from year 5 through year 23 (Rose, et al., 1974). Forty individuals died of colon cancer. Contrary to speculation, however, in 63% of cases the initial blood cholesterol levels of these individuals were well below the age-sex specific values. The authors themselves suggested that certain factors including unrecognized cancer, dietary regimens for lowering cholesterol levels, or participation of colonic microflora in controlling blood cholesterol levels could have influenced their findings.

The well-noted Framingham study (Williams, et al., 1981) (see Table 1) documented the course of CHD in 5,209 subjects (2,336 males and 2,873 females) over a period of 24 years. Cancer occurred in 692 cases (>90% histologically confirmed), 13% (88 cases) of which involved the colon. The

TABLE 1. Epidemiologic, clinical and drug intervention studies concerned with serum cholesterol and colon cancer.

Study and reference	Sample size male	female	Years of follow-up	Comment
Epidemiologic:				
Six countries (a) 1974	36,211	–	5–23	90 colon cancer deaths; inverse relationship with serum cholesterol.
Framingham Heart (b) 1981	2,336	2,873	24	88 colon cancer cases; inverse relationship with serum cholesterol in men only; risk greatest at <190 mg/dl
Honolulu Heart (c) 1980	8,006	–	9	80 colon cancer cases; inverse relationship with serum cholesterol; risk greatest at <180 mg/dl; no relationship of serum cholesterol to Dukes classification
Evans County, GA (d) 1980	948 (white) 537 (black)	970 (white) 647 (black)	12–14	Inverse relationship of serum cholesterol to cancer at all sites in men and women, black or white; excluding skin cancer, lowest cholesterol in colon cancer cases; low serum cholesterol correlated with low serum retinol.

Table 1, continued

International Collaborative Group (e) 1982	54,492	—	9-10	105 colon cancer deaths; no significant inverse relationship of serum cholesterol to colon cancer mortality.

Clinical:

Mount Sinai (f) 1981	81	51	—	133 colon cancer-case control pairs; inverse relationship with serum cholesterol in cases with both men and women; inverse relationship of serum cholesterol with Dukes classification in women only.
Sloan Kettering (g) 1983	76 men & women		—	76 colon cancer-case control pairs; inverse relationship with serum cholesterol in cases >5 years prior to detection; additional decrease as detection approaches in both men and women.

Table 1, continued

Epidemiologic Drug Intervention Trials:

WHO Cooperative (h)	15,000 (approx.)	—	9.6 ave.	Divided into three groups. Group I, high cholesterol given clofibrate; serum cholesterol at end of study 225 mg/dl. Group II, high cholesterol given placebo; serum cholesterol at end of study 247 mg/dl. Group III, low cholesterol given placebo; serum cholesterol at end of study 181 mg/dl. No increase risk for colon cancer with clofibrate.
LRC-CPPT (i) 1984	3,806	—	7.4 ave.	Approximately one half given cholestyramine, one half given placebo; both given low cholesterol diet; serum cholesterol level in cholestyramine group reduced from 292 to 257 mg/dl, placebo group from 292 to 277 mg/dl. No increase risk for colon cancer with cholestyramine.

a Rose et al., 1974
b Williams et al., 1981
c Kagan et al., 1981; Stemmerman et al., 1981
d Kark et al., 1980
e International Collaborative Group, 1982

f Miller et al., 1981
g Buchalter et al., 1983
h WHO Cooperative, 1980
i The Lipid Research Clinics Coronary Prevention Trial Results, 1984

inverse relationship between serum cholesterol levels and colon cancer was also observed in this group, but only in male patients. Colon cancer rates in men with the lowest serum cholesterol levels (<190 mg/dl) were approximately three-fold greater than in individuals with serum cholesterol levels between 190 to 279 mg/dl, and approximately 10 times greater than in individuals with serum cholesterol levels 279 mg/dl or higher. The study did not attribute the inverse relationship to pre-existing disease, since of the 88 cases of colon cancer, only 5 occurred during the first four years of the study. Furthermore, excess in colon cancer deaths among those with low serum cholesterol levels initially was cumulative throughout the period of the study. A recent reevaluation of the data (Sorlie and Feinleib, 1982) to determine whether this inverse relationship could have been the result of competing risks for other diseases related to serum cholesterol levels supported the initial conclusion.

The Honolulu Heart Program conducted a prospective study of cancer and heart disease in 8,006 Japanese-American men ranging in age from 45 to 68 years (Kagan, 1981). The group was studied initially for 9 years (Kagan, et al., 1981), and again for 5 additional years (Stemmermann, et al., 1981) (see Table 1). Baseline serum cholesterol levels showed a positive correlation with mortality due to CHD and a negative correlation with mortality due to colon cancer. The authors corrected for pre-existing or subclinical disease mortality by eliminating colon cancer cases that were diagnosed in the first two years of the study. Multivariate analyses included age, weight, systolic blood pressure, smoking, and alcohol consumption. Again in this population, a significant inverse relationship was observed between serum cholesterol levels and mortality. The subjects were divided into two groups based on age of entry: 45-54 and above 54. Across both groups the highest rates of colon cancer were associated with serum cholesterol levels below 180 mg/dl, although the results were statistically significant only in the older (above 54) group. Of interest, the strongest inverse association was found in individuals with right-sided colon cancer in comparison with transverse or descending colon cancer. This relationship persisted in cases diagnosed between 5 and 9 years after entry, discounting colon cancer due to pre-existing or subclinical disease, but was not found in cases diagnosed 10 to 14 years after entry.

A study emanating from Evans County, Georgia (Kark et al., 1980) documented colon cancer development at all sites in 3,102 white and black individuals of both sexes aged 14-74 years for a period of 14 years (see Table 1). Serum cholesterol levels at intake were compared after age adjustment between cancer and noncancer cases. Age, race, sex, weight, social class, and smoking were controlled using matched and regression residual analysis. The study excluded cases of cancer diagnosed in the first year. Of the remaining, 127 developed cancer; 6 developed colon cancer. When all cases were considered, the mean serum cholesterol levels at intake were lower in the cancer group than in the noncancer group regardless of race or sex. With the exception of skin cancer, the greatest mean decrease in serum cholesterol levels was found in patients with colon cancer. In all 14 sites were studied.

To determine whether the inverse relationship of serum cholesterol might be a secondary effect, Kark et al. (1981) decided to examine serum retinol levels in the same patient group (1981). This follow-up study showed that serum retinol levels were also inversely associated with cancer at all sites. However, the reverse correlation with retinol was even stronger than the cholesterol results. Previous studies and epidemiologic data reviewed by Peto and associates (1981) and others (Sporn and Newton, 1979; Wald, et al., 1980) had shown a protective effect of vitamin A (β-carotene) intake and cancer at numerous sites. Thus, Kark et al. (1981) suggested that we might improve our understanding of the serum cholesterol cancer relationship by studying retinol.

Bjelke (1974) observed 444 Norwegian men for dietary habits and noted that the relative risk for colon cancer increased inversely with serum cholesterol levels.

The International Collaborative Group (1982) accumulated the results of prospective studies of CHD from 15 study sites in 11 different countries (see Table 1). Assessing plasma or serum cholesterol levels in 61,567 men, aged 40-69 years, who were followed for up to 10 years, the study evaluated the relationship of entry and temporal serum or plasma cholesterol levels to cancer at all sites of the lung and colon. With the exclusion of Japan for insufficient follow-up, the combined population of males at risk totaled 54,492. There were 105 deaths due to colon cancer, representing only 7.1% of the total deaths due to cancers at all sites. The four men who died in the first year of colon cancer had serum or plasma cholesterol levels 20 to 30 mg/dl lower than the age adjusted means for their respective cancer-free study subjects. These small numbers precluded use in the statistical evaluation. By 5 years, 41 subjects had died of colon cancer and had serum or plasma cholesterol levels 7 to 11 mg/dl less than the mean of their respective cohorts. By the 10th year of follow-up, the additional 60 individuals who died of colon cancer had serum or plasma cholesterol levels 3 to 4 mg/dl greater than the means of their respective cohorts. No significant inverse relationship was detected between cholesterol and colon cancer.

English studies, which include some of the eldest populations, measured lowest mean plasma cholesterol levels at (198 mg/dl). Along with U.S. studies (Chicago Heart Association) these represented two-thirds of colonic cancer mortality in this report; the latter showed mean serum cholesterol levels of 213 mg/dl and represented the 2nd lowest levels of serum cholesterol in this group of populations. Danish studies, although small, showed the highest mean serum cholesterol levels (277 mg/dl), but no colon cancer mortality and represented the youngest population surveyed. Thus adjustments for age variations may be required to more precisely define the role of serum cholesterol in relation to colonic cancer risk.

Feinleib (1982) summarized the findings on cholesterol in noncardiovascular disease regarding the role of blood cholesterol levels (below 180 mg/dl) in mortalities resulting from something other than CHD, with a particular focus on cancer. Eight studies suggested a reciprocal relationship between cancer death and blood cholesterol levels. Four reports (The Framingham, Hawaii, Stockholm, and Hiroshima, Nagasaki) indicate this relationship was sex-specific, seen in males only. Two further studies appeared also to support these findings but were statistically insignificant. Seven studies failed to delineate the suggested relationship between blood cholesterol levels and colonic carcinogenesis. These studies were poorly controlled for additional factors implicated as oncogenic precipitants. Additionally, the reciprocity of blood cholesterol levels and occurrence of colonic cancer is diametrically opposed to that found in cardiovascular disease. Cholesterol levels below 180 mg/dl showed the most precipitous increase in colonic carcino-genesis, but displayed a lesser magnitude in risk of increased blood cholesterol in coronary heart disease and was more prevalent in older ages. Many of these population studies failed to analyze the age adjusted mortality for colon cancer. The U.S. age-adjusted colonic cancer mortality rate in Caucasian men between the ages of 40 and 49 is 3.9 per 100,000: the rate increases at 5 year intervals at nearly 100% a year to 91.5 per 100,000 between the ages of 65-69 years (Young, et al., 1981).

Clinical studies

Miller et al. (1981) looked at serum cholesterol levels in 133 white male and female cancer patients in a case controlled clinical study, both age and sex matched with the hospital control group. Results showed cholesterol levels in colonic cancer patients to be 181 ± 40 mg/dl for men and 193 ± 40 mg/dl for women which were significantly lower than those for the control group (206 ± 42 mg/dl for men and 219 ± 40 mg/dl for women). Further, tumors classified according to Dukes protocol showed that the serum cholesterol levels of those with early tumors, Dukes A, B1 and B2, did not vary significantly from the control group; however, patients exhibiting advanced tumors, Dukes C1, C2 and D, displayed serum cholesterol levels significantly reduced in women in comparison to cholesterol levels in patients with early colonic cancer. While similar findings were seen in males, the relatively small sample prevented statistically significant comparison. This study concluded that low serum cholesterol levels found in patients with colonic cancer may occur as a result of malignant metabolism in women (and perhaps men), and this decrease in serum cholesterol may well not precede the onset of disease.

In retrospective studies, Stemmerman and colleagues (1981) categorized patients by Dukes protocol and although a reciprocity between serum cholesterol levels in patients with colon cancer was seen, no alterations of serum cholesterol levels with the advancing carcinoma were observed.

Buchalter et al. (1983) in the single prospective case control study to date in this area along with Winawer and Herbert (personal communication) followed 76 patients at the

Memorial Sloane Kettering Cancer Center who ultimately developed cancer of the colon. All of these patients were subjected to blood cholesterol analysis at regular intervals for a minimum of 2 years preceding the clinical onset of colon cancer and displayed no prior history of malignancy. Age matched controls showed incremental elevation in serum cholesterol levels with age. However, in those patients with colonic cancer, blood cholesterol levels fell incrementally as the clinical onset of cancer grew near. While women displayed a statistically stronger association in this trend, males also showed statistically significant inverse relationships between colonic cancer and levels of cholesterol. Retrospectively, the intersection of data of control groups with cholesterol, with the case levels of serum cholesterol occurred 5 years or more preceding the clinical appearance of the disease. These findings caused investigators to postulate that preexisting disease would be unlikely to explain lower serum cholesterol levels in patients who eventually developed cancer of the colon, but that it was possible that preclinical events might also contribute to the lowering of serum cholesterol.

DRUG AND DIETARY INTERVENTION TRIALS TO LOWER SERUM CHOLESTEROL LEVELS

Clofibrate, an antihyperlipidemic agent, was employed to decrease serum cholesterol levels in an ischemic heart disease study (Report of the Committee of Principal Investigators, 1980)(see Table 1). The initial study of 5.3 years with a follow-up of 4.3 years showed that in males aged 30-59, those individuals with high cholesterol levels who were administered clofibrate showed a 25% increased mortality than placebo groups with either low or high serum cholesterol levels. Examination of the data revealed that preliminary concerns regarding the drug and an increase in GI tract cancers were unfounded. Further, no increase in cancer deaths in general were seen in this group. Additionally, individuals with essential low serum cholesterol (181 mg/dl or less) given placebo did not exhibit increased cancer deaths. Serum cholesterol levels were 9% lower in the clofibrate group I (225 mg/dl), than in the second placebo group (247 mg/dl).

A randomized double blind study of cholestyramine was employed to study the effects of reducing serum cholesterol levels on coronary heart disease. Asymptomatic males,

3,806, of 35-59 years of age with plasma cholesterol levels in excess of 264 mg/dl and with type II hyperlipoproteinemia were included in the study. Cholestyramine or placebo were administered in a 50:50 ratio in the experimental subjects, all of whom were placed on a cholesterol lowering diet. In the seventh year of the study, serum cholesterol levels were 257 mg/dl in the drug-treated group and 277 mg/dl in the placebo group, a reduction of 11.8% and 4.9%, respectively. Mortality risk in both groups was not significantly altered. Fifty-seven cases of cancer were detected in each group. Six of these were identified as colonic cancers, again in each group, leading investigators to conclude that modest decreases in high cholesterol levels by cholestyramine fail to increase the risk of cancer of the colon.

Experimental Studies

Experimental studies in rats on the effects of variation of serum cholesterol levels on DMH-induced bowel tumors appear to support the case control studies (Broitman, et al., 1977). Hypocholesterolemia and vascular lipidosis were induced in Sprague Dawley rats with 20% coconut oil, isocaloric diet. The second group received 20% safflower oil resulting in lower serum cholesterol levels with the expectation that cholesterol would be shunted through the bowel. The latter group displayed lower serum cholesterol levels but went on to incur a multiplicity of bowel tumors greater in number than the group with high serum cholesterol levels.

A study in Fischer 344 rats was conducted employing a high cholesterol diet containing bile salts (Klurfeld et al., 1983). Subsequently, 2 subgroups were fed a diet either without cholesterol and bile salts or one which contained bile salt but no cholesterol. Investigators observed diminished DMH tumor response in rats deprived of cholesterol as compared to those receiving it throughout the study. Additionally, as blood cholesterol levels declined in the latter group, sterol presence was maintained in the colon in that group with diet-containing bile salts. Tumorigenesis increased in this group when compared to the group deprived of cholesterol and bile salts. This suggested that sterol flux in the colon as serum cholesterol levels were reduced enhanced bowel tumorigenesis.

In further studies using cholestyramine or candicidin in Sprague Dawley rats with AOM induced tumors (Nigro, et al., 1977; Nigro, et al., 1973), both of these drugs displayed increases in tumorigenesis when compared with controls. Cholestyramine appeared to induce large bowel tumors, whereas candicidin apparently contributed to increases in distal small bowel cancers. The specificity of the action of these two drugs suggests that bile acids may be involved in large bowel carcinogenesis while cholesterol and metabolites appear to contribute to small bowel tumors.

Alterations in cholesterol flux into the bowel may be more critical in tumorigenesis than merely the presence of cholesterol per se in the colon lumen.

Reddy and Watanabe (1979) administered cholesterol and metabolites intrarectally and showed no apparent effect on bowel cancers resulting from N-methyl-N'-nitro-N-nitroso-guanidine (MNNG). These studies would appear to suggest that lower serum cholesterol levels and concomitant cholesterol bowel shunting are implicated in colonic tumorigenesis. At odds with case control epidemiologic studies in humans, these phenomena may exemplify alterations in cholesterol metabolism between rats and humans.

Discussion

Although the congregate epidemiologic evidence is largely descriptive in nature, these reports strongly suggest a direct relationship between levels of dietary cholesterol and colonic tumorigenesis (Liu et al., 1979; Jain et al., 1980). A number of more direct experimental studies support this evidence, using a wide variety of known colon carcinogens, as well as many innovations in experimental protocols (Cruse et al., 1978; Hiramatsu et al., 1983; Klurfeld et al., 1983; Broitman et al., in press). A hypothesis has been advanced which implies that dietary cholesterol affects the initiation of oncogenesis in two distinct steps. The question arises regarding the relation of these events and their order of importance and whether these are related to increases in bile acid secretion, lipid effects on promotion, or involved with other elements, including but not limited to, carcinogen absorption, persistence of adduct formation, interference with DNA repair, or whether dietary cholesterol acts as a tumor growth factor.

Inconsistent studies of this apparent, inverse association of blood cholesterol levels with cancer of the colon is a concern. The vast majority of studies cited were intended and designed to determine cardiovascular mortality and colon cancer epidemiology, with cholesterol levels incidental to the central concerns of these reports. Obviously, to resolve the issues of cholesterol and colon cancer, studies must be constructed specifically to elucidate the epidemiology of colon cancer and should include dietary assessment of individuals, including nutritional profiles, as well as serum lipids.

While the use of data from various coronary studies to explore colon cancer has limitations, it has, nevertheless, provided useful leads (Feinleib, 1981; Lowenfels AB, 1983; McMichael et al., 1984). However, because coronary heart disease is responsible for more than 35% of all mortality in the United States, and colorectal carcinoma for only 3%, it is impressive that the detection of the relationship between cholesterol and colon cancer was revealed in a number of these reports. Additionally, supportive findings are seen in patients with stratified colonic carcinoma as revealed by clinical studies primarily concerned with serum cholesterol levels as well as in patients followed for colonic cancer (Buchalter et al., 1983; Report of the Committee of Principal Investigators, WHO, 1980).

Reports indicating an association of low serum cholesterol levels with low serum retinol levels in individuals who develop colon cancer also provide additional directions for future studies. Well documented is the protective effect of retinoids on certain tumors (Kark et al., 1980; Sporn et al., 1979). Diminished occurrence for site-specific tumors has been positively associated with the consumption of foods containing vitamin A precursors (Committee on Diet, Nutrition and Cancer, 1982).

It is unclear whether the reciprocal relationship of colonic cancer to serum cholesterol levels is solely a male phenomenon. To date, epidemiologic studies point in this direction. However, relatively few reports have been published where females are well represented in the study. Other investigators, however, have reviewed clinical studies and suggest that, although the degree of risk may be altered at any given level of serum cholesterol, the relative risk of colonic cancer in this inverse association is shared by both men and women.

The hypothesis suggested is that individuals consuming diets high in fat and cholesterol but who display low serum cholesterol might well provide a marker for those people who are at increased risk for the development of colonic cancer. While clinical and epidemiologic reports would seem to support this position, it should be noted that hypocholesterolemia, as an isolated finding, may provide little evidence regarding absolute risk for the development of colon cancers. Many well-described groups, including Seventh Day Adventists, display blood cholesterol levels considerably below those exhibited in age-sex adjusted reports of study subjects fed a typical western diet (Walden et al., 1964). However, the relative risk for colonic cancer among Seventh Day Adventists is remarkably lower than individuals consuming typical western diets (Feinleib, 1982). Total nutritional analysis may therefore be necessary to elucidate if hypocholesterolemia occurs in spite of consuming a diet high in fat and cholesterol. Clearly, this gap of information may prove crucial and limiting in the interpretation of epidemiologic data regarding the relationship between serum cholesterol levels and colon cancer.

Parenthetically, this apparent contradiction is not irrational in the light of international reports of the correlation between CHD and cancer of the colon (Rose, et al., 1974). Furthermore, in most western populations, known risk factors of coronary heart disease including hypercholesterolemia, cigarette smoking, and hypertension do not parallel the development of colonic carcinoma (Wynder, 1975), suggesting that in any given group consuming diets high in fat and of necessity cholesterol, at high risk for both CHD and colon cancer there exists a large subgroup destined to develop the former while a significantly smaller group ultimately develops the latter. If diet proves to be a common etiologic factor, then within groups consuming a western diet there are individuals who remain in the normal cholesterol range and some who remain in the low cholesterol range, while others manifest hypercholesterolemia (Reiser, 1978), implying that individuals maintaining low cholesterol levels appear at increased risk to develop colon cancers.

As our understanding of the metabolism and kinetics of cholesterol changes, and as improved methods for elucidating its action are developed, it becomes clear that the effects, interactions, and pathways are exceedingly complex. As a result, its interaction in colon carcinogenesis is poorly understood. However, based on our present understanding of cholesterol and colon carcinogenesis, fecal bile acids and fecal cholesterol as well as associated metabolites are excreted in larger amounts in those individuals who eat high fat diets compared to those people with low fat diets (Committee on Diet, Nutrition and Cancer, 1982; Hill, et al., 1971). Further, individuals exhibiting bowel pathology which place them at high risk for colon cancer, and those diagnosed with colon cancer, with few exceptions (Moskowitz et al. 1979), excrete greater amounts of neutral and acid sterols than do those individuals free of disease (Hill et al., 1975; Lipkin et al., 1981; Reddy et al., 1977). It is not clear if increased sterol excretion enhances the predisposition for colonic carcinogenesis or is a consequence of the disease.

It is suggested that individuals who are hypocholesterolemic, even consuming a western diet, have a greater inherent capacity (genetic, colonic microflora?) to either absorb less dietary cholesterol or to convert cholesterol to greater quantities of bile acids or both, than do individuals who are normo- or hypercholesterolemic. There are few data on this point. However, an in-depth study in a single volunteer (Lin et al., 1980) has some bearing on this issue. In this hypocholesterolemic individual, feeding a diet containing 1000 mg of cholesterol daily for over five weeks increased the serum cholesterol level but it still remained in the hypocholesterolemic range. Balance studies indicated that fecal bile acid excretion increased about 17% but there was no increase in endogenously synthesized fecal neutral sterols. However, a 20% decrease in absorption of dietary cholesterol resulted in a net increase of fecal neutral sterols of 122%. Thus a high cholesterol diet resulted in increased fecal excretion of both neutral and acid sterols.

It has been known for some time that bile acids serve to regulate water and electrolyte flux in the bowel (Mekhjian, 1971) and participate in the control of the intestinal absorption of cholesterol (Lutton, 1976). Further bile acids exercise control on the proliferation of colonic mucosal cells (Fry et al., 1964; Ranken et al., 1971; Deshner et al., 1979; Palmer, 1979). In turn, the colonic microflora, which dehydrolate and deconjugate bile acids, modulate the effectiveness of bile acids in carrying out these processes (Palmer, 1979).

A linkage between these events and the occurrence of increased risk for colon cancer in the hypocholesterolemic individual consuming a western diet is as follows: It is suggested that the increased excretion of bile acids in the hypocholesterolemic individual enhances the colonic mucosal proliferation rate. A relative increase in the numbers of exfoliated cells into the gut under these conditions further contribute to the increased fecal excretion of cholesterol and derived metabolites. Subsequent to the increased mucosal proliferation rate, there is an enhanced susceptibility to the action of various carcinogens of unknown origin in the bowel lumen. Presumably, these effects of bile acids occur pre- and during initiation events in carcinogenesis and may be different from tumor promotional effects of bile acids which have been described in experimental animals (Narisawa et al., 1974). The colonic microflora govern the effectiveness of bile acids in mucosal cell proliferation and in turn are influenced by nutritional substrate availability - in part unabsorbed dietary and mucosal cellular cholesterol which reaches the colon.

Several other hypotheses, forwarded by others offer reasonable alternatives for the association of hypocholesterolemia and increased risk for colon cancer (Feinlieb, 1981; Lilienfeld, 1981; Lowenfels, 1983; McMichael et al., 1984).

No evidence exists that hypocholesterolemia is causal or that hypercholesterolemia obviates colonic cancer (Sidney, 1983).

Hypocholesterolemia in the patient with preclinical or symptomatic colon cancer may derive from circumstances that are different in the disease-free hypocholesterolemic individual. In a single study in which a group of patients were followed for a number of years, the Memorial Sloane Kettering Group (Buchalter et al., 1983) noted two changes in serum cholesterol levels. Upon entry into the group, individuals who later developed colon cancer, exhibited serum cholesterol levels significantly below those of an age-sex adjusted group without colon cancer. Unlike the disease-free counterpart, colon cancer cases did not exhibit an increased serum cholesterol level as they aged. A further decrease in serum cholesterol occurred as diagnosis approached. It is unlikely that this latter alteration in serum cholesterol is the consequence of malnutrition and cachexia associated with widespread metastatic disease. A mechanism to account for these observations is as yet not readily apparent. One possibility derives from animal studies (Nicolosi et al., 1983) in which NMU induced bowel tumors in rats "trapped" significantly greater quantities of isotopically labeled cholesterol from the serum than surrounding uninvolved bowel or normal bowel. Whether trapping serum cholesterol by tumors may contribute to the reduction of serum cholesterol levels remains to be proved.

Experimental and epidemiologic data exhibit marked differences regarding the risks of colon cancer in the presence of diet or drug-reduced levels of serum cholesterol. It would appear that drug-induced lowering of serum cholesterol is not associated with increased risk of colon cancer, while naturally occurring "low levels" of serum cholesterol show the converse to be true. Reduction of elevated serum cholesterol levels from 250 mg/dl by 10% to 225 is not within the range of 180 mg/dl or less where clear risk for colonic cancer has been reported in certain individuals.

In interventional trials, (LRC-CPPT) showed dietary alteration reduced the flux cholesterol and metabolites and resulting risk of colonic lesions when compared to individuals consuming a high cholesterol diet. Experimental data would appear to support this suggestion and describe bowel tumors that are enhanced in rats when serum cholesterol level is reduced but only when the flux of cholesterol and its metabolites are maintained (Broitman et al., 1977; Klurfeld et al., 1983) but not when this flux is interrupted. Clearly, if cholesterol dynamics in rats are relevant to humans, the data imply that chemotherapeutic measures aimed at reducing serum cholesterol levels should include a reduced dietary intake of cholesterol.

REFERENCES

Bjelke E (1974). Colon cancer and blood-cholesterol. Lancet 1:1116-1117.

Broitman SA (1981). Cholesterol excretion and colon cancer. Cancer Res 41:3738-3739.

Broitman SA. Dietary cholesterol, serum cholesterol and colon cancer: A review. In Poirier LA, Pariza M, Newberne P (eds): "Essential Nutrients in Carcinogenesis" New York: Plenum Press, (in press).

Broitman SA, Kupchick H, Gottlieb LS, et al.(1986). Dietary cholesterol and colon tumorigenesis induced by 1,2 dimethylhydrazine or N-methyl-N-nitrosurea in rats. In Meyskens FL, Prasad KN (eds): "Vitamins and Cancer - Human Cancer Prevention by Vitamins and Micronutrients," New Jersey: Humana Press, 1985, p. 181-197.

Broitman SA, Vitale JJ, Vavrousek-Jakuba E, et al.(1977). Polyunsaturated fat, cholesterol and large bowel tumorigenesis. Cancer 40:2455-2463.

Buchalter J, Herbert E, Flehinger B, et al.(1983). A case-control study of time-trends in serum cholesterol levels prior to detection of colon cancer. Gastroenterology 84:1403 (Abstract).

Cohen BI, Raicht RF, Fazzini E (1982). Reduction of N-methyl-N-nitrosurea-induced colon tumors in the rat by cholesterol. Cancer Res 42:5050-5052.

Committee on Diet, Nutrition, and Cancer; Assembly of Life Sciences, National Research Council (1982). Diet, nutrition, and cancer, Washington, D.C.: National Academy Press.

Cruse JP, Lewin MR, Ferulano GP, et al. (1978). Co-carcinogenic effects of dietary cholesterol in experimental colon cancer. Nature 276:822-825.

Deschner EE, Raicht RF (1979). The influence of bile on the kinetic behavior of colonic epithelial cells of the rat. Gastroenterology 76:1120 (Abstract).

Feinleib M (1981). On a possible inverse relationship between serum cholesterol and cancer mortality. Am J Epidemiol 114:5-10.

Feinleib M (1982). Summary of a workshop on cholesterol and noncardiovascular disease mortality. Prev Med 11:360-367.

Ferezou J, Coste T, Chevallier F (1981). Origins of neutral sterols in human feces studied by stable isotope labeling (D and ^{13}C). Existence of an external secretion of cholesterol. Digestion 21:232-243.

Fry RJM, Staffeldt E (1964). Effect of a diet containing sodium deoxycholate on the intestinal mucosa of the mouse. Nature 302:1396-1398.

Hill MJ, Drasar BS, Aries V, et al. (1971). Bacteria and etiology of cancer of large bowel. Lancet 1:95-100.

Hill MJ, Drasar BS, Williams REO, et al. (1975). Faecal bile-acids and Clostridia in patients with cancer of the large bowel. Lancet 1:539.

Hiramatsu Y, Takada H, Yamamura M, et al. (1983). Effect of dietary cholesterol on azoxymethane-induced colon carcinogenesis in rats. Carcinogenesis 4:553-558.

International Collaborative Group (1982). Circulating cholesterol level and risk of death from cancer in men aged 40 to 69 years. Experience of an international collaborative group. JAMA 248:2853-2859.

Jain M, Cook GM, Davis FG, et al. (1980). A case-control study of diety and colo-rectal cancer. Int J Cancer 26:757-768.

Kagan A, McGee DL, Yano K, et al. (1981). Serum cholesterol and mortality in Japanese-American population: the Honolulu Heart Program. Am J Epidemiol 114:11-20.

Kark JD, Smith AH, Hames CG (1980). The relationship of serum cholesterol to the incidence of cancer in Evans County, Georgia. J Chronic Dis 33:311-322.

Kark JD, Smith AH, Switzer BR, et al. (1981). Retinol, carotene, and the cancer/cholesterol association. Lancet 2:1371.

Klurfeld DM, Aglow E, Tepper SA, et al. (1983). Modification of dimethylhydrazine-induced carcinogenesis in rats by dietary cholesterol. Nutr Cancer 5:16-25.

Kolonel LN, Hankin JH, Lee J, et al. (1981). Nutrient intakes in relation to cancer incidence in Hawaii. Br J Cancer 44:332-339.

Lilienfeld AM (1981). The humean fog: cancer and cholesterol. Am J Epidemiol 114:1-4.

Lin DS, Connor DS (1980). The long term effects of dietary cholesterol upon the plasma lipids, lipoproteins, cholesterol absorption, and the sterol balance in man: The demonstration of feedback inhibition of cholesterol biosynthesis and increased bile acid excretion. J Lipid Res 21:1042-1052.

The Lipid Research Clinics Coronary Prevention Trial Results (1984). I. Reduction in incidence of coronary heart disease. JAMA 251:351-364.

Lipkin M, Reddy BS, Weisburger JH, et al. (1981). Nondegradation of fecal cholesterol in subjects at high risk for cancer of the large intestine. J Clin Invest 67:304-307.

Liu K, Moss D, Persky V, et al. (1979). Dietary cholesterol, fat, and fiber and colon-cancer mortality. An analysis of international data. Lancet 2:782-785.

Lowenfels AB (1983). Is increased cholesterol excretion the link between low serum cholesterol and colon cancer? Nutr Cancer 4:280-284.

Lutton C (1976). The role of the digestive tract in cholesterol metabolism. Digestion 14:342-356.

McMichael AJ, Jensen OM, Parkin DM, et al. (1984). Dietary and endogenous cholesterol and human cancer. Epidem Rev 6:192-216.

McMichael AJ, Potter JD (1980). Reproduction, endogenous and exogenous sex hormones and colon cancer: A review and hypothesis. J Natl Cancer Inst 65:1201-1207.

Mekhjian HS, Phillips SF, Hofmann AF (1971). Colonic secretion of water and electrolytes induced by bile acids in man. J Clin Invest 50:1569-1573.

Miller SR, Tartter PI, Papatestas AE, et al. (1981). Serum cholesterol and human colon cancer. J Natl Cancer Inst 67:297-300.

Moskowitz M, White C, Barnett RN, et al. (1979). Diet, faecal bile acids, and neutral sterols in carcinoma of the colon. Dig Dis Sci 39:274-278.

Narisawa T, Magadia NE, Weisburger JH, et al. (1974). Promoting effect of bile acids on colon carcinogenesis after intrarectal instillation of N-methyl-N'-nitro-N-nitrosoguandine in rats. J Natl Cancer Inst 53:1093-1097.

Nicolosi JV, Broitman SA (1983). Augmentation of colon tumorigenesis by dietary cholesterol. Cholesterol uptake and biosynthesis by rat gastrointestinal tissues and tumors. Fed Proc 42:1835 (Abstract).

Nigro ND, Bhadrachri N, Chomachai C (1973). A rat model for studying colonic cancer: Effect of cholestyramine on induced tumors. Dis Colon Rectum 16:438-443.

Nigro ND, Campbell RL, Gantt JS, et al. (1977). A comparison of the hypocholesterolemic agents, cholestyramine and candicidin on the induction of intestinal tumors in rats by azoxymethane. Cancer Res 37:3198-3203.

Palmer RH (1979). Editorial: Bile acid heterogeneity and the gastrointestinal epithelium: From diarrhea to colon cancer. J Lab Clin Med 94:655-660.

Peto R, Doll R, Buckley JD, et al. (1981). Can dietary [3]-carotene materially reduce human cancer rates. Nature 290:201-208.

Phillips RL (1975). Role of life-style and dietary habits in risk of cancer among Seventh-Day Adventists. Cancer Res 35:3513-3522.

Ranken R, Wilson R, Bealmear PM (1971). Increased turnover of intestinal mucosal cells of germfree mice induced by cholic acid. Proc Soc Exp Biol Med 138:270-272.

Reddy BS, Watanabe K (1979). Effect of cholesterol metabolites and promoting effect of lithocholic acid in colon carcinogenesis in germ-free and conventional F344 rats. Cancer Res 39:1521-1524.

Reddy BS, Wynder EL (1977). Metabolic epidemiology of colon cancer. Fecal bile acids and neutral sterols in colon cancer patients and patients with adenomatous polyps. Cancer 39:2533-2539.

Reiser R (1978). Oversimplification of diet: Coronary heart disease relationships and exaggerated diet recommendations. Am J Clin Nutr 31:865-875.

Report from the Committee of Principal Investigators (1978). A cooperative trial in the primary prevention of ischaemic heart disease using clofibrate. Br Heart J 40: 1069-1118.

Report of the Committee of Principal Investigators (1980). W.H.O. cooperative trial on primary prevention of ischaemic heart disease using clofibrate to lower serum cholesterol: mortality follow-up. Lancet 2:379-385.

Rose G, Blackburn H, Keys A, et al. (1974). Colon cancer and blood cholesterol. Lancet 1:181-183.

Sidney S, Farquar JW (1983). Cholesterol, cancer, and public health policy. Am J Med 75:494-508.

Sorlie PD, Feinleib M (1982). The serum cholesterol-cancer relationship: An analysis of time trends in the Framingham Study. J Natl Cancer Inst. 69:989-996.

Sporn MB, Newton DL (1979). Chemoprevention of cancer with retinoids. Fed Proc 38:2528-2534.

Stemmermann GN, Nomura AMY, Hellbrun LK, et al. (1981). Serum cholesterol and colon cancer incidence in Hawaii Japanese men. J Natl Cancer Inst. 67:1179-1182.

Wald N, Idle M, Boreham A, et al (1980). Low serum vitamin A and subsequent risk of cancer. Lancet 2:813-815.

Walden RT, Schaefer LE, Lemon RF, et al. (1974). Effect of the environment on the serum cholesterol-triglyceride distribution among Seventh Day Adventists. Am J Med 36:269-276.

Williams RR, Sorlie PD, Feinlieb M, et al. (1981). Cancer incidence by levels of cholesterol. JAMA 245:247-252.

Wynder EL (1975). The epidemiology of large bowel cancer. Cancer Res 35:3388-3394.

Dietary Fat and Cancer, pages 461–486
© 1986 Alan R. Liss, Inc.

FAT, LIPOTROPES, HYPOLIPIDEMIC AGENTS AND
LIVER CANCER

Hisashi Shinozuka, Sikandar L. Katyal and
Mohan I.R. Perera
Department of Pathology
University of Pittsburgh School of Medicine
750 Scaife Hall
Pittsburgh, PA 15261

INTRODUCTION:

The study of dietary factors which influence the
genesis and progression of a chronic disease such as cancer
in humans is extremely difficult because of complexities
associated with man living in a complicated environment and
society. Despite these complexities, a considerable amount
of data has been accumulated in the epidemiological studies
of diet and cancer in man implicating the close association
of certain dietary components and certain types of cancers
(Armstrong and Doll, 1975; Correa, 1981; Wynder, 1975).
Experimental studies using animal models also have provided
a wealth of information regarding the basic nature of
dietary modification of cancer development as discussed in
many chapters of this book. There are now unequivocal data
from both epidemiological and experimental studies linking
dietary fat to the causation of cancers of the breast, skin
and intestine. The association appears to be less clear in
the case of liver cancer despite the fact that the liver is
one of the organs most actively involved in fat metabolism
(Carroll, 1981). In this chapter, we will focus upon
dietary fat and liver cancer primarily based on information
derived from experimental studies. The discussion will
cover two major aspects; 1) general considerations of the
effects of dietary fat on liver cancer induction and 2)
effects of agents which modify lipid metabolism on the
induction of liver cancer. We selected lipotrope
deficiency and hypolipidemic agents.

GENERAL CONSIDERATIONS:

Progress in our understanding of chemical carcinogenesis has been considerable since the discovery of an
experimental model of skin cancer induction by coal tar
(Yamagiwa and Ichikawa,1916). The importance of dietary
fat in modifying carcinogenesis was first recognized by
Watson and Mellanby (1930) who demonstrated that dietary
fat enhanced the incidence of coal tar induced skin tumors.
The observation was further extended by the demonstration
that skin tumors of the mouse induced by ultraviolet light
or pure hydrocarbons were formed in greater number and at
an earlier time in mice receiving a high fat diet than in
control mice receiving a basal ration (Jacobi and Baumann,
1940; Lavik and Baumann, 1941). However, the early studies
also demonstrated that increasing the fat content of a
basic diet exerted diverse effects on formation of
different types of tumors. The effects ranged from an
augmentation of the formation of spontaneous breast tumors
to a possible inhibition of sarcomas induced by a
carcinogenic hydrocarbon (Tannenbaum, 1942).

The experimental induction of liver cancer in rats was
first demonstrated in the 1930's by feeding 0-amino-
azotoluene or P-dimethylaminoazobenzene (DAB) mixed in
basal rations of carrots and polished rice (Sasaki and
Yoshida, 1935; Kinoshita, 1937). Nutritionally these basal
diets were grossly deficient in several essentials such as
protein, salts and various constituents of the Vitamin B
complex. György et al (1942) compared the carcinogenic
effectiveness of diets low in protein and high in fat and
noted that Crisco and butter fat were cocarcinogenic as
compared to lard on DAB liver carcinogenesis. When
compared diets containing various levels of Crisco, high
levels of fat increased the rate of liver tumor induction
by DAB (Opie, 1944). A destruction of the carcinogen, DAB,
by unsaturated fatty acids was considered as a possible
explanation for the effect of the lard diet (György et al.,
1942). In the early 1940's a group of investigators at the
McArdle Memorial Laboratory had engaged in a series of
studies on diets and hepatic tumor induction using
nutritionally balanced semisynthetic diets adequate for
growth and maintenance of experimental animals (Miller et
al., 1941). In general, the nutritionally adequate diets
offered partial protection against hepatoma formation. The
protective supplements were usually rich in both protein

and the vitamin B complex, particularly riboflavin. It soon became apparent that as in the case of experimental skin tumor induction, dietary fats markedly influenced the chemical induction of liver tumors. Increasing the fat level of the diet enhanced the development of DAB induced hepatic tumors (Kline et al., 1946a). Not only the quantity of fat but also the quality of fat played an important role in determining the incidence of DAB-induced liver tumors (Miller et al., 1944). Thus when 0.06% DAB was fed to rats in a semi-synthetic diet containing 5% hydrogenated coconut oil, the incidence of hepatic tumors was only 8%, while feeding the same carcinogen in the diet with corn oil yielded 60% incidence of tumor induction. A further study of the effect of the fatty acid constituents of hydrogenated coconut oil and of corn oil revealed that no tumors developed when diets containing lauric acid, the major fatty acid constituents of coconut oil or the fatty acids of coconut oil were fed, while feeding the fatty acids of corn oil resulted in a high incidence of tumors (Kline et al., 1946b). The replacement of the dietary fat with olive oil or its chief constituent, oleic acid, yielded a slightly lower incidence of hepatoma than that obtained with corn oil. Crisco and lard exerted a similar effect as corn oil. These studies clearly indicate the importance of fatty acid constituents of different types of lipids in determining the effectiveness of liver tumor induction by DAB. The effects of dietary fat on liver tumor induction by carcinogens other than DAB were less well documented. The carcinogenic action of 2-acetylamino-fluorene (AAF), for instance, appeared to be much less subject to the nutritional status of animals than that of DAB (Wilson et al., 1947; Engel and Copeland, 1951). The lipase-indigestible or the nonurea adduct forming fraction isolated from heated oil obtained from commercial sources or prepared under laboratory conditions acted in synergism with AAF and enhanced its carcinogenic activity (Sugai et al., 1962). The results of many studies to test carcinogenic or co-carcinogenic actions of heated oil were somewhat ambiguous (Arffmann, 1960).

In the late 1960's, cyclopropenoid fatty acids (CPFA), natural components of lipids in cottonseed oil were shown to be the contributing factor for an epidemic of liver cancer in hatchery-reared rainbow trout fed aflatoxin-contaminated cottonseed oil (Wolf and Jackson, 1963). It was shown that naturally contaminated feedstuffs such as cottonseed meals produced a greater incidence and a more rapid growth rate of liver tumors than the control diet containing comparable levels of purified aflatoxin (Sinnhuber et al., 1968a, 1968b). CPFA contain sterculic acid and malvalic acid in a large quantity. When these acids were tested separately, sterculic acid had a slightly stronger action than malvalic acid in enhancing aflatoxin-induced hepatomas (Lee et al., 1971). Subsequent studies revealed that CPFA had a slight to marginal tumor enhancing activity on aflatoxin or diethylnitrosamine induced hepatomas in rats indicating that the response of rats to CPFA is considerably weaker than that of trout (Nixon et al., 1974).

The mechanism of CPFA-action on liver tumor induction is not known. CPFA has been shown to cause a variety of biological effects which include abnormalities in the reproductive processes and alterations of lipid metabolisms such as the shift in the fatty acid composition of the liver (Phelps et al., 1965). Sterculic acid inhibited the stearic fatty acyl desaturase enzyme system and there were high levels of stearic acid and corresponding lower levels of oleic acid in poultry and rats fed cyclopropenoids (Raju and Reiser, 1967; Johnson et al., 1967). However, a subsequent study (Wood et al., 1978) showed that saturated and monoene fatty acid percentages of liver phosphatidylcholine and phosphotidylethanolamines were not affected but the percentage of saturated fatty acids of triglycerides and cholesterol esters was increased while the monoene percentage decreased. Scarpelli (1974a, 1974b) observed mitogenic and necrogenic effects of CPFA on both rat and trout liver. However, it is not clear whether the mitogenic effects is direct or the secondary regenerative response following liver cell necrosis.

Even though the early studies in the 1940's amply demonstrated the importance of dietary fat in liver cancer induction, no systematic studies aimed at analyzing the mechanisms have been recorded. Instead, the study of liver carcinogenesis during the following 3 decades has made great progress in several aspects of mechanistic consideration. These include identification of an increasing number of hepatocarcinogens, establishment of carcinogen metabolic activation as an obligatory step in carcinogenesis (Miller, 1978), insights into the mechanism of carcinogen-macromolecular interactions (Rajalakshmi et al., 1982) and the recognition that the development of liver cancer, like that of cancer in many other organs or tissues, is a multistep phenomenon in which initiated preneoplastic hepatocytes progress towards highly malignant hepatocellular carcinomas through stages of tumor promotion (Pitot and Sirica, 1980; Farber, 1984). This conceptual advancement in our understanding of the process of chemical carcinogenesis necessitates a reevaluation of possible mechanisms by which dietary fat, or even other dietary components, modifies liver cancer induction. Several areas are of particular importance: diet-induced alterations in the drug metabolizing system, diet effects on separate stages of carcinogenesis and possible effects of diet-induced liver cell necrosis.

DIETARY FAT AND CARCINOGEN METABOLISM:

Since many hepatocarcinogens have to be metabolized to yield ultimate carcinogens, the enzyme systems involved in carcinogen activation plays one of the key roles in determining overall activity of carcinogenesis. Both phase 1 and phase 2 drug metabolizing enzymes participate in carcinogen metabolism, and it is now clear that dietary fat modifies activities of these enzyme systems (Campbell and Hayes, 1974; McDanell and McLean, 1985; Wade et al., 1978). Mixed function oxidase (MFO) systems of phase 1 enzymes are of considerable importance in the initial activation of carcinogens. Microsomal lipids of hepatocytes, particularly the phospholipid phosphatidylcholine is an integral component of the MFO system and plays a critical role in drug-metabolizing activity. Both quantity and quality of dietary lipids alter fatty acid composition of microsomes and influence the basal activity and the inducibility of the MFO system (Norred and Wade, 1972; Wade and Norred, 1976). Dietary lipids also influence component enzymes of the MFO system such as cytochrome P-450, and the activity of NADPH-cytochrome C reductase and glucose-6-phosphate dehydrogenase (Wade et al., 1978).

It has been shown that when feeding varying concentrations of 8 saturated fatty acids (C4-C18) with 1.8% safflower oil, the drug metabolizing activity of rat liver was associated with the absolute amount of fat in the diet and was independent of chain length (Caster et al., 1970). An increase in saturated fatty acid content of the diet from 15% to 35% doubled the rate of aniline hydroxylase. Dietary polyunsaturated or essential fatty acids appear to induce greater MFO activity than that obtained from rats fed fat-free diets or diet containing saturated fats (Century, 1969; Wade et al., 1969, 1972). In rats fed adequate dietary proteins, the response to phenobarbital for the induction of phase 1 enzymes is largely determined by the dietary fat content (Marshall and McLean, 1971). It is also known that the concentration of cytochrome P-450 or hexobarbital oxidase induced by phenobarbital is determined by the nature of dietary fat with the greater level of induction with more highly unsaturated fat (Century and Horwitt, 1968). In contrast to abundant data on the dietary effects on phase 1 enzymes of mostly oxidative reactions, little is known about the dietary effects on phase 2 enzymes of conjugation reactions. Since phase 2 enzymes are involved mainly in detoxification reactions of carcinogens, alterations of these enzymes may modify the activity of many carcinogens.

Despite the ample evidence of the dietary lipid effect on drug metabolism, little information is available regarding how dietary lipids alter the metabolism of specific hepatocarcinogens and modify the host response to liver tumor induction. Newberne et al. (1979) correlated the activation of hepatic drug metabolizing enzymes induced by diets containing different concentrations of beef fat or corn oil and their effects on aflatoxin-induced liver tumors. A diet high in corn oil induced the highest level of the enzymes and resulted in a higher tumor incidence when the diet was given during and after aflatoxin treatment. However, since multiple administration of the carcinogen was used, it is difficult to correlate the dietary effects on carcinogen metabolisms and the tumor incidence. It should be also stressed that many hepatocarcinogens possess, in addition to their carcinogenic activity, toxic properties to liver cells frequently leading to liver cell necrosis. Changes of drug metabolizing enzyme system induced by dietary lipids may alter the response of the liver to toxic effects of carcinogens resulting in varying degrees of liver cell necrosis. It has been known for many years that liver cell necrosis is followed by regenerative liver cell proliferation and that stimulation of liver cell proliferation enhances the development of liver tumors. Liver cell regeneration after partial hepatectomy or after repeated administration of carbon tetrachloride have been shown to enhance the induction of liver tumors by several different carcinogens (Chernozemski and Warwick, 1970; Pound and McGuire, 1978a, 1978b; Cole and Nowell, 1965). Several carcinogens that normally do not induce liver cancer in adult animals become hepatocarcinogenic when given in a single dose but coupled with liver cell proliferative stimulus such as partial hepatectomy (Craddock, 1973; Craddock and Frei, 1974). Several studies indicate that liver cell proliferation induced by partial hepatectomy or following liver cell necrosis is obligatory for the initiation of liver carcinogenesis (Cayama et al., 1978; Ying et al., 1981). Considering these facts, one has to be cautious in interpreting the modifying effects of dietary components on carcinogenesis, since toxic effects of chemicals will be modified by the dietary manipulation, and the resulting changes in the extent of liver cell necrosis and subsequent regenerative responses, will no doubt be reflected in the modification of liver cancer induction.

STAGE-SPECIFIC EFFECTS OF DIETARY FAT ON LIVER CARCINOGENESIS:

Even though the multistage theory of carcinogenesis in the skin was formulated over 40 years ago, experimental demonstration of the separate stages of tumor induction in the liver is relatively new. In the early 1970's, Peraino and his colleagues (1971) demonstrated that dietary administration of phenobarbital exerted a strong promoting action on the induction of hepatocellular carcinoma in rats initiated with a brief feeding of the carcinogen N-2 acetylaminofluorene. Since then, the concept of initiation and promotion for liver tumor induction in experimental animals has been firmly established (Pitot and Sirica, 1980; Farber, 1984). Many of the classical liver carcinogens served as an initiator and many investigators have identified liver tumor promoters of diverse properties. Since the mechanisms of tumor initiation and promotion are different, questions as to whether many of the observed effects of dietary fats on carcinogenesis are mediated through the changes during initiation or during promotion became quite important. In many organ systems, dietary fat appears to exert its modifying effects on a promotional phase of carcinogenesis. Furthermore in the organs such as breast, colon and pancreas, high fat diets or diets high in polyunsaturated fats _per_ _se_ act as promoting stimuli of tumor development (Carroll and Khor, 1975; Reddy, 1981; Roebuck et al., 1981).

Studies aimed at dissecting the stage-specific effects of dietary fat on liver carcinogenesis are only few. Since the drug metabolizing enzymes of the liver are modified by altering dietary fat compositions, it is conceivable that dietary fat may exert modifying effects on the initiation of hepatocytes by carcinogens which require metabolic activation. However, no experimental evidence exists for this. In the study by Newberne et al (1979), diets containing different levels of beef fat or corn oil were fed during and after, or only after the administration of aflatoxin. The incidence of tumors was increased when the corn oil diets were fed during and after aflatoxin administration but not when the diets were fed only after aflatoxin administration. The findings suggest that unsaturated fats influence the initiation phase of aflatoxin carcinogenesis, but a stringent distinction between effects on initiation and on promotion is difficult since multiple doses of the carcinogen were given as an initiating agent.

Using the short-term assays of the induction of enzyme altered foci in the liver, we demonstrated that the high level of polyunsaturated fat in a basal diet showed no promoting activity in the liver of rats initiated with a single dose of diethylnitrosamine (Perera et al., 1985a). Glauert and Pitot (1986) obtained similar results in their recent study. The diets high in polyunsaturated fat as supplied by corn oil, however, had a striking enhancing effect on the promoting action of a choline deficient (CD) diet (Perera et al., 1985a) and of phenobarbital (Glauert and Pitot, 1986). A CD diet with a high fat content is a more efficient promoter of the induction of enzyme altered foci than the diet with a low fat content (Shinozuka et al., 1982). Thus, although increasing the fat content or altering the proportion of saturated and polyunsaturated fat in the diet per se did not promote liver carcinogenesis, such dietary modifications may alter the efficacy of other known promoting agents or may even produce a promoting action of agents otherwise unproven for their promoting action.

CHOLINE (LIPOTROPE) DEFICIENCY AND LIVER CANCER:

Choline (β-hydroxyethyltrimethylammonium) is widely distributed in living organisms, and three major metabolic functions can be ascribed to this compound. It is an essential component of phospholipids, phosphatidylcholine and sphingomyelin, serves as a methyl donor in transmethylation reactions and is a precursor of a neurotransmitter, acetylcholine (Shinozuka and Katyal, 1985). In addition to choline, betaine and methionine serve as natural sources of labile methyl groups, and the de novo synthesis of the methyl group is dependent upon adequate dietary supply of folic acid and Vitamin B_{12}. Thus, methionine, folic acid and Vitamin B_{12} play a substantial role in the lipotropic action of choline (duVigneaud et al., 1950). As a moiety of phosphatidylcholine, choline is required for the synthesis of serum lipoproteins and cellular membranes. The lack of lipotrope factors in the diet results in severe alterations in lipid metabolisms leading to a variety of anatomical lesions in many organs of experimental animals (Shinozuka and Katyal, 1985). The liver is the most extensively studied organ affected by a dietary deficiency of choline, and the pathogenesis of choline-deficiency fatty liver has been clarified in considerable depth (Lombardi, 1966). Although direct evidence of diseases in man due to choline deficiency is lacking, the deficient state may develop in conjunction with other types of nutritional deficiencies (Post et al., 1952).

Since choline (lipotrope) deficiency fatty liver frequently progresses to cirrhosis in experimental animals (Hartraft, 1950) and since the association between preexisting liver cirrhosis and hepatocellular carcinomas is well known in human cases (Purtilo and Gottlieb, 1973; Omata et al., 1979), an experimental study of lipotrope deficiency was thought to serve as a model to investigate a causal relationship of two conditions. Occurrence of liver tumors in rats fed a choline deficient diet was reported 40 years ago (Copeland and Salmon, 1946). The finding was subsequently disputed by the demonstration of aflatoxin B_1 contamination in peanut meal used to formulate the deficient diet (Newberne et al., 1964). However, the fact remains that under the same experimental conditions, animals fed a choline supplemented diet made of the same batch of peanut meal used to make the deficient diet developed no tumors, indicating the importance of dietary choline in modifying the induction of cancers. Rogers and

Newberne (1982) summarized their extensive work on the effects of a lipotrope deficient diet on chemical carcinogenesis. Using a marginally lipotrope deficient diet that is deficient in choline, methionine and folic acid, they compared the effects of the diet on the carcinogenicity of chemicals of different classes on several target organs of rats. Although the results were quite variable depending on the target organs, when confined to the liver, the lipotrope deficient diet enhanced the tumor induction by a variety of carcinogens. The only hepatic carcinogen studied that showed no enhancing effects was dimethylnitrosamine. Our own studies using a diet devoid of only choline and different types of hepatocarcinogens showed a strong co-carcinogenic effect of the diet (Shinozuka et al., 1978a, 1978b; Lombardi and Shinozuka, 1979). Although our earlier study using the short term assays of carcinogen-induced enzyme altered foci showed no effects of a choline deficient diet on initiation of liver cells by a single injection of diethylnitrosamine (Shinozuka et al., 1979), Ghoshal and Farber (1983) demonstrated using a similar assay system that the initiating action of benzo(α)pyrene, 1,2-dimethylhydrazine and ethionine was enhanced by feeding a diet low in choline and methionine. Long term experiments using hepatocellular carcinomas as the end point are needed to obtain a definitive answer. While there are some uncertainty on the effect of choline deficiency on the initiation phase of carcinogenesis, it is reasonably clear that the deficient diet exerts a strong promoting activity (Shinozuka et al., 1986). However, there are reports indicating that as in the case of the earlier study by Copeland and Salmon (1946), long term feeding of a choline deficient diet per se resulted in the induction of hepatocellular carcinomas in rats (Ghoshal et al., 1983; Yokoyama et al., 1985). It is well appreciated that a stringent distinction between genuine promoters and weak but complete carcinogens is frequently difficult (Schulte-Hermann and Parzefall, 1981). It thus appears that a choline (lipotrope) deficient diet exerts modifying effects on the initiation of liver cells by certain carcinogens, it exerts promotional effects and may even be a complete carcinogen.

We proposed four possible mechanisms by which choline (lipotrope) deficiency modifies the induction of liver cancer (Shinozuka et al., 1986): i) Alterations in carcinogen metabolism; ii) Induction of liver cell proliferation; iii) Altered DNA methylation and; iv) Membrane lipid peroxidation. The roles of the liver drug metabolizing enzymes for carcinogen activation, their modifications by dietary fat and the effects of cell proliferation on carcinogenesis have already been discussed. In the case of choline (lipotrope) deficiency, there is abundant evidence to indicate that the activities of many phase 1 enzymes are reduced in the liver of animals fed the deficient diet (Campbell et al., 1978; Saito et al., 1975). The effects are most probably due to diet-induced changes in phospholipid metabolism leading to the alterations in the composition and physical states of membranes lipids. Both short term and chronic feeding of deficient diet have been shown to induce enhanced liver cell DNA synthesis and increased mitosis, though the underlying mechanisms are not clear (Rogers and McDonald, 1965; Abanobi et al., 1982). The enhanced cell proliferation has been implicated as a requirement in the initiation of target cells and as a component of tumor promotion. It may also be related to activation of certain types of cellular oncogenes related to cellular neoplastic transformation (Fausto and Shank, 1983).

Choline, its metabolite, betaine, and methionine constitute major sources of labile methyl groups for transmethylation reactions in animals. An adequate supply of folic acid is required for the de novo synthesis of methyl groups. Lipotrope (choline) deficient diets used in various experiments are usually low in or devoid of choline, low in methionine and, sometimes, low in folic acid. Thus, feeding the diets deficient in these components will result in disturbance of methylation patterns of important cellular macromolecules. Feeding a lipotrope-deficient diet has been shown to reduce cellular levels of s-adenosylmethionine (Poirier et al., 1977; Shivapurkar and Poirier, 1983) and such a reduction may interfere with important methyl transfer reactions in cells. The proper methylation of the DNA base, deoxycytidine, is critical in maintaining the proper status of cell differentiation (Razin and Riggs, 1980). The activation of many unexpressed genes which has been shown to occur frequently during the carcinogenic processes, is accompanied by hypomethylation of cytosine residues of DNA (Jones and Taylor, 1980). Alterations in the methylation patterns of DNA may also lead to the activation of certain oncogenes. Taking these observations together, the reduction of methyl donors in the liver by feeding a lipotrope (choline) deficient diet may lead to liver cells becoming more vulnerable to hypomethylation of DNA. Such a condition may favor enhancement of initiation and/or promotional phases of carcinogenesis.

The metabolic alterations of phospholipids induced by choline (lipotrope) deficiency may lead to the structural and functional changes of cell membranes. Membrane lipid peroxidation, which has been demonstrated in the kidney and liver of rats fed a lipotrope (choline) deficient diet may be one manifestation of the diet-induced changes in membrane phospholipids (Monserrat et al., 1969; Ugazio et al., 1967; Wilson et al., 1973). We recently confirmed the earlier observation of Ugazio et al (1967) and of Wilson et al (1973) that a choline (lipotrope) deficient diet induces lipid peroxidation of microsomal membrane lipids in the liver. By modifying the extent of lipid peroxidation induced by a choline deficient diet, we demonstrated a relatively good correlation between the extent of lipid peroxidation and the efficacy of liver tumor promotion (Shinozuka et al, 1986). Of particular interest is that the substitution of fat in a choline deficient diet with polyunsaturated fat, such as corn oil, resulted in enhanced lipid peroxidation and, at the same time, markedly enhanced the promoting activity of the deficient diet (Perera et al., 1985a). The consequence of membrane lipid peroxidation in the liver cells induced by a choline-deficient diet may be multiple. One possible effect is the functional alterations of membrane receptors. Our recent study of the surface membrane insulin receptor showed marked changes in number and affinity of the receptors in liver cells of rats fed the deficient diet (Betschart et al., 1985). The changes in insulin receptors observed in choline deficient hepatocytes may be one manifestation of broader alterations of cell membrane receptors involving cell growth regulation. It is not possible, at the present time, to single out any of four possible mechanisms discussed above as the sole mechanism underlying modification of certain phases of liver carcinogenesis due to lipotrope deficiency. The combination of two or more effects rather than a single effect may play a critical role in enhancing liver tumor induction by a lipotrope deficient diet.

HYPOLIPIDEMIC AGENTS AND LIVER CANCER:

For the past 20 years, considerable efforts have been made primarily by pharmaceutical industries to develop hypolipidemic drugs on the premise that reduction of elevated plasma cholesterol levels might decrease the incidence of cardiovascular morbidity and mortality. Even though the effectiveness of these drugs in clinical trials in reducing the overall incidence of fatal coronary heart disease in hyperlipidemic individuals is difficult to assess, the efforts in developing new potent and safe hypolipidemic agents continue (Bencze, 1978). One of the prototype hypolipidemic agents, clofibrate (ethyl-p-chlorophenoxyisobutylate) which is the most widely used drug both in the U.S.A. and in Europe has been shown to induce massive hepatomegaly in experimental animals (Hess et al., 1965; Svoboda et al., 1967). The hepatomegaly induced by the drug is characteristically associated with a marked increase of peroxisomes (microbodies) in the liver (Hess et al., 1965, Svoboda et al., 1967). Subsequent studies revealed that many of the structural analogs of clofibrate and hypolipidemic agents structurally unrelated to clofibrate shared the common properties of inducing proliferation of peroxisomes in the liver (Reddy, 1980). Not only the hypolipidemic drugs but also important industrial chemicals such as di(2-ethylhexyl)phthalate (DEHP) which has a hypolipidemic effect induce liver enlargement and peroxisome proliferation (Cohen and Grasso, 1981). DEHP is widely used as a plasticizer in many consumer plastic products including medical devices. It is also used as a dielectric and hydraulic fluid in industry. With an estimated 400 million pounds produced annually in the United States and its widespread use, there is opportunity for substantial human exposure to DEHP (Autian, 1983).

Long term toxicological effects of these chemicals on humans are of considerable importance. Svoboda and Azarnoff (1979) reported the induction of varieties of tumors in male Fisher rats given clofibrate. Tumors induced were hepatocellular carcinomas, adenocarcinoma of the stomach, papillary carcinoma of the urinary bladder, acinar cell carcinomas of the pancreas, renal carcinomas and sarcomas of the lung and parotid gland. Thus, clofibrate has a rather impressive broad spectrum of organotrophy for cancer induction. Subsequent studies by Reddy and his associates have shown that several other structurally unrelated compounds with hypolipidemic and peroxisome proliferating properties also induce liver tumors in rats and mice after chronic feeding (Reddy et al., 1980). These include nafenopin, Wy-14, 643, BR931 and tibric acid. The hepatocarcinogenicity of DEHP, although weak, was established by the National Toxicology Program sponsored bioassays (1980). As already mentioned, the common initial hepatic responses in rodents to a variety of hypolipidemic drugs/ agents are: i) liver enlargement; ii) proliferation of smooth endoplasmic reticulum; and iii) a marked increase in the number of peroxisomes and changes in the peroxisomal structure and enzyme composition. Peroxisomes are ubiquitous cytoplasmic organelles which contain catalase, several hydrogen peroxide generating oxidases, carnitine acetyltransferase as well as enzymes involved in the oxidation of long chain fatty acids (Hruban and Rechcigl, 1969; Lazarow, 1978). Whether there is a direct relation between hepatic peroxisome proliferation and hypolipidemia, or they are coincidentally related properties, has not been ascertained. Equally, the relationship between proliferation of peroxisomes and induction of cancer has not been fully elucidated. However, the development of liver tumors in animals fed several structurally diverse hypolipidemic compounds support the notion that hypolipidemic peroxisome proliferators belong to a novel class of hepatocarcinogens (Reddy et al., 1980).

There are several unique differences between carcinogenic hypolipidemic agents described above and known chemical carcinogens. Unlike most known chemical carcinogens which inhibit DNA synthesis and interact covalently with cellular macromolecules including DNA, the carcinogenic hypolipidemic agents stimulate DNA synthesis (Reddy et al., 1979), and they have not yet been found to interact chemically with DNA in target tissue (Warren et al., 1980; Gupta et al., 1985). None of these agents caused detectable mutagenic activity in Salmonella/microsome assays (Warren et al., 1980) or showed sister chromatic exchanges (Linnainmaa, 1984). Thus, their cellular and molecular modes of action as carcinogens remain unknown. The demonstrated hepatocarcinogenicity of the hypolipidemic agents and the lack of genotoxicity has led to the suggestion that these chemicals may have tumor promoting activity. WY 14,643 and clofibrate, when given after a 14 day exposure to DEN as the initiating regimes, demonstrated tumor enhancing capacity (Reddy and Rao,

1978). Mochizuki et al., (1982) reported that at low concentrations, clofibrate markedly enhanced the development of DEN induced liver tumors, although at higher concentrations, it showed an inhibitory effect. In contrast to these findings, several recent reports indicate that hypolipidemic peroxisome proliferators suppressed the induction of enzyme altered putative preneoplastic foci in carcinogen initiated rat liver (Stäubli et al., 1984; DeAngelo and Garrett, 1983; Popp et al, 1985). We observed that BR 931 suppressed the promoting effect of a choline deficient diet and failed to promote the emergence of enzyme altered foci in the liver of rats initiated with a single dose of DEN (Shinozuka et al., 1983). Furthermore, BR931 and DEHP accelerated the regression of preformed enzyme altered foci induced by DEN or by AAF (Perera and Shinozuka, 1984). A similar effect of the regression of preformed enzyme altered foci induced by a 10 week feeding of AAF by nafenopin was demonstrated by Williams and his associates (Numoto et al., 1985). It is conceivable that the short and long term effects of hypolipidemic peroxisome proliferators on the process of liver carcinogenesis may be mediated through different mechanisms.

Based on the common property of peroxisome prolifer-ation shared by many hypolipidemic agents, Reddy et al. proposed that their carcinogenicity may be related to indirect DNA damage mediated through H_2O_2 generated during increased oxidation of lipids (Reddy and Warren, 1981,). However, at the present time, there is no direct experimental evidence to support this hypothesis. Indirect evidence includes: i) accumulation of a large quantity of lipofuscin pigment (results of lipoperoxidation) in the liver after long term feeding of hypolipidemic agents (Reddy et al., 1982); ii) a greater increase in the activity of enzymes involved in β -oxidation of fatty acids as compared to catalase (Lazarow and deDuve, 1976); iii) an inhibition of the carcinogenicity of a hypolipidemic agent by antioxidants (Rao et al., 1984); and iv) DNA damage demonstrated by in vitro assays of peroxisomes and DNA (Fahl et al., 1984). Our recent studies indicate that during the short-term feeding (1-4 weeks) of BR931 or DEHP, there is no evidence of liver membrane lipid peroxidation as determined by diene conjugate formation (Perera et al., 1985b). There were no significant changes in glutathione peroxidases or glutathione S-transferases, though there was a slight increase in catalase and cellular glutathione levels. Furthermore, BR931 appears to protect against membrane lipid peroxidation induced by a choline deficient diet. It appears that a slight increase in catalase activity during the short-term feeding of hypolipidemic agents may be sufficient to cope with excess generation of H_2O_2. In the study of hypolipidemic peroxisome proliferators, the major attention has been focused on the initial hepatic response and on the carcinogenic end-points of hepatoma induction (14-25 months). But scant attention has been paid to the sequential biochemical and pathological changes that take place in the liver in the intervening period (6-12 months) and that could throw light on the mechanism by which these agents exert their carcinogenic effect. Further studies of cellular and biochemical analysis during the intermediate stages of carcinogenesis by hypolipidemic peroxisome proliferators may shed insight into their mechanistic actions.

CONCLUSIONS:

In the early era of study of experimental liver carcinogenesis, the important roles played by dietary fat in modifying the activity of carcinogens were recognized. However, no systematic studies followed in subsequent years to unravel the underlying mechanisms. Instead, the models of liver carcinogenesis have become instrumental in delineating and correlating cellular, biochemical and molecular events during the evolution of cancer. As our knowledge of carcinogenesis and lipid metabolism advances, a reevaluation of the effects of fat or of fat components on each critical step of carcinogenesis is needed.

As exemplified by choline (lipotrope) deficiency and by hypolipidemic agents, nutritional factors and chemicals which disturb lipid metabolism have been shown to exert profound effects on liver tumor induction. The enhancing effect of a choline (lipotrope) deficient diet on liver tumor induction was clearly demonstrated and its mechanistic actions have been analyzed in considerable depth. The mechanism by which hypolipidemic peroxisome proliferators induce liver tumors remains elusive. An attractive hypothesis of superoxide generation by these agents as a possible cause of liver tumor induction has emerged in recent years although experimental proof is still lacking. Further studies of the action of hypolipidemic peroxisome proliferators are important since some of the environmental contaminants belong to this class of agents.

ACKNOWLEDGMENT:

The authors wish to thank Ms. Deborah L. Newman for her secretarial work.

REFERENCES

Abanobi SE, Lombardi B, Shinozuka H (1982). Stimulation of DNA synthesis and cell proliferation in the liver of rats fed a choline-devoid diet and their suppression by phenobarbital. Cancer Res 42:412-415.

Arffmann E (1960). Heated fats and allied compounds as carcinogens: a critical review of experimental results. J Nat Cancer Inst 25:893-926.

Armstrong B, Doll R (1975). Environmental factors and cancer incidence and mortality in different countries with special reference to dietary practices. Int J Cancer 15:617-631.

Autian J (1983). Toxicity and health threats of phthalate esters: review of literature. Environ Health Perspect 4:3-26.

Bencze WL (1978). New hypolipidemic drugs in Kritchevsky D, Paoletti R, Holmes WL (eds). Drugs Affecting Lipid Metabolism, New York; Plenum pp 77-95.

Betschart JM, Virji MA, Perera MIR, Shinozuka H (1985). Modulation of hepatocyte insulin receptors in response to a tumor-promoting diet. J Cell Biol 101:479a.

Campbell TC, Hayes JR (1974). Role of nutrition in the drug-metabolizing enzyme system. Pharmacol Rev 25:171-197.

Campbell TC, Hayes JR, Newberne PM (1978). Dietary lipotropes, hepatic microsomal mixed function oxidase activities and in vivo covalent binding of aflatoxin B_1 in rats. Cancer Res 38:4569-4573.

Carroll KK (1981). Neutral fats and cancer. Cancer Res 41:3695-3699.

Carroll KK, Khar HT (1975). Dietary fat in relation to tumorigenesis. Prog Biochem Pharmacol 10:308-353.

Caster WO, Wade AE, Norred WP, Bargmann RE (1970). A differential effect of dietary saturated fat on the metabolism of aniline and hexobarbital by the rat liver. Pharmacology 3:177-186.

Cayama E, Tsuda H, Sarma DRS, Farber E (1978).

Initiation of chemical carcinogenesis requires cell proliferation. Nature 275:60-62.

Century B (1969). Lipids affecting drug metabolism and cellular functions in C.W. Holmes (ed). Drugs Affecting Lipid Metabolism, New York; Plenum Press p 629-638.

Century B, Horwitt, MK (1968). A role of dietary lipid in the ability of phenobarbitone to stimulate hexobarbitone and antipyrene metabolism. Fed Proc 27:349.

Chernozemski IN, Warwick GP (1970). Liver regeneration and induction of hepatomas in B6AF mice by urethan. Cancer Res 30:2685-2690.

Cohen AJ, Grasso P (1981). Review of the hepatic response to hypolipidemic drugs in rodents and assessment of its toxicological significance to man. Fd Cosmet Toxicol 19:585-605.

Cole LJ, Nowell PC (1965). Radiation carcinogenesis: the sequence of events. Science 150:1782-1786.

Copeland DH, Salmon WD (1946). The occurrence of neoplasms in the liver, lungs and other tissues of rats as a result of prolonged choline deficiency. Am J Path 22:1059-1081.

Correa P (1981). Epidemiologic correlations between diet and cancer frequency. Cancer Res 41:3685-3689.

Craddock VM (1973). Induction of liver tumors in rats by a single treatment with nitroso-compounds given after partial hepatectomy. Nature 245:386-388.

Craddock VM, Frei JV (1974). Induction of liver cell adenomata in the rat by a single treatment with N-methyl-N-nitrosourea given at various times after partial hepatectomy. Br J Cancer 30:503-511.

de Angelo AB, Garrett CT (1983). Inhibition of development of preneoplastic lesions in the livers of rats fed a weakly carcinogenic environmental contaminant. Cancer Letters 20:199-205.

du Vigneaud V, Ressler C, Rachele JR (1950). The biological synthesis of "labile methyl group". Science 112:267-271.

Engel RW, Copeland DH (1951). Influence of diet on the relative incidence of eye, mammary, ear duct and liver tumors in rats fed 2-acetylaminofluorene. Cancer Res 11:180-183.

Fahl WE, Lalwani ND, Watanabe T, Goel SK, Reddy JK (1984). DNA damage related to increased hydrogen peroxide generation by hypolipidemic drug-induced liver peroxisomes. Proc Nat Acad Sci 81:7827-7830.

Farber E (1984). The multistep nature of cancer

development. Cancer Res 44:4217-4223.

Fausto N, Shank PR (1983). Oncogene expression in liver regeneration and hepatocarcinogenesis. Hepatology 3:1016-1023.

Ghoshal AK, Farber E (1983). The induction of resistant hepatocytes during initiation of liver carcinogenesis with chemicals in rats fed a choline deficient methionine low diet. Carcinogenesis 4:801-804.

Ghoshal AK, Farber E (1984). The induction of liver cancer by dietary deficiency of choline and methionine without added carcinogens. Carcinongenesis 5:1367-1370.

Glauert HP, Pitot HC (1986). Influence of dietary fat on the promotion of diethylnitrosamine-induced hepato-carcinogenesis in female rats. Proc Soc Exp Biol Med (in press).

Gupta RC, Joel SK, Earley K, Singh B, Reddy JK (1985). ^{32}P-post labeling analysis of peroxisome proliferator-DNA adduct formation in rat liver in vivo and hepatocytes in vitro. Carcinogenesis 6:933-936.

György P, Tomarelli R, Ostergard RP, Brown JB (1942). Unsaturated fatty acids in the dietary destruction of N,N-dimethylaminoazobenzene (butter yellow) and in the production of anemia in rats. J Exp Med 76:413-420.

Hartroft WS (1950). Accumulation of fat in liver cells and in lipodiastaemata preceding experimental dietary cirrhosis. Anat Rec 106:61-87.

Hess R, Staubli W, Reiss W (1965). Nature of the hepatomegalic effect produced by ethyl-chlorophenoxy-isobutylate in the rat. Nature 208:856-858.

Hruban Z, Rechigl M (1969). Microbodies and related particles, morphology, biochemistry and physiology. Int Rev Cytol Suppl 1:20-72.

Jacobi HP, Baumann CA (1940). The effect of fat on tumor formation. Am J Cancer 39:338-342.

Johnson AR, Pearson JA, Shenstone FS, Fogarty AC (1967). Inhibition of the desaturation of stearic to oleic acid by cyclopropene fatty acids. Nature 214:1244-1245.

Jones PA, Taylor SM (1980). Cellular differentiation, cytidine analogs and DNA methylation. Cell 20:85-93.

Kinoshita R (1937). Special report. Studies on the carcinogenic chemical substances. Tr Soc Path Jap 27:665-727.

Kline BE, Miller JA, Rusch HP, Baumann CA (1946a). Certain effects of dietary fats on the production of liver tumors in rats fed p-dimethylaminoazobenzene. Cancer Res 6:5-7.

Kline BE, Miller JA, Rusch HP, Baumann CA (1946b). The carcinogenicity of p-dimethylaminoazobenzene in diets containing the fatty acids of hydrogenated coconut oil or of corn oil. Cancer Res 6:1-4.

Lavik PS, Baumann CA (1941). Dietary fat and tumor formation. Cancer Res 1:181-187.

Lazarow PB (1978). Rat liver peroxisomes catalyze the β -oxidation of fatty acids. J Biol Chem 253:1522-1528.

Lazarow PB, deDuve Ca (1976). A fatty acyl-CoA oxidizing system in rat liver peroxisomes: enhancement by clofibrate, a hypolipidemic drug. Proc Nat Acad Sci 73:2043-2046.

Lee DJ, Wales JH, Sinnhuber RO (1971). Promotion of aflatoxin-induced hepatoma growth in trout by methyl malvalate and sterculate. Cancer Res 31:960-963.

Linnainmaa K (1984). Induction of sister chromatid exchanges by the peroxisome proliferators, 2,4-D MCPA and clofibrate in vivo and in vitro. Carcinogenesis 5:703-707.

Lombardi B (1966). Considerations on the pathogenesis of fatty liver. Lab Invest 15:1-20.

Lombardi B, Shinozuka H (1979). Enhancement of 2-acetylaminofluorene liver carcinogenesis in rats fed a choline devoid diet. Int J Cancer 23:565-570.

Marshall WJ, McLean AEM (1971). A requirement for dietary lipids for induction of cytochrome P450 by phenobarbitone in rat liver microsomal fraction. Biochem J 122:569-573.

McDanell RE, McLean AEM (1985). Role of nutritional status in drug metabolism and toxicity in H. Sidransky (ed). Nutritional Pathology, New York; Marcel Dekker p 321-356.

Miller EC (1978). Some current perspectives on chemical carcinogenesis in humans and experimental animals. Presidential address. Cancer Res 38:1479-1496.

Miller JA, Kline BE, Rusch HP, Baumann CA (1944). The carcinogenicity of p-dimethylaminoazobenzene in diets containing hydrogenated coconut oil. Cancer res 4:153-158.

Miller JA, Miner DL, Rusch HP, Baumann CA (1941). Diet and hepatic tumor formation. Cancer Res 1:699-708.

Mochizuki Y, Furukawa K, Sawada N (1982). Effects of various concentrations of ethyl-p-chlorophenoxyisobutyrate (clofibrate) on diethylnitrosamine-induced hepatic tumorigenesis in the rat. Carcinogenesis 3:1027-1029.

Monserrat AJ, Ghoshal AK, Hartroft WS, Porta EA (1969).

Lipoperoxidation in the pathogenesis of renal necrosis in choline-deficient rats. Am J Path 55:163-190.

National Toxicology Program (1980). Carcinogenesis bioassay of di(2-ethylhexyl) phthalate (CAS No 117-81-7) in F-344 rats and B6C3F1 mice. NTP Technical Report Series No 217, National Institutes of Health, Bethesda, MD.

Newberne PM, Carlton WW, Wogan GN (1964). Hepatomas in rats and hepatorenal injury induced by peanut meal or Aspergillus flavus extract. Path Vet 1:105-132.

Newberne PM, Weigert J, Kula N (1979). Effects of dietary fat on hepatic mixed function oxidases and hepatocellular carcinoma induced by aflatoxin B_1 in rats. Cancer Res 39:3986-3991.

Nixon JE, Sinnhuber RO, Lee DJ, Landers MK, Harr JR (1974). Effect of cyclopropenoid compounds on the carcinogenic activity of diethylnitrosamine and aflatoxin B_1 in rats. J Nat Cancer Inst 53:453-458.

Norred WP, Wade AE (1972). Dietary fatty acid induced alterations of hepatic microsomal drug metabolism. Biochem Pharmacol 21:2887-2897.

Numoto S, Mori H, Furuya K, Levine WG, Williams GM (1985). Absence of a promoting or sequential syncarcinogenic effect in the rat liver by the hypolipidemic drug Nafenopin given after N-2-fluorenylacetamide. Toxicol Appl Pharmacol 77:76-85.

Opie EL (1944). The influence of diet on the production of tumors of the liver by butter yellow. J Exp Med 80:219-230.

Peraino C, Fry RJM, Staffeldt E (1971). Reduction and enhancement by phenobarbital of hepatocarcinogenesis induced in the rat by 2-acetylaminofluorene. Cancer Res 31:1506-1512.

Perera MIR, Demetris JA, Katyal SL, Shinozuka H (1985a). Lipid peroxidation of liver microsome induced by choline deficient diets and its relationship to the diet-induced promotion of the induction of γ-glutamyltranspeptidase-positive foci. Cancer Res 45:2533-2538.

Perera MIR, Katyal SL, Shinozuka H (1985b). Inhibition of choline deficient diet induced membrane lipid peroxidation by hypolipidemic peroxisome proliferators. Proc Am Assoc Cancer Res 26:131.

Perera MIR, Shinozuka H (1984). Accelerated regression of carcinogen-induced preneoplastic hepatocyte foci by peroxisome proliferators, BR931, 4-chloro-6-(2,3-xylidino)-

2-pyrimidixylthio (B- hydroxyethyl) acetamide, and di(2-ethylhexyl)phthalate. Carcinogenesis 5:1193-1198.

Phelps RA, Shenstone FS, Kemmerer AR, Evans RJ (1965). A review of cyclopropenoid compounds: biological effects of some derivatives. Poult Sci 44:359-394.

Pitot HC, Sirica AE (1980). The stages of initiation and promotion in hepatocarcinogenesis. Biochem Biophys Acta 605:191-215.

Poirier LA, Grantham PH, Rogers AE (1977). The effects of a marginally lipotrope-deficient diet on the hepatic levels of S-adenosylmethionine and on the urinary metabolites of 2 acetylaminofluorene in rats. Cancer Res 37:744-748.

Popp JA, Garvey LK, Hamm TE Jr, Swenberg JA (1985). Lack of hepatic promotional activity by the peroxisomal proliferating hepatocarcinogen di(2-ethylhexyl) phthalate. Carcinogenesis 6:141-144.

Post J, Benton JG, Breakstone R, Hoffman J (1952). The effects of diet and choline on fatty infiltration of the human liver. Gastroenterol 20:403-410.

Pound AW, McGuire LJ (1978a). Repeated partial hepatectomy as a promoting stimulus for carcinogenic response of liver to nitrosamine in rats. Br J Cancer 37:595-602.

Pound AW, McGuire LJ (1978b). Influence of repeated liver regeneration on hepatic carcinogenesis by diethylnitrosamine in mice. Br J Cancer 37:595-602.

Purtilo DT, Gottlieb LS (1973). Cirrhosis and hepatoma occurring at Boston City Hospital (1917-1968). Cancer 32:458-462.

Rajalakshmi S, Rao PM, Sarma DSR (1982). Interactions of carcinogens with nucleic acids. In F.F. Becker (ed). Cancer - A Comprehensive Treatise, New York; Plenum Press pp 335-409.

Raju PK, Reiser R (1967). Inhibition of fatty acyl desaturase by cyclopropene fatty acids. J Biol Chem 242:379-384.

Rao MS, Lalwani ND, Watanabe T, Reddy JK (1984). Inhibitory effect of antioxidants ethoxyquin and 2(3)-tert-butyl-4-hydroxyanisole on hepatic tumorigenesis in rats fed ciprofibrate, a peroxisome proliferator. Cancer Res 44:1072-1076.

Razin A, Riggs AD (1980). DNA methylation and gene function. Science 210:604-610.

Reddy BS (1981). Dietary fat and its relationship to

large bowel cancer. Cancer Res 41:3700-3705.

Reddy JK (1980). Hepatic peroxisome proliferative and carcinogenic effects of hypolipidemic drugs in Fmagalli R, Kritchevsky D, Paoletti (eds). Drugs Affecting Lipid Metabolism, New York; Elsevier pp 301-309.

Reddy JK, Azarnoff DL, Hignite CD (1980). Hypolipidemic hepatic peroxisome proliferators form a novel class of chemical carcinogens. Nature 283:397-398.

Reddy JK, Lalwani ND, Reddy MK, Qureshi SA (1982). Excessive accumulation of autofluorescent lipofuscin in the liver during hepatocarcinogenesis by methyl clofenapate and other peroxisome proliferators. Cancer Res 42:259-266.

Reddy JK, Rao MS (1978). Enhancement by Wy14,643, a hepatic peroxisome proliferator, diethylnitrosamine-initiated hepatic tumorigenesis in the rat. Br J Cancer 38:537-543.

Reddy JK, Rao MS, Azarnoff DL, Sell S (1979). Mitogenic and carcinogenic effects of a hypolipidemic peroxisome proliferator [4-chloro-6-(2,3 xylidino)-2-pyrimidinyl-thio] acetic acid (Wy14,643) in rat and mouse liver. Cancer Res 39:152-161.

Reddy JK, Warren JR (1981). Toxicological implications of hepatic peroxisome proliferation = possible role of oxygen radical toxicity in hypolipidemic drug-induced carcinogenesis. Toxicologist 1:131-142.

Roebuck BD, Yager JD Jr, Longnecker DS, Wilpone SA (1981). Promotion by unsaturated fat of azaserine-induced pancreatic carcinogenesis in the rat. Cancer Res 41:3961-3966.

Rogers AE, MacDonald RA (1965). Hepatic vasculature and cell proliferation in experimental cirrhosis. Lab Invest 14:1710-1726.

Rogers AE, Newberne PM (1982). Lipotrope deficiency in experimental carcinogenesis. Nutr Cancer 2:104-112.

Saito R, Estes LW, Lombardi B (1975). Reduced response to phenobarbital by the liver of rats fed a choline-deficient diet. Biochem Biophys Acta 381:185-194.

Sasaki T, Yoshida T (1935). Experimentelle Erzeugrind des Lebercarcinomas durch Futterung mit O-Amidoazotoluol. Virchows Arch Path Anat Physiol 295:175-200.

Scarpelli DG (1974a). Experimental modification of the mitogenic effect of methyl sterculate on rat liver. Virch Arch Cell Path 16:211-220.

Scarpelli DG (1974b). Mitogenic activity of sterculic acid, a cyclopropenoid fatty acid. Science 185:958-960.

Omata M, Ashcavai M, Liew C-T, Peters RL (1979). Hepato-cellularcarcinoma in the U.S.A. etiologic consideration. Localization of hepatitis B antigen. Gastroenterology 76:279-287.

Shinozuka H, Abanobi SE, Lombardi B (1983). Modulation of tumor promotion in liver carcinogenesis. Environ Health Perspect 50:163-168.

Shinozuka H, Lombardi B, Sell S, Iammarino RM (1978a). Enhancement of ethionine liver carcinogenesis in rats fed a choline-deficient diet. J Nat Cancer Inst 22:36-39.

Shinozuka H, Katyal SL, Lombardi B (1978b). Azaserine carcinogenesis: organ susceptibility change in rats fed a diet devoid of choline. Int J Cancer 22:36-39.

Shinozuka H, Katyal SL (1985). Pathology of choline deficiency in H Sidransky (ed). Nutritional Pathology, New York; Marcel Dekker p 279-320.

Shinozuka H, Katyal SL, Perera MIR (1986). Choline deficiency and chemical carcinogenesis. J Nat Cancer Inst Monog (in press).

Shinozuka H, Sells MA, Katyal SL, Sell S, Lombardi B (1979). Effects of a choline devoid diet on the emergence of γ-glutamyltranspeptidase positive foci in the liver of carcinogen treated rats. Cancer Res 39:2515-2521.

Shinozuka H, Takahashi S, Lombardi B, Abanobi SE (1982). Effects of varying the fat content of a choline-devoid diet on promotion of the emergence of γ-glutamyl-transpeptidase positive foci in the liver of carcinogen-treated rats. Cancer Lett 16:43-50.

Shivapurkar N, Poirier LA (1983). Tissue levels of S-adeno-sylhomocysteine in rats fed methionine-deficient, amino acid defined diet for one to five weeks. Carcinogenesis 4:1051-1057.

Sinnhuber RO, Wales JH, Ayres JL, Engebrecht RH, Amend DL (1968a). Dietary factors and hepatoma in rainbow trout (Salmo gairdneri). I. Aflatoxins in vegetable protein feedstuffs. J Nat Cancer Inst 41:711-718.

Sinnhuber RO, Lee DJ, Wales JH, Ayres JL (1968b). Dietary factors and hepatoma in rainbow trout (Salmo gairdneri). II. Cocarcinogenesis by cyclopropenoid fatty acids and the effect of gassypol and altered lipids on aflatoxin induced liver cancer. J Nat Cancer Inst 41:1293-1301.

Stäubli W, Bentley P, Bieri F, Frohlich E, Walchter F (1984). Inhibitory effect of nafenopin upon the development of diethylnitrosamine-induced altered foci within the rat liver. Carcinogenesis 5:41-46.

Sugai M, Witting LA, Tsuchiyama H, Kummerow FA (1962). The effect of heated fat on the carcinogenic activity of 2-acetylaminofluorene. Cancer Res 22:519-519.

Svoboda DJ, Azarnoff DL (1979). Tumors in male rats fed ethylchlorophenoxyisobutyrate, a hypolipidemic drug. Cancer Res 39:3419-3428.

Svoboda D, Grady H, Azarnoff D (1967). Microbodies in experimentally altered cells. J Cell Biol 35:127-152.

Tannenbaum A (1942). The genesis and growth of tumors III. Effects of a high fat diet. Cancer Res 2:468-475.

Ugazio G, Gabriel L, Burdinor E (1967). Osservazioni sperimentale sui lipidi accumulati nil fegato di ratto alimentato con dieta colino priva. Lo Sperimentale 117:1-17.

Wade AE, Caster WO, Greene FE, Meadows JS (1969). Effect of thiamine and dietary linoleate levels on hepatic drug metabolism in the male rat. Arch Int Pharmacodyn Ther 181:466-473.

Wade AE, Norred WP (1976). Effect of dietary lipid on drug metabolizing enzymes. Fed Proc 35:2475.

Wade AE, Norred, WP, Evans JS (1978). Lipids in drug detoxification in J.N. Hathcock and J. Coon (eds). Nutrition and Drug Interactions, New York; Academic Press p 475-503.

Wade AE, Wu B, Caster WO (1972). Relationship of dietary essential fatty acid consumption to drug hydroxylation. Pharmacology 7:305-314.

Warren JR, Simmon VF, Reddy JK (1980). Properties of hypolipidemic peroxisome proliferators in the lymphocyte [^{3}H]-thymidine and Salmonella mutagenesis assays. Cancer Res 40:36-41.

Watson AF, Mellanby E (1930). Tar cancer in mice. II. The condition of the skin when modified by external treatment or diet, as a factor influencing the cancerous reaction. Br J Exp Path 11:311-322.

Wilson RH, DeEds F, Cox AJ Jr (1947). The carcinogenic activity of 2-acetylaminofluorene. III. Manner of administration, age of animals and type of diet. Cancer Res 7:450-452.

Wilson RB, Kula NS, Newberne PM, Conner MW (1973). Vascular damage and lipid peroxidation in choline deficient rats. Exp Mol Path 18:357-368.

Wolf H, Jackson EW (1963). Hepatoma in rainbow trout: descriptive and experimental epidemiology. Science 142:676-678.

Wood R, Chumbler F, Wiegand RD (1978). Effect of dietary cyclopropene fatty acids on actadecenoates of individual lipid classes of rat liver and hepatoma. Lipids 13:232-238.

Wynder EL (1975). The epidemiology of large bowel cancer. Cancer Res 35:3388-3394.

Yamagiwa K, Ichikawa K (1966). Experimental studies on the pathogenesis of epithelial tumors. The first report. Toky Igakkai Zassi 30:1-43.

Ying TS, Sarma DSR, Farber E (1981). Role of acute hepatic necrosis in the induction of early steps in liver carcinogenesis by diethylnitrosamine. Cancer Res 41:2096-2101.

Yokoyama S, Sells MA, Reddy TV, Lombardi B (1985). Hepatocarcinogenic and promoting action of a choline-devoid diet in the rat. Cancer Res 45:2834-2842.

Dietary Fat and Cancer, pages 487–494
© 1986 Alan R. Liss, Inc.

EFFECT OF DIETARY CALCIUM ON THE TOXICITY OF BILE ACID
AND ORALLY ADMINISTERED FAT TO COLONIC EPITHELIUM.

R.P. Bird and W.R. Bruce

Ludwig Institute for Cancer Research,
Toronto Branch, 9 Earl Street,
Toronto, Ontario M4Y 1M4, Canada

INTRODUCTION

Free fatty acids and bile acids are detergent-like
compounds that are known to exert membrane damaging
effects in biological systems (Hagerty, 1938; Pinkerton,
1928; Butcher, 1953; Peltier, 1956; Ammon and Phillips,
1979; Gaginella et al, 1977; Vahouny et al, 1981; Bull
et al, 1983). They have been shown to be toxic to the
colonic epithelium and to lead to increased
proliferation in the colonic crypt cells (Ammon and
Phillips, 1979; Gaginella et al, 1977; Vahouny et al,
1981). In most studies that have been reported to date,
the compounds have been perfused through the colon or
instilled intra-rectally. Our studies were directed
towards determining the effects of the acidic lipids
when they were given by the oral route and when they
were given with other dietary factors.

The pathological effects of these agents on the
colonic epithelium was of interest to us because it had
been proposed that the promotional effect of a high fat
diet on colon tumorigenesis was mediated by increased
levels of these acidic lipids on the colonic lumen and
it had been hypothesized that other dietary components
could affect the toxicological properties of the lipids.
The suggestion was made after the demonstration by
Wargovich et al (1983, 1984) that orally administered
calcium salts were able to counteract the toxic effect
of intra-rectally instilled deoxycholic acids and free
fatty acids in C57BL/6J mice. Subsequently, Rafter et
al (1986) showed that an increased level of calcium in

the perfusion fluid decreased the toxic effects of
deoxycholic acid and noted that the amount of
deoxycholic acid in the solution was reduced in the
presence of additional calcium.

It was thus of interest to investigate the effect of
dietary calcium on the toxicity of bile acid and orally
administered fat to the colonic epithelium in a feeding
regimen. In these studies the index of biological
toxicity of the bile acids and orally administered fat
was determined from the compensatory proliferation which
they produced in the colonic crypts.

MATERIALS AND METHODS

Animals: In all studies, 8 to 10 week old
C57BL/6J mice (The Jackson Laboratory, Bar Harbor,
Maine) were used. The animals were housed in plastic
cages with wire tops and sawdust bedding with 12 hour
light and 12 hour dark cycles. The animals were fed ad
libitum and had free access to water.

Diets: All animals were fed standard laboratory
chow unless specified otherwise. In those studies in
which dietary effects were investigated, all diets were
formulated based on the composition of AIN-76 diet
(American Inst. of Nutrition, 1977). Dietary calcium
(0.1, 0.5 or 1.0%) was increased or decreased by
modifying the AIN-76 mineral mix (Bird, 1986). In all
diets Ca:P was approximately 1:1.

Measurement of Proliferative Indices: Animals were
either injected with colchicine (1 mg/kg body weight) or
^{3}H-thymidine (1 µCi/g body weight, specific activity
42 Ci/mmol, Amersham Corporation, Arlington Heights,
IL). The animals injected with colchicine were killed
3 hr later and their colons were removed and processed
for histology (Bird, 1986; Bird and Stamp, 1986). The
number of cells in metaphase were enumerated in complete
longitudinal sections of colonic crypts. At least 5 to
10 crypts were quantified for each animal. Those
animals which were injected with [^{3}H]-thymidine were
killed 1 hr later and their colons were processed for
autoradiography by standard procedure. Labelling
indices for whole crypts and their distribution
according to the position along the crypt height, near

the position of the uppermost labelled cells and crypt height were determined (Bird, 1986; Bird and Stamp, 1986).

EXPERIMENTAL FINDINGS

Effect of dietary calcium on the cholic acid induced proliferative response of the murine colonic epithelium: The animals were fed the test diets varying in cholic acid (0.1 or 0.25%) and calcium (0.1, 0.5 and 1.0%) over a period of two weeks. Cholic acid supplemented diet has been shown to increase the level of bile acids (primary as well as secondary) in the colonic lumen, increase colonic cell proliferation and tumorigenesis in rodent models (Deschner et al, 1981; Cohen et al, 1980). After two weeks of feeding on test and control diets the animals were injected with colchicine or [^{3}H]-thymidine. Their colons were removed after appropriate time intervals (see Materials and Methods) and processed for histology and autoradiography respectively.

The animals fed cholic acid supplemented diets exhibited lower body weights than control groups regardless of the level of calcium in their diet (Bird, 1986; Bird et al, 1986). Food consumption data indicated that the cholic acid supplemented diets were less palatable to the animals than the control diets. The values for arrested metaphase figures in the colonic crypts were significantly higher for the 0.1% Ca + cholic acid compared to the 1.0% Ca + cholic acid groups (4.92±1.06 vs 2.20±0.53).

Autoradiographic analysis of the colonic crypts clearly indicated that dietary calcium alone affects colonic cell proliferation. The low calcium diet (0.1%) was conducive to more active proliferative compartments (Bird et al, 1986). Also, the low calcium group supplemented with cholic acid exhibited a markedly higher labelling index (Table 1) and mean position of the uppermost labelled cells compared to the high calcium group (1.0% Ca) supplemented with cholic acid (13.1±1.2 vs 10.6±1.0).

Influence of Dietary Calcium on the Susceptibility of Colonic Epithelium to the Toxicity of Orally Administered Fat: In an experiment designed to determine whether orally administered fat grossly damaged the colonic epithelium, mice (C57BL/6J) were given a gavage of 0.4 ml of corn oil (commercially available), beef tallow (a gift from Canada Packers Ltd., Toronto, Canada), water or concentrated albumin solution (400 mg/animal). Each group consisted of five male and five female mice. Two, 4 or 8 hr later animals from each group were killed. Their colons were excised and cleaned gently by flushing with Kreb's Ringer solution. Microscopic examination of sections prepared at these times revealed that the tall columnar cells on the surface of the normal epithelium were replaced with cells which had flattened, pleomorphic, pyknotic and fragemented nuclei (Bird et al, 1985). This phenomenon was quantitated by scoring 100 intercrypt epithelial zones between well-defined crypts. The maximum damage, affecting 25-45% of the epithelial zones, was seen at 2-4 hr after treatment with 0.4 ml of beef tallow or corn oil and the epithelium appeared normal with 10% damage at 12 hr. The mitotic activity in the colonic crypts was unchanged up to 8 hr and then showed a marked increase of 2- to 3-fold at 12-16 hr. The severity of the epithelial damage and ensuing mitogenic response was related to the size of the fat bolus.

Autoradiographic analysis of the colons of the animals given 0.1, 0.2, or 0.4 ml of beef tallow revealed maximum number of labelled cells after approximately 12 hr of fat gavage and the 12 hr labelling indices for these groups were 10.4 ± 1.83, 24.2 ± 2.9 and 24.7 ± 2.7, respectively, whereas the control value was 4.0 ± 0.2. The labelling indices of the fat treated colons were not different from the control value after 24 hr.

In order to study the effect of dietary calcium on fat induced cell proliferative activity, 3 groups of mice were fed 0.1, 0.5 or 1.0% calcium diet for two weeks. They were then gavaged with 0.1 ml of beef tallow or corn oil. Sixteen hours later they were injected with colchicine and their colonic crypts were enumerated for number of metaphase figures per 10 crypts as described previously. In the case of beef tallow treatment the effect of dietary calcium was more pronounced and showed a definite pattern. The group given the lowest level of calcium was more susceptible to the mitogenic effect of beef tallow. In the case of corn oil a definite pattern was not seen, which indicated that the type of fat reaching the colon may be important in influencing the effect of calcium (Table 2).

DISCUSSION

The mechanism by which a high calcium diet inhibits the proliferative response induced by dietary cholic acid or by fat boluses has not been resolved. However, calcium plays an important role in mitogenic processes, and is implicated in the maintenance of epithelial structures (Reese, 1982). Recently it has been suggested that free calcium ions in the colonic lumen can counteract the toxic effects of bile acids and free fatty acids by binding with them and rendering them biologically inactive (Newmark et al, 1984). However, such an interaction between bile acids and calcium has not been demonstrated.

Since the data described in this manuscript were from short term studies and conducted on non-neoplastic colons, caution is necessary in extrapolating the findings to neoplastic events. Increased cell proliferation and proliferative abnormalities have been noted in the colonic epithelium undergoing neoplastic transformation and in people with a higher risk for colon cancer development (Lipkin, 1974; Lipkin et al, 1985). However, the role of cell proliferation in colon tumorigenesis is not well understood. Also, the role of calcium and a high fat diet in colon carcinogenesis can be assessed only when a direct link can be made between a high fat diet together with increased level of bile acids and/or free fatty acids in the colonic lumen and a concomitant increase in colon cell proliferation followed by an increase in tumor incidence.

ACKNOWLEDGEMENT:

We thank Ms. M. Magee for typing this manuscript and Mr. D. Stamp and Mr. R. Schneider for technical assistance.

TABLE 1. Effect of dietary calcium on cholic acid induced enhanced cell proliferation in the colonic epithelium (a)

Dietary Group	Labelling Index
0.1% Ca	8.5 ± 1.6
1.0% Ca	5.1 ± 0.7 (b)
0.1% Ca + CA	19.0 ± 1.6
1.0% Ca + CA	11.9 ± 1.3 (b)

(a) Mean ± SEM 6 to 10 animals/group
(b) Significantly different from the corresponding value for the low calcium group (p < 0.05)

TABLE 2. Influence of dietary calcium on the susceptibility of colonic epithelium to the mitogenic response induced by orally administered fat

		Metaphase figures/crypt	
Dietary Ca (%)	Control	0.1 ml beef tallow (a)	0.1 ml corn oil (b)
0.1	1.78±0.32	5.10±0.84	3.1 ±0.66
0.5	1.08±0.18	2.72±0.18	1.90±0.35
1.0	1.21±0.15	2.20±0.18	2.65±0.41

Animals were fed various diets for two weeks, then they were gavaged with saline (control), 0.1 ml of beef tallow or corn oil/animal. Colonic sections were enumerated for metaphase figures in the longitudinal sections of full crypts.

(a) 5 animals/group, 10 crypts/animal. The value for 0.1 Ca group given beef tallow is significantly different from the other two calcium groups.
(b) 6-9 animals/group, 10 crypts/animal.

REFERENCES

Ammon HV, Phillips S (1979). Inhibition of colonic water and electrolyte absorption by fatty acids in man. Gastroenterology 65: 744-749.

Bird RP (1986). Effect of dietary components on the pathobiology of colonic epithelium: Possible significance to colon tumorigenesis. Lipids (in press).

Bird RP, Medline A, Furrer R and Bruce WR (1985). Toxicity of orally administered fat to the colonic epithelium of mice. Carcinogenesis 6: 1063-1066.

Bird RP, Schneider R, Stamp D, Bruce WR (1986). Effect of dietary calcium and cholic acid on the proliferative indices of murine colonic epithelium. Submitted for publication.

Bird RP, Stamp D (1986). Effect of low and high fat diet on the proliferative indices of murine colonic epithelium. Cancer Lett (in press).

Bull AW, Marnett LJ, Dane EJ, Nigro ND (1983). Stimulation of deoxythymidine incorporation in the colon of rats treated with bile acids and fats. Carcinogenesis 4: 207-210.

Butcher (1953). The penetration of fat and fatty acids into the skin of the rat. J Invest Dermat 26: 43-48.

Cohen BI, Raicht RF, Deschner EE, Takahashi M, Sarwal AN and Fizzini E (1980). Effect of cholic acid feeding on N-methyl-N-nitrosourea-induced colon tumors and cell kinetics in rats. J Natl Cancer Inst 64: 573-576.

Deschner EE, Cohen BI, Raicht RF (1981). Acute and chronic effect of dietary cholic acid on colonic epithelial cell proliferation. Digestion 21: 290-296.

Gaginella TS, Chadwick VS, Debognie JC, Lewis JC, Phillips SF (1977). Perfusion of rabbit colon with ricinoleic acid: Dose related mucosal injury, fluid secretion, and increased permeability. Gastro-enterology 73: 95-101.

Hagerty CS (1938). Embolic glomerulonephritis produced with human fat, fatty acids and calcium soaps. Arch Path 25: 24-34.

Lipkin M (1974). Phase 1 and phase 2 proliferative lesions of colonic epithelial cells in premalignant diseases leading to colonic cancer. Cancer 34: 878-888.

Lipkin M, Vehara K, Winawer S, Sanchez A, Bauer C, Phillips R, Lynch HT, Blattner WA and Fraumeni Jr, JF (1985). Seventh-Day Adventist vegetarians have quiescent proliferative activity in colonic mucosa. Cancer Lett 26: 139-144.

Newmark HL, Wargovich MJ and Bruce WR. Colon cancer and dietary fat, phosphate and calcium: a hypothesis. J Natl Cancer Inst 72: 1323-1325.

Peltier (1956). The toxic properties of neutral fat and free fatty acid. Surgery 10: 665-670.

Pinkerton H (1928). The reaction to the oils and fats in the lung. Arch Path 5: 380-401.

Rafter J, Eng VWS, Furrer R, Medline A, Bruce WR (1986). The effect of calcium and pH on the mucosal damage produced by deoxycholic acid in the rat colon. Gut (in press).

Reese DH. The role of calcium in the regulation of urothelial growth. In "The Role of Calcium in Biological Systems", Anghileri L and Tuffet-Anghileri AM (eds), pp. 165-173, CRC Press Inc., Boca Raton, Florida.

Report of the American Institute of Nutrition, Ad Hoc Committee on Standards of Nutritional Studies (1977). J. Nutr : 1340-1348.

Vahouny GV, Cassidy MM, Lightfoot F, Grace L, Kritchevsky D (1981). Ultrastructural modifications of intestinal and colonic mucosa induced by free or bound bile acids. Cancer Res 41: 3764-3765.

Wargovich MJ, Eng VWS, Newmark HL, Bruce WR (1983). Calcium ameliorates the toxic effect of deoxycholic acid on colonic epithelium. Carcinogenesis 4: 1205-1207.

Wargovich MJ, Eng VWS, Newmark HL (1984). Calcium inhibits the damaging and compensatory proliferative effects of fatty acids on mouse colonic epithelium. Cancer Lett 23: 253-258.

Dietary Fat and Cancer, pages 495–515
© 1986 Alan R. Liss, Inc.

FAT, CALORIES AND FIBER

David Kritchevsky

The Wistar Institute of Anatomy and Biology,
Philadelphia, Pennsylvania 19104

INTRODUCTION

Cancer is a multifactorial disease. Armstrong and Doll (1975) cautioned that correlations between specific food items and cancer "should be taken only as suggestions for further research and not as evidence of causations or as bases for preventive action." Still, it is tempting to indict one or another dietary component as being the "prime suspect" in cancer etiology. Few investigators have been able to resist this temptation.

FAT AND CALORIES

In 1939 Baumann, Jacobi and Rusch reported that diets high in fat accelerated UV-induced epitheliomas and benzpyrene-induced skin tumors. Further work (Jacobi and Baumann, 1940) showed that diets containing more than 15% fat accelerated production of skin tumors induced by benz(a)pyrene (BP), methylcholanthrene (MC) or 7,12-dimethylbenz(a)anthracene (DMBA). Similar results were obtained using any of five fats (coconut oil, butter, lard, wheat germ oil or partially hydrogenated cottonseed oil) so that the response was considered to be a general one. Highly saturated fats such as coconut oil, hydrogenated coconut oil or trilaurin were less co-carcinogenic than corn oil in rats fed p-dimethyl-aminoazobenzene (Miller et al., 1944). A similar observation was made later with relation to fats and DMBA-induced mammary tumors (Carroll and Khor, 1971). Meat ingestion (as a source of fat and cholesterol) has been suggested as being positively correlated with colon cancer. Copeman and Greenwood (1926) commented that certain famous British medical men had suggested that "...rich abundant food, particularly meat, contributes to the production of cancer; that intestinal stasis conditioned by the diet of civilized mankind is the most important aetiological factor of malignant disease; and that increased use of preservatives in the food industries has a bearing upon the increased mortality from cancer." A survey of cancer among various religious orders did not bear out the surmise concerning meat (Copeman and Greenwood, 1926) and this finding was confirmed almost six decades later (Kinlen, 1982). For the general population, Enstrom (1975) had shown that between 1940 and 1970, meat intake in the United States had doubled while the incidence of colon cancer had not changed. A diet high in meat is usually a sign of affluence and the cancers more prevalent among affluent, Western societies (breast, colon, prostate) have long been positively correlated with dietary fat. Dietary fat is, in turn, associated with diets high in calories and Berg (1975) and Howell (1975) have indeed suggested that correlations of certain tumors with overall dietary lifestyle might be pertinent. Many aspects, probably every aspect, of dietary fat and cancer are being discussed elsewhere in this monograph. The ensuing discussion will center on the role of caloric intake in tumorigenesis.

Moreschi (1909) found that underfeeding could retard markedly the growth of transplanted sarcomas in mice. The underfed mice usually lost weight but on occasion tumor size was smaller even when the mice had gained weight. Rous (1914, 1915) examined the effect of dietary restriction on regeneration of spontaneous tumors in mice. He excised the tumors leaving a small fragment behind, recurrence of the tumor occurred in 83% of mice fed freely and in only 41% of mice who were underfed. A 67% restriction in food intake inhibited recurrence or growth of transplanted or spontaneous tumors in rats and mice (Sugiura and Benedict, 1926). Bischoff and his colleagues (1935, 1938) observed similar effects of caloric restriction on growth of Sarcoma 180 in mice.

The most thorough investigation of effects of dietary restriction on growth of spontaneous and induced tumors was carried out by Tannenbaum in the 1940's. Tannenbaum examined both underfeeding (in which the test animals were offered less of the diet fed the controls) and caloric restriction (in which specific caloric restriction is achieved by restriction of a specific nutrient). Underfeeding (Tannenbaum 1940) reduced the incidence of BP-induced skin tumors in mice by 75%; of BP-induced sarcomas by 37%; and of spontaneous mammary tumors by 95% in parous mice and by 77% in virgin mice. The underfed mice were given between one-third and one-half of the amount of diet presented to the controls.

In his experiments involving caloric restriction, Tannenbaum used a control diet containing commercial dog or fox ration, skim milk powder and corn starch. Caloric restriction was achieved by deleting various amounts of corn starch. Caloric restriction inhibited formation of induced or spontanous tumors in four different strains of mice (Tannenbaum, 1942) (Table 1). Tannenbaum (1945) also considered the effects of reduction of levels of "essential" nutrients (akin to underfeeding). He considered protein, vitamins and minerals to be the essentials. The principal effects were due to calories and, in isocaloric regimens, to fat.

TABLE 1. Caloric Restriction and Tumorigenesis in Mice*

Tumor	Mouse Strain	% of Control
Induced Epithelial	ABC	42
	Swiss	65
	DBA	34
Induced Sarcomas	C57 black	60
	Swiss	45
Spontaneous Mammary	DBA	30
Spontaneous Lung	ABC	53
	Swiss	19

*After Tannenbaum (1940)

Boutwell et al. (1949) examined the effects of fat and calories on BP-induced skin tumors in mice fed a well

defined semipurified diet. On a low fat diet the percentage of carcinomas on 12.1, 10.0, 8.0 or 6.0
calories/mouse/day were 82, 64, 49, and 18, respectively.
On a medium fat diet the percentages of carcinomas in mice
fed 10 or 6 calories/day were 72 and 33. Thus, at the same
level of caloric intake a low fat diet led to 11% fewer
tumors (10 calories/day) or 33% fewer tumors (6
calories/day). When mice were fed isocaloric amounts of
diets containing 2 or 61% fat weight gain was similar and
percent carcinomas was 64 on the 2% fat diet and 78 on the
61% fat diet. The findings were interpreted to mean that
there is a residual caloric effect of fat which leads to
increased tumor formation. Forbes et al. (1946 a, b) had
suggested that the energy expense of utilization of a diet
is reduced as fat content increases. In other words, the
metabolic energy value of fat may be more than the 9
calories/gm adduced from calorimetric measurements. A
similar suggestion has been advanced recently by Donato and
Hegsted (1985). Boutwell's data also show that at 10
calories/mouse/day, a medium fat diet leads to 12.5% more
tumors than a low fat diet and to 12.2% fewer tumors than
seen in mice fed a low fat diet at a level of 12.1
calories/mouse/day.

White (1961) summarized the literature on caloric
restriction and tumorigenesis available in 1961. More
recently, Tucker (1979) has shown that food restriction by
20% lowered incidence and onset of common tumors in mice
and rats. Incidence of radiation-induced tumors in rats
was reduced by 77% when diet was restricted by 67% (Gross
and Dreyfuss, 1984). Incidence of methylazoxymethanol-
induced tumors in rats was significantly reduced by 25-33%
reduction in calories (Pollard et al., 1984).

Lavik and Baumann (1943) altered fat and caloric content of diet fed mice in whom skin tumors were being
induced by MC. They found that a diet low in fat but high
in calories led to 93% more tumors than one high in fat but
low in calories and caused only 18% fewer tumors than a
diet high in both calories and fat (Table 2).

TABLE 2. Influence of Fat and Calories on Incidence of
Methylcholanthrene-Induced Skin Tumors in Mice*

Fat	Calories	Incidence (%)
Low	Low	0
Low	High	54
High	Low	28
High	High	66

* After Lavik and Baumann (1943)

Kritchevsky et al. (1984) approached this question by
investigating the effects of drastic caloric restriction
(by 40%) on DMBA-induced mammary tumors in rats fed more
fat than the ad libitum-fed controls. The experimental
diets were devised to provide equal levels of fiber,
minerals and vitamins. The ad libitum diet provided 3.9%
fat (2.9% coconut oil and 1.0% corn oil) (9.8% of
calories). The calorie restricted diet contained 14% fat
and, as fed, provided 8.4% fat (7.8% coconut oil, 0.6% corn
oil) (34.2% of calories). The tumor incidence in the
freely fed rats was 58% whereas no tumors were found in the
rats whose calories were restricted by 40%. We repeated
this study using a calorie restricted diet which differed
from the control diet only in level of sucrose and fat.
The dietary fat was corn oil. Calories were restricted by
40% and, while the fat content of the control diet was 4%
(10% of calories), that of the diet actually ingested by
the calorie restricted rats contained 7.9% corn oil (32.3%
of calories). The diets were used in experiments involving
DMBA-induced mammary tumors in female Sprague-Dawley rats
and 1,2-dimethylhydrazine (DMH)-induced colon tumors in
male F344 rats. The results (Table 3) show that the rats
fed the calorically restricted diet showed significantly
fewer mammary or colonic tumors.

TABLE 3. Caloric Restriction (40%) and Tumorigenesis in Rats.

Group	% Fat	Incidence (%)
Mammary Tumors[a]		
Ad Lib	3.9[c]	58
Restricted	8.4	0
Ad Lib	4.0	80
Restricted	7.9	20
Colon Tumors[b]		
Ad Lib	4.0	100
Restricted	7.9	53

[a] DMBA-induced, female Sprague-Dawley rats
[b] DMH-induced, male F344 rats
[c] 1% corn oil remainder coconut oil in first study; only corn oil used in others

Caloric restriction by 40% is drastic and the levels of fat fed was rather low and the questions of effects of more reasonable caloric restriction or of increased fat content were considered. In one study, we compared reduction of calories by 10, 20, 30 or 40%. The diets, as fed, all contained the same levels of casein, corn oil (5%), cellulose, vitamins and minerals. The effects of serial reduction of calories on DMBA-induced mammary tumors were examined. As Table 4 shows, 10% restriction of calories did not affect tumor incidence but tumors/tumor-bearing rat and tumor weight were reduced by 36 and 10%, respectively, with a 47% reduction in tumor burden. Twenty percent reduction in calories led to a 33% reduction in tumor incidence but other tumor characteristics were similar to those observed in rats whose caloric intake was reduced by 10%. Caloric restriction by 30% resulted in 42% reduction in tumor incidence and a 91% reduction in tumor burden (compared to controls); one of 20 rats whose caloric intake was reduced by 40% exhibited a single tumor.

TABLE 4. Graded Caloric Restriction and Mammary Tumors in Rats*

Restriction	Incidence[a] (%)	T/TBR	Tumor Burden[b] (g)
None	60	4.7 ± 1.3	10.1 ± 3.3
10%	60	3.0 ± 0.8	5.4 ± 3.0
20%	40	2.8 ± 0.7	4.7 ± 1.9
30%	30	1.3 ± 0.3	0.9 ± 0.8
40%	5	1.0 ± 0	

*DMBA-induced; [a] $p < 0.005$; [b] $p < 0.05$

In another experiment, calories were restricted by 25% and the level of fat ingested in the diet was 5, 15 or 20% in control rats and 15 or 20% in the calorie restricted animals. Mammary tumors were induced by DMBA administration. The control rats ingested corn oil at levels of 5% (12.4% of calories), 15% (32.5% of calories) or 20% (40.9% of calories); rats subjected to caloric restriction ingested 15% (43.0% of calories) or 20% (71.2% of calories) corn oil. The results (Table 5) show that increasing fat content in either ad libitum or restricted diet increases tumor burden but rats fed the same absolute level of corn oil as controls but restricted in calories exhibit significantly lower tumor incidence, number, weight and burden. Caloric restriction by 25% reduced weight gain by 26-28%.

TABLE 5. Effect of 25% Caloric Restriction on DMBA-Induced Mammary Tumors in Rats

Group	% Corn Oil	Incidence (%)	T/TBR[a]
Ad Lib	5	65	1.9 ± 0.3
Ad Lib	15	85	3.0 ± 0.6
Restricted	15[b]	60	1.9 ± 0.4
Ad Lib	20	80	4.1 ± 0.6
Restricted	20[c]	30	1.5 ± 0.3

[a] Tumors/tumor-bearing rat
[b] Diet contained 20% fat, effective dose 15%
[c] Diet contained 26.7% fat, effective dose 20%

Boissonneault et al. (1986) reported on tumor incidence in DMBA-treated female F344 rats who were fed a high fat diet, a low fat diet or a high fat diet in which calories were restricted by 16% compared to the ad libitum-fed high fat diet. The rats fed the high fat diet ingested 40.8 ± 1.5 kcal/day and 2.7 g of fat/day; those fed the low fat diet ate 42.4 ± 2.7 kcal/day and 0.6 g fat daily; and the restricted high fat group took 34.1 ± 1.0 kcal and 2.2 g fat per day. Tumor incidence was 73, 43 and 7%, respectively.

Caloric restriction results in reduced weight gain. Loeb et al. (1942) found a direct relationship between body weight and frequency of mammary carcinoma in several strains of mice. Modalities (hypothermia, dinitrophenol, sodium fluoride) other than caloric restriction which lead to weight loss inhibited spontaneous mammary tumor formation in mice (Tannenbaum and Silverstone, 1949). Thyroid extract, when fed, caused mice to eat more but weigh less than controls. This treatment retarded development of BP-induced skin tumors (Silverstone and Tannenbaum, 1949). Turnbull et al. (1985) studied the relationship of body weight to neoplasia in male and female Sprague-Dawley rats of both sexes observed for over two years. Eventual incidence of tumors was related to body weight. McCay and his colleagues (1935, 1938 a,b, 1943) found that rats which were underfed did not grow as large as their ad libitum-fed litter mates but lived longer and appeared healthier, exhibiting fewer chronic diseases. Carlson and Hoelzel (1946) found that rats fasted every other day lived 154 days longer (25%) and exhibited 81% fewer spontaneous tumors. Fasting one day in four reduced tumor incidence by 22%.

The most thorough lifetime studies of caloric restriction and tumorigenesis have been conducted by Ross and his associates. Ross and Bras (1971) placed 650 rats into three groups who were fed: ad libitum for their entire life span (AL); calorically restricted (by 60-70%) for their entire life span (R); or fed a restricted diet for seven weeks post weaning (21-70 days) then fed ad libitum (R-AL). Only 12% of AL rats lived beyond 800 days, none lived past 1000 days; 23% of R-AL rats lived beyond 800 days, none past 1000 days; and 76% of the R rats lived beyond 800 days and 39% lived between 1000 and 1499 days. Both restricted groups exhibited about half as many benign tumors as did group AL; groups R and R-AL exhibited 15 and 31% fewer malignant tumors than group AL. Sixty two percent of the benign tumors and 59% of the malignant tumors observed in group R appeared after 999 days. The three dietary groups were divided into lighter and heavier subgroups. The incidence of tumors in the heavier subgroup was greater in every case. Ratios of tumor incidence (heavy/light) were: AL group: all tumors - 1.62, benign - 1.98; malignant - 1.42; R group: all tumors - 2.06, benign - 1.32; malignant - 4.81; and R-AL group: all tumors - 1.95, benign - 2.14, malignant - 1.55.

Dietary practices which increased the probability of tumor development in rats were: 1) high absolute protein intake shortly after weaning; 2) high efficiency of converting food into body mass at puberty; 3) high level of protein intake relative to body weight in early adulthood; 4) high food intake in early adulthood; and 5) rapid growth during early post natal life (Ross et al., 1982). Total tumor risk was directly and exponentially related to caloric intake (Ross and Bras, 1965). Garfinkel (1985) has summarized data relating to overweight and cancer and has reported on mortality ratios for cancer sites affected by increased weight. Greenberg et al. (1985) have analyzed survival in premenopausal breast cancer as a function of body size. Quelelet index was not significantly related to survival although the tallest and most obese women fared worst. Perhaps the practices cited above (Ross et al., 1982) relate to humans as well as rats.

Fat and calories both influence tumorigenesis. Under conditions of ad libitum feeding, increased dietary fat leads to increased tumor incidence. Caloric restriction will inhibit tumor formation but even when calories are restricted, increased dietary fat will affect tumorigenesis to some extent. The experimental data suggest that caloric restriction overrides fat level of the diet.

FIBER

Dietary fiber is generally defined as plant material which defies degradation by our digestive juices or enzymes (Trowell, 1976). The major components of dietary fiber are cellulose, hemicellulose, pectin and lignin and the description has been expanded to include gums, mucilages, and algal polysaccharides. Analysis of foodstuffs for fiber is still not standardized but methodology has improved vastly in the last few years and it is becoming possible to obtain accurate assessment of all fiber components (Selvendran and DuPont, 1984; Prosky, 1986; Englyst and Cummings, 1986). A simple classification which is used with increasing frequency is into insoluble fiber (lignin, cellulose, hemicellulose) which increase fecal bulk and decreases intestinal transit time and soluble fiber (pectin, gums) which delays gastric emptying and delays glucose absorption. Cleave (1956) related diseases of the developed world to diet containing refined carbohydrates and later Burkitt (1971) based his hypothesis concerning fiber and cancer upon observations of African populations. It must be noted that the "fiber hypothesis" is based on overall dietary lifestyle.

Epidemiological data relating to diet and colon cancer date to the work of Stocks and Karns (1933) who examined dietary habits of 450 colon cancer patients and controls and found negative corelations with intake of whole meal bread, vegetables and milk. The epidemiological data have been reviewed (Cummings, 1981; Kritchevsky, 1983; Byers and Graham, 1984; Willett and MacMahon, 1984; Bingham, 1986) and do not reveal unanimity regarding a protective role for fiber. Byers and Graham (1984) discussed the strengths and weaknesses of epidemiologic investigations, but the various features of epidemiology are beyond the scope of this essay, suffice it to point out that a committee of the National Academy of Science (USA) (1982) concluded: "The committee found no conclusive evidence to indicate that dietary fiber (such as present in fruits, vegetables, grains and cereals) exerts a protective effect against colorectal cancer in humans." Bingham et al. (1979) found a negative correlation between pentose-rich fiber and colorectal cancer mortality in England, but not between total fiber and cancer mortality. Reanalysis of their earlier data using more accurate methods of fiber analysis now shows the best negative correlation to be with non-starch polysaccharides (Bingham et al., 1985). A recently published analysis of diet and cancer mortality for men in 38 countries showed, after adjustment for other dietary components, that cereals were the only form of dietary fiber negatively correlated with mortality (McKeown-Eyssen abd Bright-See, 1984). A study of diets of rural and urban populations in a country at low risk for colon cancer (Finland) and one at high risk (Denmark) showed negative correlations with carbohydrate, cereals, protein, saturated fat, starch and total dietary fiber and positive correlations with alcohol and fecal bile acid concentration (Jensen et al., 1982). Several studies discussed in the reviews which have been cited have not found correlations between dietary fiber and colon cancer. One problem is that some analyses have utilized data on fiber-rich foods. Foods are sources of more than one type of fiber and the properties of a particular fiber may be affected by its interaction with other components of the food matrix in which it is present.

Animal studies are difficult to analyze. The experiments (almost exclusively in rats) involve differences in strain, sex, carcinogen, mode of administration, diet and type and amount of fiber (Kritchevsky 1983,1984).

Not all types of fiber confer protection from chemically-induced colon cancer. Glauert et al. (1981) found agar to enhance DMH-induced colon cancer in mice. Jacobs and Lupton (1986) found a higher incidence of DMH-induced large bowel tumors in rats fed pectin, guar gum or oat bran than in fiber-free controls. Klurfeld et al. (1986) found increased incidence of DMH-induced colon tumors in   rats with increasing levels of dietary cellulose. All the data are complex and different fibers affect distribution of tumors in various parts of the large intestine.

Dietary fiber can exert a number of different effects in the human colon (Table 6). Effects on fecal weight and transit time do not appear to be important. Japanese immigrants to Hawaii and their sons exhibit similar transit time and stool weight but the fathers have a low incidence of colon cancer and that of their sons is the same as that of Hawaiian Caucasians (Glober et al., 1977). Dietary fiber will adsorb bile acids, bile salts, and other lipids, the extent of adsorption being determined by both the type of fiber and the type of bile acid or salt (Eastwood and Hamilton, 1968; Story and Kritchevsky, 1976; Vahouny et al., 1980). Cholestyramine, a potent binder of bile acids, enhances chemically-induced colon cancer in rats (Nigro et al., 1973) and it has been shown that different fibers, when fed to rats, induced varying degrees of disruption of normal intestinal mucosal topography (Cassidy et al., 1981)

TABLE 6. Influences of Dietary Fiber in the Human Colon.

Increases fecal weight

Increases frequency of defecation

Decreases transit time

Dilutes colonic contents

Increases microbial growth

Alters energy metabolism

Absorbs organic and inorganic substances

Decreases dehydroxylation of bile acids

Produces H_2, CH_4, CO_2 and short chain fatty acids

The usually observed increase in fecal bulk seen when fiber is added to the diet may be taken as evidence of dilution of colonic contents. Decreased concentration of

fecal bile acids has been shown to correlate positively
with decreased risk of colon cancer. Hill et al. (1971)
found fecal acidic steroid concentrations in developed
countries (US, UK) to be 6.15 ± 0.66 mg/g feces, whereas in
low risk countries such as Uganda, Japan and India fecal
bile acids concentrations was 0.61 ± 0.13. Crowther et al.
(1976) studied cancer and diet in three socioeconomic
groups in Hong Kong and found that concentration of bile
acids rose with increasing affluence and so did incidence
of colon cancer. It is interesting to note (Hill et al.,
1979) that the most affluent subjects ate more of
everything (calories, fats, vegetables, fiber) than the
poorest. Comparison of fecal bile acid concentration in
Danes (high risk) and Finns (low risk) shows the lowest
risk group (rural Finns) to have a 33% lower concentration
of bile acids in feces than the highest risk group (urban
Danes) (Jensen et al., 1982). The concentration of bile
acids in feces of New Yorkers is 11.7mg/g feces compared to
4.6 mg/g in residents of Kuopio, Finland (Reddy et al.,
1978).

The polysaccharides of dietary fiber are degraded in
the large intestine. Among the products of degradation are
short chain fatty acids (SCFA) - acetic, propionic and
butyric. The SCFA can be absorbed through the intestinal
wall and represent a source of energy (Cummings and Brnach,
1986). SCFA would tend to reduce colonic pH which has been
thought to inhibit tumorigenesis (Thornton, 1981). Parish
and Lupton (1986) have shown that dietary fiber does indeed
lower intestinal pH and that wheat bran leads to increased
production of butyric acid and pectin leads to more propionic acid. Jacobs and Lupton (1986) concluded that lower
luminal pH was associated with higher tumor yield. Studies
of pH effects and action of specific SCFA are only now
beginning. Data concerning effects of SCFA as a function
of their source (i.e. specific fiber) would be welcome.

Secondary bile acid, deoxycholic and lithocholic acids,
are produced by dehydroxylation of cholic and chenodeoxycholic acids, respectively. The secondary bile acids
are regarded as being mutagenic or co-carcinogenic (Hill,
1982). The dehydroxylation is carried out by the intestinal flora. Anaerobic bacteria metabolize steroids more
actively than aerobic bacteria and the ratio of anaerobes
to aerobes in countries with high incidence of colon cancer
is more than twice that seen in low risk countries (Hill et

al., 1971). One would think, then, that the ratio of primary to secondary fecal bile acids might provide clues to
risk or susceptibility but efforts to adduce such a correlation have not been successful (Kritchevsky and Klurfeld,
1981).

Dietary fiber enhances fecal energy loss (Southgate and
Durnin, 1970; Kelsay et al., 1978). Increased energy loss
results in reduced caloric availability . The loss of
calories may go unnoticed in developed countries with high
caloric intake, but in underdeveloped countries the reduction in caloric availability due to dietary fiber may be
significant. We have demonstrated (vide supra) that
caloric reduction inhibits tumori-genesis in rats and,
under certain conditions, it may do so in man. Ross and
Bras (1971) showed that deprivation of calories in rats for
only a few weeks post-weaning reduced risk of spontaneous
carcinogenesis by 40%. This observation may help to
explain some of the human migrant data. The Japanese
immigrant to Hawaii was subsisting on his indigenous diet
until he moved and then was exposed to a luxus diet; his
Hawaiian-born son, on the other hand, has always had the
rich American diet.

There are data which associate dietary differences to
different risk of colon cancer but dietary differences are
accompanied by other environmental and cultural variables.
Regional differences in colon cancer incidence in the
United States (Blot et al., 1976) remain to be examined
closely. The cancers which predominate in developed
countries are related to high fat and calories and low
fiber. Gregor et al. (1969) showed a positive correlation
between standard of living and mortalty for colon cancer.
Hakama and Saxen (1967) reported a positive association
between cereal consumption and stomach cancer mortality as
well as a negative association between per capita income
and stomach cancer mortality. Diet does not cause nor cure
cancer. However, various aspects of diet have been correlated with increased risk of certain types of cancer in
selected populations.

The cancers prevalent in the developed world may be due
to caloric excess as evidenced by high fat and low fiber
intake. There is still no universally accepted thread of
evidence linking fiber to definite protection from colon
cancer. If we go back to the earliest epidemiological

study (Stocks and Karns, 1933) we have been exploiting part of their evidence, negative association with whole grain and vegetables, but not that relating to dairy foods. More data are needed concerning the roles of various micro-nutrients, proportions of macronutrients, and interactions among macronutrients. A moderate increase in fiber-rich foods has been suggested in a number of dietary guidelines but the currently available data do not permit one to pro-mise reduced risk of cancer with confidence or comfort. Virtually every set of dietary guidelines, regardless of its disease orientation, recommends maintenance of ideal weight. This might serve as the best starting point in consideration of dietary modulation of tumorigenesis.

ACKNOWLEDGEMENTS

Supported, in part, by a Research Career Award (HL00734) from the National Institutes of Health, and by funds from the Commonwealth of Pennsylvania.

REFERENCES

Armstrong B and Doll R (1975). Enviromental factors and cancer incidence and mortality in different countries, with special reference to dietary practices. Int J Cancer 15: 617-631.

Baumann CA, Jacobi HP and Rusch HP (1939). The effect of diet on experimental tumor production. Am J Hygiene 30: 1-6.

Berg JW (1975). Can nutrition explain the pattern of international epidemiology of hormone-dependent cancers? Cancer Res 35: 3345-3350.

Bingham SA (1986). Epidemiology of dietary fiber and colorectal cancer: current status of the hypothesis. In Vahouny GV, Kritchevsky D (eds): "Dietary Fiber: Basic and Clinical Aspects," New York: Plenum Press, pp 523-542.

Bingham SA, Williams DRR, Cole TJ, James WPT (1979). Dietary fibre and regional large bowel cancer mortality in Britain. Br J Cancer 40: 456-463.

Bingham SA, Williams DRR, Cummings JH (1985). Dietary fibre consumption in Britain: new estimates and their relation to large bowel cancer mortality. Br J Cancer 52: 399-402.

Bischoff F and Long ML (1938). The influence of calories per se upon the growth of Sarcoma 180. Am J Cancer 32: 418-421.

Bischoff F, Long ML and Maxwell LC (1935). Influence of caloric intake upon the growth of Sarcoma 180. Am J Cancer 24: 549-553.

Blot WJ, Fraumeni FJ Jr, Stone BJ, McKay FW (1976). Geographic patterns of large bowel cancer in the United States. J Natl Cancer Inst 57: 1225-1231.

Boissonneault GA, Elson ED and Pariza MW (1986). Net energy effects of dietary fat on chemically-induced mammary carcinogenesis in F344 rats. J Nat Cancer Inst 76: 335-338.

Boutwell RK, Brush MK and Rusch HP (1949). The stimulating effect of dietary fat on carcinogenesis. Cancer Res 9: 741-746.

Byers T, Graham S (1984). The epidemiology of diet and cancer. Adv Cancer Res 41: 1-69.

Carlson AJ and Hoelzel F (1946). Apparent prolongation of the life span of rats by intermittent fasting. J Nutr 31: 363-375.

Carroll KK and Khor TH (1971). Effect of level and type of dietary fat on incidence of mammary tumors induced in female Sprague-Dawely rats by 7,12-dimethylbenz(a)anthracene. Lipids 6: 415-420.

Cassidy MM, Lightfoot FG, Grau LE, Story JA, Kritchevsky D, Vahouny GV (1981). Effect of intake of dietary fibers on the ultrastructural topography of rat jejunum and colon. A scanning electron microscope study. Am J Clin Nutr 34: 218-228.

Cleave TL (1956). The neglect of natural principles in current medical practice. J Roy Nav Med Serv 42: 55-82.

Committee on Diet, Nutrition and Cancer (1982). "Diet, Nutrition and Cancer," Washington, D.C., National Academy Press.

Copeman SM and Greenwood M (1926). Diet and cancer, with special reference to the incidence of cancer upon members of certain religious orders. Report on Public Health and Medical Subjects, No. 36: Ministry of Health, London, pp 1-31.

Crowther JS, Drasar BS, Hill MJ, Maclennan R, Magnin D, Peck S, Teah-Chan CH (1976). Faecal steroids and bacteria and large bowel cancer in Hong Kong by socioeconomic groups. Br J Cancer 34: 191-198.

Cummings JH (1981). Dietary fibre and large bowel cancer. Proc Nutr Soc 40: 7-14.

Cummings JH, Branch WJ (1986). Fermentation and production of short chain fatty acids in the human large intestine. In Vahouny GV, Kritchevsky D (eds): "Dietary Fiber: Basic and Clinical Aspects," New York: Plenum Press, pp 131-149.

Donato K and Hegsted DM (1985). Efficiency of utilization of various sources of energy for growth. Proc Natl Acad Sci (USA) 82: 4866-4870.

Eastwood MA, Hamilton D (1968). Studies on the adsorption of bile salts to non-absorbed components of diet. Biochim Biophys Acta 152: 165-173.

Englyst HN, Cummings JH (1986). Measurement of dietary fiber as non-starch polysaccharides. In Vahouny GV, Kritchevsky D (eds): "Dietary Fiber: Basic and Clinical Aspects," New York: Plenum Press, pp 17-34.

Enstrom JE (1975). Colorectal cancer and consumption of beef and fat. Br J Cancer 32: 432-439.

Forbes EB, Swift RW, Elliott RF and James WH (1946a). Relation of fat to economy of food utilization. II. By the mature albino rat. J Nutr 31: 213-227.

Forbes EB, Swift RW, Thacker EJ, Smith VF and French CE (1946b). Further experiments on the relation of fat to economy of food utilization. II. By the mature albino rat. J Nutr 32: 397-403.

Garfinkel L (1985). Overweight and cancer. Ann Int Med 103: 1034-1036.

Glauert HP, Bennink MR, Sander CH (1981). Enhancement of 1,2-dimethylhydrazine-induced carcinogenesis in mice by dietary agar. Food Cosmet Toxicol 19: 281-286.

Glober GA, Nomura A, Kamiyama S, Shimoda A, Abba BC (1977). Bowel transit time and stool weight in populations with different colon cancer risks. Lancet 2: 110.

Greenberg ER, Vessey MP, McPherson K, Doll R and Yeates D (1985). Body size and survival in premenopausal breast cancer. Br J Cancer 51: 691-697.

Gregor O, Toman R, Prusova F (1969). Gastrointestinal cancer and nutrition. Gut 10: 1031-1034.

Gross L and Dreyfuss Y (1984). Reduction in the incidence of radiation-induced tumors in rats after restriction of food intake. Proc Natl Acad Sci (USA) 81: 7596-7598.

Hakama M, Saxen EA (1967). Cereal consumption and gastric cancer. Int J Cancer 2: 265-268.

Hill MJ (1982). Bile acids and human colorectal cancer. In Vahouny GV, Kritchevsky D (eds): "Dietary Fiber in Health and Disease," New York: Plenum Press, pp 299-312.

Hill MJ, Drasar BS, Aries VC, Crowther JS, Hawksworth G,

Williams REO (1971). Bacteria and the aetiology of cancer of the large bowel. Lancet 1: 95-100.

Hill MJ, Maclennan R, Newcombe K (1979). Diet and large bowel cancer in three socioeconomic groups in Hong Kong. Lancet 1: 436.

Howell MA (1975). Diet as an etiological actor in the development of cancers of the colon and rectum. J Chronic Dis 28: 67-80.

Jacobi HP and Baumann CA (1940). The effect of fat on tumor formation. Am J Cancer 39: 338-342.

Jacobs LR, Lupton JR (1986.) Relations between colonic luminal pH, cell proliferation, and colon carcinogenesis in 1,2-dimethylhydrazine treated rats fed high fiber diets. Cancer Res 46: 1727-1734.

Jensen OM, Maclennan R, Wahrendorf J (1982). Diet, bowel function, fecal characteristics and large bowel cancer in Denmark and Finland. Nutr Cancer 4: 5-19.

Kelsay JL, Behall KM, Prather ES (1978). Effect of fiber from fruits and vegetables on metabolic responses of human subjects. 1. Bowel transit time, number of defecations, fecal weight, urinary excretions of energy and nitrogen and apparent digestibilities of energy, nitrogen and fat. Am J Clin Nutr 31: 1149-1153.

Kinlen MJ (1982). Meat and fat consumption and cancer mortality: a study of strict religious orders in Britain. Lancet 1: 946-949.

Klurfeld DM, Weber MM, Buck CL, Kritchevsky D (1986). Dose response of colonic carcinogenesis to different amounts and types of cellulose. Fed Proc 45: 1076.

Kritchevsky D (1983). Fiber, steroids and cancer. Cancer Res (Suppl) 43: 2419S-2495S.

Kritchevsky D (1984). Dietary fiber and cancer. Nutr Cancer 6: 213-219.

Kritchevsky D, Klurfeld DM (1981). Fat and Cancer. In Newell GR, Ellison NM (eds): "Nutrition and Cancer: Etiology and Treatment," New York: Raven Press: pp 173-188.

Kritchevsky D, Weber MM and Klurfeld DM (1984). Dietary fat versus caloric content in initiation and promotion of 7,12-dimethylbenz(a)anthracene-induced mammary tumorigenesis in rats. Cancer Res 44: 3174-3177.

Lavik PS and Baumann CA (1943). Further studies on tumor promoting action of fat. Cancer Res 3: 749-756.

Loeb L, Suntzeff V, Blumenthal HT and Kirtz MM (1942). Effect of weight on the development of mammary carcinoma in various strains of mice. Arch Path 33: 845-865.

McCay CM, Crowell MF and Maynard LA (1935). The effect of retarded growth upon the length of life span and upon the ultimate body size. J Nutr 10: 63-79.

McCay CM, Ellis GH, Barnes LL, Smith CAH and Sperling G (1939b). Chemical and pathological changes in aging and after retarded growth. J Nutr 18: 15-25.

McCay CM, Maynard LA, Sperling G and Barnes LL (1939a). Retarded growth, life span, ultimate body size and age changes in the albino rat after feeding diets restricted in calories. J Nutr 18: 1-13.

McCay CM, Sperling G and Barnes LL (1943). Growth, ageing, chronic diseases and life span in rats. Arch Biochem 2: 469-479.

McKeown-Eyssen GE, Bright-See E (1984). Dietary factors in colon cancer: International relationships. Nutr Cancer 6: 160-170.

Miller JA, Kline BE, Rusch HP and Baumann CA (1944). The effect of certain lipids on the carcinogenicity of p-dimethylamino-azobenzene. Cancer Res 4: 756-761.

Moreschi C (1909). Beziehungen zwischen ernahrung und tumorwachstum. Z f Immunitatsforsch 2: 651-675.

Nigro ND, Bhadrachari N, Chomchai C (1973). A rat model for studying colonic cancer: Effect of cholestyramine on induced tumors. Dis Colon Rectum 16: 438-443.

Parish PD, Lupton JR (1986). The effect of wheat bran and pectin supplementation on luminal pH and short chain fatty acid production in the rat large intestine. Fed Proc 45: 349.

Pollard M, Luckert PH and Pan GY (1984). Inhibition of intestinal tumorigenesis in methylazoxymethanol-treated rats by dietary restriction. Cancer Treatment Rep 58: 405-408.

Prosky L (1986). Analysis of total dietary fiber: The collaborative study. In Vahouny GV, Kritchevsky D (eds): "Dietary Fiber: Basic and Clinical Aspects," New York: Plenum Press, pp 1-16.

Reddy BS, Hedges AR, Laakso K, Wynder EL (1978). Metabolic epidemiology of large bowel cancer. Cancer 42: 2832-2838.

Ross MH and Bras G (1965). Tumor incidence patterns and nutrition in the rat. J Nutr 87: 245-260.

Ross MH and Bras G (1971). Lasting influence of early caloric restriction on prevalence of neoplasms in the rat. J Nat Cancer Inst 47: 1095-1113.

Ross MH, Lustbader ED and Bras G (1982). Dietary practices of early life and spontaneous tumors of the rat. Nutr and Cancer 3: 150-167.

Rous P (1914). The influence of diet on transplanted and spontaneous mouse tumors. J Exp Med 20: 433-451.

Rous P (1915). The influence of dieting upon the cause of cancer. Johns Hopkins Hosp Bull 26: 146-148.

Selvendran RR and DuPont MS 91984). The analysis of dietary fiber. In King RD (ed): "Food Analysis Techniques, Vol. 3," London: Applied Science, pp 1-68.

Silverstone H and Tannenbaum (1949). Influence of thyroid hormone on the formation of induced skin tumors in mice. Cancer Res 9: 684-688.

Stocks P, Karns MK (1933). A cooperative study of the habits, homelife, dietary and family histories of 450 cancer patients and an equal number of control patients. Ann Eugen (London) 5: 237-280.

Story JA, Kritchevsky D (1976). Comparison of the binding of various bile acids and bile salts by several types of fiber. J Nutr 106: 1292-1294.

Southgate DAT, Durnin JVGA (1970). Caloric conversion factors. An experimental reassessment of the factors used in the calculation of the energy value of human diets. Br J Nutr 24: 517-535.

Sugiura K and Benedict SR 91926). The influence of insufficient diets upon tumor recurrence and growth in rats and mice. Am J Cancer 10: 309-318.

Tannenbaum A (1940). The initiation and growth of tumors. I. Effects of underfeeding. Am J Cancer 38: 335-350.

Tannenbaum A (1942). The genesis and growth of tumors. II. Effects of caloric restriction per se. Cancer Res 2: 460-467.

Tannenbaum A (1945). The dependence of tumor formation on the composition of the calorie restricted diet as well as on the degree of restriction. Cancer Res 5: 616-625.

Tannenbaum A and Silverstone H (1949). Effect of low environmental temperature, dinitrophenol, or sodium fluoride on the formation of tumors in mice. Cancer Res 9: 403-410.

Thornton JR (1981). High colonic pH promotes colorectal cancer. Lancet 1: 1081-1083.

Trowell H (1976). Definition of dietary fiber and hypothesis that it is a protective factor in certain diseases. Am J Clin Nutr 29: 417-427.

Tucker MJ (1979). The effect of long term food restriction on tumors in rodents. Int J Cancer 23: 803-807.

Turnbull GJ, Lee PN and Roe FJC (1985). Relationship of body weight gain to longevity and to risk of development

of nephropathy and neoplasia in Sprague-Dawley rats.
Food Chem Toxic 23: 355-361.

Vahouny GV, Tombes R, Cassidy MM, Kritchevsky D, Gallo LL
(1980). Dietary fibers. V. Binding of bile salts,
phospholipids and cholesterol from mixed micelles by bile
acid sequestrants and dietary fibers. Lipids 15:
1012-1018.

White FR (1961). The relationship between underfeeding and
tumor formation, transplantation, and growth in rats and
mice. Cancer Res 21: 281-290.

Willett WC, MacMahon B (1984). Diet and cancer - an overview. New Engl J Med 310: 633-638, 697-703.

Dietary Fat and Cancer, pages 517-528
© 1986 Alan R. Liss, Inc.

ROLE OF ACUTE CALORIC-RESTRICTION IN MURINE TUMORIGENESIS

Paul W. Sylvester

Grace Cancer Drug Center
Roswell Park Memorial Institute
666 Elm Street, Buffalo, New York 14263

INTRODUCTION

Early studies by Tannenbaum (1940) were the first to show that caloric-restriction decreased the incidence of spontaneous mammary tumors in mice. Animals subjected to chronic food-restriction not only had fewer mammary tumors, but tumors also appeared later than in animals fed ad libitum. During the course of this work, the relationship between the degree of caloric-restriction and inhibition of mammary tumorigenesis was found to be non-linear. As caloric intake was reduced, only a gradual reduction in tumor formation was observed; when dietary restriction reached a critical level however, there was a sharp inhibition of tumor development (Tannenbaum, 1945). Furthermore, the reduction in mammary tumorigenesis by underfeeding was shown to be maximal when food-restriction was instituted prior to tumor appearance (Tannenbaum, 1944). Likewise, caloric-restriction at the time of tumor induction results in long-term inhibition of mammary carcinomas in rats (Ross and Bras, 1971).

These studies were among the first to indicate that both the degree and the timing of caloric-restriction are important determinants for the suppression of mammary tumorigenesis in rodents. Further studies revealed that intermittent caloric-restriction is not effective in suppressing mammary tumor development. When animals are fasted twice weekly for 24 hours, but allowed to feed ad libitum between fastings, the incidence and growth of spontaneous mammary tumors were not reduced, even though these animals consumed significantly less food overall than full-fed controls (Tannenbaum and Silverstone, 1950). A correlation between body weight and tumorigenesis in mice with varying degrees of caloric-restriction has also been demonstrated. Larger animals were found to be more susceptible to spontaneous mammary tumors than smaller animals, while food-restriction was more effective for the inhibition of tumorigenesis in the large mice. It was also shown that as little as a 20% reduction in food intake over a 2 year period, significantly inhibited the development of spontaneous mammary tumors in rats and mice (Tucker, 1979).

Caloric-restriction has also been shown to significantly reduce the incidence and growth of many types of non-endocrine tumors, including hepatomas, lung adenomas, leukemias, skin tumors, intestinal and colon tumors, and sarcomas (Carroll, 1975). It is possible that a common mechanism is involved in mediating the inhibitory effects of underfeeding on these diverse kinds of tumors, but at the present time it has not been identified. In general, underfed animals appear to be in good overall health, do not show signs of clinical nutritional deficiencies, and live longer than full-fed controls. It is unlikely therefore, that caloric-restriction suppression of murine tumorigenesis is due to the lack of some essential dietary component. Rather, caloric-restriction induces a wide range of physiological changes, particularly in the endocrine and immune systems, and it is possible that diverse mechanisms mediate the inhibitory effects of underfeeding on individual tumor types. The purpose of this communication will be to review the effects and discuss possible inhibitory mechanism(s) of acute caloric-restriction on tumorigenesis in rodents.

ENDOCRINOLOGY

Pituitary insufficiency as a result of underfeeding leads to decreased estrogen production, as indicated by regression in size of the ovaries, uterus, and mammary glands, similar to that seen in hypophysectomized animals (Huseby, et al., 1945). This condition has been referred to as "pseudohypophysectomy". Other investigators have demonstrated that food-restriction results in decreased secretion of anterior pituitary hormones, including prolactin and gonadotropins, as measured by radioimmunoassay (Campbell, et al., 1977). Underfeeding also diminishes gonadal steroids hormone secretion, which causes initial irregularities and finally loss of estrous cycles in rats (Piacsek and Meites, 1967). In addition to supression of pituitary hormone secretion, severe food restriction increases adrenocorticoid activity (Boutwell, et al., 1948).

Acute changes in circulating hormone levels in the rat have been shown to play a critical role in initiation and promotion of mammary carcinomas induced by aromatic hydrocarbons. Such mammary tumors arise in undifferentiated, rapidly proliferating epithelial terminal end buds and terminal ducts present in the mammary gland of young virgin females (Russo and Russo, 1978). The highest incidence of 7,12-dimethylbenz(a)anthracene (DMBA)-induced mammary tumors, arise when the carcinogen is administered between 50-55 days of age and are reduced markedly if the carcinogen is given to younger or older animals (Huggins, et al., 1961). Estrogen and prolactin induce mitosis in mammary epithelial cells. By promoting cellular replication and DNA synthesis, these hormones sensitize the mammary gland to maximal carcinogen binding around 55 days of age. Removal of estrogen and prolactin by ovariectomy inhibits hormone-dependent mitotic activity and renders the gland refractory to carcinogen action. Numerous experimental studies have shown that increased or decreased estrogen and prolactin levels prior to carcinogen administration, results in significant inhibition of mammary tumorigenesis (Meites, 1972). The decreased susceptibility of tumor induction by these hormones (the state of elevated hormone levels) is attributed to acceleration of mammary gland maturation, thus rendering the gland refractory to the carcinogen. Elevation of these hormones after carcinogen administration however, results in a significant stimulation of mammary tumor growth (Leung, et al., 1983). It has been established that the first week after carcinogen administration to Sprague-Dawley rats is critical in terms of hormonal requirements for development of mammary tumors (Dao, 1962).

Since food restriction results in decreased secretion of anterior pituitary and gonadal hormones, the hormonal deficiencies that develop during the first week after DMBA administration may be responsible for the inhibition of mammary tumorigenesis. It was of interest therefore, to determine whether administration of estrogen, prolactin, growth hormone, or all 3 together, given during the "crit-ical period" after DMBA administration, could overcome the inhibition of mammary tumors development and growth in rats.

Seven days prior to DMBA administration, virgin 50-day old female Sprague-Dawley rats were placed on a food-restricted diet (approximately 50% ad libitum controls) and continued on this regimen until 30 days after DMBA inject-ion. One day prior to and 7 days after DMBA administrat-ion, animals were given daily 0.1 ml s.c. injections of either 0.9% NaCl solution (controls), haloperidol (HAL, 0.5 mg/kg b.w.) to increase prolactin secretion, growth hormone (GH, 0.5 mg/kg b.w.), estradiol benzoate (EB, 1 ug/rat), or a combination of these three treatments. Restricted feeding continued until 30 days after DMBA administration, at which time all animals were placed on ad libitum feeding for the remainder of the 26 week experiment.

Table 1.
Effects of different treatments on development of mammary tumors at the end of 26 weeks

Treatment	% rats with tumors	No. tumors per rat	Av. latency period (days)
Full-fed	76[a]	1.94[a]	106.6 + 6.5[a]
Underfed	29	0.64	140.8 + 7.8
Underfed + HAL	60	0.84	125.5 + 6.6
Underfed + GH	33	0.46	105.9 + 8.8
Underfed + EB	71[a]	1.71[a]	126.2 + 3.0
Underfed + HAL + GH + EB	86[a]	2.35[a]	131.3 + 3.9

[a] $p < 0.05$, as compared to underfed controls. From Sylvester et al., 1981, with permission.

The effects of the various treatments on mammary tumor incidence are shown in Table 1. Food restriction for 7 days prior to and 30 days after DMBA administration significantly reduced mammary tumor incidence, number and tumor latency, as compared to full-fed controls. Food restricted rats which received daily injections of HAL or GH showed no significant differences in tumor development when compared with the food-restricted controls. However, underfed rats which received daily injections of EB or the combination of EB, GH and HAL displayed a significant increase in both mammary tumor incidence and number as compared with food-restricted controls.

The effect of drug and hormone injections on mammary tumor size in the different treatment groups are shown in Figure 1. Underfed controls showed a severe suppression in tumor burden that persisted throughout the entire 26 week experiment, as did food-restricted groups which received HAL or GH. Caloric-restricted animals which received EB, or the combination of EB, GH and HAL, 1 day prior to and 7 days after DMBA administration developed a significantly greater tumor burden as compared to food-restricted controls.

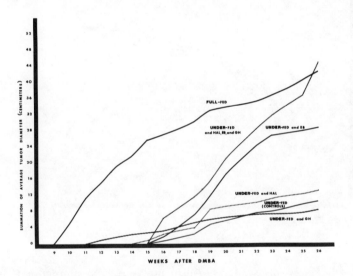

Figure 1. Summation of average tumor diameter. From Sylvester et.al., 1981, with permission.

Blood samples taken on the last day of treatment (7 days after DMBA administration) showed reduced serum prolactin levels in food-restricted controls as compared to full-fed controls. Caloric-restricted rats given HAL showed a significant elevation in serum prolactin, as did the food-restricted rats given EB. The food-restricted rats given the combination of HAL, EB, and GH showed significantly higher serum prolactin levels than any of the other groups. Serum prolactin levels in all underfed groups on the last day of caloric-restriction (30 days after DMBA administration) were significantly lower than full-fed controls. On the day the experiment was terminated (26th week after DMBA), when all animals had long since returned to ad libitum feeding, assays showed no differences in serum prolactin levels among treatment groups.

The effects of food-restriction on average body weight is shown in Figure 2. At the end of 1 week, caloric-restricted animals established a lower steady-state body weight which persisted for the duration of the period of underfeeding. When placed on ad libitum feeding 30 days after DMBA treatment, rats gradually reached body weights equal to that of full-fed controls.

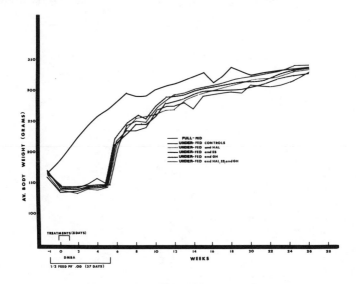

Figure 2. Average body weight during the course of the experiment. From Sylvester et.al., 1981, with permission.

These results demonstrate that the long-term inhibitory effects of caloric-restriction on the formation of DMBA-induced mammary tumors in rats was largely the result of a hormonal deficiency state at the time of tumor initiation and could be counteracted by elevation of blood estrogen and prolactin levels. Elevations in circulating levels of estrogen and prolactin for only 1 day prior to and 7 days after DMBA administration were able to prevent the inhibition of mammary tumorigenesis in rats subjected to a 50% reduction in food intake for 7 days prior to and 30 days after DMBA administration. It was of interest therefore, to determine whether food restriction begun 1 week before and continuing for only 1 week after DMBA administration, was as effective in inhibiting mammary tumor development as chronic underfeeding. It was also of interest to determine whether food restriction imposed for 2 or 4 week periods after the first critical week following DMBA treatment had any effect on mammary tumor development.

Normal cycling virgin female Sprague-Dawley rats were divided into different treatment groups and subjected to 50% ad libitum feed intake for 2 or 4 weeks at consecutive periods of time before and/or after DMBA administration, and then returned to full-fed diets. The effects of the different periods of underfeeding after DMBA administration on rat mammary tumorigenesis are shown in Table 2.

Table 2.
Effects of different periods of half-feeding on mammary tumorigenesis after DMBA administration.

Treatment	% of rats with tumors	Total No.of tumors	Av.tumor dimeter (cm)	Av. latency period (days)
Full-fed	80.9	54	2.00+0.0	103+3.6
Half-fed 1 wk prior to and 1 wk after DMBA	27.8[a]	12	1.30+0.3	125+7.0
Half-fed 2 wk starting 1 wk after DMBA	76.2	39	1.71+0.2	108+3.7
Half-fed 2 wk starting 3 wk after DMBA	75.0	44	2.09+0.2	107+3.4
Half-fed 4 wk starting 5 wk after DMBA	75.0	43	1.89+0.2	109+3.0

[a] $p < 0.05$ as compared to full-fed controls
From Sylvester et.al., 1982, with permission

Caloric-restriction for 1 week prior to and 1 week after DMBA administration showed significant reductions in mammary tumor development for the entire 21 weeks of the experiment, as compared to full-fed controls. Rats underfed for 2 weeks beginning 1 or 3 weeks after DMBA administration or underfed for 4 weeks starting 5 weeks after DMBA administration, did not show significant differences in any of the parameters used to evaluate mammary tumor development when compared with full-fed controls.

Blood was sampled from all animals on the last day of the underfeeding period for each of the individual treatment groups. All treatment groups showed a signifcant reduction in serum prolactin levels, at the end of their respective underfeeding period, as compared to all other groups at that time. In addition, during their period of food-restriction, animals displayed irregular estrous cycles, followed by cessation of cycles. When animals were returned to ad libitum feeding, all animals returned to normal 4 day estrous cycles in approximately 2 weeks.

The effects of food restriction on average body weight can be seen in Figure 3. Full-fed rats continued to gain weight throughout the entire experiment, but reached a plateau in body weight of about 300g. Rats in underfed groups showed significant reductions in body weight during their group food-restricted period. However, when these rats were returned to full-feeding, average body weight increased quickly and returned to the level of full-fed controls in only two weeks

The results of these studies demonstrate that inhibition of mammary tumor development by underfeeding during the critical first week after DMBA administration is associated with a reduction in prolactin and estrogen secretion. These rats showed a significant and perhaps permanent reduction in mammary tumor incidence, number, and growth even though they were returned to ad libitum feeding 1 week after carcinogen treatment. These findings indicate that a 30-day period of food restriction after DMBA administration is not necessary for long-term inhibition of mammary tumorigenesis. Furthermore, animals subjected to similar periods of food-restriction at various times following the critical first week after DMBA treatment also showed reduced levels of serum prolactin and disruption of regular estrous cycles, but this did not result in the inhibition of mammary tumorigenesis.

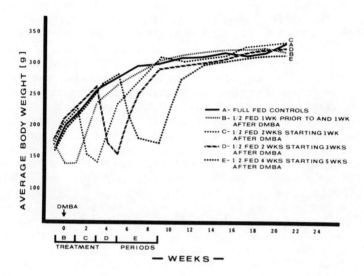

Figure 3. Average body weight of rats during the course of this study. From Sylvester et.al., 1982, with permission.

IMMUNOLOGY

Caloric-restriction has also been shown to reduce the incidence and delay the onset of many chronic non-cancerous diseases in rodents, including pneumonia and nephrosis (Ross, 1976). These effects have been associated with underfeeding-induced mechanisms which affect host immune function. It has been shown that while B-cell immunity is decreased when animals are fed restricted diets, T-cell activity is maintained or even enhanced (Good, et al., 1979). Enhancement of cell-mediated immunity by underfeeding is further evidenced by studies which have demonstrated delayed hypersensitivity, increased rate of allograft rejection, tumor immunity, proliferative responses to T-cell mitogens and production of migration inhibition factor (Fernandes, et al., 1979). The characteristic decline of thymic function which naturally occurs in aging animals can be delayed by modifications in dietary intake. Animals fed ad libitum diets display an early onset of thymic involution and an associated decline in thymus-associated immunity. In contrast, caloric-restricted animals show delayed deterioration in thymus associated immune function and extended immunocompetence during early life, which has been correlated with a decreased incidence of both cancerous and non-cancerous diseases (Fernandes, et al., 1979). This evidence supports the belief that mechanisms involved in host immune surveillance provides an important first-line defense against the establishment of many types of cancers. In addition, various chemical carcinogens have been found to have powerful immunosuppressive effects in experimental animals, while their non-carcinogenic analogues were not found to affect immune function (Ball, 1970). These studies demonstrate the importance relationship between nutrition and immune function in certain types of murine tumorigenesis.

CONCLUSIONS

Studies reviewed here demonstrate the ability of caloric-restriction to inhibit development and growth of various spontaneous, transplantable and carcinogen-induced tumors in rodents. At the present time, no common mechanism by which underfeeding is able to inhibit such a large variety of tumors has been identified. However, in the case of DMBA-induced mammary tumors, studies demonstrate that hormonal deficiencies in food-restricted rats at the time of tumor induction are responsible for long-term inhibition of tumor development. Nevertheless, in these experiments a 50% reduction in calories was used for the inhibition of mammary tumorigenesis. The severity of such a restricted diet results in drastic alterations in the basic physiology of these animals. While it is possible that the inadequate calories or malnutrition in many developing countries may explain their low incidence of breast cancer, it is obvious that severe caloric-restriction is not a practical method for the prevention of human breast cancer. Rather, the above studies illustrates a mechanism by which underfeeding inhibits breast cancer, and firmly establishes and defines the involvement of the endo-crine system. The reduction in pituitary hormone secretion by underfeeding may also influence development of non-endo-crine dependent tumors, since a decrease in these hormones results in the decline of many metabolic processes, some of which may be involved in bringing about an enhancement of thymus-associated immune function. At present however, the exact interaction between the endocrine and immune systems in underfed animals is not fully understood.

REFERENCES

Ball JK (1970). Immunosuppression and carcinogenesis: Contrasting effects with 7,12-dimethylbenz(a)anthracene, benz(a)pyrene, and 3-methylcholanthrene. JNCI 44:1-10.

Boutwell RK, Brush MK, Rusch HP (1948). Some physiological effects associated with chronic caloric-restriction. Am J Physiol 154:517-524.

Campbell GA, Kurcz M, Marshall S, Meites J (1977). Effects of starvation in rats on serum levels of follicle stimulating hormone, luteinizing hormone, thyrotropin, growth hormone and prolactin; response to luteinizing hormone-releasing hormone and thyrotropin-releasing hormone. Endocrinology 100:580-587.

Carroll KK (1975). Experimental evidence of dietary factors and hormone-dependent cancers. Cancer Res 35:3374-3383.

Dao TL (1962). The role of ovarian hormones in initiating the induction of mammary cancer in rats by polynuclear hydrocarbons. Cancer Res 22:973-981.

Fermandes G, West A, Good RA (1979). Nutrition, immunity, and cancer - a review. Part III. Effects of diet on the diseases of aging. Clin Bull 9:91-106.

Good RA, Fernandes G, West A (1979). Nutrition, Immunity, and cancer - a review. Part I. Influcence of protein or protein-calorie malnutrition and zinc deficiency on immunity function. Clin Bull 9:3-12.

Huggins G, Grand LC, Brillantes FP (1961). Mammary cancer induced by a single feeding of polynuclear hydrocarbons and its suppression. Nature 189:204-207.

Huseby RA, Ball ZB, Visscher MB (1945). Further observations on the influence of simple caloric-restriction on mammary cancer, incidence and related phemonena in C3H mice. Cancer Res 5:40-46.

Leung FC, Aylsworth CF, Meites J (1983). Counteraction of underfeeding-induced inhibition of mammary tumor growth in rats by prolactin and estrogen administration. Proc Soc Exp Biol Med 173:159-163.

Meites J (1972). Relation of prolactin and estrogen to mammary tumorigenesis in the rat. JNCI 48:1217-1224.

Piacsek BE, Meites J (1967). Reinitiation of gonadotropin release in in underfed rats by constant light or epinephrine. Endocrinology 81:535-541.

Ross MH (1976). Nutrition and longevity in experimental animals. In Winick M (ed): "Nutrition and Aging," New York: Wiley and Sons, pp 43-57.

Ross MH, Bras G (1971). Lasting influence of early caloric restriction on prevalence of neoplasm in the rat. JNCI 47:1095-1113.

Russo J, Russo IH (1978). Developmental stage of the rat mammary gland as determinant of its susceptablility to 7,12-dimethybenz(a)anthracene. JNCI 61:1439-1449.

Sylvester PW, Aylsworth CF, Meites J (1981). Relationship of hormones to inhibition of mammary tumor development by underfeeding during the "critical period" after carcinogen administration. Cancer Res 41:1384-1388.

Sylvester PW, Aylsworth CF, Van Vugt DA, Meites J (1982). Influence of underfeeding during the "critical period" of thereafter on carcinogen-induced mammary tunors in rats. Cancer Res 42:4943-4947.

Tannenbaum A (1940). The initiation and growth of tumors. Introduction. I. Effects of underfeeding. AM J Cancer 38:335-350.

Tannenbaum A (1944). The dependence of the genesis of skin tumors on the caloric intake during different stages of carcinogenesis. Cancer Res 4:673-677.

Tannenbaum A (1945). The dependence of tumor formation on the degree of caloric restriction. Cancer Res 5:609-615.

Tannenbaum A, Silverstone H (1950). Failure to inhibit the formation of mammary carcinoma in mice by intermittent fasting. Cancer Res 10:577-579.

Tucker MJ (1979). The effects of long term food restriction on tumours in rodents. Int J Cancer 23:803-807.

V. Cellular and Other Mechanisms of Fat Effects on Carcinogenesis

Dietary Fat and Cancer, pages 531–553
© 1986 Alan R. Liss, Inc.

METABOLIC ADAPTATIONS TO DIETARY FATS

Steven D. Clarke

The Upjohn Company
Kalamazoo, Michigan   49001

While it is generally agreed that diets containing a
high proportion of calories as fat are associated with
several health risks including impaired glucose metabolism,
obesity and intestinal and mammary cancer, the definition of
a high fat diet is ill-defined and arbitrary. Based upon
several metabolic anomalies, a high fat diet is defined for
the purpose of this review as one which contains greater
than 45% of the dietary energy as fat but which is adequate
in all nutrients. An essential understanding in the
discussion of dietary fat is that the metabolic outcomes of
dietary fat vary tremendously with the fatty acid
composition of the fat (Herzberg, 1983; Philipson et al.,
1985). Therefore the objective of this review is to provide
a consensus metabolic explanation for the consequences of
ingesting a high fat diet, and to contrast wherever possible
the differences between saturated and unsaturated lipids.

DIETARY FAT INTERFERES WITH GLUCOSE TOLERANCE

The most pronounced adaptation to the consumption of
diets high in fat is reduced glucose utilization by muscle,
adipose, and hepatic tissues accompanied by enhanced hepatic
glucose synthesis. This sparing of glucose is
physiologically sensible in order to provide adequate fuel
for tissues, e.g. red blood cells, which have an absolute
requirement for glucose. However, continued surfeit
consumption of a mixed diet high in fat may lead to such
poor glucose homeostasis as to be a health risk, e.g.

insulin resistance. High fat diets impair glucose tolerance in rodents, as well as humans (Romsos and Clarke, 1980). When normal young men were fed liquid diets containing various proportion of fat and carbohydrate ranging in fat content from 20 to 80% dietary energy, intakes of fat above 40% of energy as fat significantly impaired oral glucose tolerance. Intravenous glucose clearance was less suppressed than oral clearance which suggests dietary fat may alter gut hormone (insulinogenic) release or function. The impairment action of fat is not simply the result of low carbohydrate diets. When the carbohydrate component of the diet was replaced with protein rather than fat, oral glucose tolerance in young men was not impaired. Thus, deterioration in glucose clearance appears to be the specific consequence of high fat diets. However, the extent of this impairment in glucose metabolism appears to vary with the composition of the dietary fat, i.e., insulin resistance was less pronounced with dietary corn oil in contrast to lard (Tepperman and Tepperman, 1985).

The cause of dietary fat inhibition of glucose metabolism is not completely clear, but involves functions in the muscle, adipose and hepatic tissues. Within these tissues the molecular alterations involve reduced: (a) insulin binding, (b) glucose entry into cells, (c) second message production from insulin, and (d) glucose oxidation due to suppressed glycolysis, pyruvate decarboxylation, and fatty acid synthesis.

ADAPTATION OF GLUCOSE TRANSPORT TO HIGH FAT DIETS

The impairment of glucose tolerance caused by high fat diets is the product of suppressed rates of glucose oxidation and transport in muscle, adipose and hepatic tissues (Bringolf et al., 1972; Tepperman and Tepperman, 1985). Soleus and diaphragm muscles taken from rats fed a high fat diet expressed a low capacity for insulin stimulated glucose uptake and oxidation. This reduced capacity for glucose uptake is reflected in the very low concentration of muscle glycogen associated with high fat diets (Newsholme and Leech, 1984). Howard and Widder (1976) have suggested that fatty acids inhibit glycogen synthetase, but the specificity of this fatty acid effect is questionable. The more likely explanation is that high fat intakes reduce intracellular availability via (a) less cellular uptake and (b) simply, less glucose ingestion. While glycogen accumulation is decreased by a high fat diet, the overall impairment in intracellular glucose utilization appears to involve more glycolysis and pyruvate oxidation than glucose conversion to glycogen (Abumrad et al., 1978). This adaptation to dietary fat involves the activities of muscle hexokinase, phosphofructokinase and pyruvate dehydrogenase.

Adipose tissue also adapts to high fat diets by markedly decreasing its utilization of glucose (Tepperman and Tepperman, 1985). In the classic studies of the Teppermans (1985) adipocytes isolated from rats fed a high fat - carbohydrate free diet transported and oxidized 50% and 85% less glucose than adipocytes isolated from rats fed a high carbohydrate - fat free diet. While these diets differed greatly in essential fatty acid content, Lavau et al. (1979) demonstrated that dietary fat suppression of glucose uptake and oxidation was independent of essential fatty acid status.

The molecular explanation for the adaptation to reduced glucose utilization resulting from high fat diets is controversial. Hissin et al. (1982) reported that high fat diets reduced the number of glucose transport proteins in rat adipose tissue. Accompanying fewer glucose receptors, the Teppermans have presented ample evidence that glycosylation of the receptors may be altered, i.e. glycosyltransferases which participate in the latter stages of protein glycosylation (Tepperman and Tepperman, 1985). In addition to an altered glucose receptor, high fat diets have been reported to reduce insulin binding to adipocyte and hepatocyte membranes (Ip et al., 1976; Sun et al., 1977). Lavau et al. (1979) were unable to demonstrate that high fat diets altered insulin binding to adipocytes. Similarly, peripheral mononuclear cells isolated from young female subjects who had been previously adapted to a high carbohydrate (80%) vs a high fat diet (60%) displayed no differences in insulin binding or affinity. The high fat diet did impair glucose tolerance (Wigand et al., 1979). The key difference among these studies lies in the essential fatty acid (EFA) status. The high carbohydrate diet used by Ip et al. (1976) was devoid of EFA while Lavau's (1979) experimental diet containing adequate EFA. Consistent with this explanation is a recent report by the Teppermans indicating that adipocyte and hepatocyte plasma membranes isolated from rats fed a high corn oil diet bound much more insulin than membranes from rats fed a high hydrogenated coconut oil diet.

In spite of the changes in membrane functions related to glucose metabolism, the primary adaptive response which precedes reduced glucose transport and lowered insulin sensitivity is a decrease in intracellular metabolism of glucose. The challenge has become to not only decipher how dietary fat suppresses the intracellular activity of enzymes involved in glucose utilization, but also to determine how this intracellular resistance leads to a suppression of glucose transport.

ADAPTATION OF INTRACELLULAR GLUCOSE METABOLISM TO HIGH FATDIETS

An appreciation of the mechanisms by which fat spares glucose utilization requires a brief overview of the current thoughts on interorgan glucose utilization. Current information indicates that the liver metabolizes only a small percentage of absorbed glucose, i.e. <20% (Katz and McGarry, 1984). The remainder of the glucose is utilized by peripheral tissues, notably, muscle and adipose. Quantitatively muscle constitutes the largest glucose utilizing tissue. Here the glucose is stored as glycogen, and glucose in excess of glycogen synthetase capacity is metabolized to pyruvate, lactate, and alanine. These 3-carbon metabolites are released by muscle tissue and removed by hepatic tissue for gluconeogenic and lipogenic substrates (Katz and McGarry, 1984). With a high carbohydrate diet hepatic glucose-6-phosphate synthesized from pyruvate is used for glycogen synthesis while with a high fat diet the glucose-6-phosphate hydrolysis to glucose by hepatic glucose-6-phosphatase is favored (Hems and Whitton, 1980). Glucose removed by human adipose tissue is largely utilized for glyceride-glycerol formation but in rodent and porcine adipose, glucose is a substrate for de novo fatty acid synthesis (Romsos and Leveille, 1974).

Obviously, if dietary fat suppressed muscle and adipose glucose uptake, glycolytic flux, and glycogen synthesis, then glucose clearance and hepatic substrate availability for glycogen and fatty acid synthesis would be compromised. Moreover, inhibition of liver pyruvate decarboxylation by a high fat diet would favor glucose synthesis and output. Suppression of adipose glycolysis and stimulation of hepatic gluconeogenesis by dietary fat is well established, but regulation of muscle glucose uptake and glycolysis by dietary fat is equivocal. Inhibition of glucose utilization by high fat diets appears to occur in cardiac muscle and slow-twitch red fiber (e.g. soleus) but glucose utilization by white fiber muscle, which functions during intense exercise, appears unaffected by fatty acids (Ruderman et al., 1979). However, high fat diets may limit the glycogen stores of the white fibers. There appears to be consistent agreement that cardiac and skeletal muscle, adipose, and hepatic pyruvate dehydrogenase activity is suppressed by fatty acids and high fat diets (Harris et al., 1973; Ruderman et al., 1979; Tepperman and Tepperman, 1985). Thus, pyruvate dehydrogenase likely plays a pivotal role in fatty acid - sparing of glucose and possibly in the development of glucose intolerance associated with high fat diets.

A. Adaptation of Glycolytic Enzymes.

     Initiation of intracellular glucose metabolism is depen-dent upon ATP-phosphorylation of glucose catalyzed by low K_m hexokinase II of muscle and adipose and high K_m hexokinase IV (glucokinase) of liver. Dietary fat decreases the maximal activity of adipose hexokinase II, but the muscle enzyme is unchanged (Romsos and Leveille, 1974). In addition to decreasing the amount of hexokinases, high fat diets increase the concentration of glucose-6-phosphate by reducing glycolytic flux presumably at the level of phosphofructokinase (Hems and Whitton, 1980). Glucose-6-phosphate is an inhibitor of hexokinase II. Such feedback regulation may be the mode of control of glucose phosphorylation in red fiber muscle. Hepatic tissue not only has a loss of glucokinase, but also displays an increase in glucose-6-phosphate conversion to glucose with a high fat diet (Romsos and Clarke, 1980).

     A fascinating regulatory characteristic of hexokinase, but not glucokinase, is its ability to change its catalytic efficiency by associating and dissociating from the mitochondrial membrane. The membrane-bound hexokinase is more active, has a lower Km for ATP, and greater resistance to glucose-6-phosphate inhibition (Parry and Pedersen, 1983). Cancer cells, such as Novikoff ascites and Ehrlich-lettre hyperdiploid ascites tumor cells (Kurokawa et al., 1982; Parry and Pedersen, 1983), have a high proportion of mitochondrial-bound hexokinase which likely determines the high rate of glucose utilization by tumor cells. The ability of dietary fat to alter the proportion of bound/free hexokinase in normal or tumor cells is unexplored. However, since dietary lipids will alter membrane characteristics (Teppermanand Tepperman, 1985), and decrease glucose utilization, one may speculate that dietary fats may regulate muscle and adipose glycolysis via control of the amount of membrane bound hexokinase.

Several studies with cardiac muscle, red fiber skeletal muscle, and liver (Newsholme and Leech, 1984) indicate that increased availability of fatty acids and ketones as metabolic fuels during fasting or diabetes inhibits glucose-6-phosphate flux to pyruvate primarily at the level of phosphofructokinase activity (PFK). These data imply that such a glycolytic adaptation should occur with a high fat diet, but evidence supporting this contention is lacking. We found no decrease in hepatic PFK activity with either saturating or subsaturating concentrations of fructose-6-phosphate in rats fed saturated or polyunsaturated fats (Toussant et al.,1981). Clark et al. (1982) reported that long-term feeding (200 days) of a high fat diet did not decrease the amount of immunoprecipitable rat heart PFK. However, the enzymatic activity at sub-maximal fructose-6-phosphate concentrationswas 20% of that occurring in rats fed a high carbohydrate diet. This indicates a high fat diet may decrease PFK catalytic efficiency by either metabolite (Pilkis et al., 1982) or covalent modification (Narabayshi et al., 1985).

Decreased fructose-2,6-bisphosphate concentrations in liver and muscle may potentially be the pivotal adaptation to a high fat diet which governs PFK activity and glycolyticrate. Fructose-2,6-bisphosphate in micromolar amounts greatly stimulates liver PFK activity, reduces PFK sensitivity to ATP inhibition, and accelerates hepatic glycolytic flux (Pilkis et al., 1982). In addition, fructose-1,6-bisphosphatase which catalyzes the opposing gluconeogenic reaction is inhibited by fructose-2,6-bisphosphate (Pilkis et al., 1982). The concentration of hepatic fructose-2,6-bisphosphate is increased by insulin, decreased by glucagon, and raised by refeeding carbohydrate. Although unreported, it can be anticipated that a high fat diet would decrease the hepatic content of fructose-2,6-bisphosphate and thereby lower PFK catalytic efficiency and glycolytic flux. Fructose-2,6-bisphosphate is found in cancer cells. It is tempting to speculate that the high rate of glycolysis in cancer cells is caused by high levels of fructose-2,6-bisphosphate.

The impact of fructose-2,6-bisphosphate on muscle PFK activity and its interaction with dietary composition is unclear. The concentration of fructose-2,6-bisphosphate in rat gastrocnemius may be too low to be a physiological activator (Tornheim, 1985) and does not correlate to glycolytic rate either at rest or upon electrical stimulation (Hue etal., 1982). On the other hand insulin increased muscle fructose-2,6-bisphosphate and the kinetic behavior of purified muscle PFK is affected by the metabolite (Narabayashi et al., 1985). A more important regulator of muscle PFK and muscle glycolytic rate, especially with high fat diets, may be fructose-1,6-bisphosphate (Tornheim, 1985). This metabolite decreases with a high fat diet, is at a physiologically relevant concentration, and is a potent activator (increases Vmax) of muscle PFK.

Sommercorn and Freedland (1982, 1984) have questioned the role of fructose-2,6-bisphosphate and have proposed 6-phosphogluconate may be a more likely regulator of PFK and glycolysis. 6-Phosphogluconate varied in concentration with amount and type of carbohydrate and was highly correlated to rates of glycolysis and lipogenesis. The effect of dietary fat has been unexplored. It is interesting that glucose-6-phosphate dehydrogenase which forms 6-phosphogluconate greatly increases during malignant transformation of hepatomas (Selmeci and Weber, 1976).

The adaptation of glycolysis, particularly in skeletal muscle, is unclear. Certainly, skeletal muscle quantitatively plays the greatest role in glucose clearance. Thus, establishing the influence of free fatty acids upon the regulators of glycolysis is essential to deciphering the mechanism of the development of glucose intolerance resulting from a high fat diet.

B. Adaptation of Pyruvate Dehydrogenase.

The utilization of pyruvate, derived from alanine, lactate or pyruvate per se, as an energy source or lipogenic substrate in muscle, adipose, and hepatic tissues is suppressed by the ingestion of a high fat diet (Ruderman et al.,1979; Begum et al., 1982; Begum et al., 1983). Using are constituted in vitro lipogenic system consisting of isolated cytosol and mitochondria, Harris and coworkers (1983) have uniquely demonstrated that mitochondria isolated from rats fed a high fat diet have a very limited capability to oxidize ^{14}C-alanine and convert alanine to fatty acids. This mitochondrial adaptation to dietary fat primarily involves inhibition of pyruvate dehydrogenase activity, but may also reflect inhibited pyruvate translocase, citrate translocase, and ATP/ADP translocase (Romsos and Leveille, 1974; Sul et al., 1979).

Pyruvate dehydrogenase (PDH) in normal tissue is regulated by phosphorylation and dephosphorylation, i.e., the active form (PDHa) is dephosphorylated. Perfusing liver with oleate significantly decreases pyruvate decarboxylation and the proportion of active PDH. Similarly, the amount of PDHa in perfused rat heart decreased from 57% to 27% upon addition of palmitate to the perfusate (Wieland et al., 1971). Refeeding fasted rats with glucose or fructose increased PDH activity 5-fold in heart muscle and kidney, but refeeding with olive oil maintained the low proportion of PDHa resulting from fasting (Wieland et al., 1971). Muscle taken from rats fed a high fat diet have low rates of pyruvate oxidation (Bringolf et al., 1972) and marked reductions in the amount of PDHa. Like the other organs, adipose tissue PDH is also inhibited by diets high in fat (Tepperman and Tepperman, 1985). In fact, the amount of PDHa in adipose tissue of rats fed a high fat diet was comparable to that found in severely diabetic rats.

The mechanism by which fatty acids suppress PDH involves an increase in NADH/NAD and acetyl CoA/CoA ratios which activate PDH kinase and inhibit PDH phosphatase

(Stansbie et al., 1976). When a high fat diet is consumed, mitochondrial oxidation of fatty acids is increased. This increases the mitochondrial content of NADH and acetyl CoA which leads to inactivation of PDH and activation of pyruvate carboxylase. The metabolic result is partitioning of pyruvate away from decarboxylation and toward oxaloacetate and ultimately glucose. NADH and acetyl CoA inhibition of PDH also occurs in tumor cells (Lazo and Sols, 1980), but the inhibition may be directly upon PDH rather than via changes in phosphorylation state because tumor cell PDH appears not to be under phosphorylation control.

While increased fatty acid oxidation appears to be one mechanism by which high fat diets decrease pyruvate conversion to acetyl CoA, the Teppermans (1985) have convincingly demonstrated that high fat diets decrease insulin activation of pyruvate dehydrogenase. Treatment of adipose and liver plasma membranes with insulin releases a factor which stimulates PDH activity (Begum et al., 1982,1983). This ill-defined factor is considered the second messenger for insulin. Interestingly, plasma membranes isolated from rats fed a high fat diet produce much less of this PDH activating factor upon insulin stimulation. Apparently high fat diets decrease the production of insulin's second message which may potentially explain many of the intracellular adaptations to high fat diets.

C. Adaptation of the De Novo Fatty Acid Biosynthetic Pathway

Glucose consumed in excess of immediate need is stored as glycogen and fatty acids. Conversion of excess carbohydrate to fatty acids occurs primarily in the liver of humans and chicks, liver and adipose of rodents, and adipose of pigs and ruminants. De novo fatty acid synthesis also occurs in mammary gland for synthesis of milk fat especially short-chain fatty acids; and lung for synthesis of palmitate for surfactant phosphatidylcholine. Dietary fats interfere with hepatic and adipose fatty acid synthesis (Romsos and Leveille, 1974). However, mammary gland (Abraham et al.,1983) and lung (Clarke et al., 1984) are very resistant to dietary fat inhibition of lipogenesis. Dietary polyunsaturated lipids, particularly marine oils, are more

effective inhibitors of hepatic fatty acid biosynthesis than
are saturated fats, but adipose tissue lipogenesis appears
less dependent upon type of fat (Herzberg, 1983). This
unique action of polyunsaturated fats extends to nursing
animals (Abrahamet al., 1983). Furthermore the
hypolipogenic behavior of polyunsaturates may carry-over
into adulthood even if the high polyunsaturated fat intake
is discontinued (O'Brien et al., 1983). Unlike newborns and
adults, fetal liver lipogenesis is not influenced by fat
content or composition of the maternal diet (Miguel and
Abraham, 1976).

Dietary fat suppression of liver and adipose fatty
acid biosynthesis is both an acute (e.g. fat intubation) and
long-term (i.e., adaptive decrease in content of lipogenic
enzymes) response. The rapid, short-term inhibition likely
involves a reduced proportion of active PDH, and an
inactivation of acetyl CoA carboxylase (Clarke and Clarke,
1982). Fatty acids impair acetyl CoA conversion to malonyl
CoA by altering the conformation of acetyl CoA carboxylase
which results in decreased catalytic efficiency (Clarke and
Clarke, 1982). Acute suppression of fatty acid biosynthesis
by fat ingestion does not differ significantly between
saturated and polyunsaturated fats (Clarke and Salati,
1985). In contrast,the decrease in hepatic content of
lipogenic enzymes associated with dietary fats is highly
dependent upon the polyunsaturated fatty acid content of the
diet (Herzberg, 1983),i.e. polyunsaturates act with greater
efficacy than saturates. The decrease in lipogenic enzymes
is the result of an inhibited enzyme protein synthesis. The
intracellular mechanism and the mediator of the
polyunsaturated fat action are unknown. Utilizing malic
enzyme as a model, Abraham's group has reported that
polyunsaturated fats inhibit translation rate (Schwartz and
Abraham, 1983). However, confirmation of this observation
will require cDNA-hybridization methodologies. The mediator
of polyunsaturated fat suppression of enzyme production is
not likely a prostanoid and appears to be independent of
insulin function (Wilson et al., 1986). Furthermore
extensive studies from our laboratory utilizing rat
hepatocytes cultured in a serum-free, defined medium
indicate fatty acids have little ability to directly block
the insulin or T_3 induction of lipogenic enzymes (Salati and
Clarke, 1986). The in vivo inhibition of enzyme synthesis
by dietary fat, especially polyunsaturates, appears to

involve altered responsiveness to a hormonal signal which is
not insulin. The hormones involved can only be speculated.
Data from Berdanier's laboratory suggests polyunsaturated
fats interfere with glucocorticoid induction of lipogenic
enzymes (Williams and Berdainier, 1982). Our own data
indicated dietary fat especially polyunsaturated fat blocks
T_3-stimulation of malic enzyme, fatty acid synthetase and
glucose-6-phosphate dehydrogenase. These two events may be
related. Naito et al. (1985) recently reported that
thyroxine administration to rats increased liver
glucocorticoid binding capacity. Thus, the level of
polyunsaturated fat action may involve suppression of
glucocorticoid function or receptor binding. Alternatively,
dietary fats, especially polyunsaturates, could possibly
increase hepatic sensitivity to antilipogenic hormones such
as glucagon by increasing membrane binding or affinity, or
enhancing adenylate cyclase activity (Houslay, 1985).

FATTY ACID OXIDATION AND TRIGLYCERIDE SYNTHESIS

The respiratory quotient of an individual on a high
fat diet approaches 0.7 which indicates the primary
metabolic fuels are fatty acids and ketones. When adapted
to a high carbohydrate diet, the primary source of
intracellular fatty acids for nonhepatic tissues originates
from lipoprotein lipase hydrolysis of VLDL-triglyceride and
albumin-bound fatty acids. On a high fat diet much of the
fatty acid for oxidation in red fiber muscle, e.g. soleus
and diaphragm, is actually derived from intracellular
triglyceride stores (Abumard et al., 1978). Rats fed a high
lard diet (vs high glucose) increased their diaphragm
triglyceride content 3-fold. When these rats were fasted
the muscle and plasma triglyceride concentrations decreased.
Plasma free fatty acids did not increase which was due to an
adipose resistance to glucagon and epinephrine activation of
adenylate cyclase and subsequently lipolysis (Abumard et
al., 1978). High fat diets appear not only to shift the
type of metabolic fuel utilized by muscle, but also shift
the location from which fatty acids are mobilized.

Free fatty acids require albumin for plasma transport.
Thus, their availability to peripheral tissues are limited
by the amount of albumin and the access of albumin to the
tissues. In this respect fatty acids are a poor fuel for

brain and neural tissues. In order to provide a fuel which is water soluble and available to nearly all tissues, fatty acids are used as a substrate by the liver for ketone production. Since the liver is also the primary site of free fatty acid recycling to triglycerides, regulation of the trafficking of fatty acids between triglyceride synthesis and oxidation will determine the relative production and availability of plasma ketones vs triglycerides.

Consumption of a high fat diet, particularly polyunsaturated fish oils, leads to increased partitioning of hepatic free fatty acids into mitochondrial and peroxisomal oxidation and away from triglyceride synthesis (Thomassen et al., 1982; Kalopissis et al., 1981). The origin of free fatty acids for ketogenesis on a high fat diet are from albumin-bound fatty acids and from chylomicron remnant uptake and hydrolysis. The intracellular adaptations to a high fat diet which favor fatty acid flux to ketogenesis include: (1) reduced availability of glycerol-3-phosphate for triglyceride synthesis (Declercq et al., 1982), (2) higher K_i of carnitine palmitoyl transferase for malonyl CoA (Wong et al., 1984), and (3) lower activities of the triglyceride synthesizing enzymes (Stewart and Briggs, 1981).

Glycerol, derived from glycerol-3-phosphate, is the backbone of triglycerides and phospholipids. The origin of hepatic glycerol-3-phosphate is glycolysis and adipose glycerol release during lipolysis. When fatty acids are the primary metabolic fuel, hepatic gluconeogenesis from 3-carbon substrates, (e.g. glycerol) is accelerated. Under these conditions glycerol-3-phosphate availability could become a limiting substrate for triglyceride production. McGarry and Foster (1979) have argued that malonyl CoA inhibition of fatty acid entry into the mitochondria is the key mechanism regulating fatty acid oxidation and partitioning away from triglycerides. Malonyl CoA inhibits carnitine palmitoyl transferase of liver mitochondria isolated from fed rats at a K_i of physiological concentrations (McGarry and Foster, 1979). The concentration of hepatic malonyl CoA is low in diabetic and fasted rats and increases 10-fold with carbohydrate refeeding (McGarry and Foster, 1979; Clarke and Clarke, 1982). Incubating rat hepatocytes from fed donors with 1 mM palmitate, oleate or linoleate inactivates acetyl CoA carboxylase, decreases malonyl CoA concentrations, inhibits fatty acid synthesis and increases ketone production (Clarke and Salati, 1985; McGarry and Foster, 1979). This effect of fatty acid appears to be synergistic with glucagon (Clarke and Salati, 1985). Thus a logical hypothesis would be that the elevation in hepatic free fatty acids plus a higher glucagon/insulin ratio associated with a high fat diet, would inactivate acetyl CoA carboxylase, decrease malonyl CoA level, and enhance mitochondrial fatty acid oxidation. Consequently ketone production is increased as a result of greater hepatic oxidation of free fatty acids to acetyl CoA which in turn increases mitochondrial substrate availability for ketone synthesis.

In opposition to this theory we have found that polyunsaturated fat inhibition of liver triglyceride synthesis, fatty acid synthesis, and acetyl CoA carboxylase are not accompanied by a decrease in hepatic malonyl CoA concentration (Toussant et al., 1981). Furthermore, Cook and associates have questioned the malonyl CoA hypothesis because the high rate of ketogenesis in mitochondria from fasted rats was very insensitive to malonyl CoA regulation (1984). Some resolution of these conflicting data has come with a recent report indicating the Ki of carnitine palmitoyl transferase for malonyl CoA is greatly dependent upon the fatty acid composition of the diet (Wong et al., 1984). For example, diets high in 20- and 22-carbon polyenoic omega-3 fatty acids inhibit triglyceride synthesis, promote ketogenesis, and increase the Ki of carnitine palmitoyl transferase for malonyl CoA (Wong et al., 1984).

The fact that high fat diets reduce hepatic triglyceride synthesis and VLDL output is unquestionable. In addition, polyenoic dietary fats are more effective inhibitors than saturated fats, and oils rich in 20- and 22-carbon omega-3 fatty acids are better than omega-6 lipids (Pillipson et al.,1985). The suppression of lipogenesis appears in part to be regulated by changes in glycerol-phosphate and malonyl CoA. It is tempting to also propose that high fat diets decreased the concentration and/or catalytic efficiency of the triglyceride synthesizing enzymes. However, such adaptations to dietary fat are poorly defined. Wong et al. (1984) found no effect of

dietary fat on liver glycerol-phosphate acyltransferase
activity. Stewart and Briggs (1981) did report that liver
phosphatidic acid phosphohydrolase activity was 2-3 fold
higher in essential fatty acid deficient rats than in rats
fed 15% corn oil. Similarly, a diet containing lard tended
to result in higher phosphohydrolase activity in rat liver
than a diet containing corn oil. On the other hand,
increasing the concentration of corn oil from 0.5% to 10%
had no effect on phosphatidic acid phosphohydrolase activity
but did suppress hepatic triglyceride production (Stewart
and Briggs, 1981). We have found that in cultured
hepatocytes the flux of diglyceride to triglyceride was
reduced 50% in cells enriched with eicosapentaenoic acid and
30% in cells enriched with arachidonate, but palmitate and
linoleate has no effect. These data indicate a fatty acid
inhibition of diacylglycerol acyltransferase, but enzymatic
activity measurements have not been conducted.

Both phosphatidic acid phosphohydrolase and
diacylglycerol acyltransferase undergo short-term acute
changes in catalytic efficiency. Diacylglycerol
acyltransferase is activated by fatty acids and inhibited by
phosphorylation (Haagsman et al., 1982). In the case of
phosphohydrolase it associates and dissociates from the
microsomal membrane with the active form being membrane
bound (Cascales et al., 1984). It seems feasible that high
fat diets, especially polyunsaturated marine oils, may
enhance phoshorylation inhibition in the liver, or change
membrane composition such that membrane binding of these
enzymes is reduced. The consequence would be decreased
triglyceride synthesis without decreased enzyme content.
Such behavior awaits verification.

At this time the adaptation of triglyceride
synthesizing enzymes in liver, as well as in other tissue,
to high fat intakes awaits definition. Clearly, such
definition is fundamental to explaining the decrease in
hepatic triglyceride production associated with high fat
diets. Furthermore, elucidation of the adaptive mechanisms
of triglyceride production will provide information as to
the causative factors in cancer associated
hypertriglyceridemia and the ability of dietary fats to
lower blood lipids in cancer bearing organisms (Kannan et
al., 1978). This hypolipemic action of dietary fats may be
beneficial in that fatty acid and cholesterol availability

for cancer cell membrane growth and development might be lessened in the hypolipemic state.

ADAPTATIONS IN CHOLESTEROL METABOLISM TO DIETARY FAT

Although nearly all cell types have the capacity to synthesize cholesterol to some degree, the majority of cholesterol synthesis occurs in the liver and small intestine. The capacity of cholesterol production in both tissues varies with type and amount of dietary fat (Ide et al., 1978; Bochenek and Rodgers, 1979). The site of regulation of this pathway by dietary fat appears to primarily involve the rate-determining enzyme, hydroxymethylglutaryl CoA (HMG CoA)reductase.

Hepatic cholesterol synthesis and HMG CoA reductase activity doubled when the amount of dietary fat was increased from 10% of energy to 40% (Ide et al., 1978). Similarly, adding 10% corn oil (w/w) to a high sucrose, fat-free diet increased jejunal and ileal villi HMG CoA reductase activity 25% (Bochenek and Rodgers, 1979). The hepatic response to corn oil likely reflects the accelerated loss of cholesterol from the liver due to enhanced bile flow and increased cholesterol content of the bile (Balamubramaniam et al., 1985). The intestinal response reflects the requirement of cholesterol for assembly dietary lipid into chylomicrons for absorption and transport. In addition, dietary fats increase fecal losses of sterols and bile acids which alleviates cholesterol and bile acid feedback inhibition of liver cholesterolgenesis (Balamubramaniam et al., 1985).

Several studies indicate that dietary hydrogenated triglycerides increase hepatic and intestinal HMG CoA reductase activity and cholesterol synthesis (Ide et al.,1978; Bochnek and Rogers, 1979). Rats fed a diet containing 10% tristearin (w/w) had hepatic and intestinal HMG CoA reductase activities 3-fold higher than rats fed equal amounts safflower oil (Ide et al., 1978; Bochenek and Rodgers, 1979). The difficulty with trial which use tristearin, tripalmitin,or hydrogenated oils is that their absorbability is very low and fecal lipid losses are very high (Clarke et al.,1977). Consequently, their stimulation of cholesterol synthesis may reflect the poor reabsorption

of bile acids into the enterohepatic circulation plus
greater bile acid and cholesterol losses in the feces
(Balamubramaniam et al., 1985). When dietary saturated and
unsaturated fats of comparable absorbability are utilized,
the saturated fat diet tended to result in higher rates of
hepatic cholesterol synthesis than the diet containing
safflower oil (Spady and Dietschy, 1985) but the differences
were not nearly as great as those which occur with
tristearin. This unique study by Spady and Dietschy (1985)
also demonstrated that dietary fat control of cholesterol
synthesis is not likely caused by the fatty acids per se, but
relates more to the regulation of cholesterol uptake and its
feedback inhibition of HMG CoA reductase. When a diet
containing 20% (w/w) safflower oil plus 0.12% cholesterol
was fed to rats, hepatic receptor-mediated LDL-cholesterol
uptake was reduced 30%. In contrast a diet of 20%
hydrogenated coconut oil plus 0.12% cholesterol decreased
liver LDL receptors by 90%. The less extensive cholesterol
uptake with saturated fat would be expected to lower the
cholesterol mediated suppression of HMG CoA reductase
synthesis and thereby promote higher rates of cholesterol
synthesis. Such a mechanism appears to be in play. What is
of continued interest is the mechanism by which a high
linoleate diet maintains LDL receptors. This action of
polyunsaturated fats may not extend to all oils.

Cholesterol is an essential component of cell
membranes. Preventing cholesterol synthesis or uptake by
cultured cells often inhibits cell proliferation.
Furthermore, cholesterol often accumulates in many types of
cancer cells. Thus, regulation of cholesterol synthesis
and/or uptake by dietary fat could have significant
ramifications with regard to cancer cell growth rate.
However, several studies indicate that transplanted rodent
and human hepatomas are unable to alter their rate of
cholesterol synthesis in response to dietary manipulations
including cholesterol (Mitchell et al.,1978).
Interestingly, these cells when grown in culture express
feedback inhibition in response to exogenous cholesterol
(Beirne and Watson, 1976). Apparently the resistance to
feedback inhibition involves an in vivo factor, e.g.
hormone, which may regulate receptor behavior and
cholesterol control of HMG CoA reductase gene expression.
It would appear that management of dietary lipid would have

minimal impact on cholesterol metabolism in tumor tissue.

CONCLUSION

Dietary fats, particularly omega-3 fatty acids inhibit hepatic production of fatty acids and triglycerides while promoting gluconeogenesis. In muscle and adipose tissues high fat diets impair glucose utilization by reducing insulin sensitivity which suppresses pyruvate dehydrogenase, and possibly inhibits glycolysis. The interaction of other hormones is likely. The changes in hormone responsiveness likely involves membrane lipid compositional changes induced by dietary fats. Such membrane alterations have already been associated with changes in norepinephrine turnover, adenylate cyclase activity, insulin binding, and LDL-receptor number. To date dietary manipulations have not affected the high rate of glucose metabolism and cholesterol synthesis occurring in cancer cells. However, hepatoma cells enriched with unsaturated fatty acids do exhibit greater susceptibility to natural killer cell-mediator cytolysis (Yoo et al., 1982). Furthermore diets rich in omega-3 fats decreased cancer growth in mice (O'Conner,1985). It is tempting to propose that omega-3 fatty acids (e.g., salmon oil) may have unique effects on cancer cell metabolism because of their potent capacity to alter carbohydrate and lipid metabolism (Phillipson et al.,1985) and their extensive enrichment of cell membranes (Odinet al.,1986). This aspect of lipid metabolism provides a significant area for productive study.

REFERENCES

Abraham S, Hillyard LA, Lin CY, Schwartz RS (1983). Specific dietary fatty acids on lipogenesis in the livers and mammary glands of lactating mice. Lipids 18:820-829.
Abumrad NA, Stearns SB, Tepperman HM, Tepperman J (1978). Studies on serum lipids, insulin, and glucagon and on muscle triglyceride in rats adapted to high fat and high carbohydrate diets. J Lipid Res 19:423-432.
Balasubramanian S, Simons LA, Chang S, Hickie JB (1985). Reduction in plasma cholesterol and increase in biliary cholesterol by a diet rich in n-3 fatty acids in the rat. J Lipid Res 26:684-689.

Begum N, Tepperman HM, Tepperman J (1982). Effect of high fat and high carbohydrate diets on adipose tissue pyruvate dehydrogenase and its activation by a plasma membrane-enriched fraction and insulin. Endocrinology 110:1914-1921.

Begum N, Tepperman HM, Tepperman J (1983). Effects of high fat and high carbohydrate diets on liver pyruvate dehydrogenase and its activation by a chemical mediator released from insulin-treated liver particulate fraction: Effect of neuraminidase treatment on the chemical mediator. Endocrinology 112:50-59.

Beirne OR, Watson JA (1976). Comparison of regulation of 3-hydroxy-3-methylglutaryl coenzyme A reductase in hepatoma cells grown in vivo and in vitro. Proc Natl Acad Sci (USA):2735-2739.

Bochenek WJ, Rodgers JB (1979). Dietary regulation of 3-hydroxy-3-methylglutaryl-CoA reductase from rat intestine. Biochim Biophys Acta 575:57-62.

Bringolf M, Zaragoza N, Rivier D, Felber JP (1972). Studies on the metabolic effects induced in the rat by a high fat diet. Eur J Biochem 26:360-369.

Cascales C, Mangiapane EH, Brindley DN (1984). Oleic acid promotes the activation and translocation of phosphatidate and phosphohydrolase from the cytosol to particulate fractions of isolated rat hepatocytes. Biochem J 219:911-916.

Clark M, Patten G S, Filsell OH (1982). An effect of diet on the activity of phosphofructokinase in rat heart. Biochem Biophys Res Comm 105:44-50.

Clarke BA, Clarke SD (1982). Polymer-protomer transition of acetyl-CoA carboxylase as a regulator of lipogenesis in rat liver. Arch Biochem Biophys 218:92-100.

Clarke SD, Romsos DR, Leveille GA (1977). The differential effects of dietary methylesters of long chain saturated and polyunsaturated fatty acids on rat liver and adipose tissue lipogenesis. J Nutr 107:1170-1180.

Clarke SD, Salati LM (1985). Fatty acid mediated disaggregation of acetyl-CoA carboxylase in isolated liver cells using avidin-inactivation technique. Fed Proc 44:2458-2462.

Clarke SD, Wilson, MD, Ibnhoughazala T (1984). Resistance of lung fatty acid synthesis to inhibition by dietary fat in the meal-fed rat. J Nutr 114:598-605.

Cook GA, Stephens TW, Harris RA (1984). Altered sensitivity of carnitine palmitoyltransferase to inhibition by malonyl-CoA in ketotic diabetic rats. Biochem J 219:337-339.

Cushman SW, Zarnowski J, Fransusoff AJ, Salans LB (1978). Alterations in glucose metabolism and its stimulation by insulin in isolated adipose cells during the development of genetic obesity in the Zucker fatty rat. Metabolism 27:1930-1940.

Declercq PE, Debeer LJ, Mannaerts GP (1982). Role of glycerol-phosphate and glycerophosphate acyltransferase in the nutritional control of hepatic triacylglycerol synthesis. Biochem J 204:247-256.

Haagsman HP, DeHaas CGM, Geelen MJH, Van Golde LMG (1982). Regulation of triacylglycerol synthesis in the liver. Biochem J 198:373-377.

Harris RA, Leland MC, Mahoney JM Mapes JP (1973). Regulatory function of mitochondria in lipogenesis. Lipids 8:711-716.

Hems DA, Whitton PD (1980). Control of hepatic glycogenolysis. Physiol Rev 60:1-49.

Herzberg GR (1983). The influence of dietary fatty acid composition on lipogenesis. Advan Nutr Res 5:221-253.

Howard RB, Widder DJ (1976). Substrate control of glycogenlevels in isolated hepatocytes. Biochem Biophys Res Comm 68:262-269.

Houslay MD (1985). Regulation of adenylate cyclase activityby its lipid environment. Proc Nutr Soc 44:157-165.

Hue L, Blackmore PG, Shikama H, Robinson-Steiner A, Exton JH(1982). Regulation of fructose-2,6-bisphosphate content in rat hepatocytes, perfused hearts, and perfused hindlimbs. J Biol Chem 257:4308-4313.

Ide T, Okamatsu H, Sugano M (1978). Regulation by dietary fats of 3-hydroxy-3-methylglutaryl CoA reductase in rat liver. J Nutr 108:601-612.

Ip C, Tepperman HM, Holohan P, Tepperman J (1976). Insulin binding and insulin response of adipocytes from rats adapted to fat feeding. J Lipid Res 17:588)599.

Kalopissis AD, Griglio S, Maswiak MI, Rozen R, Liepvie XL (1981). Very-low density lipoprotein secretion by isolated hepatocytes of fat-fed rats. Biochem J 198:373-377.

Kannan R, Wilson L, Baker N (1978). The role of dietary fat and hepatic triglyceride secretion in cancer-induced hypertriglyceridemia. Lipids 13:887-891.

Katz J, McGarry JD (1984). The glucose paradox- Is glucose a substrate for liver metabolism. J Clin Invest 74:1901-1909.

Kurokawa M, Oda S, Tsubotani E, Fujiwara H, Yokoyama K Ishibashi S (1982). Characterization of hexokinase isoenzyme types I and II in ascites tumor cells by an interaction with mitochondrial membrane. Molec Cell Biochem 45:151-157.

Lavau M, Fried SK, Susini C, Freychet P (1979). Mechanism of insulin resistance in adipocytes of rats fed a high fat diet. J Lipid Res 20:8-16.

Lawson N, Jennings RJ, Pollard AD, Sturton RG, Ralph SJ, Marsden CA, Fears R, Brindley DN (1982). Effects of chronic modification of dietary fat and carbohydrate in rats. Biochem J 200:265-273.

Lazo PA, Sols A (1980). Pyruvate dehydrogenase complex of ascites tumor. Biochem J 190:705-710.

McGarry JD, Foster DW (1979). In support of the roles of malonyl-CoA and carnitine acyltransferase I in the regulation of hepatic fatty acid oxidation and ketogenesis. J Biol Chem 254:8163-8168.

Miguel SG, Abraham S (1976). Effect of maternal diet on fetal hepatic lipogenesis. Biochim Biophys Acta 424:213-234.

Naito K, Isohashi F, Tsukanaka K, Horiuchi M, Okamoto K, Matsunaga T, Sakamoto Y (1985). Effects of D- and L-thyroxine on the glucocorticoid binding capacity of adult rat liver. Biochem Biophys Res Comm 129:447-452.

Narabayashi H, Lawson JWR, Uyeda K (1985). Regulation of phosphofructokinase in perfused rat heart. Requirement for fructose 2,6)bisphosphate and a covalent modification. J Biol Chem 260: 9750-9758.

Newsholme EA, Leech AR (1984). "Biochemistry for the Medical Sciences." New York: John Wiley, pp 336.

O'Brien BC, McMurray DN, Reiser R (1983). The influence of premature weaning and the nature of the fat in the diet during development on adult plasma lipids and adipose cellularity in pair-fed rats. J Nutr 113:602-609.

O'Connor TP, (1985). Dietary fat, calories and cancer. Contemporary Nutr 10:#7.

Parry DM, Pederson PL (1983). Intracellular localization and properties of particulate hexokinase in the Novikoff ascites tumor. J Biol Chem 258:10904-10912.

Phillipson BE, Rothrock DW, Connor WE, Harris WS, Illingworth DR (1985). Reduction of plasma lipids,

Lipoproteins, and apoproteins by dietary fish oils in patients with hypertriglyceridemia. New Engl J Med 312:1210-1216.

Pilkis SJ, El-Maghrabi MR, McGrane M, Pilkis J, Fox E, Claus TH (1982). Fructose 2,6-bisphosphate: A mediator of hormone action at the fructose-6-phosphate\fructose-1,6-bisphosphate substrate cycle. Molec Cell Endo 25:245-266.

Romsos DR, Clarke SD (1980). Suppliers of energy: Carbohydrate-fat interrelationships. Human Nutr 3A:141-158.

Romsos DR, Leveille GA (1974). Effect of diet on activity of enzymes involved in fatty acid and cholesterol synthesis. Advan Lipid Res 12:97-145.

Ruderman NB, Goodman MN, Conover CA, Berger M (1979). Substrate utilization in perfused skeletal muscle. Diabetes 28:1317.

Salati LM, Clarke SD (1986). Fatty acid inhibition of hormonal induction of acetyl-CoA carboxylase in hepatocyte monolayers. Arch Biochem Biophys 246:82-89.

Schwartz RS, Abraham S (1983). The effect of dietary fat on the activity, content, rates of synthesis and degradation and translation of messenger RNA coding for malic enzyme in mouse liver. Arch Biochem Biophys 221:206-215.

Selmeci LE, Weber G (1976). Increased glucose-6-phosphate dehydrogenase concentration in hepatoma 3924A: enzymic and immunological evidence. FEBS Lett 61:63-67.

Sommercorn J, Freedland RA (1982). Regulation of hepatic phosphofructokinase by 6-phosphogluconate. J Biol Chem 257:9424-9428.

Sommercorn J, Freedland RA (1984). Effects of diets on concentration of 6-phosphogluconate and fructose 26-bisphosphate in rat livers and an assay of fructose 26-bisphosphate with an improved method. J Nutr 114:1462-1469.

Spady DK, Dietschy JM (1985). Dietary saturated triacyglycerols suppressed hepatic low density lipoprotein receptor activity in the hamster. Proc Natl Acad Sci (USA) 82:4526-4530.

Stansbie D, Denton RM, Bridges BJ, Pask HT, Ramdle PJ (1976). Regulation of pyruvate dehydrogenase and pyruvate dehydrogenase phosphate phosphatase activity in rat epididymal fat pads. Biochem J 154:225-236.

Stewart JH, Briggs GM (1981). The effect of essential-
fatty acid deficiency on the activity of liver
phosphatidate phosphatase in rats. Biochem J 198:413-
416.
Sul HS, Shrago E, Goldfarb S, Rose F (1979). Comparison of
the adenine nucleotide translocase in hepatomas and rat
liver mitochondria. Biochem Biophys Acta 551:148-156.
Sun JV, Tepperman HM, Tepperman J (1977). A comparison of
insulin binding by liver plasma membranes of rats fed a
high glucose or a high fat diet. J Lipid Res 18:533-
539.
Tepperman HM, Tepperman J (1985). Membranes and the
response to insulin. Proc Nutr Soc 44:211-220.
Thomassen MS, Christinsian EN, Norum KR (1982).
Characterization of the stimulatory effect of high fat
diets on peroxisomal B-oxidation in rat liver. Biochem
J 206:195-202.
Tornheim K (1985). Activation of muscle phosphofructokinase
by fructose 2,6-bisphosphate and fructose 1,6-
bisphosphate is differently affected by other regulatory
metabolites. J Biol Chem 260:7985-7989.
Toussant WJ, Wilson MD, Clarke SD (1981). Coordinated
suppression of liver acetyl-CoA carboxylase and fatty
acid synthetase by polyunsaturated fat. J Nutr 111:146-
153.
Wieland O, Siess E, Schulze Z, Wethmar FH, Funcke HG,
WintonB (1971). Active and inactive forms of pyruvate
dehydrogenase in rat heart and kidney: Effects of
diabetes, fasting and refeeding on pyruvate
dehydrogenase interconversion. Arch Biochem Biophys
143:593-601.
Wigand JP, Anderson JH, Jennings SS, Blackard WG (1979).
Effect of dietary composition on insulin receptors in
normal subjects. Amer J Clin Nutr 32:6-9.
Williams BH, Berdanier CD (1982). Effects of diet
composition and adrenalectomy on the lipogenic responses
of rats to starvation-refeeding. J Nutr 112:534-541.
Wilson MD, Hays R, Clarke SD (1986). Inhibition of liver
lipogenesis by dietary polyunsaturated fat in severely
diabetic rats. J Nutr (in press).
Wong SH, Nestel PJ, Trimble RP, Storer GB, Illman RJ,
Topping DL (1984). The adaptive effects of dietary fish
and safflower oil on lipid and lipoprotein metabolism in
perfused rat liver. Biochem Biophys Acta 792:103-109.

Yoo TJ, Kuo CY, Spector AA, Denning GM, Floyd R, Whiteaker S, Kim H, Abbas M, Budd TW (1982). Effect of fatty acid modification of cultured hepatoma cells on susceptibility to natural killer cells. Cancer Res 42:3596-3600.

Dietary Fat and Cancer, pages 555–586
© 1986 Alan R. Liss, Inc.

MECHANISMS OF DIETARY FAT MODULATION OF TUMORIGENESIS:
CHANGES IN IMMUNE RESPONSE

Kent L. Erickson

Department of Human Anatomy, University of
California, School of Medicine, Davis,
California 95616

INTRODUCTION

The concept that fatty acids could play a role in
modulation of the immune response is not new. Over a
decade ago investigators demonstrated that addition of
exogenous fatty acids to lymphocytes in vitro influenced
immune function (reviewed by Meade and Mertin, 1978).
Both enhancement and suppression of T- and B-cell
responses have been reported depending on how fatty acids
were introduced. Other studies have used direct injection
of lipids into animals. Besides those types of studies
numerous other observations support the concept that fatty
acids, especially polyunsaturated ones, may take part in
immunoregulatory mechanisms and that will be discussed in
this review. However, the addition of fatty acids in
organic solvents to lymphocyte cultures or direct
injection of fatty acids into animals is
nonphysiological. Moreover, changes in immune response
after manipulation of fatty acids in vitro may not relate
to changes in vivo because of the complexity of cellular
and humoral interactions observed in vivo.

In general when rodents are fed a high-fat diet,
mammary tumor incidence is sharply increased and the
latency period of mammary tumor appearancy is reduced when
compared to the same parameters in animals fed low or
moderate levels of dietary fat (Welsch and Aylsworth,
1983). One possible mechanism is that dietary fat may
influence mammary tumorigenesis by suppression of the
immune response. Consequently we, as well as others, have

undertaken experiments to assess the influences of dietary fat on immune response. This review will thus focus first on how dietary fat influences lymphocytes and immune responsiveness. Accordingly the mode of action of dietary fats may be divided into two categories: 1) structural and 2) functional alterations. Examples of structural changes would include alteration in fatty acid composition, receptor binding sites and mobility, membrane rigidity and other biophysical parameters. Functional changes would include modification of any immunological response such as cytolysis of tumor targets by T lymphocytes or antibody and complement. Second, some of the possible mechanisms by which dietary fat may influence immunity will be discussed.

Compared to the number of studies which have used in vitro fatty acid manipulation very few have used a dietary approach. Although the focus of this review is on dietary fats, a summary of in vitro fatty acid effects on lymphocytes and macrophages may be helpful for hypothesis formulation and for explaining the possible mechanisms by which dietary fatty acids may influence immune responsiveness. A general review of immune response especially as it relates to nutrition has been given by Gershwin and coworkers (1985). Recently the role of eicosanoids in immunity has been reviewed (Johnston, 1985).

IN VITRO FATTY ACID INFLUENCES ON STRUCTURAL FEATURES OF LYMPHOCYTES

Lymphocytes, like other cells, contain a variety of fatty acids, some of which are essential, such as linoleic acid (18:2n-6) and others which are nonessential. Essential fatty acid(s) (EFA) must be present for many normal physiological functions. Not only do lymphocytes incorporate in vitro derived fatty acids into the cell membranes (Mandel et al, 1978; Klausner, et al 1980a; 1980b) but they may also undergo morphological changes as a result (Horwitz, et al, 1974). Lymphocytes, however, maintain a relatively constant degree of fatty acid saturation in the membrane phospholipids when grown in the presence of unsaturated fatty acids as demonstrated by the unsaturated:saturated fatty acid ratio (Mandel and Clark, 1978; Trail and Wick, 1984). It cannot be stated with certainty whether membrane fatty acid modification includes phospholipid fatty acyl substitution or intercalation into the membrane. In addition, changes in membrane lipid structure may involve either bulk lipids, localized changes in specific lipid domains, or a combination of both (Spector and Yorek, 1985). Cultured cells may also accumulate triglycerides as lipid droplets when they are exposed to excessive amounts of fatty acids relative to their immediate needs (Horwitz, 1977). In contrast, when fatty acids are limited in culture most of the exogenous fatty acids are incorporated into phospholipids for new membrane synthesis (King and Spector, 1981). Several other factors may influence fatty acid incorporation.

The lymphocyte has a membrane consisting chiefly of proteins and lipids in which the latter are constantly in a fluid state. Fatty acyl modification can influence the degree of ordering and motion in the hydrocarbon core of the lipid bilayer, a property that commonly is referred to as membrane fluidity. One factor that contributes to membrane fluidity is the ratio of polyunsaturated to saturated fatty acids; those cells having a lower ratio are generally less fluid than those cells having a higher ratio (Overath and Trauble, 1973; Trail and Wick, 1984; Stubbs and Smith, 1984). Fluidity will be markedly dependent on the number and position of the double bonds. On that basis, cells from animals in which their level of dietary fat concentration or saturation had been modified would be expected to either stiffen or fluidize their plasma membrane (Burns, et al, 1979). In addition, a relationship between membrane lipid composition and surface protein mobility may exist such that the less fluid membrane lipids would result in less mobility of the surface proteins particularly those that have a segment that passes through the lipid bilayer. For example, modification of membrane lipids affected patching and capping of murine histocompatability (H-2) antigens (Mandel and Clark, 1978). Changes in fluidity may depend on substitution of several fatty acids, as is the case with dietary fat manipulation, and not simply on substitution of a single fatty acid. For example, no difference was observed in electron spin resonance motional parameters between unsubstituted control murine leukemia cells and ones substituted with a single fatty acid, suggesting that incorporation of exogenous fatty acids induces compensatory changes in the membrane lipid

composition (Poon and Clark, 1982). Electron spin
resonance, however, may not be sufficiently sensitive to
detect changes due to modifications of the acyl chain
composition in complex biological membrane.

Fluidity can be assessed in several ways and one
method has been to measure the depolarization of a
hydrophobic probe molecule. Although controversial, the
use of 1,6-diphenyl 1,3,5-hexatriene (DPH) allows for the
assessments of environmental constraints upon the rotation
of the DPH molecule inserted between the acyl chains of
membrane phospholipids. In contrast to unsaturated fatty
acids which incorporate into the lymphocyte membrane when
added to the culture and reduce the polarization of DPH,
saturated fatty acids had no effect on DPH polarization
(Klausner et al, 1980a). They (Klausner et al, 1980a,
1980b) believe that based on difference in fluorescent
lifetimes, unsaturated free fatty acids partition
preferentially into the fluid-phase lipid domains whereas
saturated fatty acids partition into the gel-phase lipid
domains. However, other investigators have shown that
extensive changes in the fatty acid composition of
malignant murine T-cells did not lead to any biophysical
changes that could be detected by DPH. They suggested
that fatty acid alterations caused dramatic changes in the
function of plasma membrane-associated enzymes (McVey et
al, 1981).

Cross-linking and rearrangement of cell surface
antibody receptor molecules is one event that can trigger
an immune response. Receptor proteins in the plasmalemma
are mobile and may be cross-linked by divalent ligands
such as antibodies. These form aggregations called
patches which coalesce into a cap. The latter is shed or
internalized by the cell. Although low levels of
unsaturated free fatty acids added to the lymphocyte
plasma membrane were associated with inhibition of capping
no effect was observed with saturated fatty acids
(Klausner et al, 1980b; Hoover et al, 1982).

In addition to change in fatty acid composition by
exogenous lipids, lymphocyte stimulation by antigen or
mitogen may result in a change of the membrane fatty acid
composition (Ferber et al, 1975). These changes include a
rapid fatty acid turnover and an increase in select
acids. Membrane-associated acyl CoA lysolecithin

acyltransferases increase the incorporation of coenzyme A derivatives into the membrane with a high affinity for polyunsaturated fatty acids especially arachidonic acid (Ferber and Resch, 1976; Trotter et al, 1982). The increased fatty acid turnover can also be due to phospholipase generation of lysophosphatides in the cell membrane. Phospholipid methylation and the associated change in membrane fluidity may also play an important role in lymphocyte response to mitogens (Hirata and Axelrod, 1980). In vitro modification of the membrane phospholipid composition of plasmacytoma cells can cause a reduction in the intracellular transport and secretion of IgG1 (Nakano et al, 1982). In view of these observations, we hypothesize that the response of lymphocyte to antigens may be modified depending on the fatty acid substrate availability and the incorporation of those compounds into the cell membranes or the intracellular substrate storage pools.

IN VIVO FATTY ACID INFLUENCES ON STRUCTURAL FEATURES OF LYMPHOCYTES

Alteration of dietary fat concentration or saturation can result in alteration of the fatty acid composition of the cell itself. This has been demonstrated for a number of cells including lymphocytes from lymph nodes (Meade et al, 1978) and spleen (Tsang et al 1976; Erickson et al, 1983). Diets varying in either the concentration or saturation of fat changed the fatty acid composition of total splenic lymphocytes (Fig. 1) and the serum. For example, when the diets were supplemented with 20% polyunsaturated fat (PUF), safflower oil, the levels of linoleic acid increased in the lymphocytes with a concomitant decrease in both palmitoleic and oleic acids. Mice fed a diet with 20% saturated fat (SF), coconut oil, had decreased levels of oleic and linoleic acid in the lymphocytes (Erickson et al, 1983). In mice fed 8 and 20% PUF the levels of serum linoleic acid were higher and oleic and palmitoleic levels were lower as compared to mice fed a diet containing the minimum of EFA. Thus, only changes in serum unsaturated fatty acid levels were observed after varying dietary fat concentration and saturation (Thomas and Erickson, 1985b).

Besides changes in the fatty acid composition of the whole lymphocyte with dietary fat, the composition of cell

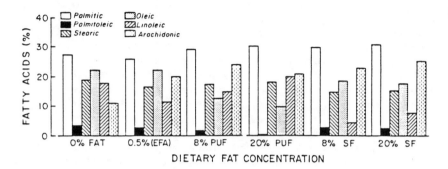

Figure 1. Fatty acid composition of splenic lymphocytes from mice fed differing amounts and types of fat. Diets contained either 0% fat (EFA deficient) or minimum EFA (0.5% corn oil). To test the influence of saturation 4 diets contained addition 8 or 20% safflower oil (PUF) or 8 or 20% coconut oil (SF) besides the EFA. Data shown represents triplicate samples for each group with six mice per group. Data from Erickson et al (1983).

membranes can also be modified (Burns et al, 1979). Specifically, lymphoid phospholipid composition may change as a function of dietary fat. For example, Marshall and Johnston (1983) reported that increasing the dietary α-linoleic to linoleic acid ratios resulted in an increase of n-3 fatty acids and a decrease in the n-6 fatty acids of phosphatidyl choline and phosphatidyl ethanolamine obtained from total nucleated spleen and thymus cells and peripheral blood lymphocytes. The magnitude of the change and the specific fatty acids altered varied with the cell populations and the dietary fat.

One potential problem when determining dietary fat influences on fatty acid composition of cells after culture is the flux of lipids. After culture the composition of cellular membranes may reflect the fatty acid composition of the serum (Horwitz, 1977). High levels of exogenously added fatty acids in the plasma membrane of the lymphocyte may flux into the culture medium when those cells are grown without high levels of the same exogenous fatty acid (Mandel et al, 1978; Poon & Clark, 1981). More recently, investigators have demonstrated a similar phenomenon with respect to changes

in the phospholipid composition of cells taken from
dietarily-manipulated animals and placed into culture
(Loomis et al, 1983). From these studies we may conclude
that lymphocytes from animals fed on high fat diets may
change their fatty acid composition to generally reflect
dietary intake. Which specific fatty acids are usually
involved as well as the kinetics of the change remain
poorly defined at this time.

INFLUENCE OF EXOGENOUS FATTY ACIDS ON IMMUNE RESPONSE

Manipulation of lymphocytes with fatty acids by
introduction into culture or subcutaneous injection has
been shown to influence cell-mediated immunity (review by
Meade & Mertin, 1978; Trail & Wick, 1984). Nevertheless,
a controversial issue is the exact influence of those
fatty acids; both an increase or decrease of immune
response have been reported. Experimental results,
however, depend upon how the fatty acids were delivered
into culture. For example, some investigators have
reported that polyunsaturated fatty acids dissolved in
ethanol inhibited lymphocyte transformation in response to
phytohemagglutinin while the same fatty acids injected
subcutaneously caused the prolongation of skin allograft
survival (Mertin et al, 1974; Ring et al, 1974) of both
the primary and secondary responses (Mertin, 1976; Mertin
and Hunt, 1976). Arachidonic acid dissolved in hexane,
however, has been reported to slightly enhance, whereas
the same fatty acid dissolved in ethanol has inhibited
phytohemagglutinin induced human lymphocyte blastogenesis
(Mikas et al, 1975; Kelly and Parker, 1979). Exposure of
cytotoxic memory cells to exogenous fatty acids during
their lectin-driven maturation to cytotoxic effector cells
markedly altered their cytotoxic potential (Gill and
Clark, 1980). Unsaturated fatty acids lead to an increase
in cytolytic capacity whereas saturated fatty acids lead
to a decreased function. The fatty acid alteration of
cytolytic capacity did not seem to be simply altering the
general metabolic activity of lymphocytes such as rates of
DNA and protein synthesis. These effects occurred in the
absence of cell division and, therefore, investigators
have suggested that this effect was mediated at the level
of the individual lymphocyte rather than through an
alteration of lymphocyte frequency in the effector cell
populations (Bialick, et al, 1984) Thus, it may be
hypothesized that polyunsaturated fatty acids take part in

immunoregulatory mechanisms and that the concentration of
these fatty acids could affect the interaction of lipids
and binding glycoproteins within the membrane of the cells
involved in cell-mediated immunity. However, changes in
immune response after manipulation of fatty acids in
culture, may not relate to changes of immune
responsiveness in vivo because of the complexity of cell
interactions.

Select tumor target cells cultured in certain fatty
acids may be more susceptible to complement-mediated
cytolysis than control cells cultured without fatty acids
supplements. Generally, fluidity of the tumor cell target
regulates the cell's susceptibility to complement attack;
increased susceptibility correlates with decreased
cholesterol:phospholipid ratios. For example, hepatoma
cells which were enriched with linoleic and oleic acid and
contained an increased amount of those fatty acids in
their cellular lipids were more susceptible to complement-
mediated cytolysis than control cells (Yoo et al, 1980;
Schlager, 1979; Schlager and Ohanian, 1979). To
investigate different parameters influencing the
susceptibility of target cells to lysis by antibody and
complement or cytotoxic T cells, Schlager and Ohanian
(1983) used a panel of drugs to block various metabolic
functions. Tumor cells with an increased sensitivity to
complement killing exhibited an increase in plasma
membrane fluidity whereas cells with an increased
susceptibility to cytotoxic T-lymphocyte attack showed an
increase in their net negative cell surface charge density
(Schlager and Ohanian, 1983). Cytotoxic T-cell
lympholysis also directly correlated with the synthesis
and content of highly polar lipids. In contrast, culture
of tumor target cells in other fatty acids usually not
found in mammalian cells such as nonadecanoic or elaidic
or found at low levels such as linolenic acid, were not
effected by complement-mediated lysis (Mandel et al,
1978). However, substitution of those same fatty acids
into the plasma membrane of the tumor target influenced
the rate of patching of H-2 surface antigens.

Changes in the susceptibility of target cells to
complement-mediated lysis may not only depend on the fatty
acids used for enrichment but also on the target cell and
the vehicle used to present the fatty acid (Erickson and
Thomas, 1985). The susceptibility of murine mammary tumor

cells to complement-mediated lysis by anti H-2 antibody
was tested after in vitro treatment with selected
unsaturated or saturated fatty acids dissolved in the
solvents, hexane or ethanol, or presented to the cells in
the form of micelles. The lytic susceptibility of those
cells was compared to similar targets grown in mice fed
diets containing different concentrations of safflower or
coconut oil or cultured with serum obtained from tumor-
free control mice fed pair matched diets. Alterations in
dietary fat resulted in changes of the tumor target cell
fatty acid composition but did not influence the
susceptibility of target cells to complement-mediated
lysis. In contrast, unsaturated fatty acids dissolved in
ethanol but not saturated fatty acids, reduced the lytic
susceptibility of tumor cells in vitro (Fig. 2).

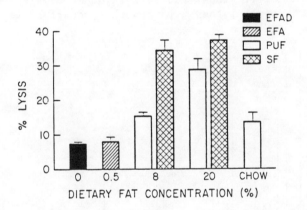

Figure 2. Complement-mediated cytolysis of mammary tumor
cells treated in vitro with serum from mice fed differing
amounts and types of fat. Line 168 tumor cells were
cultured with 5% serum obtained from normal mice
maintained on experimental diets as described for Fig.
1. Serum from mice fed 8% PUF, 8% SF, 20% PUF, and 20% SF
were significantly different than minimum EFA (0.5%)
control diet. Data from Erickson et al (1985).

Alterations in dietary fat resulted in changes of the
tumor target cell fatty acid composition but did not
influence the susceptibility of target cells to
complement-mediated lysis. In contrast, a combination of
unsaturated fatty acids dissolved in ethanol reduced the

lytic susceptibility of tumor cells in vitro whereas
saturated fatty acids increased the susceptibility (Fig.
3). When hexane was used as a carrier for fatty acids no
differences were observed among treatments with the
individual fatty acids at several concentrations. Lack of
differences may be due to the hexane and fatty acid
modification of target cell fragility. Thus, in vitro
fatty acids manipulation has a differential effect on the
lytic susceptibility of mammary cells to complement and
this appears to depend on the method used in the
presentation of fatty acids to the cell. The same pattern
of cytolysis after incubation with various dilutions of
antibody or complement suggests that incubation of target
cells in solvent plus fatty acids does not influence the
binding of anti-H2 or complement that mediates an effect
directly on the cell. Thus, the pattern of cytolysis in
vitro does not parallel the situation that occurs in vivo.

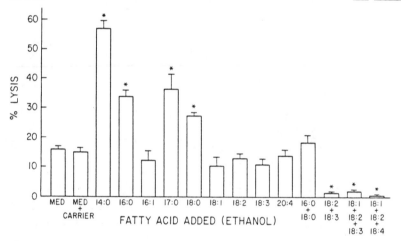

Figure 3. Complement-mediated cytolysis of mammary tumor
cells after culture with fatty acids. Line 168 tumor
cells from culture were incubated for 24 hr in medium plus
fatty acids delivered in ethanol. Cytolysis was measured
by incubation of diluted anti-H2^d antibody with
radiolabeled tumor cells followed by
complement. *Significantly different than carrier
control. Data from Erickson et al (1985).

Fatty acids in culture may be rapidly incorporated
into macrophages and can selectively alter the fatty acyl

composition of the macrophage phospholipids (Schroit and Gallily, 1979). Such fatty acid modification may influence functional characteristics. For example incorporation of the fatty acids, elaidic or nonadecanoic acid, decreased fluid-phase pinocytosis and receptor mediated phagocytosis. Macrophages containing a higher proportion of cis unsaturated fatty acids (cis-18:1) had higher phagocytic potentials than macrophages containing higher proportions of trans-unsaturated fatty acids (trans-18:1) (Schroit et al, 1976). No correlation between nonreceptor-mediated phagocytic activity and membrane fluidity was observed. Mahoney and coworkers (1977) have suggested that the degree of lipid fluidity of the macrophage membrane influenced receptor-mediated phagocytosis as well as the ability of the cell to interiorize its plasma membrane. Culture of macrophages with lymphokines and their resulting tumoricidal activation may be associated with changes in cellular cholesterol and polyunsaturated fatty acid composition (Schlager et al, 1983). When macrophages lost their tumoricidal activity cellular lipid content returned to normal. To mimic lymphokine activation macrophages were enriched with linolenic acid which resulted in tumoricidal activity. Thus, it appears that exogenously added fatty acids may influence select parameters of macrophage function.

DIETARY FAT MODULATION OF IMMUNE RESPONSE

Generally diets either deficient in essential fatty acid(s) (EFA) or containing high levels of fat can influence host immune status. Changes of those fatty acids during the prenatal and postnatal period may have an important influence on parameters of immune status in neonatal mice (Erickson et al, 1980). For example, lymphocyte transformation induced by concanavalin A (Con A) a polyclonal T-cell activator, was significantly decreased as levels of PUF increased from 2-24% whereas dietary fat did not influence the response to lipopolysaccharide, a B-cell mitogen. In that experiment the number of immunoglobulin-positive cells and serum IgG1 and IgG2 levels also decreased with increasing fat concentration. The drawback of that study was that some of the differences ascribed to the saturation of the dietary fat may be caused by EFA deficiency. Thus, with mice fed diets containing low or moderate amounts of coconut oil one cannot differentiate whether the effects were SF versus PUF or EFA deficiency versus EFA sufficiency. Nevertheless, high levels of PUF have been generally shown to depress the response of lymphocytes to mitogens. However, that effect is not the same for all sources of cells.

The fat content of the early postweaning diet may have an impact on the immune response which persists into adulthood (Carlomagno et al, 1983). Thus, interpretation of dietary effects may depend upon the duration of feeding and the organs examined. For example, rats fed a high fat diet showed evidence of splenic hyperplasia but no histopathological changes in the mesenteric lymph nodes (Locniskar et al, 1983). However, lack of quantitative data in that experiment makes interpretation of the extent of change difficult. When cultured with 10% fetal bovine serum (FBS) spleen cells of animals fed high PUF diets had a reduced level of blastogenesis in response to the mitogens Con A, phytohemagglutinin, and pokeweed. Supplementing the culture medium with 10% rat serum altered responses but the addition of serum from rats fed high fat diets did not have a suppressive effect on blastogenosis. The latter observation is in direct contrast to results obtained by others (Olson and Visek, 1984) who also used homologous serum in their cultures. However, because fatty acid composition of the cells was not reported it is difficult to know to what extend fatty acid were incorporated into or fluxed from the cells.

Interpretation of dietary fat influences on lymphoid cell function is tenuous when in vitro assays longer than 24 hrs are used. That is because of the potential change in cellular fatty acid composition to reflect that fatty acid composition of the culture medium. Although the kinetics of lipid flux from lymphocytes of dietary fat manipulated mice has not been reported, based on culture of leukemia cells with exogenous fatty acids the exchange requires about 24 hrs to reach an equilibrium (Mandel et al, 1978). Therefore, the addition of autologous or homologous serum may help to reduce the problem but certainly will not mimic the in vivo conditions with respect to lipid concentration. Besides a 3-5 day culture period, mitogen assays add the additional problem of circumventing a number of the early events in lymphocyte recognition. Therefore, use of that assay does not allow for assessment of either mechanisms of how lipid can modulate immune response or all events of specific immune response.

Effects on T-Cell Responses

Besides impairment of effector functions such as reduced allograft rejection, and response to T-cell mitogens dietary fats may also modulate lymphocyte response to defined antigens (Mertin & Hunt, 1976, Erickson, et al 1980). To assess that influence lymphocyte blastogenesis to alloantigens was measured. Spleen cells from mice fed experimental fat diets were used as responders to stimulation by spleen cells from mice fed a stock diet (table 1). Blastogenesis of responder lymphocytes was significantly greater for those mice fed a diet containing minimal EFA than those fed an EFA-deficient diet (Erickson, et al, 1983). When the dietary fat concentration was increased (20%), blastogenic responses decreased compared to the EFA control diet. To test whether dietary fats influenced the ability of histocompatability antigens to stimulate lymphocyte blastogensis, spleen cells from dietarily manipulated mice acted as stimulator cells for responding splenic lymphocytes from mice fed a stock diet. Blastogenesis of control lymphocytes in response to lymphocytes from mice fed a fat-free diet were significantly greater than responses to lymphocytes from mice fed a diet containing additional fat. The only exception was those stimulating cells from mice fed a high level of PUF (Erickson et al, 1983). Thus, dietary fats may differentially influence both the antigen stimulation and the lymphocyte resonse phase of lymphocyte blastogenesis.

The cell-mediated cytotoxic T-cell reaction, perhaps more than any other type of immune response, might be expected to be sensitive to changes in the biochemical composition and physical properties of the cell membrane because such an interaction involves significant numbers of receptors and antigenic determinants (Sanderson and Glauert, 1977; Kalina and Berke, 1976). Thus, the physical state of the cell membrane could affect the outcome of cytolysis in a number of ways. Exogenous free unsaturated fatty acids in ethanol increased whereas saturated fatty acids in the same vehicle decreased the in vitro cytotoxic capability of effector lymphocytes (Gill

TABLE 1. Blastogenesis of lymphocytes in response to alloantigens*

Dietary fat	Lymphocytes from dietary fat manipulated mice in response to alloantigens from control mice	Lymphocytes from control mice in response to alloantigens from dietary fat manipulated mice
0%	9,200 ± 1,000**	52,500 ± 1,740**
0.5%	24,700 ± 3,300	26,500 ± 5,000
8% PUF	18,800 ± 2,800	23,600 ± 4,000
8% SF	15,700 ± 2,600	28,000 ± 6,000
20% PUF	14,500 ± 2,400**	42,000 ± 4,100**
20% SF	14,200 ± 1,000**	25,000 ± 3,000

*CPM ± SEM for one way mixed lymphocyte culture. The diets contained either no fat (EFA deficient) or at least the minimum of EFA (0.5% corn oil). Two diets contained addition PUF (safflower oil) and two contained SF (coconut oil).
**Significantly (P< 0.05) different than the control (EFA) diet.

and Clark, 1980). To understand the possible mechanism(s) by which dietary fat may influence cytolysis, both effector and target cells were examined in an allogeneic anti-tumor cell-mediated immune response (Erickson, 1984; Thomas and Erickson, 1985a). Cytotoxicity mediated by murine splenic or peritoneal lymphocytes against tumor targets after a primary immunization decreased when moderate or high levels of fat (more than 8%) were fed. Generally, lymphocyte-mediated lysis was inversely proportional to the amount of fat present in the diet (table 2). Similar dietary influences were observed after a secondary immunization. This effect was directly mediated by the cytotoxic T-lymphocyte and not through a change in the number of suppressor or helper cells (Thomas and Erickson, 1985a). That, however, does not preclude

TABLE 2. Cytotoxicity of mammary tumor cells mediated by lymphocytes from dietary fat-manipulated mice*

Dietary fat	Cytotoxicity (%)	
	E:T = 20:1	E:T = 50:1
0	27.8 ± 1.6	45.6 ± 4.6
0.5%	28.2 ± 1.6	53.3 ± 5.3
8% PUF	14.4 ± 0.7**	32.6 ± 2.1**
8% SF	15.3 ± 1.4**	36.9 ± 1.9**
20% PUF	11.9 ± 1.2**	13.0 ± 0.9**
20% SF	8.9 ± 1.5**	36.2 ± 1.5**

*Splenic lymphocytes obtained from immunized mice fed experimental diets were used as effector (E) cells and line 168 mammary tumor cells (T) from culture were used as targets. Each value represents the mean ± SEM for 6 mice in each group. The diets used were the same as indicated for table 1; the experiment was repeated twice.
**Significantly ($P < 0.05$) less cytotoxicity than in the control (EFA) group.

that dietary fat could have an influence on suppressor or helper cell function. To determine the influence of dietary fat on mammary tumors as targets for immune cytolysis, tumor cells were either obtained from mice fed the experimental diets or cultured with serum from tumor-free control mice fed pair-matched diets. Dietary change of the fatty acid environment of the target mammary tumor cells in vivo or in vitro had no detectable effect on their susceptibility to lymphocyte-mediated cytotoxicity. Thus, we (Thomas and Erickson, 1985a) believe that lipids do not act by increasing or decreasing the number of T-cells or frequency of subpopulations or by altering susceptibility of the mammary target cell membrane to cytolysis. The fatty acid effects appear to be limited to immunocompetent cells and are qualitative through alteration at the levels of the individual cytotoxic lymphocyte.

To circumvent the problem of fatty acid flux into the culture medium when lymphocytes are grown without high levels of the same exogenous fatty acid, in vivo assays of T-cell functions have been used (DeWille et al, 1981; Thomas and Erickson, 1985b). Changing dietary fat concentration or degree of saturation has impaired effector functions such as reduced allograft rejection and delayed type hypersensitivity (DTH). For example, DTH responsiveness of mice fed an EFA deficient diet was less than for mice fed a diet containing a minimum amount of EFA (Fig. 4).

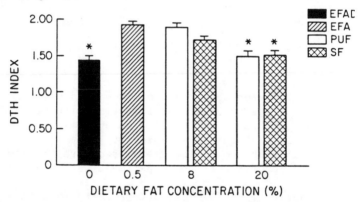

Figure 4. Dietary fat influences on delayed-type hypersensitivity (DTH) to allogeneic tumor cells. The diets used were same as indicated for figure 1. Mice fed the 0, 20% PUF, and 20% SF diets had a reduced level of responsiveness compared to mice fed the EFA control diet. Data from Thomas and Erickson (1985).

The suppressive effect of feeding an EFA deficient diet required a significant period of time but was reversed by feeding an EFA sufficient diet (DeWille et al, 1981). Likewise, the DTH reaction was reduced for mice fed a high level of total fat. Apparently, higher (20%) but not moderate (13%) concentrations of fat are required to mediate a suppressive effect. Thus, the usual level of fat in a murine diet (8% concentration) does not effect the Lyt 1[+] cells in mediating the DTH reaction. Another measure of T-cell responsiveness, the graft-versus-host reaction of spleen cells injected into irradiated mice, was suppressed in those mice fed similar high levels (20%) of PUF (Fig. 5). In those same animals, serum linoleic acid levels increased commensurate with increasing levels of PUF in the diets (Thomas and Erickson, 1985b). Likewise, levels of linoleic acid in whole lymphocytes appear to change in direct relation to serum fatty acid levels (Erickson et al, 1983). Thus, we conclude that linoleic acid plays a pivotal role in modulating cellular immune responses.

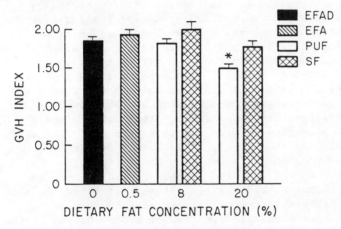

Figure 5. The influence of dietary fat on the graft-versus-host (GVH) reaction of spleen cells to allogeneic hosts. C57BL/6 spleen cells from mice fed the experimental fat diets were injected into the footpad of irradiated BALB/c mice previously fed the same diet as the donor mice. The GVH index was calculated by the ^{125}I-iododeoxyuridine radioactivity in the experimental/control popliteal lymph node. Mice fed the 20% PUF diet had a significantly lower response than mice fed the control (EFA only) diet. Data from Thomas and Erickson (1985).

Effect on B-Cell Responses

Early work has indicated that changes in dietary lipids during prenatal and postnatal development could influence several parameters of immune status in neonatal mice such as serum IgG1 and IgG2 levels (Erickson et al, 1980). Investigators have also shown that exogenous free fatty acids in culture had little effect on B-cell response to mitogens in vitro (Buttke, 1984). In contrast, dietary fat concentration and saturation may differentially modulate the level of antibody response to a defined antigen. High concentrations of dietary fat, particularly PUF, suppressed IgM and IgG plaque-forming cell (PFC) responses as long as minimal EFA were available (Erickson, et al, 1983) (Table 3). Mice fed a high level of SF exhibited increased IgM PFC responses. Other investigators have also demonstrated that a 20% PUF diet decreased antibody response in guinea pigs after a primary immunization (Friend et al, 1980). After a secondary immunization the number of IgG producing cells followed a similar response pattern. Those changes associated with dietary fat were also reflected in serum anti-SRBC IgM and IgG levels. We conclude that the differential in the number of antibody forming cells appears to be inversely related to the levels of linoleic acid in the lymphocyte components other than the plasmalemma. This is based on the observation that levels of linoleic acid in whole lymphocytes changed in direct relation to the serum fatty acid level (Erickson et al, 1983; Thomas and Erickson, 1985b) however, no differences in the fatty acid composition of the isolated lymphocyte plasmalemma was observed (Adams et al, 1985). Although it is possible that the fatty acid composition is altered in certain membrane lipid domains, detection of gross changes in the fatty acid composition is not possible. Homeostatic regulation of lipid composition appears to be relatively strict (Trait and Wick, 1984). We conclude that changes in immune function appear to be manifested at the single cell level as an alteration in the frequency of cell responding to antigen.

EFA deficiency has been shown to either increase B-cell response (Boissonneault and Johnston, 1983) or depress (DeWille et al, 1979) it depending upon the route of injection of antigen. For example, after an i.v. injection of SRBC, EFA deficiency resulted in stimulation of PFC responses observed compared to controls of mice fed an EFA adequate diet. In addition, EFA deficiency resulted in a diminution in PGE and PGF levels in spleen and liver (Boissonneault and Johnston, 1983). They concluded that an inverse relationship existed between hepatic arachidonic acid levels and capacity for PG synthesis and an inverse relationship between splenic PGF1 levels and PFC responses. However, without direct measurements of fatty acid levels of the splenic B cells the exact relationship, if any, among dietary fat, arachidonic acid, and B-cell response remains obscure.

TABLE 3. Antibody-forming cell response of lymphocytes from mice fed various amounts of dietary fat*

Dietary fat	PFC/10^6 spleen cells	
	direct	indirect
0	187 ± 64	416 ± 113
0.5%	336 ± 56	685 ± 123
8% PUF	237 ± 70	738 ± 19
8% SF	381 ± 51	798 ± 120
20% PUF	155 ± 42**	480 ± 70**
20% SF	422 ± 40	782 ± 97

*Mice were fed the experimental diets for 6 weeks before primary immunization with SRBC then maintained on the same diet until assay on day 6 for the number of plaque forming cells (PFC). The diets used were the same as indicated for table 1.
**Significantly ($P < 0.05$) different than for mice fed the 0.5% (minimal EFA) diet.

Effects on Macrophages

Fatty acids introduced in vivo may influence some parameters of macrophage function but have no effect on others. For example, Intralipid, a soybean emulsion used in total parenteral nutrition, is removed from circulation by macrophages and suppresses functional activities such as the production of C2 and C4 in guinea pig macrophages (Strunk et al, 1983). After direct incubation with

Intralipid, macrophage phospholipids had an increased
level of palmitic, oleic, and linoleic acids and a
decreased level of arachidonic acid. The reduced
production of C2 by macrophages was reversed after
incubating with both Intralipid and arachidonic acid. The
influence of dietary fat on other select macrophage
functions has also been examined (Magrum and Johnston,
1983). The relationship of dietary fat to PG production
and macrophage activity is an important one as PG,
particularly PGE, have a very important role in the down
regulation of macrophage effector function such as
macrophage-mediated cytolysis of tumor targets (Taffet and
Russell, 1981). Phagocytosis by peritoneal macrophages
was significantly decreased in mice fed high fat diets,
particularly lard, (Morrow et al, 1985). Phagocytosis has
also been shown to be accompanied by the synthesis of PG
by the macrophage. In contrast, the feeding of n-3 fatty
acids did not appear to affect the phagocytosis of yeast
cells or carbon particles. However, arginase activity in
macrophages from rats fed linseed oil was found to be
greater when compared to macrophages from rats fed corn
oil. Change in arginase activity correlated with a
decrease in PGE production. Chemiluminescence, an
activity resulting from the synthesis of reactive oxygen,
was reduced in macrophages cultured with arachidonic acid
(Magrum and Johnston, 1985). Whether dietary fats
directly effect macrophage functions which are associated
with immune response such as antigenic processing and
presentation remains to be determined.

MECHANISMS OF DIETARY FAT INDUCED IMMUNOMODULATION

There are two principal mechanisms by which dietary
fat may influence immune responsiveness: by alteration of
cell membrane structure and function, by modulation of
prostaglandin synthesis, or both. These will be discussed
with consideration to the _in vivo_ and _in vitro_ effects of
lipids mentioned above.

Modulation of Membrane Structure

Cross-linking and rearrangement of cell surface
antibody receptor molecules may be an event that triggers
an immune response. Receptor proteins in the plasmalemma
are mobile and may be cross-linked by divalent ligands
such as antibodies. Changes in the composition of the

local lipid environment of a receptor molecule may affect both binding and cross-linking events. Thus, lipid fluidity may play a role in protein mobility by an influence on rotational or lateral diffusion within the lipid bilayer or their interactions with other membrane components. This has been demonstrated by the observation that fluidity of membrane lipids affects patching and capping of H-2 antigens (Mandel et al, 1978). Lipids surrounding receptors or antigens may affect the conformation, thereby enhancing or reducing the accessibility of the binding sites. If that is the case then only certain protein segments which pass through the lipid bilayer would be potentially affected by lipid modification. Alternatively, the receptor or antigen may be located in a lipid domain that is or is not affected by a particular type of lipid modification.

Fluidity is usually decreased by increasing the ratios of saturated:unsaturated fatty acids, cholesterol:phospholipids, and spingomyelin:lecithin (Trail & Wick, 1984). Modulation of membrane cholesterol and fatty acid content has been used to study the effect of altered fluidity on membrane protein lateral and rotational mobility and membrane function. Although polarization of DPH is commonly used, criticism of the technique centers around the meaningfulness of average fluidity measurements when the probe may partition into different domains or exhibit different lifetimes in different environments. Our studies of fluorescent polarization with DPH in total splenic lymphocytes indicated a shift in the motional restriction of DPH with changes in dietary fat (Adams, et al, 1985). Polarization values of DPH were reduced in whole splenic lymphocytes from mice fed the 20% PUF diet compared to lymphocytes from mice fed the minimal EFA diet (Fig. 6). Polarization values of lymphocytes from mice fed the 20% SF diets were increased. To determine whether changes in polarization values were a function of changes in membrane fluidity or uptake of the probe into several hydrophobic domains within the whole cell, fluorescent lifetimes were measured. More than one lifetime indicates the presence of more than one molecular environment. Fluorescent lifetime measurements of control lymphocytes indicated two lifetime components. This shows that the polarization values for the intact cell are an average of molecular motion in more than one domain. Accordingly, fluorescent

polarization analysis has been carried out on isolated
plasma membranes. Kleinfeld and coworkers (1981) have
found a decrease in polarization of DPH in the plasmalemma
isolated from lymphocytes cultured with free linoleic acid
as compared to controls without exogenous fatty acids.
More pronounced changes in fluidity may also depend on
substitution of several fatty acids as in the case of
dietary fat manipulation not simply on substitution of a
single fatty acid. We (Adams et al 1985) have observed
that isolated lymphocyte plasmalemmas from mice fed 20%
PUF diet had a lower polarization value than mice fed a
diet with minimal EFA implying greater mobility of the
probe in the plasma membrane (Fig. 6). Most observed
changes, however, in the polarization values of DPH in
splenic lymphocytes probably arise from components other
than the plasmalemma. Other workers believe that the
effect on rotational relaxation time of lymphocytes
cultured with unsaturated fatty acids was due to the
formation of lipid droplets in the cytoplasm (Stubbs et
al, 1980). Lack of pronounced change in the total cell
may also be due to offsetting differences in lymphocyte
subpopulations. For example, we have observed a
differential polarization response in T and B cells to
dietary fat manipulation; the B-cell membrane from
lymphocytes of mice fed high fat diets was more rigid than
B-cell membranes from mice fed a diet containing the
minimum of EFA. These observations could represent an
uncoupling of the receptors in the B cell from the enzyme
systems which must confer changes upon specific membrane
domains to allow for the production of immunoglobulins.

   Shortly after binding of ligand to receptor membrane
enzymes may become activated. Before Ca^{++} influx is
observed two methyl transferase enzymes may be activated
to methylate phosphatidyl ethanolamine to become
phosphatidyl choline (PC) and cause a transfer from the
inner leaflet to the outer leaflet of the plasmalemma.
This has been associated with an increase in fluidity
(Hirata & Axelrod, 1980). Concomitant activation of the
acyl CoA lysolecithin acyltransferase enzymes with
incorporation of unsaturated fatty acids into
phospholipids may account for the increase in fluidity
observed shortly after stimulation of a lymphocyte by
mitogen. Our preliminary evidence with proton nuclear
magnetic resonance indicates that the relative ratios of
PC of the inside and outside membrane bilayer shifts in

lymphocytes from animals fed high levels of PUF (Fig. 7). Position of the PC was identified by incubation of the cells with increasing concentrations of $GdCl_3$. With that compound the external phospholipid in the bilayer is

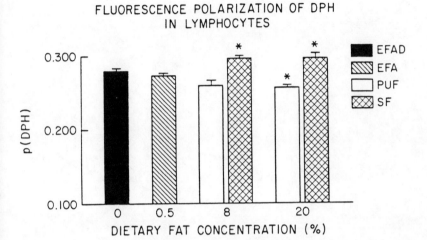

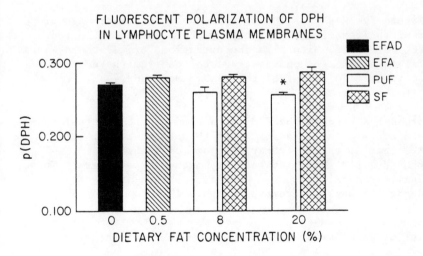

Figure 6. Polarization values of DPH in whole cells and plasma membrane of lymphocytes from mice fed experimental diets. Values are mean p ± SD.

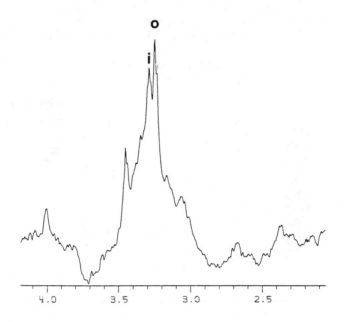

Figure 7. High resolution (500 mHz) [1]H-nuclear magnetic resonance spectra of splenic lymphocytes from mice fed a 20% PUF diet. With high concentrations of PUF there was a relative shift of phosphatidylcholine from the outer (O) to inner (I) leaflet of the plasma membrane.

broadened because the Gd^{3+} ions bind to the external face and are unable to pass through (Mountford et al, 1982). In light of this, further analysis of membrane phospholipid and fatty acid asymmetry is necessary. This analysis should also use purified subpopulations to determine any differential effect.

Influence of Prostaglandins on Immune Function

Linoleic acid is one of the unsaturated fatty acids which can be a precursor for PG. T cells appear to be influenced by PG (Goodwin and Webb, 1980). For example, PGE added to culture caused a reduction in the ability to phytohemmagglutinin to stimulate lymphocyte blastogenesis. PGE_1 and E_2 are also known to be T-cell feedback inhibitors and are formed in the cell membrane from the incorporation of dihomo-γ-linoleic and arachidonic acids in membrane phospholipids. PG are capable of inhibiting T-cell responses such as T-cell proliferation, lymphokine production, and cytotoxicity as well as the differentiation of lymphocyte destined to become helper, cytotoxic, or suppressor cells. A close correlation between increased cAMP levels and inhibition of cytolysis by lymphocytes have been observed when PG are present (Henney et al, 1972). With the addition of the PG inhibitor, indomethacin, to cultures, increased antibody dependent cellular cytotoxicity (Droller et al, 1978) as well as inhibition of the suppressive effect of T cells (Fulton and Levy, 1980) have resulted. Since high levels of PUF are associated with high levels of PG, and PG has been shown to suppress the immune response through an increase in cAMP then one possible mechanism of dietary fat modulation of immune responsivenss may be mediated through PG. Decreased PG synthesis in correlation with an increased humoral response are consistent with the immunosuppressive effects of PG (Boissonneault and Johnston, 1983).

Modification of the phospholipid fatty acyl composition can affect PG production by cultured cells. This may be due to increased availability of arachidonic acid in the intercellular phospholipid storage pools that provide substrate for PG synthesis. The arachidonic content may vary considerably because the pools are very labile. Thus, PG effects may be explained by changes in the polyunsaturated fatty acid composition of the intercellular substrate pools. Then the primary effect would be mediated through a change in substrate availability. Most studies of dietary fat, eicosanoids, and immune response, however, have mainly been concerned with stable PG. It is possible that PG precursors, like arachidonic acid, when diverted from one pathway will follow another path such as that of the leukotrienes. Certainly future investigation should pursue studies on the relationship between dietary fat and lipoxygenase products on specific immune responsiveness.

CONCLUSIONS

We are just starting to understand the role that

lipids can play in regulation of immune response. Sufficient evidence indicates that dietary fat can modulate immune responsiveness. Dietary fat modulation of immune response has generally been demonstrated with high levels of one fat type. Because diets consumed by animals and humans usually contain a blend of fats and some which may be processed, e.g., hydrogenated, it will be important to assess the effects of varying ratios or those blends on immune function. Other potentially important factors which effect the dietary fat include fatty acid concentration, chain length, number and position of the double bond(s). Studies of dietary effects on immune response present a challenge because many of the assay systems use longer term in vitro cultures which may allow the fatty acid composition of the lymphocyte to reflect the composition of the culture medium rather than the diet. One solution would be to use short term (less than 4 hr) in vitro or in vivo assays. Nevertheless, dietary lipid associated changes may influence one or several of the necessary events in lymphocyte activation. Such parameters as antigen binding, receptor modulation, signal transduction, and antibody secretion may all be sensitive to the lipid composition of the cell. Whether the same or different mechanisms are operational for T and B cells and macrophages is not known at this time. In addition, the exact relationship among dietary lipids, immune response, and mammary tumorigenesis remains to be determined. It does appear, however, that dietary fat effects are mediated through changes in the effector lymphocyte and not the tumor target. We believe that responses of lymphocyte to antigen may be modified depending upon the available fatty acids and that dietary fat manipulation will change that availability.

ACKNOWLEDGEMENTS

The authors work cited in this review was supported by grant CA 30273 from the National Cancer Institute and a grant from the National Live Stock Meat Board, Chicago, IL.

REFERENCES

Adams DA, Freauff SJ, Erickson KL (1985). Biophysical characterization of dietary lipid influences on lymphocytes. In Kabara J (ed): "Pharmacological Role

of Lipids", Vol. 2, Champaign, IL: American Oil
   Chemists Society, pp 11-22.
Bialick R, Gill R, Berke G, Clark WR (1984). Modulation
   of cell-mediated cytotoxicity function after
   alteration of fatty acid composition in vitro. J
   Immunol 132:81-87.
Boissonneault GA, Johnston PV (1983). Essential fatty
   acid deficiency, prostaglandin synthesis and humoral
   immunity in Lewis rats. J Nutr 113:1187-1194.
Boissonneault GA, Johnston PV (1984). Humoral immunity in
   essential fatty acid deficient rats and mice: effect
   on route of injection of antigen. J Nutr 114:89-94.
Burns CP, Luttenegger DG, Dudley DT, Buetter GR, Spector
   AA (1979). Effect of modification of plasma membrane
   fatty acid composition on fluidity and methotrexate
   transport in L1210 murine leukemia cells. Cancer Res
   39:1726-1732.
Buttke TM (1984). Inhibition of lymphocyte proliferation
   by free fatty acids. I. Differential effects on
   mouse B and T lymphocytes. Immunology 53:235-242.
Carlomango MA, O'Brien BC, McMurray DN (1983). Influence
   of early weaning and dietary fat on immmune responses
   in adult rats. J Nutr 113:610-617.
DeWille JW, Fraker PJ, Romsos DR (1981). Effects of
   dietary fatty acids on delayed-type hypersensitivity
   in mice. J Nutr 111:2039-2043.
DeWille JW, Fraker PJ, Romsos DR (1979). Effects of
   essential fatty acid deficiency, and various levels of
   dietary polyunsaturated fatty acids on humoral
   immunity in mice. J Nutr 109:1018-1027.
Droller MJ, Perlmann P, Schneider MU (1978). Enhancement
   of natural and antibody-dependent lymphocyte
   cytotoxicity by drugs which inhibit prostaglandin
   production by tumor target cells. Cell Immunol
   39:154-164.
Erickson KL (1984). Dietary fat influences on murine
   melanoma growth and lymphocyte-mediated
   cytotoxicity. J Natl Cancer Inst 72:115-120.
Erickson KL, Adams DA, McNeill CJ (1983). Dietary lipid
   modulation of immune responsiveness. Lipids 18:468-
   474.
Erickson KL, McNeill CJ, Gershwin ME, Ossman JB (1980).
   The influence of dietary fat concentration and
   saturation on immune ontogeny in mice. J Nutr
   110:1555-1572.
Erickson K, Thomas IK (1985). Susceptibility of mammary

tumor cells to complement-mediated cytolysis after in vitro and in vivo fatty acid manipulation. J Natl Cancer Inst 75:333-340.

Ferber E, DePasquale GG, Resch K (1975). Phospholipid metabolism of stimulated lymphocytes composition of phospholipid fatty acids. Biochim Biophys Acta 398:364-376.

Ferber E, Resch K (1976). Phospholipidstoffwechsel stimuliester Lymphozyten, Unterschungen zum molekularen Mechanisms der Aktivierung. Naturwissenshaften 63:375-381

Friend JV, Lock SO, Gurr MI, Parish WE (1980). Effect of different dietary lipids on the immune responses of Hartley strain guinea pigs. Int Archs Allergy Appl Immunol 62:292-301.

Fulton AM, Levy JG (1980). The possible role of prostaglandins in mediating immune suppression by non-specific suppressor cells. Cell Immunol 52:29-37.

Gershwin ME, Beach RS, Hurley LS (1985). "Nutrition and Immunity". New York: Academic Press, pp 1-417.

Gill R, Clark W (1980). Membrane structure-function relationships in cell-mediated cytolysis. I. Effect of exogenously incorporated fatty acids on effector cell function in cell-mediated cytolysis. J Immunol 125:689-695.

Goodwin JS, Webb DR (1980). Regulation of the immune response by prostaglandins. Clin Immunol Immunopathol 15:106-122.

Henney CS, Bourne HE, Licktenstein CM (1972). The role of cyclic 3',5'-adenosine monophosphate in the specific cytolytic activity of lymphocytes. J Immunol 108:1526-1534.

Hirata F, Axelrod J (1980). Phospholipid methylation and biological signal transmission. Science 209:1082-1090.

Hoover RL, Klausner R, Karnovsky MJ (1982). Inhibition of cap formation on lymphocytes by free fatty acids is not mediated by a depletion of ATP. J Biol Chem 257:2151-2154.

Horwitz AF (1977). Manipulation of the lipid composition of cultured animal cells. In Poste G, Nicolson GL (eds): "Dynamic Aspects of Cell Surface Organization" Amsterdam: Elseiver pp 295-305.

Horwitz AF, Hatten ME, Burger MN (1974). Membrane fatty acid replacements and their effect on growth and lectin-induced agglutinability. Proc Natl Acad Sci

USA 71:3115-3119.

Johnston PV (1985). Dietary fat, eicosanoids, and immunity. Adv Lipid Res 21:103-140.

Kalina M, Berke G (1976). Contact regions of cytotoxic T lymphocyte-target cell conjugates. Cell Immunol 25:41-51.

Kelly JP, Parker CW (1979). Effects of arachidonic acid on mitogenesis in human lymphocytes. J Immunol 122:1556-1562.

King ME, Spector AA (1981). Lipid metabolism in cultured cells. In Waymouth C, Ham R, Chapple PJ (eds), "Growth Requirements of Vetebrate Cells" New York: Cambridge Univ. Press, pp 293-312.

Klausner RD, Bhalla DK, Dragsten P, Hoover RL, Karnovsky MJ (1980a). Model for capping derived from inhibition of surface receptor capping by free fatty acids. Proc Natl Acad Sci U.S.A. 77:437-441.

Klausner RD, Kleinfeld AM, Hoover RL, Karnovsky MJ (1980b). Lipid domains in membranes. J Biol Chem 255:1286-1295.

Kleinfeld AM, Dragsten P, Klausner RD, Pjura WJ, Matayoshi ED (1981). The lack of relationship between fluorescence polarization and lateral diffusion in biological membrnaes. Biochim Biophys Acta 649:471-480.

Locniskar M, Nauss KM, Newberne PM (1983). The effect of quality and quantity of dietary fat on the imnmune system. J Nutr 113:951-961.

Loomis RJ, Marshall LA, Johnston PV (1983). Sera fatty acid effects on cutlured rat splenocytes. J Nutr 113:1292-1298.

Magrum LJ, Johnston PV (1983). Modulation of prostaglandin synthesis in rat peritoneal macrophages with $\omega 6$ fatty acids. Lipids 18:514-521.

Magrum LJ, Johnston PV (1985). Effect of culture in vitro with eicosatetraenoic and eicosapentaenoic acid on fatty acid composition, prostaglandin synthesis and chemiluminescence of rat peritoneal macrophages. Biochim Biophys Acta 836:354-360.

Mahoney EM, Hamill AL, Scott WA, Cohn ZA (1977). Response of endocytosis to altered fatty acyl composition of macrophage phospholipids. Proc Natl Acad Sci USA 74:4895-4899.

Mandel G, Clark W (1978). Functional properties of EL-4 tumor cells with lipid altered memranes. J Immunol 120:1637-1643.

Mandel G, Shimizu S, Gill R, Clark W (1978). Alteration of the fatty acid composition of membrane phospholipids in mouse lymphoid cells. J Immunol 120:1631-1636.

Marshall LA, Johnston PV (1983). The effect of dietary α-linolenic acid in the rat on fatty acid profiles of immunocompetent cell populations. Lipids 18:737-742.

McVey E, Yguerabide J, Hanson DC, Clark WR (1981). The relationship between plasma membrane lipid composition and physical-chemical properties. Biochim. Biophys Acta 642:106-118.

Meade CJ, Mertin J (1978). Fatty acids and immunity. Adv Lipid Res 16:127-165.

Meade CJ, Mertin J, Sheena H, Hunt R (1978). Reduction by linoleic acid of the severity of experimental allergic encephalomyelitis in the guinea pig. J Neurol Sci 35:291-308.

Mertin J, Hunt R (1976). Influence of polyunsaturated fatty acids on survival of skin allografts and tumor incidence in mice. Proc Natl Acad Sci USA 73:928-931.

Mikas AD, Gibson RG, Herschowitz BI (1975). Suppression of lymphocyte transformation by 16,(16) dimethyl prostaglandin E_2 and unsaturated fatty acids. Proc Soc Exp Biol Med 149:1026-1028.

Morrow WJW, Ohashi Y, Hall J, Pribnow J, Hirose S, Shirai T, Levy JA (1985). Dietary fat and immune function I. Antibody responses, lymphocyte and accessory cell function in (NZB X NZW)F_1 mice. J Immunol 135:3857-3863.

Mountford CE, Grossman G, Reid G, Fox RM (1982). Characterization of transformed cells and tumors by proton nuclear magnetic resonance spectroscopy. Cancer Res 42:2270-2276.

Nakano A, Maeda M, Nishijima M, Akamatsu Y (1982). Phospholipid modification retards intracellular transport and secretion of immunoglobulin G1 by mouse MOPC-31C plasmacytoma cells. Biochim Biophys Acta 692:177-186.

Olson LM, Visek WJ (1984). Influence of dietary protein level and fat type on lymphocyte activation. Fed Proc 43:475.

Overath P, Trauble H (1973). Phase transition in cells, membranes and lipids of Escherichia coli. Detection by fluorescent probes, light scattering, and dilatometry. Biochem 12:2625-2634.

Poon R, Clark WR (1982). The relationship between plasma

membrane lipid composition and physical-chemical properties. III. Detailed physical and biochemical analysis of fatty acid-substituted EL-4 plasma membranes. Biochim Biophys Acta 689:230-240.

Poon R, Richards JM, Clark WR (1981). The relationship between plasma-membrane lipid composition and physical-chemical properties. II. Effect of phospholipid fatty acid modulation on plasma membrane physical properties and enzymatic activity. Biochim Biophys Acta 649:58-66.

Ring J, Serfeit J, Mertin J, Brendel W (1974). Prolongation of skin allografts in rats treated with linoleic acid. Lancet 2:1331.

Sanderson CJ, Glauert AM (1977). The mechanisms of T-cell mediated cytotoxicity. Proc R Soc Lond (Biol) 198:315-323.

Schlager SI (1979). Specific ^{125}I-iodination of cell surface lipids: plasma membrane alterations induced during humoral immune attack. J Immunol 123:2108-2113.

Schlager SI, Meltzer MS, Madden LD (1983). Role of membrane lipids in the immunological killing of tumor cells: II. Effector cell lipids. Lipids 18:483-488.

Schlager SI, Ohanian SH (1983). Role of membrane lipids in the immunological killing of tumor cells: I. Target cell lipids. Lipids 18:475-482.

Schlager SI, Ohanian SH (1979). A role for fatty acid composition of complex cellular lipids in the susceptibility of tumor cells to humoral killing. J Immunol 123:146-152.

Schroit AJ, Gallily R (1979). Macrophage fatty acid composition and phagocytosis: effect of unsaturation on cellular phagocytic activity. Immunology 36:199-205.

Schroit AJ, Rottem S, Gallily R (1976). Motion of spin-labeled fatty acids in murine macrophages: relation to cellular phagocytic activity. Biochim Biophys Acta 426:499-512.

Spector AA, Yorek MA (1985). Membrane lipid composition and cellular function. J Lipid Res 26:1015-1035.

Strunk RC, Kunke KS, Kolski GB, Revsin BK (1983). Intralipid alters macrophage membrane fatty acid composition and inhibits complement (C2) synthesis. Lipids 18:493-500.

Stubbs CD, Smith AD (1984). The modification of mammalian membrane polyunsaturated fatty aicd composition in relation to membrane fluidity and function. Biochim Biophys Acta 779:89–137.

Stubbs CD, Tsang WM, Belin J, Smith AD, Johnson SM (1980). Incubation of exogenous fatty acids with lymphocytes. Changes in fatty acid composition and effects on the rotational relaxation time of 1,6-diphenyl-1,3,5-hexatriene. Biochem 19:2756–2762.

Taffet SM, Russell SW (1981). Macrophage-mediated tumor cell killing: regulation of expresion of cytolytic activity by prostaglandin E. J Immunol 126:424–427.

Thomas IK, Erickson KL (1985a). Lipid modulation of mammary tumor cell cytolysis: direct influence of dietary fats on the effector component of cell-mediated cytotoxicity. J Natl Cancer Inst 74:675–680.

Thomas IK, Erickson KL (1985b). Dietary fatty acid modulation of murine T-cell responses in vivo. J Nutr 115:1528–1534.

Trail KN, Wick G (1984). Lipids and lymphocyte function. Immunol Today 5:70–76.

Trotter J, Flesch I, Schmidt B, Ferber E (1982). Acyltransferase-catalyzed cleavage of arachidonic acid from phospholipids and transfer to lysophosphatides in lymphocytes and macrophages. J Biol Chem 257:1816–1823.

Tsang WM, Belin J, Monro JA, Smith AD, Tompson RH, Zlkha KJ (1976). Relationship between plasma and lymphocyte linoleate in multiple sclerosis. J Neurol Neurosurg Psychiat 39:767–771.

Welsch CW, Aylsworth CF (1983). Enhancement of murine mammary tumorigenesis by feeding high levels of dietary fat: a hormonal mechanism? JNCI 70:215–221.

Yoo TJ, Chiu HC, Spector AA, Whiteaker RS, Denning GM, Lee NF (1980). Effect of fatty acid modification on cultural hepatoma cells on susceptibility to complement-mediated cytolysis. Cancer Res 40:1084–1090.

Dietary Fat and Cancer, pages 587–606
© 1986 Alan R. Liss, Inc.

Metabolic Activation of Carcinogens

Adelbert E. Wade and Suniti Dharwadkar

Department of Pharmacology and Toxicology
College of Pharmacy, Univ. of Georgia
Athens, Georgia 30602

It has been suggested that a large proportion of human cancers results from exposure to chemical procarcinogens. Most procarcinogens are inert when exposure occurs but become reactive when activated metabolically following entrance into the body. Dietary fat has been associated with increased incidence of several human cancers, and laboratory evidence suggests that the major influence of fat occurs during the promotional phases of chemically induced carcinogenesis. The fact that human exposure to chemical carcinogens generally occurs over several years and involves very low doses of multiple carcinogens and/or promoters suggests that carcinogenic processes are occurring repeatedly. The influence of dietary fat on the initial events such as activation of the carcinogen as a contributing factor in human carcinogenesis cannot therefore be dismissed.

ACTIVATION/DETOXIFICATION SYSTEMS

The Mixed Function Oxidases in Carcinogen Activation

One of the most important enzyme systems for metabolically activating carcinogens is a group of enzymes known as the mixed function oxidases (MFO) located in the endoplasmic reticulum of most cells. This membrane bound system requires cytochromes P-450 (P-450), NADPH cytochrome P-450 reductase and phosphatidylcholine for its maximal catalytic activity. Molecular oxygen and NADPH are essential for this system to function. Most procarcinogens

undergo metabolism in the body and the resulting
metabolites may have greater or lesser potential to
initiate cancer depending upon the enzyme or its location
in the body. Benzo(a)pyrene [B(a)P], the most thoroughly
studied prototype of the polycyclic aromatic hydrocarbon
(PAH) carcinogens, is metabolized by the MFO to several
products including phenols, quinones and epoxides. Of
these metabolites, the epoxides are most reactive with
nucleophilic moieties of cellular macromolecules such as
DNA (Singer and Grunberger, 1983). Primary epoxides may
undergo hydration by epoxide hydrolase. The location of
epoxide hydrolase in the endoplasmic reticulum allows it to
act in conjunction with the MFO as a detoxifying enzyme.
(Fig. 1) For example, Oesch et al. (1976) reported that
epoxide hydrolase decreased the mutagenic action of B(a)P
when added to the microsome mediated Ames reverse mutation
assay. However, epoxide hydrolase may also produce
dihydrodiols which serve as substrates for the formation of
the ultimate carcinogenic diolepoxides, and thus this
enzyme also plays an important role in chemical carcinogenicity. The balance between activating and detoxifying
enzymes is often the determining factor in the expression
of carcinogenicity, and this balance may be altered by
factors such as age and nutrition, as well as by the
selective induction of one or more components of the MFO.

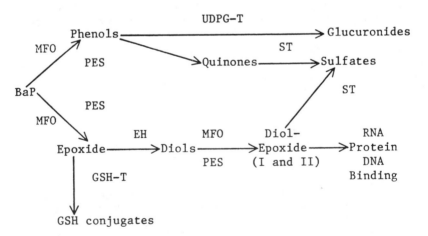

Fig. 1 Metabolism of B(a)P. EH = epoxide hydrolase; GSHT=
glutathione S-transferase; ST = sulfotransferase; UDPG-T =
UDP glucuronyl transferase

Jerina and Daly (1977), Jerina et al. (1980) and Levin
et al. (1977) reported that oxygenation of the conformationally hindered "bay regions" of PAH, such as B(a)P leads
to formation of epoxides that are resistant to epoxide
hydrolase and subsequent glucuronide conjugation. As a
result, these bay region epoxides tend to form highly
reactive carbonium ions capable of reacting with critical
intracellular nucleophiles such as DNA. These bay regions
are probably oxidized by one of two mechanisms a)
oxygenation by hydroxyl radicals, such as the trans-
oxygenation during prostaglandin formation (Reed and
Marnett, 1982), or b) oxygenation by a P-450 species having
an active site that can accomodate this conformation.
Among the different molecular species of the cytochrome
isolated, those induced by phenobarbital (P-450) and
3-methylcholanthrene (P-448) appear to exhibit the most
widely contrasting stereo specificities toward several
substrates including B(a)P. Although P-450 inserts oxygen
into conformationally unhindered positions, P-448
oxygenates conformationally hindered positions or bay
regions (Thakker et al., 1977; Deutsch et al., 1978).
Levin et al. (1977) using solubilized preparations
demonstrated that P-448 is more efficient than P-450 in
forming mutagenic products from B(a)P and in converting the
± trans B(a)P-7,8 dihydrodiol to the 7,8-dihydrodiol-
9,10-epoxide, the ultimate carcinogen. Ioannides et al.
(1984) suggest that compounds which induce P-448 should be
suspect carcinogens.

The extent of covalent binding to DNA and RNA but not
to proteins has been reported to correlate with carcinogenic potency of the compound. The major adduct of B(a)P
metabolites to DNA is the d-guanine B(a)P diol epoxide I
adduct where the N-2 of guanine is bound to the C-10
position of the B(a)P metabolite.

Although the greatest MFO activity occurs in liver,
the activity is not evenly distributed throughout all cells
of this organ. Several PAH including B(a)P, are hydroxyl-
ated most extensively within centrilobular regions in
livers of untreated rats (Wattenberg and Leong, 1962).
These authors also reported that B(a)P hydroxylase (AHH)
activity appears to be enhanced to the greatest degree
within the central portion of the liver lobule following
the treatment of rats with 3-methylcholanthrene (3-MC).
Others have reported that MFO activities associated with
drug and carcinogen metabolism are also unequally
distributed within tissues such as the lung and skin (Baron

and Kawabata, 1983). Differences in the concentrations and activities of xenobiotic activating and detoxicating enzymes within either discrete cell types or morphologically similar cells may account for the relatively selective nature of chemically induced carcinogenicity.

Prostaglandin Endoperoxide Synthase in Carcinogen Activation

Marnett et al. (1975, 1981) showed that several chemicals, including B(a)P, were metabolized during the conversion of arachidonic acid to prostaglandins. Two enzymatic steps are involved in the conversion of arachidonic acid to prostaglandin H_2. One, catalyzed by cyclooxygenase, converts arachidonic acid to the hydroperoxy endoperoxide PGG_2 while the other, catalyzed by hydroperoxidase, reduces PGG_2 to the alcohol PGH_2. During this reduction the carcinogen is oxidized by a cooxidation process. Both enzyme functions are carried out by a single protein called prostaglandin endoperoxide synthase (PES). Since PES activity is high in many extrahepatic tissues which have low MFO activity, this enzyme may play a major role in the activation of carcinogens in these tissues. Although cooxidation of B(a)P during prostaglandin biosynthesis leads to the stable metabolites 1,6, 3,6 and 6,12 quinones which are generally considered detoxication products, cooxidation of the proximate carcinogen B(a)P-7,8-dihydrodiol forms the anti-diolepoxide. Both isomers of B(a)P-7,8-dihydrodiol are converted by PES to the anti-diol epoxide while the MFO convert the positive isomer to the syn-diol epoxide and the negative isomer to the anti-diol epoxide (Thakker et al., 1977; Deutsch et al., 1975; Krauss and Eling, 1984). The anti-diol epoxide is considered the most potent carcinogenic metabolite of B(a)P.

Several kinds of chemical carcinogens besides B(a)P have been shown to undergo activation by PES through cooxidation reactions (Amstad and Cerutti, 1983; Robertson et al., 1983; and Zenser et al., 1983). When cooxidation with PES was the apparent activating system, a decreased incidence of resulting tumors was generally observed following the administration of PES inhibitors (Zenser et al., 1983); however, when both systems (PES and MFO) were involved in the activation, inhibition of PES did not alter resultant DNA adduct formation or tumorigenesis (Anderson et al., 1983). Nemoto and Takayama (1984) showed that the addition of arachidonic acid and other unsaturated fatty acids such as linoleic, were effective in activating B(a)P with both lung and liver microsomes and cytosols. Linolenic acid activated B(a)P less efficiently but oleic acid was ineffective. In contrast, they reported that addition of polyunsaturated fatty acids to incubation mixtures inhibited the MFO catalyzed metabolic activation and resultant binding of B(a)P metabolites to DNA (Nemoto and Takayama, 1983). Negishi and Hayatsu (1984) demonstrated that polyunsaturated fatty acids inhibited the in vitro mutagenic activation of N-nitrosodimethylamine (DMN).

Detoxifying Conjugation Reactions

Metabolites generated by the MFO or PES systems can be conjugated enzymatically to form products which are usually more polar, less lipid soluble and thus more readily excreted from the organism. Primary epoxides such as those from the PAH can be conjugated by the glutathione S-transferases, whereas the phenols and quinones are conjugated principally by UDP-Glucuronyl transferase and/or sulfotransferases (Singer and Grunberger, 1983).

Wattenburg (1983) suggested that one approach to inhibiting carcinogenesis might be to enhance the level of activity of the glutathione S-transferases and thus prevent the carcinogen from reaching or reacting with critical target sites. Induction of glutathione S-transferase by extracts of the green coffee bean were shown to inhibit mammary neoplasia in the rat resulting from the administration of 7,12 dimethylbenzanthracene (DMBA). In another study, Wattenberg (1979) reported that enhancement of glutathione-S-transferase was associated with reduced carcinogenic response of the forestomach to B(a)P administration.

ROLE OF DIETARY FAT IN CARCINOGEN ACTIVATION

Changes in Carcinogen Metabolism Mediated by Dietary Fat

Although the mechanism by which dietary fat enhances cancer incidence in response to carcinogens is unknown, it has been suggested that dietary factors such as fat may affect the rate(s) of carcinogen activation or detoxification.

A source of polyenoic fatty acids is necessary for optimal activities of the microsomal MFO system. Deprivation of dietary lipid results in changes in relative content of microsomal phospholipid fatty acids, and associated with these changes are decreased metabolism of various xenobiotics, decreased content of P-450 and decreased binding of substrates to microsomal P-450 (Norred and Wade, 1972). Qualitative alterations, as evidenced by changes in the apparent Michaelis constant (Km) for several substrates, may also occur. Cheng et al. (1980) reported that P-450 content of microsomes, as quantitated by sodium dodecylsulfate polyacrylamide gel electrophoresis, was not altered by dietary corn oil nor were there significant differences in the quantity of protein representing each of the four isolated species of P-450. Therefore, we concluded that dietary fats may cause selective pertubations in the membrane which in turn alter the intra-membrane positioning of P-450. These alterations in P-450 orientation may increase its reactivity with carbon monoxide and thus result in an apparent increase in P-450 content as measured by the intensity of the carbon monoxide-induced spectral change. Thus dietary polyenoic acids may be necessary for the synthesis of endoplasmic reticulum phospholipids which facilitate electron transfer (Strobel et al., 1970; Coon et al., 1971), and which are capable of maintaining a full complement of P-450. These phosopholipids also support this hemeprotein in its proper conformation to effect maximal xenobiotic oxidation reactions.

We have shown that the MFO inducer, phenobarbital (PB), increases liver weight to body weight ratio and the content of microsomal P-450 to a greater extent in rats fed diet containing corn oil than in those fed diets devoid of polyunsaturated fats (Norred and Wade, 1973). Although PB significantly increased the concentrations of the 43,000, 45,000 and 48,000 molecular weight P-450's in rats fed both diets, this effect was significantly more pronounced in rats fed the corn oil diet (Cheng et al., 1980). Feeding a diet containing coconut oil (largely saturated fatty acids) failed to permit the degree of PB induction afforded by the diet containing corn oil. These findings imply that dietary polyunsaturated fatty acids have a central role in promoting maximal induction of the MFO by PB.

Lam and Wade (1981) studied the rate of metabolism of B(a)P in the isolated perfused livers of 3-methyl-cholanthrene (3-MC) treated rats fed a diet for 21 days devoid of or containing 10% corn oil. Significantly higher concentrations of the B(a)P dihydrodiols and 3-hydroxy B(a)P were recovered in perfusates of livers from rats fed the diet containing 10% corn oil than from perfusates of livers of rats fed the fat-free diet. The fact that only the 7,8- and 9,10-dihydrodiols could be recovered from the perfusate in the unconjugated form and that the concentrations of these two metabolites were the only ones to decline with time (after reaching a peak at about 30-40 minutes), suggested that they were (1) resistant to conjugative detoxication and (2) could serve as substrate for further metabolism to the highly reactive diol epoxides. These dihydrodiols which are resistant to conjugative detoxification may be distributed to other organs for further metabolic activation by MFO or PES. The enhanced rate of production of B(a)P metabolites by livers of rats fed high fat diets might thus be expected to increase the carcinogenicity of B(a)P.

Wade et al. (1985) reported that microsomal metabolism of the procarcinogens, DMN and B(a)P, increased as the level of dietary corn oil increased from 0 to 20% by weight. The apparent Vmax of these substrates was increased in relation to microsomal P-450 content. Since essential fatty acid deficiency evokes changes in fatty acid composition of the endoplasmic reticulum within four days (for example, decrease in linoleic and arachidonic acids and an increase in palmitic acids, Brenner et al., 1982), it seems reasonable to postulate a probable causal relationship based on these membrane changes. Although induction of several drug metabolizing enzymes and P-450 by PB is dependent upon a dietary source of fat, this fat dependence was not observed for induction of B(a)P or DMN metabolism. That the level of fat, although important in determining basal activities, failed to alter AHH inducibility by PB may be in part related to the multiple pathways of B(a)P degradation and to the fact that we measured only the production of phenols. The administration of PB for 4 days prior to harvesting microsomes resulted in significant induction of the Vmax for DMN N-demethylase I (substrate concentrations od 0.125 to 8 mmolar) in rats fed the fat-free diet, but resulted in no induction (females) or suppression (males) of this enzyme in rats fed the diet containing corn oil.

    Male rats fed fat-free diet for 21 days responded to
3-MC induction of P-448 content equally to those fed a diet
containing 3% corn oil although the basal and induced
levels of enzyme activity were both lower in those animals
fed the fat-free diet (Wade et al., 1978). Using a
starvation/refeeding protocol we reported similar effects
(Wade and Bellows, In Press). In both 4 and 21 day feeding
studies P-450 induction due to 3-MC was more pronounced
than that due to PB in rats fed fat-free diet. For
example, PB resulted in about 10% induction of P-450 in
rats refed a fat-free diet, while 3-MC resulted in 112%
induction in P-448 in liver microsomes of rats refed that
diet. Although final concentrations of 3-MC-induced P-448
were higher in rats fed the 3% and 20% corn oil diets, the
percentage induction was inversely related to dietary fat.
The dependency on a dietary source of fat for the synthesis
of new P-450 therefore, appears to vary with the form of
cytochrome being synthesized in response to different
inducers. As shown previously, basal level of DMN
demethylase I was elevated with increasing concentration of
corn oil in the diet. Although DMN N-demethylase I is
generally not induced by 3-MC, those animals fed the
fat-free diet exhibited increased activity in a manner
similar to their response to PB. Rats fed diets containing
corn oil responded to the 3-MC and PB with the expected
depression of this N-demethylase.
    Roebuck et al., 1985, 1985a reported that increasing
concentration of corn oil (rich in n-6 fatty acids)
increased the incidence of L-azaserine induced pancreatic
preneoplastic lesions and the growth of visible tumors in
male Wistar rats while diets containing 5% corn oil or 20%
menhaden fish oil (rich in n-3 fatty acids) under otherwise
identical experimental conditions reduced the number and
size of pre-neoplastic lesions (O'Conner et al., 1985).
These findings suggest that manipulating dietary fat type
may be important in altering incidence of certain types of
tumors. Wade et al. (In Press) found that an increase in
menhaden oil content of the diet from 0.5% to 20% was
correlated with an increase in hepatic microsomal P-450
content. The apparent Vmax for microsomal DMN N-demethylase
likewise was increased as menhaden oil content of the diet
was increased. Not only was total liver P-450 increased by
menhaden oil but the specific activity of the P-450 for
metabolizing DMN (metabolized per unit of P-450) was also
increased. Although corn oil also enhanced Vmax of DMN
N-demethylase in a dose dependent manner, the specific

activity of P-450 mediating this reaction was not elevated. The apparent Vmax for microsomal AHH was increased in rats fed the menhaden oil diet; however, the increase did not appear to be dose dependent as observed for corn oil.

Phenobarbital induced the microsomal P-450 content significantly only in rats refed diets containing 10% or 20% menhaden oil and the induced levels of P-450 were elevated in proportion to the menhaden oil concentration in the diet. The apparent Vmax for DMN N-demethylase, although enhanced by dietary menhaden oil in a dose related manner, was not induced by PB in rats fed this oil. In the menhaden oil fed rats the specific activity of P-450 for DMN-N- demethylase decreased as the amount of P-450 increased. Thus PB-induced P-450's in menhaden oil fed animals did not support the oxidative demethylation of DMN. This PB-induced repression of DMN N-demethylase has been reported for animals fed corn oil (Wade et al., 1985) as well as laboratory chow (Arcos et al., 1975). Induction of the apparent Vmax for AHH by PB was similar in all dietary groups and does not appear to depend upon the level of coconut oil (saturated fatty acids), corn oil (unsaturated n-6 fatty acids) or menhaden oil (unsaturated n-3 fatty acids).

Although PB induction of the apparent Vmax for AHH is not fat dependent there were fat-related changes in the kinetics of this reaction. Recent experiments conducted in our laboratory show that the apparent Km for this reaction was increased by PB in menhaden oil fed rats. This increase in Km was due to a progressive decrease in hydroxylation of B(a)P below control values as concentrations of substrate were lowered. These findings may explain some of the inconsistencies which appear in the literature concerning the influence of dietary fat on B(a)P activation, mutagenicity and carcinogenicity in the presence of inducers.

Martin et al. (1980) reported that feeding a high fat diet did not change the activity of AHH regardless of whether they used an unsaturated vegetable fat, such as corn oil or a saturated animal fat such as beef tallow. Although Gaillard et al. (1977) observed that in male rats, AHH activity was related to the quantity and not the quality of fat in the diet, others have shown that quality of fat is important. Lambert and Wills (1977, 1977a) and Wills (1980) demonstrated that the activity of AHH was enhanced by feeding a 10% corn oil diet or a 10% herring oil diet when compared to values from a 10% lard group.

Agradi et al. (1975) reported that B(a)P metabolism by liver microsomes from rats fed a 10% saturated fat diet was reduced to about 50% of that of microsomes from rats fed diets containing olive, rapeseed or sunflower oils.

Martin et al. (1980) and Smith-Barbaro et al. (1981) reported that increasing the amount of dietary vegetable fat caused an increase in the level of P-450 present in small intestine and colon. This increase was much more significant in female rats than in male rats. Increasing the amount of saturated fat, however, caused no change in small intestine mucosal P-450 levels in male rats while a 30% increase in the small intestine of female rats fed a high saturated fat diet has been reported. Martin et al. (1980) also reported a sex related stimulation of AHH activity in the small intestine of male rats fed a high vegetable fat diet but Chhabra and Fouts (1974) could not detect a sex related difference in the metabolism of B(a)P by microsomes of the small intestine from rats fed laboratory chow.

The relation between dietary intake of polyunsaturated fatty acids and the formation of biologically active products derived from them is complex. Galli et al. (1981) showed that feeding corn oil significantly reduced arachidonate levels of phospholipids of platelets and aorta but increased linoleate and arachidonate levels of phospholipids in hepatocytes. Their findings that dietary manipulations selectively affected the cyclooxygenase component of PES depending upon the tissue suggests that activation of carcinogens may be different under various dietary states and in various tissues. Little is known about the influence of dietary fat on carcinogen activation by the PES system.

Although the MFO may in certain circumstances perform detoxification functions and in other circumstances activate compounds to highly reactive metabolites, the functions of the glutathione S-transferases are restricted to detoxification. Using two substrates, Norred and Marzuki (1984) reported that feeding a diet containing 20% corn oil resulted in a 25% to 40% increase in cytosolic glutathione S-transferase activities compared to those of rats fed 20% coconut oil (saturated fat) diet. Associated with these increased Vmax's were a 3 fold decrease in the Michaelis constants (Km) for these reactions. We have shown that cytosolic glutathione S-transferases which have the potential for detoxifying or trapping enzymatically generated reactive metabolites are induced by PB only in rats fed a source of polyunsaturated fatty acids (Wade et al., in press). Thus the potential for dietary fat to qualitatively or quantitatively alter the ratio of these activating and detoxifying systems may be extremely important in understanding the role of diet in the initial steps in drug detoxification or carcinogen activation. The final effect in vivo thus is dependent on the balance between the activities of these two systems in various environmental and/or dietary conditions.

Relation of Metabolism to Carcinogen-DNA Binding

Baker et al. (1983) measured rates of B(a)P metabolite formation and the metabolism of B(a)P to products which covalently bind with macromolecules using hepatic nuclei in an in vitro microsomal preparation. They reported that microsomes from male ICR Swiss mice fed diet containing corn oil metabolized B(a)P to products that bound to DNA more extensively than those from mice fed a fat-free diet. At a high B(a)P concentration (96 µmolar), microsomes from the corn oil fed untreated mice produced 26% more extractable metabolites and covalent binding to exogenous DNA was increased by 58%. However at lower substrate concentrations (.94 to 15 µmolar) B(a)P-DNA and B(a)P protein binding were 300 to 400 percent greater when incubated with microsomes from the corn oil fed mice than when incubated with microsomes from rats fed the fat-free diet. The apparent Vmaxs determined for the formation of each extractable metabolite were increased 1.5 to 3 times by the corn oil diet. Hepatic nuclear AHH and nuclear activation of B(a)P to products which covalently bind to DNA in both non-induced and 3-MC pretreated animals fed the corn oil diet were also greater. The increase in protein and DNA adduct formation may have resulted not only from increases in metabolism but also from selective alterations of those pathways which lead to the formation of reactive metabolites.

At saturating substrate concentrations the B(a)P metabolites which bind to DNA represent approximately 1% of the total metabolites extracted. Thus small to moderate alterations of activation pathways as determined by extracted metabolite formation may not be detectable in this system. At lower substrate concentrations, however, metabolic profile changes may be more evident since they are reflected in alterations of their apparent kinetic parameters. For example, the apparent Vmax for the formation of 7,8-dihydroxy-7,8-dihydro-B(a)P was increased and its apparent Km decreased by feeding the corn oil diet. This metabolite is the precursor of the ultimate carcinogen 7,8-dihydroxy-9,10-epoxy 7,8,9,10-tetrahydro B(a)P. The fact that this product has a lower Km than all other substrates measured suggests that in in vivo situations, where the substrate concentrations are low, this 7,8-dihydroxy-7,8-dihydro-B(a)P may be preferentially formed.

The ability of dietary corn oil to selectively enhance B(a)P metabolism indicates that certain forms of P-450 are responsive to changes in dietary fats. Dietary corn oil had little effect on the degree of hepatic microsomal AHH activity following induction with 3-MC. Differences in responsiveness may be due to the presence of forms of P-450 which differ in their dependence upon membrane phospholipids for optimal activity. Therefore, modulation of carcinogen activation by dietary lipids with respect to target tissue and carcinogen type should be considered as a factor in chemical carcinogenesis. Our recent studies on the interrelationship of dietary fat type and content to B(a)P metabolism, indicate that dietary corn oil and menhaden oil enhanced the microsomal capacity to catalyze in vitro covalent binding of B(a)P to exogenously added DNA (Dharwadkar et al., 1985). Further, PB induced this capacity to metabolize B(a)P to those forms which bind to DNA only in rats fed a source of these dietary fats. Since increases in B(a)P-DNA binding were accompanied with reduced levels of AHH (measured by phenolic products formed), the fat-related increase in in vitro B(a)P-DNA binding may be due to a selective increase in the formation of diol epoxides. It has been reported that MFO inducers increase in vitro DNA-adduct formation (Boobis et al., 1979; Sykora, 1984) but decrease subsequent tumor formation in vivo (Slaga, 1980).

Marzuki and Norred (1984) found no difference in biliary excretion of aflatoxin metabolites or their in vivo binding to nucleic acids when male rats were fed diets containing either 20% corn oil, 20% coconut oil or 18% coconut oil plus 2% corn oil for three weeks and adminstered a single dose of tritiated aflatoxin B_1. As expected, the corn oil diet resulted in higher hepatic microsomal P-450 levels than the coconut oil diet. Although there was increased in vitro conversion of aflatoxin B_1 to aflatoxin Q_1 and M_1, the in vitro production of water soluble metabolites and the covalent binding of metabolites to protein were unaffected by corn

oil in the diet. The authors suggest that the formation of
the putative carcinogenic metabolite, aflatoxin B_1 epoxide,
which undergoes detoxication through glutathione
conjugation is not affected by the type of dietary fat.
Thus unsaturated fat enhances aflatoxin B_1 carcinogenesis
through a mechanism other than by alterating the metabolic
activation of aflatoxin B_1.

Relation of Metabolism to Mutagenicity

Wade et al. (1982), in looking at the effects of
dietary corn oil on the metabolism and mutagenic activation
of DMN by hepatic microsomes found that feeding a diet
containing 10% corn oil resulted in microsomes from both
male and female rats capable of metabolizing DMN more
rapidly than microsomes recovered from rats fed a similar
diet but devoid of corn oil. Using concentrations of DMN
ranging from 12 to 100 mM, microsomes from rats fed the
high fat diet activated DMN to produce mutagenesis in
S-typhimurium TA 100 more rapidly than those from rats fed
the fat-free diet. Phenobarbital administration induced
this activation more effectively in rats fed the corn oil
diet than in rats fed the fat-free diet. Phenobarbital
induces DMN N-demethylation in rats fed both fat-free and
10% corn oil diets when the DMN concentration is above 10
mM and explains at least in part this enhanced mutagenic
activation.

Castro et al. (1978) recovered microsomes from rats
fed up to 21 days on diets containing high polyunsaturated
fats or low fat diets and demonstrated that microsomes from
animals fed high fat diets provided greater mutagenic
capabilities to acetylaminofluorene (AAF) than rats fed low
fat or saturated fat diets. Ponder (1984) and Ponder and
Greene (1984) evaluated the influence of trans fatty acids
in diets of rats on the mutagenic potential of several
carcinogens using rat hepatocytes and liver cell
homogenates as metabolic activating systems in the Ames
Assay. The mutagenic potential of B(a)P and AAF were
significantly decreased in the S-9 assay from arachlor
induced animals fed the trans fatty acid diet when compared
to animals fed a control diet. In the hepatocyte assay
B(a)P, 2-anthramene, and aminofluorene (AF) did not produce
a mutagenic response. The incorporation of butylated
hydroxy toluene (BHT) in the diet of rats enhanced
mutagenic potential of AAF and AF but not B(a)P. This

effect was independent of the lipid composition of the diet. The most significant increment in the production of mutagenic metabolites was observed with AAF when BHT and hydrogenated fats were included in the diet of rats. Dietary hydrogenated fats appeared to potentiate the effects of BHT on AAF mutagenicity.

Relation of Metabolism to Tumorigenicity

Rikans et al. (1979) found a positive correlation between the incidence of DMBA induced mammary tumors in rats fed diets of different lipid compositions with different MFO activities, and suggested that metabolism in this target tissue may be involved in DMBA induced carcinogenesis. Clinton et al. (1984) fed isoenergetic diets containing 20% corn oil, 20% beef tallow or an equal mixture of 10% corn oil and 10% beef tallow to rats for 4 weeks following weaning. A higher incidence of DMBA induced mammary tumors was accompanied by increased levels of P-450. However no significant differences in AHH or glutathione S-transferase activities were observed. Although these authors did not measure the formation of the ultimate carcinogen they concluded that the higher incidence of mammary tumors in rats fed unsaturated fat diets was not associated with changes in AHH activity. Bunce et al. (1983) studied the effect of dietary fat on tumor promotion in DMN treated mice. There was a significantly greater number of lung tumors in DMN treated animals than in controls. Lung tumor incidence in DMN treated animals varied significantly among the dietary regimens, with those receiving the fat-free diet having more tumors than those receiving the tallow diet and these in turn had more tumors than the mice fed the diet containing corn oil. Although the incidence of liver tumors was low in DMN treated animals, the following trends were noted; fat free > tallow > corn oil. These and earlier results suggest that lung tumor incidence following DMN administration is inversely related to the metabolic rate of DMN by hepatic microsomes.

Since humans are exposed repeatedly to relatively low concentrations of carcinogens and continuously to inducers present in diet and environment, these findings may have significant implications on the potential for human carcinogenesis. The fact that AHH activity was decreased by PB at low substrate concentrations in the presence of the n-3 fatty acids of menhaden fish oil suggests that manipulating dietary fat could decrease carcinogen activation. Also the fact that glutathione S-transferase activity was induced only in the presence of fat suggests that dietary manipulation of type and/or quantity of fat may enhance the potential for detoxication and the resultant reduction of the concentration of ultimate electrophilic carcinogenic forms.

ACKNOWLEDGEMENTS

Portions of this research were supported by NIH BRGS RR 07025-17 and grant no. 83B21C84B from the American Institute for Cancer Research. The authors express their appreciation to Ms. Judy Bates for her expert preparation of the manuscript and to Ms. Jenella Bellows for her technical assistance.

REFERENCES

Agradi E, Spagnuolo C, Galli C (1975). Dietary lipids and aniline and benzpyrene hydroxylations in liver microsomes. Pharmacol Res Commun 7: 469-480.

Amstad P, Cerutti P (1983). DNA binding of aflatoxin B_1 by cooxygenation in mouse embryo fibroblasts C3H/10T½. Biochem Biophys Res Commun 112: 1034-1040.

Anderson MW, Sivarajah K, Adriaenssens PI, Boorman GA, Eling TE (1983). Effect of prostaglandin endoperoxide synthetase (PES) inhibitors on the formation of benzo(a)pyrene (BP)-induced pulmonary adenomas and on the binding of BP metabolites to DNA. Proc Am Assoc Cancer Res 24: 86.

Arcos JC, Bryant GM, Venkatesan N, Argus MF (1975). Repression of dimethylnitrosamine-demethylase by typical inducers of microsomal mixed function oxidases. Biochem Pharmacol 24: 1544-1547.

Baker MT, Karr SW, Wade AE (1983). The effects of dietary corn oil on the metabolism and activation of benzo(a)pyrene by benzo(a)pyrene metabolizing enzymes of the mouse. Carcinogenesis 4: 9-15.

Baron J, Kawabata TT (1983). Intratissue distribution of activating and detoxicating enzymes. In Biological Basis of Detoxication. (ed Caldwell J and Jakoby WB, Academic Press, New York)

Boobis AR, Nebert DW, Pelkonen O (1979). Effects of

microsomal enzyme inducers in vivo and inhibitors in vitro on the covalent binding of benzo(a)pyrene metabolites to DNA catalysed by liver microsomes from genetically responsive and nonresponsive mice. Biochem Pharmacol 28: 111-121.

Brenner RR, Garda H, de Gomez Dumm INT, Pezzano H (1982). Early effects of EFA deficiency on the structure and enzymatic activity of rat liver microsomes. In progress in Lipid Research, Vol 20 (ed Holman RT, Pergamon Press, New York) pp 315-325.

Bunce OR, Mattingly E, Ragland WR, Evans B, Wade AE (1983). Effect of dietary fat on tumor promotion in N-nitrosodimethylamine (DMN)-treated mice. Ga J Sci 41: 33.

Castro CE, Felkner IC, Yang SP (1978). Dietary lipid-dependent activation of carcinogen N-2 fluorenylacetamide in rats as monitored by Salmonella typhimurium. Cancer Res 38: 2836-2841.

Cheng K-C, Ragland WL, Wade AE (1980). Effects of lipid ingestion on the induction of drug metabolizing enzymes of nuclear envelope and microsomes by phenobarbital. J Environ Pathol Toxicol 4: 219-235.

Chhabra RS, Fouts JR (1974). Sex differences in the metabolism of xenobiotics by extrahepatic tissue in rats. Drug Metab Dispos 2: 375-379.

Clinton SK, Mulloy AL, Visek WJ (1984). Effects of dietary lipid saturation on prolactin secretion, carcinogen metabolism and mammary carcinogenesis in rats. J Nutr 114: 1630-1639.

Coon MJ, Autor AP, Strobel HW (1971). Role of phospholipid in electron transfer in a reconstituted liver microsomal enzyme system containing cytochrome P-450. Chem Biol Interact 3: 248-250.

Deutsch J, Leutz JC, Yang SK, Gelboin HV, Chiang YL, Vatis KP, Coon MJ (1978). Regio- and stereoselectivity of various forms of purified cytochrome P-450 in the metabolism of benzo(a)pyrene and (-) trans-7,8-dihydroxy-7,8 dihydrobenzo(a)pyrene as shown by product formation and binding to DNA. Proc Natl Acad Sci 75: 3123-3127.

Dharwadkar SM, Bellows JT, Ramanathan R, Wade AE (1985). Influence of dietary fat on liver mixed function oxidases and on the in vitro formation of benzo(a)pyrene-DNA adducts. Soc Exp Biol Med SE Sect 10: 8.

Gaillard D, Chamoiseau G, Derachi L (1977). Dietary effects on inhibition of rat hepatic microsomal drug metabolizing enzymes by a pesticide (Morestan®). Toxicology 8: 23-32.

Galli C, Agradi E, Petroni A, Tremoli E (1981).
  Differential effects of dietary fatty acids on the
  accumulation of arachidonic acid and its metabolic
  conversion through cyclooxygenase and lipooxygenase in
  platelets and vascular tissue. Lipids 16: 165-172.
Ioannides C, Lum PY, Park DV (1984). Cytochrome P-448 and
  the activation of toxic chemicals and carcinogens.
  Xenobiotica 14: 119-137.
Jerina DM, Daly JW (1977). Oxidation at carbon. In Drug
  Metabolism from Microbe to Man. (ed Park DV and Smith RL,
  Taylor and Francis, London) pp. 13-32.
Jerina DM, Yagi H, Thakkar DR, Lehr RE, Wood AE, Levin W,
  Conney AH (1980). Bay region activation of polycyclic
  aromatic hydrocarbons to ultimate mutagens and
  carcinogens. In Microsomes and Drug Oxidations and
  Chemical Carcinogenesis. (ed Coon MJ, Conney AH,
  Estabrook RW, Gelboin HV, Gillette JR, O'Brien PJ,
  Academic Press, NY) pp 1041-1051.
Krauss RS, Eling TE (1984). Arachidonic acid-dependent
  cooxidation. A potential pathway for activation of
  chemical carcinogens in vivo. Biochem Pharmacol 33:
  3319-3324.
Lam T-C, Wade AE (1981). Effect of dietary lipid on
  benzo(a)pyrene metabolism by perfused rat liver.
  Drug-Nutr Interact 1: 31-44.
Lambert L, Wills ED (1977). The effect of dietary lipid
  peroxides, sterols and oxidized sterols on cytochrome
  P450 and oxidative demethylation in endoplasmic
  reticulum. Biochem Pharmacol 26: 1417-1421.
Lambert L, Wills ED (1977a). The effect of dietary
  lipids on 3,4,benzo(a)pyrene metabolism in the hepatic
  endoplasmic reticulum. Biochem Pharmacol 26: 1423-1477.
Levin W, Wood AW, Lu AYH, Ryan D, West S, Conney AH,
  Thakkar DR, Yagi H, Jerina DM (1977). Role of purified
  cytochrome P-448 and epoxide hydrase in the activation
  and detoxification of benzo(a)pyrene. In Drug Metabolism
  Concepts. Vol 6 (ed Jerina DM, American Chemical Society)
  pp 99-125.
Marnett LJ, Wlodawer P, Samuelsson B (1975). Cooxygenation
  of organic substrates by prostaglandin synthetase of
  sheep vesicular gland. J Biol Chem 250: 8510-8157.
Marnett LJ (1981). Polycyclic aromatic hydrocarbon
  oxidation during prostaglandin biosynthesis. Life
  Sciences 29: 531-546.
Martin CW, Fjermestad J, Smith-Barbaro P, Reddy BS
  (1980). Dietary modifications of mixed function

oxidases. Nutr Rep Int 22: 395–407.

Marzuki A, Norred WP (1984). Effect of saturated and unsaturated dietary fat on aflatoxin B metabolism. Food and Chem Toxicol 22: 383–389.

Negishi T, Hayatsu H (1984). Inhibitory effect of saturated fatty acids on the mutagenicity of N–nitrosodimethylamine. Mut Res 135: 87–96.

Nemoto N, Takayama S (1983). Effects of unsaturated fatty acids on metabolism of benzo(a)pyrene in an NADPH–fortified rat liver microsomal system. Carcinogenesis 4: 1253–1257.

Nemoto N, Takayama S (1984). Arachidonic acid–dependent activation of benzo(a)pyrene to bind to proteins with cytosolic and microsomal fractions from rat liver and lung. Carcinogenesis 5: 961–964.

Norred WP, Marzuki A (1984). Effects of dietary saturated or polyunsaturated fat on hepatic glutathione S–transferase activity. Drug–Nutr Interact 33: 11–20.

Norred WP, Wade AE (1972). Dietary fatty acid–induced alterations of hepatic microsomal drug metabolism. Biochem Pharmacol 21: 2887–2897.

Norred WP, Wade AE (1973). Effect of dietary lipid ingestion on the induction of drug–metabolizing enzymes by phenobarbital. Biochem Pharmacol 22: 432–436.

O'Conner TP, Roebuck BD, Peterson F, Campbell TC (1985). Effect of dietary intake of fish oil and fish protein on the development of L–azaserine induced prenoeoplastic lesions in rat pancreas. Fed Proc 44: 769.

Oesch F, Bentley P, Glatt H (1976). Prevention of benzo(a)pyrene induced mutagenicity by homogenous epoxide hydratase. Int J Cancer 18: 448–452.

Parke DV, Ioannides C (1980). The role of nutrition in toxicology. Ann Rev Nutr 1: 207–234.

Ponder DL (1984). The co–mutagenic potential of trans– fatty acids in the metabolism of benzo(a)pyrene, 2– amthramine, 2–acetylaminofluorene and 2–aminofluorene. Diss Abstr Int (B) 44: 3042–B.

Ponder DL, Green NR (1984). Effects of dietary fats and butylated hydroxytoluene (BHT) on hepatic activation of benzo(a)pyrene, 2–acetylaminofluorene and 2–aminofluorene. Fed Proc 43: 580.

Reed GA, Marnett LJ (1982). Metabolism and activation of 7,8–dihydrobenzo(a)pyrene during prostaglandin biosynthesis. J Biol Chem 257: 11368–11376.

Rikans LE, Gibson DD, McCay PB (1979). Influence of dietary fat on microsomal monooxygenases: Possible

relationship to 7,12-dimethylbenzanthracene
(DMBA)-induced mammary cancer. Fed Proc 38: 365.
Robertson IGC, Sivarajah K, Eling TE, Zeiger E (1983):
Activation of some aromatic amines to mutagenic products
by prostaglandin synthetase. Cancer Res 43: 476-480.
Roebuck BD, O'Conner TP, Campbell TC (1985). Dietary fat
intervention during the post-initiation phase of
L-azaserine-induced pancreatic preneoplastic lesions.
Fed Proc 44: 769.
Roebuck BD, Longnecker DS, Baumgartner KJ, Thron CD
(1985a). Carcinogen-induced lesions in the rat pancreas:
Effects of varying levels of essential fatty acid.
Cancer Res 45: 5252-5256.
Singer B, Grunberger D (1983). Metabolic activation of
carcinogens and mutagens. Chapter V. Molecular Biology of
Mutagens and Carcinogens (Plenum Press, New York).
Slaga TJ (1980). Cancer: Etiology, Mechanism and
Prevention. A Summary. In Carcinogenesis: Theory and
Discussion. (ed Slaga TJ, Raven Press, New York) pp
243-263.
Smith-Barbaro P, Hanson D, Reddy BS (1981). Effect of fat
and microflora on hepatic, small intestinal and colonic
HMB CoA reductase, cytochrome P-450 and cytochrome b_5.
Lipids 16: 183-188.
Strobel HW, Lu AYH, Heidema J, Coon MJ (1970).
Phosphatidylcholine requirement in the enzymatic
reduction of hemoprotein P-450 and in fatty acid,
hydrocarbon and drug hydroxylation. J Biol Chem 245:
4851-4854.
Sykora P (1984). The discrepancy between in vivo and in
vitro experiments with polycyclic aromatic hydrocarbon
(PAH) carcinogens: A hypothetical explanation. J Theor
Biol 110: 59-66.
Thakker DR, Yagi H, Akagi H, Koreeda M, Lu AYH, Levin W,
Wood AW, Conney AH, Jerina DM (1977). Metabolism of
benzo(a)pyrene VI stereoselective metabolism of
benzo(a)pyrene and benzo(a)pyrene 7,8-dihydrodiol to diol
epoxides. Chem Biol Interact 16: 281-300.
Wade AE, Bellows J (In Press). Role of dietary corn oil in
the function of hepatic drug and carcinogen metabolizing
enzymes of starved-refed rats: Response to the mixed
function oxidase inducer, 3-methylcholanthrene. J
Environ Path Toxicol and Oncol.
Wade AE, Bellows J, Dharwadkar S (In Press). Influences of
dietary menhaden oil on the enzymes metabolizing drugs
and carcinogens. Drug Nutrient Interact.

Wade AE, Harley W, Bunce OR (1982). The effects of dietary corn oil on the metabolism and mutagenic activation on N-nitrosodimethylamine (DMN) by hepatic microsomes from male and female rats. Mutation Res 102: 113-121.

Wade AE, Norred WP, Evans JS (1978). Lipids in Drug Detoxication In Nutrition and Drug Interrelations, (ed Hathcock JN and Coon J, Academic Press, New York) pp. 475-503.

Wade AE, White RA, Walton LC, Bellows JT (1985). Dietary fat-a requirement for induction of mixed function oxidase activities in starved-refed rats. Biochem Pharmacol 34: 3747-3754.

Wattenberg LW (1979). Inhibitors of chemical carcinogens. In Environmental Carcinogenesis. (ed Emmelot P, Kriek E, Elsevier/North-Holland, Amsterdam) pp 214-263.

Wattenberg LW (1983). Inhibition of neoplasia by minor dietary constituents. Cancer Res 43: 2448s-2453s.

Wattenberg LW, Leong JL (1962). Histochemical demonstration of reduced pyridine nucleotide dependent polycyclic hydrocarbon metabolizing systems. J Histochem Cytochem 10: 412-420.

Wills ED (1980). The role of the polyunsaturated fatty acid composition of the endoplasmic reticulum in regulation of the rate of oxidative drug and carcinogen metabolism. In Microsomes and Drug Oxidations and Chemical Carcinogenesis. Vol I (ed Coon MJ, Conney AH, Estabrook RW, Gelboin HV, Gillette JR, O'Brien PJ Academic Press, NY) pp 545-548.

Zenser TV, Cohen SM, Mattammal MB, Rice JR, Murasaki G, Davis BB, Greenfield RE (1983). Prostaglandin endoperoxide synthetase involvement in 5-nitrofuran-induced bladder cancer. Proc Am Assoc Cancer Res 24: 76.

Zenser TV, Palmier MO, Mattammal MB, Davis BB (1984). Metabolic activation of the carcinogen N[4-(t-Nitro-2-furyl)-2-furyl)-2-thiazolyl]acetamide by prostaglandin H synthase. Carcinogenesis 5: 1225-1230.

Dietary Fat and Cancer, pages 607–622
© 1986 Alan R. Liss, Inc.

EFFECTS OF LIPIDS ON GAP JUNCTIONALLY-MEDIATED
INTERCELLULAR COMMUNICATION: POSSIBLE ROLE IN THE
PROMOTION OF TUMORIGENESIS BY DIETARY FAT

Charles F. Aylsworth

Department of Anatomy, Michigan State University,
East Lansing, Michigan, 48824-1101

INTRODUCTION

It has been suggested that environmental factors and
conditions may be causally related to the occurrence of
many types of cancers in humans (Wynder, 1976; Wynder and
Gori, 1977). In recent years the nutritional aspects of
cancer causation have proven to be among the most
intriguing and extensively examined environmental factor(s)
in cancer research. Epidemiological evidence has indicated
that the incidence of breast cancer among women is related
to many nutritional components; in particular, the intake
of dietary fat. (For reviews, see Chapters by Mettlin and
Miller in this volume). Such epidemiological evidence has
been substantiated by widespread reports that high levels
of dietary fat stimulate tumor development in many
experimental cancer systems (for reviews, see Chapters by
Birt and Rogers in this volume). The tumor-promoting
capacity of high fat diets has been examined extensively in
experimental animals, particularly in models designed to
study mammary gland, colon and pancreatic carcinogenesis.
However, the mechanism(s) to explain these promotional
effects remain controversial. Recently, a mechanism has
been suggested in which unsaturated fatty acids directly
influence tumor cell growth processes by inhibiting gap
junction-mediated intercellular communication, i.e.,
metabolic cooperation (Aylsworth, et al., 1984). In this
communication the effects of lipids on metabolic
cooperation will be reviewed and the possible role of
inhibition of gap junctionally-mediated intercellular
communication in high fat diet-induced tumor promotion will
be addressed.

THE ROLE OF GAP JUNCTIONALLY-MEDIATED INTERCELLULAR
COMMUNICATION IN TUMOR PROMOTION

The development of many types of experimental tumors
following the application of a carcinogen (initiator) at
sub-threshold levels depends upon the subsequent treatment
with a "non-carcinogenic" tumor promoter. Classically,
when a chemical carcinogen such as DMBA is applied to mouse
skin at sub-threshold doses a high incidence of local
tumors is observed only in those animals which are
subsequently treated with a tumor promoter which, when
applied alone, is non-carcinogenic (Berenblum and Shubik,
1949; Van Duuren et al., 1975). This classic observation
has been expanded and adapted to include promotion of
tumors in other tissues, including the mammary gland. For
example, in mammary carcinogenesis the development of
tumors following DMBA or MNU treatment is dependent upon
subsequent exposure to mammotrophic hormones (Huggins et
al., 1959; Dao, 1962). Removal of pituitary or ovarian
influences results in a near complete suppression of
mammary tumor development (Welsch and Nagasawa, 1977;
Meites, 1972). An understanding of how the growth of
initiated, potentially tumorigenic cells are suppressed or,
conversely, how tumor promoters are able to reverse this
suppression and allow for the development of a tumor, would
contribute to our understanding of the tumorigenic process.

One proposal to explain how the proliferation of
initiated, latent tumor cells are suppressed theorizes that
normal cells surrounding the transformed or initiated foci
exert a growth inhibitory influence on these cells.
Indeed, the growth of transformed C3H10T1/2 cells is
inhibited when co-cultured with non-tumorigenic "normal"
cells in vitro (Bertram, 1977; Bertram, 1979). This growth
inhibitory effect is overcome when a tumor promoter (TPA)
is added to the culture medium (Sivak and Van Duuren, 1967;
Sivak and Van Duuren, 1970).

Intercellular communication is thought to be involved
in a wide variety of developmental processes and in the
control of cellular growth and differentiation (Weinstein,
et al., 1976; Azarnia and Loewenstein, 1977; Loewenstein,
1981). Recently it has been suggested that intercellular
communication may also have a role in tumor promotion
(Trosko, et al., 1982). A specific type of intercellular
communication, metabolic cooperation, involves the passage

of low molecular weight, possibly growth regulatory, molecules through membrane structures called gap junctions. In 1979, Yotti et al. and Murray and Fitzgerald independently reported that metabolic cooperation between cells in culture is blocked by the classical tumor promoter 12-O-tetradecanoyl-phorbol-13-acetate (TPA). Since these initial reports, many other tumor promoting compounds have been shown to inhibit metabolic cooperation (for review see Trosko et al., 1982). Table 1 lists some of the tumor-promoting compounds that inhibit gap junction-mediated intercellular communication. It should be noted that a diverse range of compounds are listed, including naturally occurring compounds, environmental toxicants and/or pollutants, drugs, food additives and nutritionally-related compounds. Thus, inhibition of intercellular communication by tumor promoters is not limited to related compounds nor is it specific to a certain class of compounds. Also, correlations linking the efficacy of these compounds as tumor promoters with their ability to block metabolic cooperation in vitro have been described (Trosko et al., 1982; Jenson et al., 1982). Accordingly, a hypothesis has been evolved whereby the enhanced proliferation of "initiated" cells and subsequent tumor development induced by tumor promoters (e.g., TPA) is caused by an inhibition of intercellular communication resulting in a blockade of the transfer of growth inhibitory signals via gap junctions. Increased proliferation of initiated cells, in the presence of tumor promoters, allows for these cells to gain a selective growth advantage and increases the probability for further mutational events to occur resulting in autonomous, promoter-independent growth (i.e., tumor progression).

IN VITRO ASSAY TO MEASURE METABOLIC COOPERATION

An in vitro assay system to examine the influence of various environmental compounds on gap junctionally-mediated intercellular communication and to study the mechanism(s) of tumor promotion has been developed by Trosko and colleagues (Trosko et al., 1979; Trosko et al., 1981; Trosko et al., 1985a). Metabolic cooperation is the phenomenon in which small molecular weight, possibly growth regulatory, molecules are passed from the cytoplasm of one cell to an adjacent cell via membrane structures called gap junctions. Hypoxanthine

Table 1: TUMOR PROMOTERS THAT INHIBIT INTERCELLULAR COMMUNICATION (compiled in part from Trosko et al., 1982).

NATURALLY OCCURRING COMPOUNDS	TUMOR-PROMOTED TISSUE
TPA (AND OTHER TUMOR-PROMOTING PHORBOL ESTERS)	SKIN
TELEOCIDIN	SKIN
BILE ACIDS (DEOXYCHOLIC, LITHOCHOLIC ACIDS)	COLON
T-2 TOXIN	ESOPHAGUS
APLASIATOXIN	SKIN

ENVIRONMENTAL TOXICANTS AND/OR POLLUTANTS	
2,4,5,2',4',5' HEXABROMOBIPHENYL	LIVER
2,4,5,2',4',5' HEXACHLOROBIPHENYL	LIVER
BENZOYL PEROXIDE	SKIN
ANTHRALIN	SKIN
DI-(2-ETHYLREXYL)-PHTHALATE	LIVER
CHLORDANE	LIVER
CIGARETTE SMOKE CONDENSATES	SKIN
LINDANE	LIVER
2,4-DINITROFLUOROBENZENE	SKIN
LINDANE	LIVER
2,4-DINITROFLUOROBENZENE	SKIN
DDT-(1.1.1-TRICHLORO-2,2-BIS p-CHLOROPHENYL ETHANE)	LIVER
KEPONE	LIVER
ALDRIN	LIVER
DIELDRIN	LIVER
MIREX	LIVER
NTA-(TRISODIUM NITRILOTRIACETATE MONOHYDRATE)	KIDNEY

DRUGS, FOOD ADDITIVES	
PHENOBARBITOL	LIVER
CHLORPROMAZINE	LIVER
BHT (BUTYLATED HYDROXTOLUENE)	LIVER

NUTRITIONALLY-RELATED COMPOUNDS	
SACCHARIN	URINARY BLADDER
CYCLAMATES	URINARY BLADDER
UNSATURATED FATTY ACIDS	MAMMARY GLAND, OTHERS
RETINOIC ACID (HIGH CONCENTRATIONS)	SKIN

guanine phosphoribosyltransferase (HG-PRT) is a non-essential enzyme involved in the purine salvage pathway. Normal, wild-type, V79 Chinese hamster cells that contain HG-PRT (HG-PRT$^+$), which are grown in vitro in culture medium containing 6-thioguanine (6-TG), take up 6-TG, phosphoribosylate it to a lethal metabolite (6-thioguanosine monophosphate), and then, unable to proliferate, die. However, V79 Chinese hamster cells which have been mutated by x-irradiation or UV-radiation and lack HG-PRT (HG-PRT$^-$) are unable to metabolize 6-TG contained in the medium. (Since HG-PRT is a nonessential enzyme, the metabolism of these cells is otherwise essentially normal.) When wild-type HG-PRT$^+$ V79 cells are co-cultivated with mutant HG-PRT$^-$ V79 cells in medium containing 6-TG, the wild-type HG-PRT$^+$ cells take up the 6-TG, phosphoribosylate it and transfer the lethal metabolite (6-thioguanosine monophosphate) via gap junctions to the mutant HG-PRT$^-$ cells if they are in physical contact. Transfer of 6-thioguanine monophosphate is dependent upon the presence and proper functioning of gap junctions. Transfer of sufficient amounts of 6-thioguanine monophosphate will kill HG-PRT$^-$ cells. Therefore, the recovery of the mutant HG-PRT$^-$, V79 cells is inversely related to the amount of metabolic cooperation between HG-PRT$^+$, 6-TG sensitive (6-TG^S) and HG-PRT$^-$, 6-TG resistant (6-TG^R) cells (i.e. an increase in the recovery of HG-PRT$^-$, 6-TG^R, cells indicates a decrease in metabolic cooperation). Addition of chemicals to the culture medium that decrease metabolic cooperation will result in an increase in the recovery of 6-TG^R cells. As stated previously, a number of known tumor promoters inhibit the transfer of 6-thioguanosine monophosphate from 6-TG^S to 6-TG^R V79 Chinese hamster cells and increase the recovery of HG-PRT$^-$ cells (i.e. inhibit metabolic cooperation).

Details of this metabolic cooperation assay system have been published elsewhere (Trosko et al., 1979; Trosko et al., 1981; Trosko et al., 1985a) and are summarized as follows: Wild type 6-TG sensitive (6-TG^S, HG-PRT$^+$) cells are seeded in 6 cm dishes at a density of 4×10^5 cells per plate with 100 6-TG resistant (6-TG^R, HG-PRT$^-$) cells in 5 mls of culture medium. After approximately 3-4 hrs various doses of the test lipid, dissolved and diluted in 100% ethanol are added. Ethanol alone is added (final concentration 0.5%) to a series of plates as a solvent control. TPA (1-2 ng/ml) is added to another series of plates as a positive control. After the test chemicals have been added, 6-TG (10 µg/ml) is added to all plates. Cells are cultured for 3 days, after which the culture medium is changed and replaced with selective culture medium containing only 6-TG (10 µg/ml). Culture medium is changed once again at day 6. Cytotoxicity is determined by testing the effect of the same concentrations of the lipid on the colony forming ability of 100 6-TG^R metabolic cooperation deficient (MC$^-$) mutants (Chang et al., 1982) co-cultured with 4 x 10^5 6-TG cells in 6 cm tissue culture dishes in the presence of 6-TG (10 µg/ml). This method allows for a more accurate assessment of cytotoxicity since, unlike the previous cytotoxicity evaluation (i.e. 100 6-TG^R cells cultured alone), the cell density conditions are similar to those used in the metabolic cooperation determinations.

EFFECT OF LIPIDS ON METABOLIC COOPERATION

In view of the well-established promotional influences of high levels of unsaturated dietary fat on experimental tumorigenesis and the possible role of inhibition of gap junction-mediated intercellular communication in tumor promotion, a series of experiments were conducted to assess the influence of lipids on metabolic cooperation. The results of these experiments have been published previously (Aylsworth et al., 1984; Aylsworth et al., 1986). From the data presented in figures 1-2, it is readily apparent that unsaturated fatty acids inhibit metabolic cooperation at noncytotoxic concentrations whereas saturated fatty acids fail to do so at both noncytotoxic and cytotoxic concentrations. The unsaturated fatty acids linoleic acid (18:2; fig 1A), palmitoleic acid (16:1; fig. 1B), myristoleic acid (14:1; fig. 2A) and arachidonic acid (20:4; fig. 2B) significantly increase the recovery of 6-TG^R cells cocultured with 6-TG^S cells in a concentration-dependent manner at non-cytotoxic concentrations. However, the saturated fatty acids stearic acid (18:0; fig. 1A), palmitic acid (16:0; fig. 1B), myristic acid (14:0; fig. 2A) and arachidic acid (20:0; fig. 2B) failed to significantly influence the recovery of 6-TG^R cells at non-cytotoxic concentrations. Other unsaturated 18-carbon fatty acids, linolenic acid (18:3) and oleic acid (18:1), also inhibit metabolic cooperation, resulting in an increase in the recovery of 6-TG^R cells (Fig. 3A).

In order to assess the importance of the degree of unsaturated fatty acids, the relative capacity of 18:1, 18:2 and 18:3 to increase 6-TG^R cell recovery was evaluated. Fig. 3A shows that no relationship exists between the degree of unsaturation of fatty acids and their ability to inhibit metabolic cooperation. Oleic acid (18:1) appears to be slightly more efficacious than linoleic (18:2) and linolenic (18:3) acids in increasing 6-TG^R cell recovery (i.e. inhibiting metabolic cooperation). Linoleic (18:2) and linolenic (18:3) acids are approximately equal in their ability to inhibit metabolic cooperation.

There is an apparent association between the ability of unsaturated fatty acids to inhibit metabolic cooperation and the carbon chain length. When fatty acids with the same degree of unsaturation (i.e. one double bond) and differing chain lengths are compared, the longer the carbon chain length monounsaturated fatty acids inhibit metabolic cooperation to a greater degree than the shorter carbon chain length monounsaturated fatty acids. Fig. 3B shows

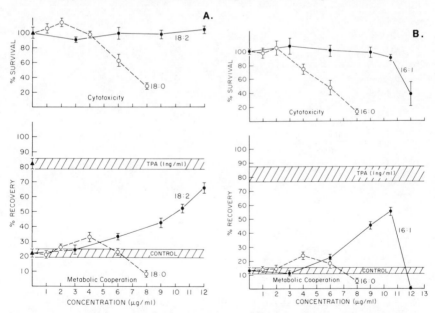

Figure 1. (A) Effect of linoleic (18:2) and stearic (18:0) acids and (B) effect of palmitoleic (16:1) and palmitic (16:0) acids on metabolic cooperation and cytotoxicity. Reprinted with permisstion from Cancer Research (from Aylsworth et al., 1986).

that oleic acid (18:1) is more efficacious than palmitoleic (16:1) and myristoleic (14:1) acids in inhibiting metabolic cooperation. Also, palmitoleic acid (16:1) appears to be slightly more effective than myristoleic acid (14:1) in inhibiting metabolic cooperation.

The geometric isomerism also appears to be of importance in determining the effect of unsaturated fatty acids on metabolic cooperation. Fatty acids with the cis-double bond orientation are more efficacious than the corresponding trans-oriented fatty acids. Fig. 4A shows that cis-oleic acid (cis 18:1) is much more effective than elaidic acid (trans 18:1) in inhibiting metabolic cooperation. Also cis-palmitoleic (cis 16:1) is more effective than palmitelaidic acid (trans 16:1) in inhibiting metabolic cooperation (Fig. 4B). However the differences between cis-16:1 and trans 16:1 are much less dramatic than the differences between cis 18:1 and trans

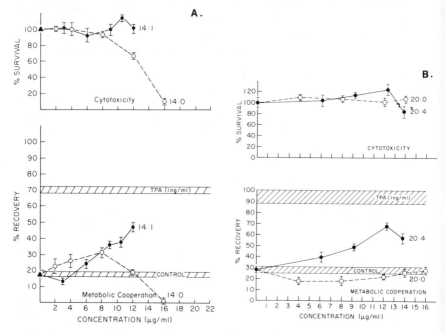

Figure 2.(A) Effect of myristoleic (14:1) and myristic (14:0) acids and (B) effect of arachidonic (20:4) and arachidic (20:0) acids on metabolic cooperation and cytotoxicity. Reprinted with permission from Cancer Research (from Aylsworth et al., 1986).

18:1.   Therefore, these data suggest that while the
cis-double bond orientation appears to be of importance for
the inhibition of metabolic cooperation by some unsaturated
fatty acids, it is of lesser importance for other fatty
acids.   These results correlate well with in vivo data from
Ip and colleagues that diets containing trans-fatty acids
are less efficacious in promoting mammary carcinogenesis
than similar diets which contain cis- fatty acids
(Selenskas et al., 1984).   Diets containing trans-fatty
acids are also less efficacious in promoting small
intestine and colon tumors in rats (Reddy et al., 1985).

Similar results are obtained when diacylglycerol
compounds are examined.   From figs. 5A and 5B it is clear
that diacylglycerol compounds containing unsaturated fatty
acids inhibit metabolic cooperation at non-cytotoxic
concentrations, whereas diacylglycerol compounds containing
only saturated fatty acids do not.   1,3-dilinolein (fig.

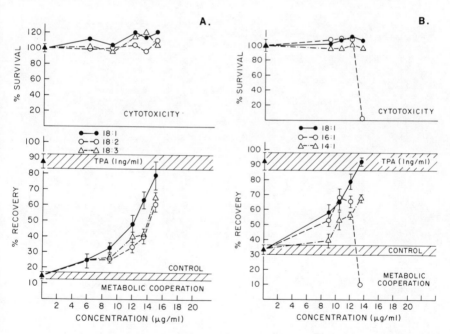

Figure 3.(A) Effect of oleic (18:1), linoleic (18:2), and
linolenic (18:3) acids and (B) effect of myristoleic (14:1),
palmitoleic (16:1) and oleic (18:1) acids on metabolic
cooperation and cytotoxicity.   Reprinted with permission
from Cancer Research (from Aylsworth et al., 1986).

5A), 1-oleoyl-2-acetylglycerol (OAG) and 1,2-diolein (fig. 5B) significantly increase 6-TG^R cell recovery. 1,3-distearin had no effect on 6-TG^R cell recovery (fig. 5A).

CONCLUSIONS

High levels of dietary fat clearly promote many types of experimental cancers and are implicated in the etiology of some human cancers. Many mechanisms have been proposed to explain the promoting influence of high polyunsaturated fat diets on mammary tumorigenesis including endocrine-related and immune-mediated mechanisms. In reviewing the current literature, a direct influence of unsaturated dietary fat to promote the growth of incipient mammary tumor tissue appears to be the most favorable interpretation (Welsch and Aylsworth, 1982; Welsch and Aylsworth, 1983).

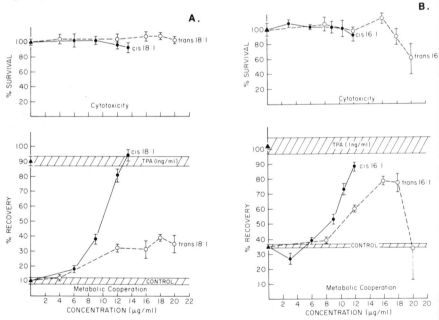

Figure 4. (A) Effect of cis-oleic (cis 18:1) and elaidic (trans 18:1) and (B) effect of cis-palmitoleic (cis 16:1) and palmitelaidic (trans 16:1) on metabolic cooperation and cytotoxicity. Reprinted with permission from Cancer Research (from Ayslworth et al., 1986).

Kidwell and colleagues have reported that unsaturated fatty acids (linoleate, oleate, linolenate and arachidonate) promote, whereas saturated fatty acids inhibit, the growth of normal and neoplastic mammary epithelial cells in vitro. (Kidwell et al., 1978; Kidwell et al., 1982; Wicha et al., 1979) Similar in vitro growth promoting effects of unsaturated fatty acids also have been described in X563.5 mouse melonoma cells (Holley et al., 1974) and in V79 Chinese hamster cells (unpublished data).

Clearly, it is apparent from the data included in this review that one way in which unsaturated fatty acids may directly influence the growth regulation of mammary tumor tissue in vivo and in vitro, and thereby promote tumor development, is by inhibiting gap junction-mediated intercellular communication. Inhibition of gap junction-mediated intercellular communication is an effect associated with many known tumor promoters. Indeed, unsaturated fatty acids such as oleate, linoleate,

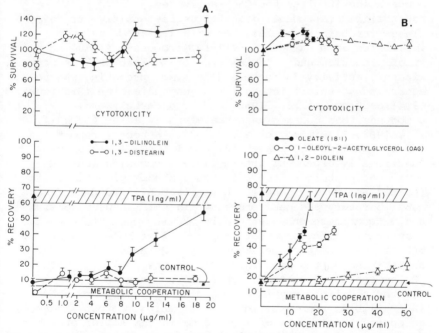

Figure 5. (A) Effect of 1,3-dilinolein and 1,3-distearin and (B) effect of oleate (18:1), 1-oleoyl-2-acetylglycerol (OAG) and 1,2-diolein on metabolic cooperation and cytotoxicity. Reprinted with permission from Cancer Research (from Aylsworth et al., 1986).

linolenate, palmitoleate and myristoleate inhibit metabolic cooperation, a process that depends on gap junction-mediated intercellular communication.

While the inhibition of metabolic cooperation by unsaturated, long-chain fatty acids is now established, a mechanism which can explain these effects remains to be clarified. Since gap junctions are membrane-associated structures it is not difficult to conceive that lipids may have an important role in the structure and function of gap junctions. Many mechanisms are currently being investigated to explain the inhibition of metabolic cooperation by unsaturated fatty acids. These include lipid peroxidation, mediation by prostaglandins (Trosko et al., 1985b) and alterations in membrane biophysical properties including membrane fluidity.

However, one of the most convincing explanations for the inhibitory effects of unsaturated lipids on metabolic cooperation involves the Ca^{2+}-activated, phospholipid-dependent, diacylglycerol-sensitive protein kinase (protein kinase C). Protein kinase C has been implicated in a number of cellular processes including tumor promotion and intercellular communication. Protein kinase C activity is increased by tumor-promoting phorbol esters that inhibit intercellular communication (Nishizuka, 1984; Castagna et al., 1982) and by diacylglycerol compounds that contain unsaturated fatty acids (McPhail, et al., 1984; Kishimoto, et al., 1980). A recent report has shown that 1-oleoyl-2-acetylglycerol (OAG) inhibits gap junctionally dependent intercellular communication and activates protein kinase C in HEL-3 mouse epidermal cells (Gainer and Murray, 1985). Recently published data from our laboratory and data presented in this chapter confirm and extend these observations by showing that OAG and other unsaturated diacylglycerol compounds (dilinolein, diolein) inhibit metabolic cooperation in V79 Chinese hamster cells, and that saturated diacylglycerol (distearin) does not (Aylsworth et al., 1986). Thus, it appears that unsaturated lipid may inhibit gap junctionally-mediated intercellular communication by activating protein kinase C, an enzyme that may be of importance in the action of tumor promoters in general. Studies currently are underway to examine the influence of unsaturated lipids on protein kinase C activity and to correlate these with their effects on metabolic cooperation.

ACKNOWLEDGEMENTS

The author would like to acknowledge Dr. Clifford W. Welsch and Dr. James E. Trosko for their financial and intellectual support which made many of the results included in this chapter possible. The work included in this report was supported by grants from the National Institutes of Health, National Cancer Institute (CA36364-02 and CA21104).

REFERENCES

Aylsworth CF, Jone C, Trosko JE, Meites J, Welsch CW (1984). Promotion of 7,12-dimethylbenz(a)anthracene-induced mammary tumorigenesis by high dietary fat in the rat: Possible role of intercellular communication. J Natl Cancer Inst 72:637-645.
Aylsworth CF, Trosko JE, Welsch CW (1986). Influence of lipids on gap junctionally-mediated intercellular communication between Chinese hamster cells in vitro. Cancer Res, in press.
Azarnia R, Loewenstein WR (1977). Intercellular communication and tissue growth: VII. A genetic analysis of junctional communication and cancerous growth. J Membr Biol 34:1-25.
Berenblum I, Shubik P (1949). The persistence of latent tumour cells induced in the mouse skin by a single application of 9:10-dimethyl-1:2-benzanthracene. Br J Cancer 3:384-386.
Bertram JS (1977). Effect of serum concentrations on the expression of carcinogen-induced transformation in the C3H-10T 1/2 CL8 cell line. Cancer Res 37:514-523.
Bertram JS (1979). Modulation of cellular interactions between C3H-10T 1/2 cells and their transformed counterparts by phosphodiesterase inhibitors. Cancer Res 39:3502-3508.
Castagna M, Takai Y, Kaibuchi K, Sano K, Kikkawa U, Nishizuka Y (1982). Direct activation of calcium-activated protein kinase by tumor-promoting phorbol esters. J Biol Chem 257:7847-7851.
Chang CC, Trosko JE, Dawson B (1982). Isolation of metabolic cooperation deficient mutants of Chinese hamster V79 cells. In Proceedings of the 33rd Annual Tissue Culture Association Meeting, San Diego, CA.

Dao TL (1962). The role of ovarian hormones in initiating the induction of mammary cancer in rats by polynuclear hydrocarbons. Cancer Res 22:973-981.

Gainer H, Murray A (1985). Diacylglycerol inhibits gap junctional communication in cultured epidermal cells: Evidence for a role of protein kinase C. Biochem Biophys Res Commun 126:1109-1113.

Holley RW, Baldwin JH, Kiernan JA (1974). Control of growth of a tumor cell line by linoleic acid. Proc Natl Acad Sci USA 71:3967-3978.

Huggins C, Briziarelli G, Sutton H (1959). Rapid induction of mammary carcinoma in the rat and the influence of hormones on the tumors. J Exp Med 109:25-42.

Kidwell WR, Monaco WE, Wicha WS, Smith GS (1978). Unsaturated fatty acid requirements for growth and survival of a rat mammary tumor cell line. Cancer Res 38:4091-4100.

Kidwell WR, Knazek RA, Vonderharr BK, Losonczy I (1982). Effects of unsaturated fatty acids on the development and proliferation of normal and neoplastic breast epithelium. In Arnott MS, Van Eyes J, Wang Y (eds): "Molecular Interactions of Nutrition and Cancer," New York: Raven Press, pp 219-236.

Kishimoto A, Takai Y, Mori T, Kikkawa V, Nishizuka Y (1980). Activation of calcium and phospholipid-dependent protein kinase by diacylglycerol, its possible relation to phosphatidylinositol turnover. J Biol Chem 255:2273-2276.

Jenson RK, Sleight SD, Goodman JI, Aust SD, Trosko JE (1982). Polybrominated biphenyls as promoters in experimental hepatocarcinogenesis in rats. Carcinogenesis 3:1183-1186.

Loewenstein WR (1981). Junctional intercellular communication: The cell-to-cell membrane channel. Physiological Reviews 61:829-913.

McPhail LC, Clayton CC, Snyderman R (1984). A potential second messenger role for unsaturated fatty acids: Activation of Ca^{2+}-dependent protein kinase. Science 224:622-625.

Meites J (1972). Relation of prolactin and estrogen to mammary tumorigenesis in the rat. J Natl Cancer Inst 48:1217-1224.

Murray AW, Fitzgerald DJ (1979). Tumor promoters inhibit metabolic cooperation in coculture of epidermal and 3T3 cells. Biochem Biophys Res Commun 91:395-401.

Nishizuka Y (1984). The role of protein kinase C in cell surface signal transduction and tumour promotion. Nature 308:693-698.

Reddy BS, Tanaka T, Simi B (1985). Effect of different levels of dietary trans fat or corn oil on axoxymethane-induced colon carcinogenesis in F344 rats. J Natl Cancer Inst 75:791-798.

Selenskas SL, Ip MM, Ip C (1984). Similarity between trans fat and saturated fat in the modification of rat mammary carcinogenesis. Cancer Res 44:1321-1326.

Sivak A, Van Duuren BL (1967). Phenotypic expression of transformation: Induction in cell culture by a phorbol ester. Science 157:1443-1444.

Sivak A, Van Duuren BL (1970). A cell culture system for the assessment of tumor promoting activity. J Natl Cancer Inst 44:1091-1097.

Trosko JE, Yotti LP, Warren ST, Chang CC (1979). In vitro detection of potential tumor promoters. In Santi L, Parodi S (eds): "Short Term Tests for Prescreening of Potential Carcinogens," Genoa: Instituto Scientifico per lo Studio e la Cura dei Tumori, pp 45-53.

Trosko JE, Yotti LP, Dawson B, Chang CC (1981). In vitro assay for tumor promoters. In Stich H, San RH (eds): "Short Term Tests for Chemical Carcinogens," New York: Springer-Verlag, pp 420-427.

Trosko JE, Yotti LP, Warren ST, Tsushimoto G, Chang CC (1982). Inhibition of cell-cell communication by tumor promoters. In Hecker E, Fusenig NE, Kunz W, Marks F, Thielmann HW (eds): "Carcinogenesis - A Comprehensive Survey Vol 7: Cocarcinogenesis and Biological Effects of Tumor Promoters," New York: Raven Press, pp 565-585.

Trosko JE, Jone C, Aylsworth CF, Chang CC (1985). In vitro assay to detect inhibitors of intercellular communication. In Milman HA, Weisburger (eds): "Handbook of Carcinogen Testing," Park Ridge, NY: Noyes Publications, pp 422-437.

Trosko JE, Aylsworth CF, Jone C, Chang CC (1985b). Possible inhibition of arachidonate products in tumor promoter involvement of cell-cell communication. In Fischer SM, Slaga TJ (eds): "Arachidonic acid metabolism and tumor promotion," Boston: Martinus Nijhoff Publishing, pp 170-197.

Van Duuren BL, Sivak A, Katz C, Sudman I, Melchionne S (1975). The effect of aging and interval between primary and secondary treatment in two-stage carcinogenesis on mouse skin. Cancer Res 35:502-505.

Weinstein RS, Merk FB, Alroy J (1976). The structure and function of intercellular junctions in cancer. Adv Cancer Res 23:23-89.

Welsch CW, Nagasawa H (1977). Prolactin and murine mammary tumorigenesis: A review. Cancer Res 37:951-963.

Welsch CW, Aylsworth CF (1982). The interrelationship between dietary lipids, endocrine activity and the development of mammary tumors in experimental animals. In Perkins EG, Visek WJ: "Dietary Fats and Health, Monograph No 10," Champaign, IL: American Oil Chemists Society, pp 790-816.

Welsch CW, Aylsworth CF (1983). Enhancement of murine mammary tumorigenesis by feeding high levels of dietary fat: A hormonal mechanism? J Natl Cancer Inst 70:215-221.

Wicha MS, Liotta LA, Kidwell WR (1979). Effects of free fatty acids on the growth of normal and neoplastic rat mammary epithelial cells. Cancer Res 39:426-435.

Wynder EL (1976). Nutrition and Cancer. Fed Proc 35:1309-1315.

Wynder EL, Gori GB (1977). Contribution of the environment to cancer incidence: An epidemiological exercise. J Natl Cancer Inst 58:825-832.

Yotti LP, Chang CC, Trosko JE (1979). Elimination of metabolic cooperation in Chinese hamster cells by a tumor promoter. Science 206:1089-1091.

Dietary Fat and Cancer, pages 623–654
© 1986 Alan R. Liss, Inc.

INTERRELATIONSHIP BETWEEN DIETARY FAT AND ENDOCRINE
PROCESSES IN MAMMARY GLAND TUMORIGENESIS

Clifford W. Welsch

Department of Anatomy, Michigan State University
East Lansing, Michigan 48824

In 1942, Tannenbaum reported a high incidence of
mammary carcinomas in nulliparous and multiparous DBA mice
fed a diet containing 12% fat (hydrogenated cottonseed oil),
a level of fat six times greater than that which was fed to
control mice (Tannenbaum, 1942). Since this report,
numerous laboratories have confirmed and extended this
important observation. Enhanced mammary tumorigenesis as a
result of increasing and/or altering the composition of
dietary fat, has now been demonstrated in the following
experimental rodent mammary tumor models: spontaneous
mammary carcinomas in DBA (Tannenbaum, 1945), A (Szepsenwol,
1957), A/St (Bennett, 1984), C3H (Silverstone and
Tannenbaum, 1950), C3H/HeJ (Waxler et al., 1979; Gridley et
al., 1983), C3H/St (Tinsley et al., 1981) and TM
(Szepsenwol, 1963; Szepsenwol, 1964) mice; spontaneous
mammary carcinomas in obese (gold-thioglucose treated)
C3H/HeJ mice (Waxler et al., 1979); DMBA-induced mammary
carcinomas in Balb/c mice (Lane et al., 1985);
transplantable mammary carcinomas in Balb/c (Hillyard and
Abraham, 1979; Giovarelli et al., 1980; Abraham and
Hillyard, 1983; Abraham et al., 1984), DBA/2 (Giovarelli et
al., 1980), C3H/Crgl (Rao and Abraham, 1976; Hillyard and
Abraham, 1979; Abraham and Hillyard, 1983) and C3H-A^{Vy}fB
mice (Hopkins and West, 1977); spontaneous mammary
fibroadenomas in Sprague-Dawley rats (Benson et al., 1956;
Davis et al., 1956); diethylstilbestrol-induced mammary
carcinomas in AxC rats (Dunning et al., 1949); DMBA-induced
mammary carcimomas in Sprague-Dawley rats (Gammal et al.,
1967); DMBA-induced mammary fibroadenomas in Sprague-Dawley
rats (Ip, 1980; Ip et al., 1980); MNU-induced mammary
carcinomas in Fischer, Long-Evans, Sprague-Dawley and BUF

rats (Chan and Dao, 1981; Jurkowski and Cave, 1985); AAF-induced mammary carcinomas in AES rats (Engel and Copeland, 1951); X-ray-induced mammary carcinomas in Sprague-Dawley rats (Silverman et al., 1980); transplantable DMBA-induced mammary carcinomas in Wistar/Furth rats (Ip and Sinha, 1981; Kollmorgen et al., 1983) and the R3230AC transplantable mammary carcinoma in Fischer rats (Hillyard and Abraham, 1979; Ghayar and Horrobin, 1981). In general, when these animals are fed a high fat diet, mammary tumor incidence is sharply increased and/or the latent period of mammary tumor appearance is markedly reduced when compared with mammary tumor incidence and the latency period in animals fed a low or moderate (standard) level of dietary fat. Thus, the effect of dietary fat in enhancing mammary tumorigenesis is not confined to a particular type of rodent mammary tumor model as the enhancing effect of this dietary constituent is seen in an impressive array of spontaneous, carcinogen-induced, transplantable, benign and carcinomatous experimental rodent mammary tumor systems.

The type of fat important for enhancement of mammary tumorigenesis in mice and rats has been examined by a number of laboratories (Carroll and Khor, 1971; Rao and Abraham, 1976; Hopkins and Carroll, 1979; Tinsley et al., 1981; Gridley et al., 1983). In general, diets rich in unsaturated fatty acids (e.g., corn oil, soybean oil, sunflowerseed oil, olive oil, cottonseed oil) are considerably more efficacious in enhancing mammary tumorigenesis than are diets rich in saturated fatty acids (e.g., coconut oil, beef tallows, butter). The unsaturated fatty acids which appear to be most important in the enhancement of mammary tumorigenesis in rodents appears to be linoleic acid (18:2) and perhaps oleic acid (18:1) and linolenic acid (18:3) (Kidwell et al., 1978; Wicha et al., 1979; Hopkins and Carroll, 1979; Tinsley et al., 1981). Cis-isomerization of the fatty acids appears to be prerequisite for enhancement of mammary tumorigenesis; diets rich in unsaturated fatty acids with a large proportion of trans-isomerization behave much like saturated fat diets in the enhancement of mammary gland tumorigenesis (Selenskas et al., 1984). In contrast, diets rich in long-chain polyunsaturated fatty acids such as eicosapentaenoic acid (20:5) and decosahexaenoic acid (22:6) which are uniquely found in many fish oils (e.g., menhaden oil) do not appear to enhance (and may inhibit) mammary gland tumorigenesis (Jurkowski and Cave, 1985).

The question as to whether or not the mammary tumorigenic activities of high fat diets act at the initiation stage or promotional stage (or both) of this tumorigenic process has also been addressed by several laboratories. Clearly, high levels of dietary fat can act on the promotion stage of mammary tumorigenesis; the increasement of size of transplantable mammary tumors in rodents fed high fat diets is unequivocal evidence for an effect on this stage of tumorigenesis (Rao and Abraham, 1976; Hopkins and West, 1977; Ip and Sinha, 1981). Furthermore, rats treated with mammary gland chemical carcinogens (e.g., DMBA, MNU) have a high yield of mammary tumors when the high fat diets are fed commencing several days to several weeks after carcinogen treatment (Carroll and Khor, 1975; Ip, 1980). On the other hand, whether or not high fat diets can influence the initiating phase of this tumorigenic process has not been resolved. Earlier studies by Carroll and colleagues (Carroll and Khor, 1970) could not demonstrate an effect on this stage of mammary tumorigenesis, i.e., when rats were fed the high fat diet before and/or during carcinogen feeding, no effect of the high fat diets on mammary tumorigenesis was observed. Very recently, however, in studies reported by Rogers (Wetsel et al., 1981; Rogers, 1983), the Ip's (Sylvester et al., 1985) and Kritchevsky (Kritchevsky et al., 1984) and their colleagues, evidence is presented indicating that high levels of dietary fat can influence the initiating phase of rat mammary gland tumorigenesis, i.e., when the high fat diets were fed before and/or during carcinogen treatment, an increase in mammary tumor incidence was observed. Very interestingly, the type of fat which appears to effect the initiating phase of this carcinogenic process appears to be the animal fats, i.e., lard and beef tallow (rich in saturated fatty acids), not the vegetable oils (e.g., corn oil) which are clearly more important in influencing the promoting phase of mammary gland tumorigenesis.

INFLUENCE OF THE ENDOCRINE SYSTEM ON MAMMARY GLAND TUMORIGENESIS

It has been known for nearly 70 years that the secretory activity of the endocrine system, particularly the pituitary and the ovaries, has a profound influence on the genesis, progression and growth of rodent mammary tumors. This subject has been the focus of a number of comprehensive reviews and therefore it is not our intention in this communication to provide an exhaustive survey of this important subject. Instead, we wish to summarize only the pertinent and salient features of the hormonal control of this tumorigenic process. For a more comprehensive disquisition of the subject, we refer the reader to a number of recent reviews (Welsch and Nagasawa, 1977; Welsch, 1981; Welsch, 1983; Welsch, 1985). The hormones which appear to be most relevant to mammary neoplasia and those which have been most extensively examined, are prolactin, growth hormone, estrogen, progesterone, glucocorticoids, insulin and thyroxine; these hormones will be addressed separately and in the sequence indicated.

Prolactin

Prolactin is an important hormone in rodent mammary gland tumorigenesis. In female mice, transplantation of multiple pituitaries to intact, ovariectomized or ovariectomized-adrenalectomized animals results in a sharp increase in the incidence of mammary carcinomas (Muhlbock and Boot, 1959; Bittner and Cole, 1961; Yanai and Nagasawa, 1972). The transplanted pituitary, being free from direct hypothalamic influence, secretes large amounts of prolactin and reduced amounts of all other anterior pituitary hormones. In addition, the administration of prolactin-releasing neuroleptic drugs (e.g., reserpine), or the placement of hypothalamic lesions which enhance the release of prolactin, results in a sharp increase in the genesis of these neoplasms in mice (Lacassagne and Duplan, 1959; Bruni and Montemurro, 1971). The chronic injection of prolactin in mice increases mammary tumor incidence (Boot et al., 1962). In accord, the chronic suppression of prolactin secretion by the administration of dopamine agonists (e.g., certain ergot alkaloids) virtually completely blocks the development of mammary carcinomas in certain strains of mice (Welsch and Gribler, 1973). Once the mouse mammary tumors become large and palpable, in most strains, these tumors lose their pituitary and ovarian hormone responsiveness. Mice treated with chemical carcinogens also develop mammary carcinomas which are, on occasion, pituitary and ovarian hormone responsive (Medina et al., 1980). The growth of most (but not all) transplantable mouse mammary tumors is hormone-independent.

In female rats, grafting of prolactin-secreting multiple pituitaries or placement of prolactin-releasing hypothalamic lesions also significantly increases the incidence of mammary tumors (Welsch et al., 1970a; Welsch et al., 1970b). Mammary tumors that arise in rats spontaneously or those which are induced by a hyperprolactinemia are mostly benign fibroadenomas. The growth of these neoplasms can also be reduced by chronic, drug-induced inhibition of prolactin secretion (Quadri and Meites, 1971). Early intermittent suppression of prolactin secretion reduces the incidence of these neoplasms (Nagasawa and Morii, 1981). In female rats treated with chemical carcinogens (e.g., DMBA), a hyperprolactinemia induced shortly after carcinogen treatment almost invariably causes a striking increase in the development and growth of mammary tumors (Welsch and Nagasawa, 1977). Carcinogen-treated rats develop primarily mammary carcinomas rather than benign fibroadenomas. Enhanced growth of these neoplasms by hyperprolactinemia can occur not only in intact animals (Welsch et al., 1969) but in ovariectomized (Welsch et al., 1969) or ovariectomized-adrenalectomized (Pearson et al., 1969; Nagasawa and Yanai, 1970) animals, as well. An exception to this is during lactation, a physiological condition in which blood levels of prolactin are high and regression of mammary tumors are known to occur (Dao, 1969; Welsch and Nagasawa, 1977). An induced hyperprolactinemia prior to carcinogen exposure, however, inhibits chemical carcinogenesis of the rat mammary gland (Welsch et al., 1968). Thus, in rats, a hyperprolactinemia after carcinogen treatment usually enhances mammary carcinoma development and growth, whereas a hypersecretion of prolactin prior to carcinogen treatment inhibits this neoplastic process. Most transplantable rat mammary tumors (e.g., MTW9, 13762-MT, MRMT-1) are stimulated to grow by enhancing prolactin secretion (Welsch, 1981). The growth of a few transplantable tumors (e.g., R3230AC, 35-MT) is inhibited by increased prolactin secretion (Hilf et al., 1965; Hilf et al., 1971; Welsch, 1981).

Growth Hormone

A critical role for growth hormone in the development and growth of rodent mammary tumors has not been demonstrated. Mammary tumors in carcinogen-treated rats grow progressively after placement of hypothalamic lesions

which cause increased secretion of prolactin and reduced
secretion of growth hormone (Welsch et al., 1969). Chronic
injections of growth hormone in rats bearing carcinogen-
induced mammary tumors do not significantly increase the
growth of the tumors (Pearson et al., 1969; Nagasawa and
Yanai, 1970). A slight stimulatory effect of growth hormone
on growth of these tumors has been reported but this effect
was quantitatively much smaller than that observed following
prolactin injections (Li and Yang, 1974). Growth hormone
may stimulate DNA synthesis in organ cultures of carcinogen-
induced rat mammary tumors, although this stimulatory effect
was considerably less than that shown for prolactin (Calaf
de Iturri and Welsch, 1976). A prominent role for growth
hormone in the genesis or growth of spontaneous or
transplantable mammary tumors in rats or mice has not been
reported.

Estrogens

The estrogens, in particular, 17β -estradiol and
estrone, have been known to be mammary tumorigenic in a
variety of strains of mice and rats for many years. Thus,
the chronic treatment of mice and rats with estrogens
sharply increases the frequency and decreases the latency
period of spontaneously developing mammary carcinomas
whereas early ovariectomy or ovariectomy-adrenalectomy
inhibits this tumorigenic process (Durbin et al., 1966;
Welsch et al., 1977; Welsch, 1983). In general, chronic,
rather than intermittent, administration of the steroids
favors the induction of these tumors. 17β -estradiol is
usually more effective than estrone.

In carcinogen (DMBA)-treated rats, estrogens are
critical for the development and prolonged growth of these
tumors (Huggins et al., 1959; Dao, 1962; Dao, 1969; Welsch
and Nagasawa, 1977). Ovariectomy of rats prior to
carcinogen treatment can block this neoplastic process;
administration of estrogens to these animals restores
tumorigenesis. Ovariectomy of rats after carcinogen
treatment results in a sharp reduction in the development of
mammary tumors and/or causes a significant regression of
existing tumors. The administration of estrogen to these
animals prevents tumor regression. In intact animals, the
administration of estrogens after carcinogen treatment
enhances tumor development and growth. Estrogen-induced

growth of these tumors, however, does not occur in hypophysectomized rats, providing evidence for a pituitary-dependent growth process (Sterental et al., 1963). Thus, a significant interaction between estrogen and pituitary hormones (prolactin) in the genesis, progression and growth of carcinogen (DMBA)-induced rat mammary carcinomas is certain; such an interaction no doubt applies to the developmental phase (and in some cases, the growth phase) of many other rodent models of mammary tumorigenesis.

Progesterone

Chronic administration of progesterone has been reported to enhance, inhibit or to have no effect on the spontaneous development of mammary carcinomas in mice (Heiman, 1945; Burrows and Hoch-Ligeti, 1946; Poel, 1966). A role for this hormone in the genesis and/or growth of carcinogen-induced mammary tumors in mice has not been established. In strains of mice which develop pregnancy-dependent mammary tumors, progesterone appears to be an important hormone for tumor development and growth (Welsch et al., 1979).

Progesterone does not appear to enhance the spontaneous development of mammary tumors in female rats (Geschickter and Byrnes, 1942; Welsch, 1983). Administration of progesterone to intact rats that had been treated with carcinogens appears to enhance the development of mammary tumors (Huggins et al., 1959). When progesterone is administered in high doses prior to carcinogen treatment, mammary tumorigenesis is inhibited (Welsch et al., 1968). Progesterone has been reported to be a potent stimulator of growth of certain transplantable rat mammary tumors (e.g., MTW9) (Diamond et al., 1980). Thus, unlike the estrogens, an important role for progesterone in the development and growth of rodent mammary tumors has not been unequivocally established. Not knowing the degree to which administered progesterone is converted to estrogens in vivo further contributes to our lack of understanding of the function of this steroid in this tumorigenic process.

Glucocorticoids

Considerably less attention has been directed toward

the role of glucocorticoids in the development and growth of rodent mammary tumors. In rats treated with chemical carcinogens, adrenalectomy appears to enhance mammary tumor development and growth whereas administration of glucocorticoids inhibits this process (Chen et al., 1976; Aylsworth et al., 1979; Aylsworth et al., 1980). Glucocorticoids have also been reported to inhibit the growth of transplantable rat mammary carcinomas (Hilf et al., 1965; Hilf et al., 1971). Treatment of mice with glucocorticoids has been reported to suppress the growth of spontaneous or transplantable mammary carcinomas (Martinez et al., 1952; Sparks et al., 1955).

Insulin

Few laboratories have investigated the role of insulin in rodent mammary gland tumorigenesis. Induction of diabetes by alloxan or streptozotocin after carcinogen (DMBA) treatment in rats sharply reduces the development of mammary tumors and causes regression of existing tumors (Heuson and Legros, 1972; Heuson et al., 1972; Cohen and Hilf, 1974). In accord, the administration of insulin to rats bearing DMBA-induced mammary carcinomas causes a slight, but significant, increase in tumor growth (Heuson et al., 1972). The growth of the R3230AC transplantable rat mammary carcinoma, however, appears to be inhibited by insulin administration (Cohen and Hilf, 1975). This experimental model of mammary cancer is considerably different than most models as its growth is also inhibited by estrogens and prolactin (Hilf et al., 1965; Hilf et al., 1971).

Thyroid Hormones

Induction of hypothyroidism by chronic ingestion of thiouracil or thiourea has been reported to have no effect or to inhibit spontaneous mammary carcinoma incidence in mice (Vazquez-Lopez, 1949; Dubnik et al., 1950). The growth of a transplantable mouse mammary carcinoma has been reported to be reduced by hypothyroidism (Jacobs and Huseby, 1959). Mild hyperthyroidism appears to stimulate the growth of spontaneous mammary tumors in mice (Sellitti et al., 1981). Spontaneous mammary tumorigenesis in rats appears to be delayed by throidectomy (Durbin et al., 1966). In rats treated with chemical carcinogens, hypothyroidism induced by thyroidectomy or chronic administration of thiouracil resulted in a significant decrease in mammary carcinoma incidence; chronic administration of a moderate dose of thyroxine to intact rats hastened the induction of these tumors (Jull and Huggins, 1960; Helfenstein et al., 1962). Carcinogen-induced mammary tumors appear to develop much more readily in hyperthyroid rats than in hypothyroid rats (Newman and Moon, 1968; Goodman et al., 1980). Others have reported that mild hypothyroidism enhances the development of carcinogen-induced rat mammary tumors (Milmore et al., 1982). Most of these reports imply a stimulatory role for thyroid hormones in rodent mammary tumorigenesis. Unfortunately, a definitive interpretation of these results is compromised because of the influence of altered thyroid status on total caloric consumption of the animals in a number of these studies.

INFLUENCE OF DIETARY FAT ON ENDOCRINE SECRETION

It is apparent that the endocrine system and/or the endocrine target tissues are influenced by dietary fat. In 1947, it was reported that rats fed moderate to high levels of dietary fat showed better reproductive and lactational performance than rats fed minimal amounts of fat (Deuel et al., 1947). Subsequently, it was reported that a diet containing 23% fat when compared to a control diet (5% fat), reduced reproductive performance in rats but had no effect on lactation (French et al., 1952). Prolonged estrous cycles (Innami et al., 1973) and early puberty (Frisch et al., 1975; Frisch et al., 1977) have been induced in rats by feeding diets high in fat. Furthermore, essential fatty acids appear to be critical for the optimal development and growth of the rodent mammary gland (Knazek et al., 1980; Knazek and Liu, 1981; Mlyamoto-Tiaven et al, 1981).

The effect of varying levels of dietary fat on the activity of endocrine secretion has been the focus of a number of studies. Rats fed a high-fat diet have been reported to have varying serum levels of insulin (Carmel et al., 1975; Rabolli and Martin, 1977; Abumrad et al., 1978) and increased serum levels of thyroxine (Blazquez and Quijada, 1968). A lack of an effect of high dietary fat on serum growth hormone and corticosterone levels has been reported (Blazquez and Quijada, 1968). Pituitary growth hormone synthesis and secretion, examined in vitro, does not appear to be altered in rats fed a high-fat diet (Cave et al., 1979).

Considerably more attention, however, has been directed toward determining whether dietary fat influences ovarian hormone and/or prolactin blood levels. Chan et al. (1977) have reported a slight, but significant, increase in total serum estrogens at metestrus-diestrus in Fischer rats fed a high-fat diet (20% lard). Total serum estrogen levels at proestrus-estrus were not altered by fat intake. Ip and Ip (1981) measured serum estrone and estradiol levels at proestrus in female Sprague-Dawley rats fed a low (0.5%), moderate (5.0%) and high (20%) level of dietary fat (corn oil). Levels of the steroids were significantly reduced in the animals fed the low-fat diet; no effect of the high-fat diet on the level of these hormones was observed. Hopkins et al. (1981) and Wetsel et al. (1984) have reported that high dietary fat does not influence serum estradiol or progesterone levels in female Sprague-Dawley rats.

In 1975, Chan et al. (1975) reported that female Sprague-Dawley rats fed a high-fat diet (20% lard) had serum prolactin levels at proestrus-estrus four to five times higher than that observed in rats fed a 0.5% lard diet. No effect of fat intake on metestrus-diestrus serum prolactin levels was observed. Since this report, Chan et al. (1977), Hill et al. (1977), Cohen (1979) and Ip et al. (1980) have reported that high dietary fat increases serum prolactin levels in female rats whereas Cave et al. (1979), Carroll (1981), Hopkins et al. (1981), Rogers and Wetsel (1981), Aylsworth et al. (1984b) and Wetsel et al. (1984) have failed to show this elevation of serum prolactin by fat. In the studies by Aylsworth et al. (1984b) and Wetsel et al. (1984), rats were fitted with atrial cannulas that allowed frequent blood sampling throughout the estrous cycle with minimal stress (e.g., lack of handling, etherization, etc.) to the animal. Failure to demonstrate a difference in prolactin synthesis and secretion in vitro from explants of pituitaries derived from female rats fed a high or moderate level of dietary fat (Cave et al., 1979) provides support for those studies which reported no effect of dietary fat on serum levels of prolactin. The basis for this apparent discrepancy among various laboratories is not readily apparent. It is germane to point out, however, that most of the studies demonstrating an increased blood level of prolactin by dietary fat are based on the comparison of low-fat diets (i.e., 0.5%) with high-fat diets (e.g., 20%). Laboratories reporting "no effect" most often compared "normal" fat diets (e.g., 3-5%) with high-fat (i.e., 20%) diets. Diets containing only 0.5% fat may be marginally deficient in essential fatty acids. Furthermore, in some of these studies, increased blood levels of prolactin were only observed in proestrus-estrus and not during the predominant time span of the rat estrus cycle, i.e., metestrus-diestrus. Whether this purported short spurt of secreted prolactin, once during the 4-5-day estrus cycle, is of quantitative significance is open to conjecture.

It is apparent from the foregoing that the concept that high levels of dietary fat (when compared to standard levels) enhance mammary tumorigenesis by increasing blood levels of critical pituitary and/or ovarian hormones lacks consistent support. This concept is further weakened by the following phenomena. High-fat diets are known to stimulate development of a number of rodent mammary tumors that are known to be hormone (prolactin and estrogen)-nonresponsive. For example, mammary tumors that are transplanted into Balb/c or C3H mice and those which are induced in Balb/c mice with DMBA are most often hormone-(pituitary and ovarian) independent, yet their growth is stimulated by hyperalimentation of dietary fat (Hillyard and Abraham, 1979; Giovarelli et al., 1980; Abraham and Hillyard, 1983; Abraham et al., 1984; Lane et al., 1985). The growth of ovarian hormone-independent, DMBA-induced rat mammary carcinomas (i.e., those mammary carcinomas which continue to grow following ovariectomy) are also stimulated by increasing levels of dietary fat (Cohen et al., 1981). Moreover, the growth of the R3230AC rat mammary carcinoma is inhibited by hypersecretion of prolactin and/or estrogen (Hilf et al., 1965; Hilf et al., 1971) yet, the growth of this neoplasm is stimulated by a high-fat diet (Hillyard and Abraham, 1979). Thus, hormone-dependent and -independent rodent mammary tumors are similarly stimulated by a high-fat diet. In addition, in rats with extremely high secretory rates of prolactin (i.e., placement of median eminence hypothalamic lesions), high-fat diets are still able to enhance the development of mammary carcinomas (Ip et al., 1980). Furthermore when circulating levels of estradiol and prolactin are controlled by endocrine and drug manipulations, high-fat diets are still capable of stimulating DMBA-induced mammary tumorigenesis

(Aylsworth et al., 1984c). These results strongly suggest that proposed alterations in estrogen and/or prolactin secretion cannot account for the stimulatory effects of dietary fat on mammary tumor development.

The influence of dietary fat on secretion of endocrine organs other than the pituitary and ovaries has received considerably less attention. Increased adrenocortical hormone secretion results in decreased growth of rodent mammary tumors (Martinez et al., 1952; Sparks et al., 1955; Aylsworth et al., 1980); the secretion of these hormones, however, does not appear to be influenced by high dietary fat levels (Rabolli and Martin, 1977). Administration of insulin to rats slightly increases DMBA-induced mammary tumor growth (Heuson et al., 1972); this hormone has been reported to be reduced (Blazquez and Quijada, 1968; Rabolli and Martin, 1977), to be unaltered (Carmel et al., 1975; Abumrad et al., 1978) and increased (Carmel et al., 1975) in the blood of rats during hyperalimentation of fat. An intriguing, yet unevaluated, relationship is that of high dietary fat, thyroid hormone secretion and rodent mammary gland tumorigenesis. High dietary fat levels may increase blood thyroxine levels in rodents ((Rabolli and Martin, 1977). Increased growth of the mouse mammary gland (Vonderhaar and Greco, 1979) and increased mammary tumor incidence in mice (Sellitti et al., 1981) have been noted in mild hyperthyroidism. Enhanced chemical carcinogenesis of the rat mammary gland also has been reported in rats that were chronically treated with thyroxine (Newman and Moon, 1968). It should be noted, however, that the relationship between thyroid status and the development of mammary tumors in rodents has not been consistent (Welsch, 1983; Welsch, 1985).

Hyperalimentation of fat also stimulates the development and growth of other experimental tumor models that are not regarded to be as dependent on or responsive to the pituitary-ovarian axis as are many rodent mammary gland tumors. High fat diets enhance colon carcinogenesis induced in rats by a variety of chemical carcinogens (Reddy et al., 1977). Spontaneous development of colon tumors in mice has also been reported to be enhanced by diets rich in fat (El-Khatib and Cora, 1981). Diets high in fat also stimulate azaserine and N-nitrosobis (2-oxopropyl)amine-induced pancreatic carcinogenesis in rats and hamsters (Roebuck et al., 1981; Birt et al., 1981). The growth in mice of the sarcoma cell line AK3T3 (Corwin et al., 1979) and B16 melanoma (Erickson, 1984) is also stimulated by high levels of dietary fat. Tumors of the integument (Watson and Mellanby, 1930), kidney (Birt and Pour, 1983a), lung (Szepsenwol, 1964; Birt and Pour, 1983a; Beems and vanBeek, 1984), lymphatic system (Szepsenwol, 1964), stomach (Szepsenwol, 1978), central nervous system ((Szepsenwol, 1971), liver (Miller and Miller, 1953; Birt and Pour, 1983a), adrenals (Birt and Pour, 1983b), thyroid (Birt and Pour, 1983b) and salivary glands (Birt and Pour, 1983b) have also been reported to be increased in experimental animals fed altered fat diets. There is no convincing evidence indicating that tumorigenesis in these organ sites or tissues is dependent upon a chronic hypersecretion of the pituitary - ovarian axis. Thus, these results and the aforementioned studies provide compelling evidence that mechanisms other than enhanced endocrine secretion are involved in the promotion of rodent mammary tumorigenesis by hyperalimentation of fat.

INFLUENCE OF DIETARY FAT ON HORMONE RESPONSIVENESS

Hormone responsiveness of a target tissue is frequently assessed by a qualitative and/or quantitative measurement of the receptor for the hormone in question. Ip and Ip (1981a) examined estrogen and progesterone receptor levels in DMBA induced mammary carcinomas in Sprague-Dawley rats fed a low (0.5%), moderate (%5) or high (20%) level of dietary fat (corn oil). Estrogen receptor levels in the tumors were the same in groups of rats fed the moderate and high levels of dietary fat but reduced in those fed the low level of fat. Levels of progesterone receptor were not affected by dietary fat consumption. In a subsequent study, they reported that the induction of progesterone receptor by estrogen in normal uterii of Wistar-Furth rats was not quantitatively altered in rats fed a low or high fat diet (Ip and Ip, 1981b). Aylsworth (1981) has provided evidence that the quantity of prolactin receptors in DMBA-induced mammary carcinomas in Sprague-Dawley rats fed a high fat (20%) (corn oil) diet, when compared to those fed a moderate level of the fat (4.5%), was not significantly altered. Subsequently, Cave and Erickson-Lucas (1982) reported that prolactin receptors were increased in carcinogen (MNU)-induced mammary tumors of female rats fed a high fat (20%) (corn oil) diet when compared to rats fed a low fat (0.5%) diet. Cave and

Jurkowski (1984), more recently, confirmed the study by Aylsworth (1981) when they observed that prolactin receptor concentrations in MNU-induced rat mammary carcinomas did not significantly vary among groups of rats fed high fat (20%) (corn oil) diets and those fed moderate (3%) levels of this dietary constituent. Wetsel and Rogers (1984), in addition, could not demonstrate any quantitative differences in hepatic prolactin binding in groups of rats fed high levels of dietary fat (24%) (corn oil) and those fed moderate or standard levels of fat (5%). In mice, it has been reported by Knazek and Liu (1979) that the quantity of hepatic prolactin receptors and their induction by prolactin is sharply reduced when the animals are fed diets deficient in essential fatty acids. Clearly, hormonal induced normal and neoplastic mammae developmental processes are suppressed in mice fed diets deficient in essential fatty acids (Rao and Abraham, 1976; Knazek et al., 1980; Knazek et al., 1980; Knazek and Liu, 1981; Mlyamoto-Tiaven et al., 1981; Abraham and Hillyard, 1983; Abraham et al., 1984). Thus, it appears that animals fed low levels of dietary fat have reduced hormone receptor levels. When comparing moderate fat consumption with high fat consumption, differences in hormone receptor levels are not readily apparent.

In an effort to determine whether or not the rodent mammary gland can be altered in its hormone responsiveness during hyperalimentation of fat, we recently performed the following experiment (Welsch et al., 1985). Twenty-one day old female Balb/c mice were divided into 3 groups and fed a diet containing 0%, 5% and 20% fat (corn oil). Ten days prior to sacrifice, one-half of the mice were injected daily with saline, the remaining half with 17β-estradiol and progesterone (E/P). After 3 months on diet and 10 days of saline or E/P treatments, all mice were sacrificed, mammary glands were excised and prepared for wholemount evaluation (#4 glands), $[^3H]$-thymidine-autoradiographic analysis (#2 glands) and organ culture analysis (#2 glands). Wholemount evaluation involved a rating for ductal and alveolar development on a scale of 1-6. $[^3H]$-thymidine autoradiographic analysis consisted of determining the total number of labelled epithelial cells per anterior 3 mm of gland. Organ culture analysis consisted of placing one gland of each gland pair in basal tissue culture media, the contralateral gland was placed in basal media + mammogenic hormones. These glands were cultured for 6 days, then analyzed for development by wholemount evaluation (scale 1-

6) and for epithelial area (mm^2) (via computer image analysis). In saline and E/P treated mice, there was a significant linear increase in number of [^{3}H]-thymidine labelled mammary epithelial cells as the fat content of the diet increased from 0% to 5% to 20% (P<0.05). In saline and E/P treated mice, mammary gland development (assessed by wholemount evaluation) was increased as the fat content of the diet increased from 0% to 5% (P<0.05). In saline treated mice, no significant difference in mammae development was observed between mice fed 5% or 20% fat diets; in E/P treated mice, mammae development was marginally increased in mice fed the 20% fat diet compared to mice fed the 5% fat diet. When the mammary glands from saline or E/P treated mice were analyzed for hormone responsiveness in organ culture, the response of these glands to mammogenic hormones was significantly increased (assessed by mammae development and mammae epithelial area), as the fat content of the diet was increased from 0% to 5% (P<0.05); as the fat content of the diet was increased from 5% to 20%, there was an increase in responsiveness to mammogenic hormones but this increase was not nearly so pronounced. Thus, the results of our study provide evidence that the level of dietary fat can effect in situ mammary gland development and growth responsiveness to mammogenic hormones. The effect of dietary fat is quite striking when comparing mice fed 0% and 5% fat diets, less pronounced, but still present, when comparing mice fed 5% and 20% fat diets.

CELLULAR MECHANISMS BY WHICH DIETARY FAT MAY ENHANCE HORMONE AND/OR GROWTH FACTOR RESPONSIVENESS

A number of mechanisms have been proposed to explain the enhancement of mammary tumorigenesis by high levels of dietary fat. For example, suppression of immune system activity (Kollmorgen et al., 1979), influencing prostaglandin production (Abraham and Hillyard, 1983; Kollmorgen et al., 1983; Carter et al., 1983), inhibiting intercellular communication (Aylsworth et al., 1984a) and generation of lipid peroxy radicals and/or oxygen radicals (King et al., 1979) are all possible biological processes which could, at least in part, explain this interesting and important phenomenon. An additional mechanism, which may be dependent upon or independent of a number of the above cited mechanisms, is that high levels of dietary fat may enhance mammary tumor developmental processes by simply an enhancement of mammary tumor cell proliferation. A number of laboratories have provided evidence that the fat content of the diet markedly affects fatty acid composition of cell membranes of host cells, i.e., the feeding of high levels of unsaturated fatty acids, for example, is reflected in a substantial increase in the amount of unsaturated fatty acids in mammae cell membranes (Hopkins et al., 1981; Chan et al., 1983; Selenskas et al., 1984; Cave and Jurkowski, 1984). The relatively recent work by Kidwell and associates (Kidwell et al., 1978; Wicha et al., 1979), showing that the addition of certain unsaturated fatty acids (i.e., linoleic, linolenic and oleic acids) to the culture media of rat mammary tumor cells significantly stimulates cell proliferation whereas the addition of certain saturated fatty acids (i.e., stearic acid) to the media was without a stimulatory effect, provides evidence that certain fats (but not others) possess the ability to directly stimulate mammary tumor cell proliferative processes. Although it has yet to be demonstrated that high levels of dietary fat can indeed stimulate mammary tumor cell proliferation in vivo, (increasement of mammary tumor development and/or size by hyperalimentation of fat may be due to a decrease in cell removal, see Hillyard and Abraham, 1979), this conceptual scheme still remains one of the more attractive theorectical processes by which to explain the dietary fat-tumor cell interrelationship. In this communication, I wish to suggest an enzymatic mechanism by which alteration of dietary fat may affect mammary tumor cell proliferative processes. Succinctly, it is proposed that hyperalimentation of fat enhances normal or neoplastic mammary cell proliferation by an increasement of mammary cell hormone and/or growth factor responsiveness; such a phenomenon could conceivably occur via a recently described enzyme system, i.e., protein kinase C.

In 1977, Nizhizuka and coworkers (Inoue et al., 1977; Takai et al., 1977a; Takai et al., 1977b) provided the first description of protein kinase C, a cyclic nucleotide independent, proteolytically activated, protein kinase. Subsequently, they demonstrated that the enzyme was calcium (Ca^{++}), phospholipid and diacylglycerol (DAG) dependent (Takai et al., 1979a; Takai et al., 1979b; Kishimoto et al., 1980). The interrelationship between protein kinase C and extracellular signal transduction appears to be the activation by DAG. In response to extracellular hormone and/or growth factor signals, phosphatidylinositol undergoes an active metabolism that gives rise to DAG. Phosphatidyl-inositol turnover is also linked to mobilization of Ca^{++}. Thus, two intracellular signals, DAG and Ca^{++}, can be produced in response to an array of extracellular signals (Nishizuka, 1984).

Protein kinase C, widely distributed in tissues and organs, consist of a single polypeptide of 78,000 molecular weight (Inoue et al., 1977). The enzyme appears to possess two functionally distinct domains which can be segmented by a Ca^{++}-dependent thiol protease (Kishimoto et al., 1983). The 58,000 molecular weight hydrophilic portion contains the active site and appears to be Ca^{++}, DAG and phopholipid independent (Inoue et al., 1977; Kishimoto et al., 1983). The 20,000 molecular weight portion interacts with phospholipid, DAG and Ca^{++}. Activation of the enzyme requires the formation of a quarternary complex comprised of DAG, phospholipid, Ca^{++} and protein kinase; such a complex causes the inactive kinase to undergo translocation from the cytosol to the cell membrane (Castagna et al., 1982; Kikkawa et al., 1982; Kikkawa et al., 1983). In physiological processes, the enzyme appears to be activated by interaction with a locus in the membrane phospholipid bilayer. DAG, in addition, markedly increases the affinity of the enzyme for Ca^{++} (Takai et al., 1979c). Phosphatidylserine is the most effective phopholipid in activating protein kinase C (Kaibuchi et al, 1981).

Most commonly, DAG contains a 1-stearoyl-2-arachidonyl backbone (Nishizuka, 1984). DAG is present in cell membranes only transiently; within a minute of formation it disappears, either returning to inositol phospholipids or becoming further catabolized to arachidonic acid for thromboxane and prostaglandin synthesis. The transient appearance of DAG in the cell membrane is consistently associated with protein kinase C activation. Unfortunately, little is known about the physiological target proteins of protein kinase C. In in vitro systems, the enzyme has broad substrate specificity and phospharylates seryl and threonyl residues, but not tyrosyl residues, of many endogenous proteins. In vivo, protein kinase C has been identified as the enzyme that is responsible for phosphorylation of a 40,000 molecular weight protein. The function of this phosphoprotein is unknown.

Importantly, DAG's containing unsaturated fatty acids are considerably more effective than DAG's containing saturated fatty acids (Kishimoto et al., 1980; Mori et al., 1982). For example, diolein, dilinolein, diarachidonin are equally effective in activating protein kinase C whereas dipalmitin and distearin (saturated fatty acids) are far less active. For DAG activation, there appears to be a need for only one unsaturated fatty acid, either at position 1 or 2. The other position can be occupied by a short chain fatty acid or by acetate. 1-Oleoyl-2-acetylglycerol, e.g., activates protein kinase C. 1,3-DAG may also be active in enhancing this enzyme system. Triacylglycerols, monoacylglycerols and free fatty acids have no effect on protein kinase C activation (Mori et al., 1982).

Figure 1 is a schematic model depicting the activation of protein kinase C by alterations in membrane lipid composition and extracellular hormone and/or growth factor stimuli. A wide variety of extracellular hormonal and/or growth factor signals induce inositol phospholipid turnover in an array of target tissues (Nishizuka, 1984). If the membrane lipid (phospholipid) composition of the target cells in these tissues were enriched with critical unsaturated fatty acids (e.g., linoleic, linolenic, oleic acids via feeding diets rich in unsaturated fatty acids), the DAG produced via phospholipase C would, upon combining with protein kinase C, increase the activity of this enzyme system. In contrast, if the cellular membrane lipids (phospholipids) of these tissues were enriched with saturated fatty acids (e.g., stearic, palmitic acids), protein kinase C would be substantially less sensitive or perhaps totally refractory to an extracellular hormone and/or growth factor stimulus. Thus, this biochemical scenario has the potential of explaining the profound differential effect of unsaturated and saturated fat diets in tumorigenic processes, i.e., diets rich in unsaturated fats are far more efficacious in enhancing mammary tumorigenesis than are diets rich in saturated fats.

Although the role of the phosphoprotein products of protein kinase C in cellular processes has not been definitively determined, there have been recent reports describing a direct relationship between protein kinase C activity and cellular proliferation (Donnelly et al., 1985; Nel et al., 1985). Furthermore, phorbol esters (e.g., 12-0-tetradecanoylphorbol 13-acetate, TPA), known tumor promoters, can act as a substitute for DAG and can directly activate protein kinase C both in vitro and in vivo (Castagna et al., 1982; Kikkawa et al., 1983). The structural requirements of phorbol-related diterpenes for tumor promotion are very similar to those for the activation of protein kinase C. The increasing interest in DAG as an important intracellular bioregulator (second messenger, analogous to cAMP, cGMP) will no doubt continue to emerge; such a cellular molecule conceivably could play a key role, via protein kinase C, in the enhancement of tumorigenesis by hyperalimentation of fat.

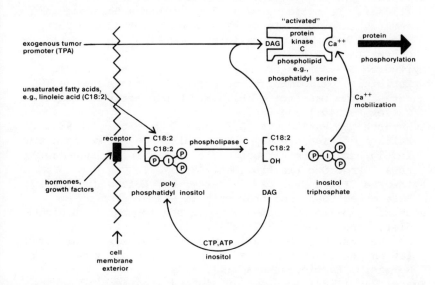

Figure 1. Activation of protein kinase C by alterations in membrane lipid composition and extracellular hormone and/or growth factor stimuli.

REFERENCES

Abraham S, Faulkin LJ, Hillyard LA, Mitchell DJ (1984). Effect of dietary fat on tumorigenesis in the mouse mammary gland. J Natl Cancer Inst 72:1421-1429.

Abraham S, Hillyard LA (1983). Effect of dietary 18-carbon fatty acids on growth of transplantable mammary adenocarcinomas in mice. J Natl Cancer Inst 71:601-605.

Abumrad NA, Stearns SB, Tepperman HM (1978). Studies on serum lipids, insulin and glucagon and on muscle triglyceride in rats adapted to high-fat and high-carbohydrate diet. J Lipid Res 19:423-432.

Aylsworth CF (1981). Effect of dietary fat on mammary tumor development and growth; relation to the endocrine system. PhD thesis. East Lansing, Mich: Michigan State University.

Aylsworth CF, Hodson CA, Berg G, Kledzik G, Meites J (1979). Role of adrenals and estrogen in regression of mammary tumors during postpartum lactation in the rat. Cancer Res 39:2436-2439.

Aylsworth CF, Jone C, Trosko JE, Meites J, Welsch CW (1984a). Promotion of 7,12-dimethylbenzanthracene-induced mammary tumorigenesis by high dietary fat in the rat: possible role of intercellular communication. J Natl Cancer Inst 72:637-645.

Aylsworth CF, Sylvester PW, Leung FC, Meites J (1980). Inhibition of mammary tumor growth by dexamethasone in rats in the presence of high serum prolactin levels. Cancer Res 40:1863-1866.

Aylsworth CF, VanVugt DA, Sylvester PW, Meites J (1984b). Failure of high dietary fat to influence serum prolactin levels during the estrous cycle in female Sprague-Dawley rats. Proc Soc Exp Biol Med 175:25-29.

Aylsworth CF, VanVugt DA, Sylvester PW, Meites J (1984c). Role of estrogen and prolactin in stimulation of carcinogen-induced mammary tumor development by a high-fat diet. Cancer Res 44:2835-2840.

Beems RB, van Beek L (1984). Modifying effect of dietary fat on benzopyrene-induced respiratory tract tumours in hamsters. Carcinogenesis 5:413-417.

Bennett AS (1984). Effect of dietary stearic acid on the genesis of spontaneous mammary adenocarcinomas in strain A/St mice. Int J Cancer 34:529-533.

Benson J, Lew M, Grand CG (1956). Enhancement of mammary fibroadenomas in the female rat by a high fat diet. Cancer Res 16:135-137.

Birt DF, Pour PM (1983a). Increased tumorigenesis induced by N-nitrosobis(2-oxopropyl)amine in Syrian golden hamsters fed high fat diets. J Natl Cancer Inst 70:1135-1138.

Birt DF, Pour PM (1983b). Influence of dietary fat on spontaneous lesions of Syrian golden hamsters. J Natl Cancer Inst 71:401-406.

Birt DF, Salmasi S, Pour PM (1981). Enhancement of experimental pancreatic cancer in Syrian golden hamsters by dietary fat. J Natl Cancer Inst 67:1327-1332.

Bittner JJ, Cole HL (1961). Induction of mammary cancer in agent free mice bearing pituitary isografts correlated with inherited hormonal mechanisms. J Natl Cancer Inst 27:1273-1284.

Blazquez E, Quijada CL (1968). The effect of a high fat diet on glucose, insulin sensitivity and plasma insulin in rats. J Endocrinol 42:489-494.

Boot LM, Muhlbock O, Ropcke G (1962). Prolactin and the induction of mammary tumors in mice. Gen Comp Endocrinol 2:601-603.

Bruni JE, Montemurro DG (1971). Effect of hypothalamic lesions on the genesis of spontaneous mammary gland tumors in the mouse. Cancer Res 31:854-863.

Burrows H, Hoch-Ligeti C (1946). Effect of progesterone on the development of mammary cancer in C3H mice. Cancer Res 6:608-609.

Calaf de Iturri G, Welsch CW (1976). Effect of prolactin and growth hormone on DNA synthesis of rat mammary carcinomas in vitro. Experientia 32:1045-1046.

Carmel N, Konijn AM, Kaufmann NA, Guggenheim K (1975). Effects of carbohydrate-free diet on the insulin-carbohydrate relationships in rats. J Nutr 105:1141-1149.

Carrol KK (1981). Neutral fats and cancer. Cancer Res 41:3695-3699.

Carroll KK, Khor HT (1970). Effects of dietary fat and dose level of 7,12-dimethylbenzanthracene on mammary tumor incidence in rats. Cancer Res 30:2260-2264.

Carroll KK, Khor HT (1971). Effects of level and type of dietary fat on incidence of mammary tumors induced in female Sprague-Dawley rats by 7,12-dimethylbenzanthracene. Lipids 64:415-420.

Carroll KK, Khor HT (1975). Dietary fat in relation to tumorigenesis. Prog Biochem Pharmacol 10:308-353.

Carter CA, Milholland RJ, Shea W, Ip MM (1983). Effect of the prostaglandin synthetase inhibitor indomethacin on 7,12-dimethylbenzanthracene-induced mammary tumorigenesis in rats fed different levels of fat. Cancer Res 43:3559-3562.

Castagna M, Takai Y, Kaibuchi K, Sano K, Kikkawa U, Nishizuka Y (1982). Direct activation of calcium activated, phospholipid-dependent protein kinase by tumor-promoting phorbolesters. J Biol Chem 257:7847-7851.

Cave WT, Dunn JT, MacLeod RM (1979). Effects of iodine deficiency and high-fat diet on N-nitrosomethylurea induced mammary cancers in rats. Cancer Res 729-734.

Cave WT, Erickson-Lucas MJ (1982). Effects of dietary lipids on lactogenic hormone receptor binding in rat mammary tumors. J Natl Cancer Inst 68:319-324.

Cave WT, Jurkowski JJ (1984). Dietary lipid effects on the growth, membrane composition, and prolactin-binding capacity of rat mammary tumors. J Natl Cancer Inst 73:185-191.

Chan PC, Dao TL (1981). Enhancement of mammary carcinogenesis by a high-fat diet in Fischer, Long-Evans and Sprague-Dawley rats. Cancer Res 41:164-167.

Chan PC, Didato F, Cohen LA (1975). High dietary fat elevation of rat serum prolactin and mammary cancer. Proc Soc Exp Biol Med 149:133-135.

Chan PC, Ferguson KA, Dao TL (1983). Effects of different dietary fats on mammary carcinogenesis. Cancer Res 43:1079-1083.

Chan PC, Head JF, Cohen LA, Wynder EL (1977). Influence of dietary fat on the induction of mammary tumors by N-nitrosomethylurea: associated hormone changes and differences between Sprague-Dawley and F344 rats. J Natl Cancer Inst 59:1279-1283.

Chen HJ, Bradley CJ, Meites J (1976). Stimulation of carcinogen induced mammary tumor growth in rats by adrenalectomy. Cancer Res 36:1414-1417.

Cohen LA (1979). The influence of dietary fat on plasma and pituitary prolactin in male rats. 61st Annual Meeting of the Endocrine Society, Anaheim, CA, The Endocrine Society, Bethesda, MD, pp 291.

Cohen LA, Chan PC, Wynder EL (1981). The role of a high fat diet in enhancing the development of mammary tumors in ovariectomized rats. Cancer 47:66-71.

Cohen ND, Hilf R (1974). Influence of insulin on growth and metabolism of 7,12-dimethylbenzanthracene-induced mammary tumors. Cancer Res 34:3245-3252.

Cohen ND, Hilf R (1975). Influence of insulin on estrogen-induced responses in the R3230AC mammary carcinoma. Cancer Res 35:560-567.

Corwin LM, Varshavsky-Rose F, Broitman SA (1979). Effect of dietary fats on tumorigenicity of two sarcoma cell lines. Cancer Res 39:4350-4355.

Dao TL (1962). The role of ovarian hormones in initiating the induction of mammary cancer in rats by polynuclear hydrocarbons. Cancer Res 22:973-981.

Dao TL (1969). Studies on mechanisms of carcinogenesis in the mammary gland. Prog Exp Tumor Res 11:235-261.

Davis RK, Stevenson GT, Busch KA (1956). Tumor incidence in normal Sprague-Dawley female rats. Cancer Res 16:194-197.

Deuel HJ, Meserve ER, Straub E, Hendrick C, Scheir BT (1947). The effect of fat level of the diet on general nutrition. J Nutr 33:569-582.

Diamond EJ, Koprak S, Hollander VP (1980). Effect of high-dose progesterone on growth of rat mammary carcinoma Cancer Res 40:1091-1096.

Donnelly TE, Sittler R, Scholar EM (1985). Relationship between membrane-bound protein kinase C activity and calcium-dependent proliferation of Balb/c 3T3 cells. Biochem Biophys Res Comm 126:741-747.

Dubnik CS, Morris HP, Dalton AJ (1950). Inhibition of mammary gland development and mammary tumor formation in female C3H mice following ingestion of thiouracil. J Natl Cancer Inst 10:815-839.

Dunning WF, Curtiss MR, Maun ME (1949). The effect of dietary fat and carbohydrate on diethylstilbesterol induced mammary cancer in rats. Cancer Res 9:354-361.

Durbin PW, Williams MH, Jeung N, Arnold JS (1966). Development of spontaneous mammary tumors over the life-span of the female Charles River (Sprague-Dawley) rat: The influence of ovariectomy, thyroidectomy and adrenalectomy-ovariectomy. Cancer Res 26:400-411.

El-Khatib SM, Cora EM (1981). Role of high-fat diet in tumorigenesis in C57BL/1 mice. J Natl Cancer Inst 66:297-301.

Engel RW, Copeland DH (1951). Influence of diet on the relative incidence of eye, mammary, ear-duct and liver tumors in rats fed 2-acetylaminofluorine. Cancer Res 11:180-183.

Erickson KL (1984). Dietary fat influences on murine melanoma growth and lymphocyte-mediated cytotoxicity. J Natl Cancer Inst 72:115-120.

French CE, Ingram RH, Knoebel LK, Swift RW (1952). The influence of dietary fat and carbohydrate on reproduction and lactation in rats. J Nutr 48:91-102.

Frisch RE, Hegsted DM, Yoshinoga K (1975). Body weight and food intake at early estrus of rats on a high-fat diet. Proc Natl Acad Sci (USA) 72:4171-4176.

Frisch RE, Hegsted DM, Yoshinaga K (1977). Carcass components at first estrus of rats on high-fat and low-fat diets: Body water, protein and fat. Proc Natl Acad Sci (USA) 74:379-383.

Gammal EB, Carroll KK, Plunkett ER (1967). Effects of dietary fat on mammary carcinogenesis by 7,12-dimethylbenzanthracene in rats. Cancer Res 27:1737-1742.

Geschickter CF, Byrnes EW (1942). Factors influencing the development and time of appearance of mammary cancer in the rat in response to estrogen. Arch Pathol 33:334-356.

Ghayur T, Horrobin DF (1981). Effects of essential fatty acids in the form of evening primrose oil on the growth of the rat R3230AC transplantable mammary tumour. IRCS Med Sci 9:582.

Giovarelli M, Podula E, Ugazio G, Forni G, Cavallo G (1980). Strain- and sex-linked effects of dietary polyunsaturated fatty acids on tumor growth and immune functions in mice. Cancer Res 40:3745-3749.

Goodman AD, Hoekstra SJ, Marsh PS (1980). Effects of hypothyroidism on the induction and growth of mammary cancer induced by 7,12-dimethylbenzanthracene in the rat. Cancer Res 40:2336-2342.

Gridley DS, Kettering JD, Slater JM, Nutter RL (1983). Modification of spontaneous mammary tumors in mice fed different sources of protein, fat and carbohydrate. Cancer Letters 19:133-146.

Herman J (1945). The effect of progesterone and testosterone propionate on the incidence of mammary cancer in mice. Cancer Res 5:426-430.

Helfenstein JE, Young S, Currie AR (1962). Effect of thiouracil on the development of mammary tumors in rats induced with 9,10-dimethyl-1,2-benzanthracene. Nature 196:1108.

Heuson JC, Legros N (1972). Influence of insulin deprivation on growth of the 7,12-dimethylbenzanthracene-induced mammary carcinoma in rats subjected to alloxan diabetes and food restriction. Cancer Res 32:226-232.

Heuson JC, Legros N, Helman R (1972). Influence of insulin administration on growth of the 7,12-dimethylbenzanthracene-induced mammary carcinoma in intact, oophorectomized and hypophysectomized rats. Cancer Res 32:233-238.

Hilf R, Bell C, Goldenberg H, Michel I (1971). Effect of fluphenazine HCl on R3230AC mammary carcinoma and mammary glands of the rat. Cancer Res 31:1111-1117.

Hilf R, Michel I, Bell C, Freeman JJ, Borman A (1965). Biochemical and morphological properties of a new lactating mammary tumor line in the rat. Cancer Res 25:286-299.

Hill P, Chan P, Cohen L, Wynder E, Kuno K (1977). Diet and endocrine related cancer. Cancer 39:1820-1826.

Hillyard LA, Abraham S (1979). Effect of dietary polyunsaturated fatty acids on growth of mammary adenocarcinomas in mice and rats. Cancer Res 39:4430-4437.

Hopkins GJ, Carroll KK (1979). Relationship between the amount and type of dietary fat in promotion of mammary carcinogenesis induced by 7,12-dimethylbenzanthracene. J Natl Cancer Inst 62:1009-1012.

Hopkins GJ, Kennedy TG, Carroll KK (1981). Polyunsaturated fatty acids as promoters of mammary carcinogenesis induced in Sprague-Dawley rats by 7,12-dimethylbenzanthracene. J Natl Cancer Inst 66:517-522.

Hopkins GJ, West CE (1977). Effect of dietary polyunsaturated fat on the growth of a transplantable adenocarcinoma in C3HAvyfB mice. J Natl Cancer Inst 58:753-756.

Huggins C, Briziarelli G, Sutton H (1959). Rapid induction of mammary carcinoma in the rat and the influence of hormones on the tumors. J Exp Med 109:25-42.

Innami S, Yang MG, Mickelsen O, Hafs HD (1973). The influence of high fat diets on estrous cycles, sperm production and fertility of rats. Proc Soc Exp Biol Med 143:63-68.

Inoue M, Kishimoto A, Takai Y, Nishizuka Y (1977). Studies on a cyclic nucleotide-independent protein kinase and its proenzyme in mammalian tissues. II. Proenzyme and its activation by calcium dependent protease from rat brain. J Biol Chem 252:7610-7616.

Ip C (1980). Ability of dietary fat to overcome the resistance of mature female rats to 7,12-dimethylbenzanthracene-induced mammary tumorigenesis. Cancer Res 40:2785-2789.

Ip C, Ip MM (1981a). Serum estrogens and estrogen responsiveness in 7,12-dimethylbenzanthracene-induced mammary tumors as influenced by dietary fat. J Natl Cancer Inst 66:291-295.

Ip C, Sinha D (1981). Neoplastic growth of carcinogen-treated mammary transplants as influenced by fat intake of donor and host. Cancer Letters 11:277-283.

Ip C, Yip P, Bernardes LL (1980). Role of prolactin in the promotion of dimethylbenzanthracene-induced mammary tumors by dietary fat. Cancer Res 40:374-378.

Ip MM, Ip C (1981b). Lack of effect of dietary fat on the growth and estrogen sensitivity of the MT-W9B transplantable mammary tumor. Nutr Cancer 3:27-34.

Jacobs BB, Huseby RA (1959). Hormonal influences on the growth of a transplantable mammary adenocarcinoma in C3H mice. J Natl Cancer Inst 23:1107-1121.

Jull JW, Huggins C (1960). Influence of hyperthyroidism and of thyroidectomy on induced mammary cancer. Nature 188:73.

Jurkowski JJ, Cave WT (1985). Dietary effects of menhaden oil on the growth and membrane lipid composition of rat mammary tumors. J Natl Cancer Inst 74:1145-1150.

Karbuchi K, Tokai Y, Nishizuka Y (1981). Cooperative roles of various membrane phospholipids in the activation of calcium-activated, phospholipid-dependent protein kinase. J Biol Chem 256:7146-7149.

Kidwell WR, Monaco ME, Wicha MS, Smith GS (1978). Unsaturated fatty acid requirements for growth and survival of a rat mammary tumor cell line. Cancer Res 38:4091-4100.

Kikkawa U, Takai Y, Minakuchi R, Inohara S, Nishizuka Y (1982). Calcium-activated, phospholipid-dependent protein kinase from rat brain. J Biol Chem 257:13341-13348.

Kikkawa U, Takai Y, Tanaka Y, Miyake R, Nishizuka Y (1983). Protein kinase C as a possible receptor protein of tumor promoting phorbol esters. J Biol Chem 258:11442-11445.

King MM, Baily DM, Gibson DD, Pitha JV, McCay PB (1979). Incidence and growth of mammary tumors induced by 7,12-dimethylbenzanthracene as related to the dietary content of fat and antioxidant. J Natl Cancer Inst 63:657-663.

Kishimoto A, Kajikawa N, Shiota M, Nishizuka Y (1983). Proteolytic activation of calcium-activated, phospholipid-dependent protein kinase by calcium-dependent neutral protease. J Biol Chem 258:1156-1164.

Kishimoto A, Takai Y, Mori T, Kikkawa U, Nishizuka Y (1980). Activation of calcium and phospholipid-dependent protein kinase by diacylglycerol, its possible relation to phosphatidylinositol turnover. J Biol Chem 255:2273-2276.

Knazek RA, Liu SC (1979). Dietary essential fatty acids are required for maintenance and induction of prolactin receptors. Proc Soc Exp Biol Med 162:346-350.

Knazek RA, Liu SC (1981). Effects of dietary essential
fatty acids on murine mammary gland development. Cancer
Res 41:3750-3751.
Knazek RA, Liu SC, Bodwin JS, Vonderhaar BK (1980).
Requirement of essential fatty acids in the diet for
development of the mouse mammary gland. J Natl Cancer Inst
64:377-382.
Kollmorgen GM, King MM, Kosanke SD, Do C (1983). Influence
of dietary fat and indomethacin on the growth of
transplantable mammary tumors in rats. Cancer Res 43:4714-
4719.
Kollmorgen GM, Sansing WA, Lehman AA, Fischer G, Longley RE,
Alexander SS, King MM, McCay PB (1979). Inhibition of
lymphocyte function in rats fed high-fat diets. Cancer Res
39:3458-3462.
Kritchevsky D, Weber MM, Klurfeld DM (1984). Dietary fat
versus caloric content in initiation and promotion of
7,12-dimethylbenzanthracene-induced mammary tumorigenesis
in rats. Cancer Res 44:3174-3177.
Lacassagne A, Duplan JF (1959). Le mecanisme de la
cancerisation de la mamelle chiz la souris considere
d'apres les resultats d'experiences au moyen de la
reserpine. Compt Rend 249:810-812.
Lane HW, Butel JS, Howard C, Shepherd F, Halligan R, Medina
D (1985). The role of high levels of dietary fat in 7,12-
dimethylbenzanthracene-induced mouse mammary
tumorigenesis: lack of an effect on lipid peroxidation.
Carcinogenesis 6:403-407.
Li CH, Yang W (1974). The effect of bovine growth hormone
on growth of mammary tumors in hypophysectomized rats.
Life Sci 15:761-764.
Martinez C, Visscher MB, King JT, Bittner JJ (1952).
Induction of necrosis in mouse mammary carcinoma by
cortisone. Proc Soc Exp Biol Med 80:81-83.
Medina D, Butel JS, Socher SH, Miller FL (1980). Mammary
tumorigenesis in 7,12-dimethylbenzanthracene-treated C57BL
x DBA/2fF mice. Cancer Res 40:368-373.
Miller JA, Miller EC (1953). The carcinogenic aminoazo
dyes. Adv Cancer Res 1:339-396.
Milmore JE, Chandrasekaran V, Weisburger JH (1982). Effects
of hypothyroidism on development of nitrosomethylurea-
induced tumors of the mammary gland, thyroid gland and
other tissues. Proc Soc Exp Biol Med 169:487-493.
Mlyamoto-Tiaven MJ, Hillyard LA, Abraham S (1981).
Influence of dietary fat on the growth of mammary ducts in
Balb/c mice. J Natl Cancer Inst 67:179-185.

Mori T, Takai Y, Yu B, Takahashi J, Nishizuka Y, Fujikura T (1982). Specificity of fatty acyl moieties of diacylglycerol for the activation of calcium-activated, phospholipid-dependent protein kinase. J Biochem 91:427-431.

Muhlbock O, Boot LM (1959). Induction of mammary cancer in mice without the mammary tumor agent by isografts of hypophyses. Cancer Res 19:402-412.

Nagasawa H, Morii S (1981). Prophylaxis of spontaneous mammary tumorigenesis by temporal inhibition of prolactin secretion in rats at young ages. Cancer Res 41:1935-1937.

Nagasawa H, Yanai R (1970). Effects of prolactin or growth hormone on growth of carcinogen-induced mammary tumors of adreno-ovariectomized rats. Int J Cancer 6:488-495.

Nel AE, Wooten MW, Goldschmidt-Clermont PJ, Miller PJ, Stevenson HC, Galbraith RM (1985). Polymyxin B causes coordinate inhibition of phorbol ester-induced C-kinase activity and proliferation of B-lymphocytes. Biochem Biophys Res Comm 128:1364-1372.

Newman WC, Moon RC (1968). Chemically induced mammary cancer in rats with altered thyroid function. Cancer Res 28:864-868.

Nishizuka Y (1984). Turnover of inositol phospholipids and signal transduction. Science 225:1365-1370.

Pearson OH, Llerena O, Llerena L, Molina A, Butler T (1969). Prolactin dependent rat mammary cancer. A model for man? Trans Assoc Am Physicians 82:225-238.

Poll WE (1966). The co-carcinogenic effect of exogenous progesterone in C3H mice. Proc Amer Assoc Cancer Res 7:56.

Quadri SK, Meites J (1971). Regression of spontaneous mammary tumors in rats by ergot drugs. Proc Soc Exp Biol Med 138:999-1001.

Rabolli D, Martin RJ (1977). Effects of diet composition on serum levels of insulin, thyroxine, triiodothyronine, growth hormone and corticosterone in rats. J Nutr 107:1068-1074.

Rao GA, Abraham S (1976). Enhanced growth rate of transplanted mammary adenocarcinoma induced in C3H mice by dietary lineolate. J Natl Cancer Inst 56:431-432.

Reddy BS, Watanabe K, Weisburger JH (1977). Effect of high-fat diet on colon carcinogenesis in F344 rats treated with 1,2-dimethylhydrazine, methylazoxymethanol acetate or methylnitrosourea. Cancer Res 37:4156-4159.

Roebuck BD, Yager JD, Longnecker DS, Wilpone SA (1981). Promotion by unsaturated fat of azaserine-induced pancreatic carcinogenesis in the rat. Cancer Res 41:3961-3966.

Rogers AE (1983). Influence of dietary content of lipids and lipotropic nutrients on chemical carcinogenesis in rats. Cancer Res 43:2477-2484.

Rogers AE, Wetsel WC (1981). Mammary carcinogenesis in rat fed different amounts and types of fat. Cancer Res 41:3735-3737.

Selenskas SL, Ip MM, Ip C (1984). Similarity between trans fat and saturated fat in the modification of rat mammary carcinogenesis. Cancer Res 44:1321-1326.

Sellitti DF, Tseng YL, Latham KR (1981). Effect of 3,5,3'-triiodo-L-thyronine on the incidence and growth kinetics of spontaneous mammary tumors in C3H/HeN mice. Cancer Res 41:5015-5019.

Silverman J, Shellabarger CJ, Holtzman S, Stone JP, Weisburger JH (1980). Effect of dietary fat on x-ray-induced mammary cancer in Sprague-Dawley rats. J Natl Cancer Inst 64:631-634.

Silverstone H, Tannenbaum A (1950). The effect of the proportion of dietary fat on the rate of formation of mammary carcinoma in mice. Cancer Res 10:448-453.

Sparks LL, Daane TA, Hayashida T, Cole RD, Lyons WR, Li CH (1955). The effects of pituitary and adrenal hormones on the growth of a transplantable mammary adenocarcinoma in C3H mice. Cancer 8:271-284.

Sterental A, Dominguez JM, Weissman C, Pearson OH (1963). Pituitary role in the estrogen dependency of experimental mammary cancer. Cancer Res 23:481-484.

Sylvester PW, Russell M, Ip MM, Ip C (1985). Comparative effects of animal and vegetable fats fed before and during carcinogen administration on mammary tumorigenesis, puberty and hormone levels in rats. Proc Amer Assoc Cancer Res 26:126.

Szepsenwol J (1957). Presence of a carcinogenic substance in hens' eggs. Proc Soc Exp Biol Med 96:332-335.

Szepsenwol J (1963). Carcinogenic effect of egg white, egg yolk and lipids in mice. Proc Soc Exp Biol Med 112:1073-1076.

Szepsenwol J (1964). Carcinogenic effect of ether extract of whole egg, alcohol extract of egg yolk and powdered egg free of the ether extractable part in mice. Proc Soc Exp Biol Med 116:1136-1139.

Szepsenwol J (1971). Intracranial tumors in mice of two different strains maintained on fat enriched diets. Europ J Cancer 7:529-532.

Szepsenwol J (1978). Gastrointestinal tumors in mice of three strains maintained on fat enriched diets. Oncology 35:143-152.

Takai Y, Kishimoto A, Inoue M, Nishizuka Y (1977a). Studies on a cyclic nucleolide-independent protein kinase and its proenzyme in mammalian tissues. I. Purification and Characterization of an active enzyme from bovine cerebellum. J Biol Chem 252:7603-7609.

Takai Y, Kishimoto A, Iwasa Y, Kowhara Y, Mori T, Nishizuka Y (1979a). Calcium-dependent activation of a multifunctional protein kinase by membrane phospholipids. J Biol Chem 254:3692-3695.

Takai Y, Kishimoto A, Iwasa Y, Kawhara Y, Mori T, Nishizuka Y, Tamura A, Fujii T (1979b). A role of membranes in the activation of a new multifunctional protein kinase system. J Biochem 86:575-578.

Takai Y, Kishimoto A, Kikkawa U, Mori T, Nishizuka Y (1979c). Unsaturated diacylglycerol as a possible messenger for the activation of calcium-activated, phospholipid-dependent protein kinase system. Biochem Biophys Res Comm 91:1218-1224.

Takai Y, Yamamoto M, Inoue M, Kishimoto A, Nishizuka Y (1977b). A proenzyme of cyclic nucleotide-independent protein kinase and its activation by calcium-dependent neutral protease from rat liver. Biochem Biophys Res Comm 77:542-550.

Tannenbaum A (1942). The genesis and growth of tumors. III. Effects of a high fat diet. Cancer Res 2:468-475.

Tannenbaum A (1945). The dependence of tumor formation on the composition of the calorie-restricted diet as well as on the degree of restriction. Cancer Res 5:616-625.

Tinsley IJ, Schmitz JA, Pierce DA (1981). Influence of dietary fatty acids on the incidence of mammary tumors in the C3H mouse. Cancer Res 41:1460-1465.

Vazquez-Lopez E (1949). The effects of thiourea on the development of spontaneous tumours in mice. Brit J Cancer 3:401-414.

Vonderhaar BK, Greco AE (1979). Lobulo-alveolar development of mouse mammary glands is regulated by thyroid hormones. Endocrinology 104:409-418.

Watson AF, Mellanby E (1930). Tar cancer in mice. II. The condition of the skin when modified by external treatment or diet, as a factor in influencing the cancerous reaction. Brit J Exp Pathol 11:311-322.

Waxler SH, Brecher G, Beal SL (1979). The effect of fat-enriched diet on the incidence of spontaneous mammary tumors in obese mice. Proc Soc Exp Biol Med 162:365-368.

Welsch CW (1981). Prolactin and growth hormone in the development, progression and growth of murine mammary tumors. In Pike MC, Siiteri PK, Welsch CW (eds): "Banbury Report #8: Hormones and Breast Cancer," Cold Spring, New York: Cold Spring Harbor Laboratory, pp 288-315.

Welsch CW (1983). Hormones and murine mammary tumorigenesis: an historical perspective. In Leung BS (ed): "Hormonal Regulation of Experimental Mammary Tumors," Montreal: Eden Press, pp 1-29.

Welsch CW (1985). Host factors affecting the growth of carcinogen-induced rat mammary carcinomas: a review and tribute to Charles Brenton Huggins. Cancer Res 45:3415-3443.

Welsch CW, Adams C, Lambrecht LK, Hassett CC, Brooks CL (1977). 17β-estradiol and enovid mammary tumorigenesis in C3H/HeJ female mice: counteraction by concurrent 2-bromo-α-ergocriptine. Brit J Cancer 35:322-328.

Welsch CW, Clemens JA, Meites J (1968). Effects of multiple pituitary homografts or progesterone on 7,12-dimethylbenzanthracene-induced mammary tumors in rats. J Natl Cancer Inst 41:465-471.

Welsch CW, Clemens JA, Meites J (1969). Effects of hypothalamic and amygdaloid lesions on development and growth of carcinogen-induced mammary tumors in the female rat. Cancer Res 29:1541-1549.

Welsch CW, DeHoog JV, O'Connor DH, Sheffield LG (1985). Influence of dietary fat levels on development and hormone responsiveness of the mouse mammary gland. Cancer Res 45:6147-6154.

Welsch CW, Goodrich-Smith M, Brown CK, Wilson M (1979). Inhibition of mammary tumorigenesis in GR mice with 2-bromo-α-ergocryptine. Int J Cancer 24:92-96.

Welsch CW, Gribler C (1973). Prophylaxis of spontaneously developing mammary carcinoma in C3H/HeJ female mice by suppression of prolactin. Cancer Res 33:2939-2946.

Welsch CW, Jenkins TW, Meites J (1970a). Increased incidence of mammary tumors in the female rat grafted with multiple pituitaries. Cancer Res 30:1024-1029.

Welsch CW, Nagasawa H (1977). Prolactin and murine mammary tumorigenesis: a review. Cancer Res 37:951-963.

Welsch CW, Nagasawa H, Meites J (1970b). Increased incidence of spontaneous mammary tumors in female rats with induced hypothalamic lesions. Cancer Res 30:2310-2313.

Wetsel WC, Rogers AE (1984). Hepatic prolactin binding in female Sprague-Dawley rats fed a diet high in corn oil. J Natl Cancer Inst 73:531-536.

Wetsel WC, Rogers AE, Newberne PM (1981). Dietary fat and DMBA mammary carcinogenesis in rats. Cancer Detect Prev 4:535-543.

Wetsel WC, Rogers AE, Rutledge A, Leavitt WW (1984). Absence of an effect of dietary corn oil content on plasma prolactin, progesterone, and 17β-estradiol in female Sprague-Dawley rats. Cancer Res 44:1420-1425.

Wicha MS, Liotta LA, Kidwell WR (1979). Effects of free fatty acids on the growth of normal and neoplastic rat mammary epithelial cells. Cancer Res 39:426-435.

Yanai R, Nagasawa H (1972). Inhibition of mammary tumorigenesis by ergot alkaloids and promotion of mammary tumorigenesis by pituitary isografts in adreno-ovariectomized mice. J Natl Cancer Inst 48:715-719.

Dietary Fat and Cancer, pages 655–685
© 1986 Alan R. Liss, Inc.

THE METABOLISM OF THE INTESTINAL MICROFLORA AND ITS
RELATIONSHIP TO DIETARY FAT, COLON AND BREAST CANCER

Barry R. Goldin

Department of Medicine, Infectious Disease Division,
Tufts-New England Medical Center Hospitals, Boston,
Massachusetts 02111

INTRODUCTION

Epidemiologic studies have shown that the incidence of
colon cancer is higher among North Americans and Western
Europeans than among residents of Africa, Asia and South
America (Armstrong and Doll, 1975; Burkitt, 1971; Doll,
1969; Drasar and Irving, 1973; Wynder and Shigimatsu,
1967). These observed differences are not genetically
related, but rather appear to be based on environmental
factors. The critical element may be the characteristic
Western diet, which is high in beef, fat, and protein.
Several lines of evidence support this hypothesis. In
Japan, the overall incidence of colon cancer is low, but
those Japanese who develop this malignancy tend to be in a
higher socioeconomic class and eat a more Westernized diet
than the general populance. In a study of large bowel
cancers of Japanese migrants in Hawaii, Haenszel et al.
(1973), found an increased incidence among those who
adopted a Western-style diet when compared to immigrants
who maintained a more traditional Japanese diet.
Multinational studies have revealed a direct correlation
between animal fat and protein and the incidence of colon
cancer (Armstrong and Doll, 1975; Drasar and Irving, 1973).

Studies of migrant populations indicate that their
cancer incidence approximates the prevailing rates in the
place of residence, rather than the place of birth. Dunn
(1975), has compared the incidence of stomach cancer in
Japan with that among Japanese in California. The
occurrence of this tumor undergoes a stepwise reduction

from high rates in Japan to intermediate rates in immigrant Japanese to lower rates in American-born Japanese. On the other hand, cancers of the colon, breast, uterine cavity, ovary, and prostate show the opposite trends, and among American-born Japanese the incidence of these tumors are approaching those observed in native Caucasians.

There have been several hypotheses to explain the effects of diet on the development of neoplasms. It has been suggested that carcinogenes or procarcinogens may exist in food products. In contrast, the effect of diet on colon caner may be indirect, namely by regulating a critical carcinogen activation step. In this regard, it is currently known that many classic carcinogens are not tumorigenic per se, but must be metabolically converted to the chemical species, which are the actual carcinogens. The liver and other host tissues usually are implicated in these transformations. However, in the case of colon cancer, the metabolic changes may be mediated by the "fermenatation pot" formed in the large bowel by its luxuriant microflora.

COMPOSITION AND DISTRIBUTION OF THE GASTROINTESTINAL FLORA

The bacterial inhabitants of the human gastrointestinal tract constitute a complex ecosystem. More than 400 bacterial species have been identified in feces of a single subject (Finegold et al., 1974; Moore and Holdeman, 1974). Anaerobic bacteria are the predominant microorganisms in the gastrointestinal tract outnumbering aerobes by a factor of 10^2 to 10^4. The most prevalent anaerobic bacteria, are Bacteroides, Bifidobacterium, Fusobacterium, Clostridium, Eubacterium, Peptococcus and Peptostreptococcus. Numerous species are present to varying but lesser degrees.

In healthy humans the upper gastrointestinal tract is sparsely populated with microorganisms. Bacteria from the oral cavity are washed along with saliva into the stomach where the vast majority of microoogranisms are destroyed by gastric juice (Drasar, 1974). The most commonly isolated bacteria in the stomach are gram-positive faculative forms such as Streptococcus, Staphyloccus and Lactobacillius.

The small intestine constitutes a zone of transition between the sparsely populated stomach and the luxuriant bacterial flora of the distal ileum and colon. The microflora of the proximal small bowel is similar to that of the stomach. The concentration of bacteria increases to between 10^3 and 10^4 colony forming units (CFU) per ml of intestinal contents. The most common organisms are gram-positive aerobes, although coliform and anaerobic bacteria can be isolated in low concentrations. In the distal ileum the concentration of bacteria increases to between 10^6 and 10^7 CFU per ml and gram-negative bacteria outnumber gram-positive organisms. Coliforms are consistently present, and anaerobic bacteria, such as Bacteroides, Bifidobacterium, Fusobacterium and Clostridium, are found in substantial concentrations (Drasar et al., 1969).

Distal to the ileocecal sphincter, bacterial concentrations increase sharply. Within the colon the bacterial concentration is between 10^{11} and 10^{12} microorganisms per ml of fecal material. One third of the fecal dry weight consists of viable bacteria.

THE ROLE OF THE INTESTINAL FLORA IN THE FORMATION OF TUMOR PROMOTORS, MUTAGENS AND CARCINOGENS

Bacterial Enzymes

Several bacterial enzymes have been implicated in generating mutagens, carcinogens, and various tumor promoters: β-glucuronidase, β-glucosidase, β-galacto-sidase, nitroreductase, azoreductase, 7-α-steroid dehydrogenase and 7-α-hydroxysteroid dehydroxylase (Goldin and Gorbach, 1976; Goldin et al., 1980; Wilkins and Van Tassel, 1983).

The carcinogenic potential of bacterial enzymes in the intestinal microflora has been illustrated in series of studies following experimental colon cancer induced by cycasin. This is a naturally-occurring β-glucoside of the methelazoxymethanol, extractable from the seeds and roots of cyad plants. Laqueur and Spatz (1975) discovered that feeding cycasin to infant rats caused hepatomas, renal sarcomas, squamous cell carcinomas of the ear duct and, in greatest frequency, intestinal adenocarcinomas that were almost exclusively located in the large bowel. The genetic strain of rat had little influence on the carcinogenic effect of cycasin, since similar tumors were induced in Osborne-Mendel, Sprague-Dawley, Fischer, and

Wistar rats (Laqueur and Spatz, 1975). It was also noted that the intestinal flora was required for the carcinogenic activity of cycasin since the compound was completely inactive when given orally to germfree rats.

The age of the animal was a critical factor. Cycasin was inactive when given parenterelly to adult conventional animals. Newborn conventional and newborn germfree rats, however, developed tumors after subcutaneous or intra-peritoneal injection of cycasin. A tissue (host) or bacterial (microflora) β-glucosidase is required to hydrolyze the glucolytic bound in cycasin in order to release the active aglycone, methylazoxymethanol. The observation that subcutaneous or intraperitoneal injections of cycasin caused tumors in infant rats, but not in older rats, supported the view that young animals have a tissue β-glucoidase which disappears by the third week of life. An additional supposition was that cycasin did not enter the bile in significant quantities since older animals did not develop intestinal adenocarcinomas when given a cycasin by the subcutaneous route.

The discovery of the carcinogenicity of cycasin led Druckery et al. (1967), to test the prescursors, azoxymethane, azomethane, and dimethylhydrazine. These compounds were carcinogenic in conventional and germfree animals (Miller an Miller, 1969). The route of administration was not critical since tumors developed after oral or subcutaneous administration (Laqeur and Spatz, 1975).

Many plant natural products occur as glycosides. These glycosides are not mutagenic in tests such as the Salmonella test however upon hydrolysis of the glycosidic linkages they become mutagenic. Several studies have reported that mixed fecal cultures (Tamura, 1980) or fecal isolates, such as, Streptococcus faecium (MacDonald, 1984) can convert rutin (quercetin-3-D-β-D-glucose-α-L-rhamnose) to quercetin a compound that is mutagenic in the Salmonella liver homogenate test. Beverages, such as red wine and tea contain glycosides of quercetin. It has also been demonstrated that cell-free extracts from fecal cultures grown in the presence of bile acids have increased ability to form quercetin from rutin (Mader and MacDonald, 1985).

Bacterial β-glucuronidase seems to play an important role in colon carcinogenesis. β-glucuronidase has a wide substrate specificity and, consequently, can hydrolyze a large number of different glucuronides. These reactions are potentially important in the generation of carcinogenic and toxic substances, inasmuch as many compounds are detoxified by glucuronide formation in the liver and subsequently enter the bowel via bile. Deconjugation in the intestine then regenerates the carcinogenic or toxic compound. Several studies have shown that intestinal β-glucuronidase can alter or amplify the biological activity of exogenous and endogenous compounds. For example, toxic aglycones can be regenerated in situ in the bowel by bacterial β-glucuronidase. Fisher et al. (1966) have carried out investigations on the metabolic fate of diethylstilbestrol-β-D-glucuronide. When given orally to germfree rats, the compound was rapidly recovered in the feces as a result of poor absorption of the glucuronide in the intestine. In contrast, when this compound was fed to conventional animals, there was a decrease in both the rate and the amount of compound recovered in the feces. These changes were accounted for by intestinal absorption of free diethylstilbestrol. In animals with a conventional microflora, diethylstilbestrol makes approximately 1.5 passes through the enterohepatic circulation. This increased exposure can amplify the biological activity of this compound, which is believed to be a carcinogen for vaginal and mammary tissue.

Weisburger et al. (1970), have studied the metabolism of the carcinogen, N-hydroxyfluorenylacetamide, administered parenterally to conventional and germfree rats. Germ-free rats excreted appreciably larger amounts of the glucuronide of N-hydroxyfluorenylacetamide in their feces than conventional animals. The cecal and fecal metabolites in conventional rats were mostly free, unconjugated compounds, whereas the major fraction in germfree animals was conjugated with glucuronic or sulfuric acid.

Morotomi et al. (1985) reported that cell free extracts of some strains of intestinal bacteria including: Bacteroides fragilis, B. vulgatus, B. thetaiotamicron, Eubacterium eligens, Peptostreptococcus and Escherichia coli enhanced the mutagenicity of bile from rats give 1-nitropyrene via stomach tube. These bacterial cell-free extracts hydrolzyed the synthetic β-D-glucuronidase of phenolphthalein and/or P-nitrophenol. Cell free extracts of bacteria not capable of increasing mutagenicity did not hydrolyze the glucuronides. These

data indicate that the glucuronides of 1-nitropyrene
metabolites secreted into bile can be hydrolyzed in the
intestine by bacterial β-glucuronidases to potent
aglycones.

Nitroreductase and azoreductase are responsible for
reducing nitro and azo compounds, respectively, to
aromatic amines. The highly reactive intermediates and
end products are known mutagens and carcinogens with
animals, these enzymes are mostly confined to bacteria
residing in the bowel.

Azo dyes are widely used in the textile printing, and
food dye industries and in laboratories. Water-soluble
azo dyes are degraded by intestinal microorganisms in the
gastrointestinal tract (Chung, 1983). Large bowel cancer
occurs more commonly in highly industrialized countries
and the extent of the use of azo dyes is related to the
degree of industrialization of the country, a possible
connection may exist between the number of cancer cases
and the use of azo dyes.

There is a 90 per cent correlation between
carcinogenicity and mutagenicity for aromatic amines and
azo dyes tested with the Salmonella/microsome mutagenicity
test. The transformation of azo dyes by intestinal
bacteria may be a necessary prerequiste of carcinogenicity.

The reduction of azo compounds by azoreductase is
believed to be mediated through a free radical mechanism,
which produces intermediates that react with proteins and
nucleic acids. Azoreductase also can reduce food dyes,
releasing phenyl- and naphthyl-substituted amines. These
compounds have been implicated as chemical carcingoens
(Weisburger and Weisburger, 1973). The amines generated
in the bowel via the azoreductase reaction are probably
further oxidized by microsomal enzymes in the intestinal
mucosa to proximal carcinogens.

The role of bacteria in the generation of mutagens
from a number of azo dyes is reviewed in this section
Trypan blue is widely used as biological stain and is not
mutagenic, but reduction by a cell-free extract of
Fusobacterium SP.2 produces a mutagen, O-tolidine
(Hartman, 1978) which is mutagenic in the Ames assay and
is also carcinogenic (Weisbuger and Weisburger, 1966).
Pancreau 3 R another biological stain is reduced in vitro
by Fusobacterium SP.2 to 2,4,5-trimethylailine which has

been determined to be mutagenic (Hartman, 1979). Incubation of methyl orange or methyl yellow with intestinal anaerobes and then tested with Salmonella TA 1538 in the presence of a microsomal activating system proved positive for mutagenicity. Both dyes are reductively cleaved to the mutagen N,N-dimethyl-P-phehylenediamine (Chung et al., 1978). Other azodyes that have been shown to undergo bacterial reduction to mutagenic or carcinogenic products are direct black 38, direct red 2 and direct blue 15 these dyes are converted to benzidine, 3-3-dimethylbenzidine and 3,3-dimethyoxybenzidine respectively. Congo red is also reduced by rat cecal bacteria to benzidine (Reid, 1983). In the absence of a bacterial reductase system congo red is not mutagenic toward Salmonella TA 1538 in the presence of a liver activating system. However, preincubation of Congo red with cecal bacteria resulted in a positive mutagenic response.

Nitroreductase causes the formation of reactive nitroso and N-hydroxy intermediates in the course of converting aromatic nitro compounds to aromatic amines. The precursor aromatic nitro compounds are commonly found in factory effluents as industrial chemical pollutants. Wheeler et al. (1975), studied a similar reaction, the reduction of p-nitrobenzoic acid, in conventional and germfree rats. Conventional animals rapidly converted p-nitrobenzoic acid, while germfree reduced very little of the nitrocompound. 1-Nitropyrene is a nitrated polynuclear aromatic hydrocarbon readily formed by reaction of nitrogen oxides with the combustion product pyrene. Its presence in diesel enzyme exhaust, represents a potential health hazard because of its high mutagenicity in bacterial test systems and its carcinogenicity in rats (El-Bayoumy, 1983). When 1-nitropyrine was administered orally to conventional rats, 5-6 per cent of the dose was detected in the feces as 1-aminopyrene. When a similar experiment was performed on germ free rats no 1-aminopyrene appeared in the feces. Since reductions of 1-nitropyrene to 1-aminopyrene is an activation process, the results indicate that intestinal microflora are important in the metabolic activation of 1-nitropyrene. Miller and Miller (1964), and Weisburger and Weisburger (1973), after reviewing the evidence, have suggested that the products of these reactions, namely the aromatic amines are extremely important in chemical carcinogenesis.

A number of investigators have studied the mutagenicity of nitrated compounds with nitroreductase-positive and nitroreductase-deficicent strains of the Salmonella used in the Ames test. The mutagenicity of compounds that did not require liver microsome activation, such as 2-nitrofluorene, 1,8-dinitropyrne, and metronidazole resulted from activation within the parent tester strains themselves (McCoy, 1981). When these mutagens were plated with the nitroreductase deficient strains, mutagenic activity was not observed. Thus, activation to a mutagen is presumed to occur by the mechanism of bacterial nitro reductin (Lindermark and Muller, 1976)

Several studies have demonstrated that strains of individual species of intestinal anaerobes are capable of activating mutagens in vitro. Cell-free extracts of strains of Bacteroides fragilis, Bacteroides vulgatus. Bacteroides thetaiotamicron, and Clostridium perfringens are capable of activating several polycyclic aromatic hydrocarbons, such as 2-aminofluorene and 2-amino-anthracene, to mutagens in the Ames test (Karpinsky and Rosenberg, 1980; McCoy et al., 1979; McCoy et al., 1977). Also, 2-nitrofluorene, which was described above as being inactive in the nitroreductase-deficient strains of Salmonella, can be activated to a mutagenic form in these strains if preincubated with cell-free extracts of the Bacteroides species mentioned above (Karpinsky and Rosenberg, 1980). The nitroreductase activity of these anaerobes replaces that of the mutant tester strains.

Nitrosamines. It has been thirty years since Magee and Barnes (1956) reported the induction of liver cancer in rats by feeding dimethylnitrosamine. Since this first report, at least 80 different N-nitroso compounds have been found to produce tumors at different organ sites. Nitrosamines form readily by the reaction of secondary amines with nitrite in an acidic medium. Nitrosation can occur in the mammalian stomach if both nitrites and amines are present (Mirvish, 1970). The potential danger of this reaction is somewhat reduced by the relatively short residence time of these compounds in the stomach. Nitrite is added to cured meat and fish, and nitroso compounds have been found in these and other sources (Ender and Ceh, 1968).

Bacteria have also been implicated in the formation of N-nitroso compounds. Nitrite is produced through the reduction of nitrate by many common microbial species.

Certain leafy vegetables may accumulate high concentrations of nitrate that can then be converted to nitrite by bacteria during storage. Tannenbaum et al (1974), reported that the oral microbial flora of humans can reduce nitrate to nitrite, producing levels in saliva as high as 6-10 ppm.

Klubes et al (1972) reported that dimethylamine and sodium nitrite, when incubated together with rat intestinal bacteria under anaerobic conditions at pH 7.0, gave rise to dimethylnitrosamide. The formation was enhanced by the presence of riboflavin. The major implication of these findings lies in the possibility of generating nitrosamines in the intestine, where the pH is nearly neutral and where the reaction could be expected to occur nonenzymatically at a very slow rate. Potentially, this reaction could be of importance since secondary amines can come from many dietary sources and nitrates are present as food additives. Although rapid transit in the stomach may prevent some extent nonenzymatic nitrosamine formation, the bacterially catalyzed reaction in the large bowel could lead to significant N-nitroso formation.

Amino Acids

Tyrosine and tryptophan can be converted to toxin and carcinogenic microflora. Tryptophaphase catalyzes the conversion of tryptophan to the known carcinogen indole. Chung et al. (1975) showed that Bacteroides thetaiotamicron, an organism commonly found in the intestine, has high levels of tryptophanase when grown in the presence of tryptophan. Rats fed a high-meat diet have higher levels of tryptophanase then animals maintained on a grain diet.

Tyrosine is converted to phenol by aerobic intestinal organisms and to P-cresol by intestinal anaerobes. Both of these metabolites are absent in the urine of germ-free mice and are present in the urine from conventional mice. Phenol and cresol are tumor promoters in a mouse strain cancer model. There role in the etiology of colon cancer is not known.

THE EFFECT OF DIET ON THE COMPOSITION OF THE INTESTINAL MICROFLORA

There have been a large number of animal and human studies concerning the effect of diet on the composition of the intestinal microflora.

The data are conflicting regarding the ability of diet to alter specific microbial components of the human adult flora. Moore et al. (1975), reported no change in the predominant organisms in the fecal flor of individuals shifted from an omnivore to a vegetarian diet. In another study Maier et al, (1974) investigated four subjects fed a meatless diet for four weeks, then shifted to a high-meat diet for four weeks; an increase in fecal counts of Bacteroides and lower counts of coliforms were noted when subjects were eating the high-meat diet. However, a statistical analysis was not performed and the changes were not great. Reddy et al. (1974), reported a similar study in which eight volunteers, initially consuming a high-meat diet, were shifted for four weeks to a non-met diet. The shift resulted in a lower number of total anaerobic bacteria, including decreased counts of Bacteroides, Bifdobacterium and Peptococcus, when consuming the non-meat diet.

Intercountry studies performed in the early 1970's (Hill et al., 1971) showed that people living in Britain or the United States eating a "Western" diet had more Bacteroides and fewer enterococci and other aerobic organisms than people eating a largely vegetarian diet in Uganda, India and Japan. In such large cross-cultural studies, however, it is difficult to eliminate factors other than diet than may influence the microflora.

The most detailed studies of the human microflora have been performed in the laboratory of Finegold. Subjects eating a "Western" diet were compared with subjects eating a Japanese diet, and with vegetarian and non-vegetarian Seventh Day Adventists (Finegold et al., 1974; Finegold et al., 1977). The subjects eating a Japanese diet had significantly higher fecal counts of S. faecalis, Eubacterium lentum, and E. contortum; they also had lower counts of Bacteroides, although the values were not significantly different. The data were also evaluated in terms of populations at low and high risk for colon cancer (Finegold et al., 1977). The low risk group included subjects eating a Japanese diet and the vegetarian and non-vegetarian Seventh Day Adventists; the high risk group included people eating a "Western" diet and patients with colonic polyps. The low risk group had higher counts in their feces of Klebsiella pneumoniae, various Lactobacillus species, while the high risk group had greater numbers of Bifidobacterium, Peptococcus and Clostridum.

Drasar et al. (1976), studied the effect of fiber on the fecal flora of four volunteers. Crude wheat fiber was increased from 3.6 grams to 11.7 grams per day by adding wheat bran to the diet. These investigators reported no change in the microbial composition of the fecal flora as a result of this dietary modification.

In summary, studies of dietary influence on specific bacteria in intestinal flora indicate that people eat low meat, high complex-carbohydrate diets have higher fecal counts of aerobic bacteria and lower numbers of certain anaerobic bacteria. The overall shifts in the composition of the flora are hardly dramatic, and in some studies, no alterations are seen.

These studies of fecal microflora are based on classic principles of bacterial taxonomy, by which bacteria are named for their morphologic characteristics and their ability to perform certain biochemical reactions, usually having no relation to the physiology of the host. Since the flora is so complex consisting of over 400 species, based on standard taxonomy, with a concentration of 10^{11} bacteria per gm, it is difficult to show changes in any specific bacterium. Another approach, discussed in a subsequent section, deals with the metabolic activity of the microflora as a whole, in relation to specific substrates. By this criterion diet can, indeed, alter the metabolic activity of the flora, and these changes may be more relevant to the host than the Latin of Greek name of the microorganisms.

EFFECTS OF DIET ON INTESTINAL BACTERIAL REACTIONS

Although variations in diet appear to exert little effect on the bacterial composition of feces, studies of the metabolic activity of the microflora have shown to be quite labile and greatly influenced by dietary factors. Many bacterial enzyme systems are inducible, so that continued exposure of colonic bacteria to substrate results in increased enzymatic activity. If the substrate is a procarcinogen, continued exposure results in increased synthesis of the carcinogen.

Bile acids have been studied extensively as candidate carcinogens because of these structural similarity to the carcinogenic polycyclic aromatic hydrocarbons (Kay, 1981). The concentration of fecal bile acids is increased in people eating a high fat diet, and this increase induces colonic bacteria to produce large amounts of 7-α-dehydroxylase, an enzyme involved in the conversion of primary to secondary bile acids (Weisburger, 1971). This finding has been confirmed by adding chenodeoxycholic acid to a growing culture of eubacteria which resulted in a striking increase in 7-α-dehydroxylase activity (White et al., 1980).

Demographic studies have demonstrated a correlation between high fecal concentrations of secondary bile acids and the Western-style, high-beef diet. Americans on a Western diet had higher levels of total fecal bile acids, as well as deoxycholic and lithocholic acid, but not cholic acid, when compared to American vegetarians, American Seventh-Day Adventists, Japanese or Chinese immigrants (Reddy and Wynder, 1973). The fecal microflora of North Americans and Western Europeans contained more bacterial strains capable of 7-α-dehydroxylation than did those from Ugandans or Indians (Hill et al., 1971). Japanese living in Akita, Japan were compared with Japanese living in Hawaii (Mower et al., 1979). The latter group had high levels of fecal deoxycholic acid, but little difference was noted in the other bile acids.

The fecal concentrations of coprostanol and coprostanone, degradation products of cholesterol, also are higher in individuals who consume the Western-style diet. In a study of patients with colon cancer, Mastramarino and coworkers found elevated levels in the feces of both 7-α-dehydroxylase and cholesterol dehydrogenase compared with normal controls (Mastramorino et al., 1976). Elevations of both these fecal bacterial enzymes were also noted in patients with nonhereditary large bowel polyps (Mastromorino et al., 1978). Higher fecal NAD- and NADP-dependent 7-α-hydroxysteroid dehydrogenase activity were associated with the Western-style diet (MacDonald et al., 1978). This enzyme converts hydroxy-bile acids to keto-bile acids.

Bacterial beta-glucuaronidase has wide substrate specificity and can hydrolyze a large number of glucuronides. This enzyme's activity was studied in volunteers on high meat diets and non-meat diets; high fecal enzyme activity noted in subjects eating the meat diet (Reddy et al., 1974). Shifting from a high-beef diet to a non-meat diet was associated with a decrease in fecal beat-glucuronidase activity.

Lindop et al. (1985), have compared intestinal bacterial β-glucuronidase activities in rats given a fibre-free diet or a diet containing pectin or cellulose. They found pectin and cellulose significantly reduced β-glucuronidase activity of the cecal contents. Cellulose also lowered the β-glucuronidase activity of the jejunal and ileal contents while pectin reduced the activity in the ileum. Dietary fibre components had no effect on jejunal or ileal mucosal β-gluronidase activity.

The effect of diets on fecal bacterial nitroreductase and azoreductase activity has been studied in rats (Goldin and Gorbach, 1976). Rats initially maintained on a grain diet, then shifted after several weeks to a meat diet, showed a tow-fold rise in fecal nitroreductase activity on the meat diet. This increase started within 6 days, though the total effect required 12-17 days. Fecal azoreductase also increased approximately two-fold when rats were shifted to the meat diet. An increase in specific activity of this enzyme was noted between 4 and 10 days after the dietary change.

Variations in diet influence fecal bacterial enzyme activity in humans in a manner similar to that reported in rats. Fecal bacterial enzymes were studied in ominvores who ate a mixed Western diet, lactovegetarians who consumed a diet that excluded all animal foods except milk products, and a group of strict vegetarians (Goldin et al., 1980). Omnivores had considerably higher levels of fecal beta-glucuronidase, nitroreductase, and 7-α-dehydroxylase than did lactovegetarians or strict vegetarians. Azoreductase was significantly lower among the strict vegetarians when compared to omnivores. Elimination of red meat from the diet of omnivores and fiber supplemetation of the mixed Western diet produced no significant change in any enzyme activity except that of 7-α-dhydroxylase. In both cases, this enzyme fell significantly during the period of diet adjustment.

The results cited above indicate that bacterial enzyme levels in the gastrointestinal tract can be altered by diet and other factors and these alternativies may effect the formation of carcinogens and the concentration of tumor promoting substances. The connection between bacterial metabolism and tumorigenesis will be discussed in subsequent sections of this chapter.

BREAST CANCER FAT, ESTROGENS AND THE ENTEROHEPATIC CIRCULATION OF STEROID HORMONES

A complex interaction exists between diet, hormonal status and breast cancer. The evidence is based on cross-country epidemiological studies of the incidence and mortality of breast cancer and dietary consumption, case-control studies, clinical observations, animal studies, endocrine studies of groups at risk and breast cancer patients, and analysis of women's reproductive histories. But because some of the findings are contradictory the physiological mechanisms by which these factors affect the etiology and pathogensis of the disease remains obscure.

Epidemiological studies show a positive correlation between fat intake and breast cancer incidence in different populations (Carroll et al., 1968; Armstrong and Doll, 1975; Lea, 1966; Gray et al., 1978). For example, Japanese women who consume 40-50 grams of fat per day and have an annual breast cancer incidence of 30-35 cases per 100,000 women (Hiryama, 1978), whereas American women who consumed three times that level (about 145 grams of fat per day) have a rate which is three times higher; approximately 100 per 100,000 women per year (Carroll, 1975; Howell, 1976; Hiryama, 1978). Secular trends are also revealing. Rates of breast cancer in Japan have been increasing dramatically in the past two decades, and this change seems to be associated with a marked shift in dietary patterns. In 1957 the average consumption of fat for Japanese people was 23 grams per day, and there were 1,500 deaths due to breast cancer. By 1973 the fat intake had more than doubled to 52 grams per day and there has been a two-fold increase in the number of breast cancer deaths, about 3,200 in 1975.

Howell (1976) reported on the relationship between consumption of foodstuffs and incidence of breast cancer in 36 countries. There were significant positive correlations for meat (r=0.70) and fat (r=0.60), and inverse correlations for cereals (r=-0.62) and pulses and legumes (r=-0.54). Gray et al. (1978) reported, in a similar study from 26 countries, a positive correlation (r=0.91) between breast cancer mortality and consumption of total fat. Similar results have also been reported by Armstrong and Doll (1975), Drasar and Irving (1973), Carroll et al. (1968, 1975) and Lea (1966).

Three case-control studies of breast cancer provide support for diet-breast cancer relationships. Among Seventh-Day Adventists (SDA) the deaths from breast cancer are about one-third less than the average American population (Phillips, 1975). SDA women who developed breast cancer, had higher intakes of dietary fat particularly fried foods and hard fats, than SDA women who did not develop cancer. Miller (1977) showed an association between total fat consumption and breast cancer in premenopausal and postmenopausal Canadian women. Lubin et al. (1981), found diet intake of animal fat and protein were higher in women with breast cancer than among healthy controls.

Dietary fat may influence the initiation and growth of breast tumors through several mechanisms including effects on the endocrine system, cellular immunity, mixed function oxidases, and the intestinal flora. Effects of estrogen metabolism are especially interesting, and considerable evidence exists that suggest a role for estrogens in human breast cancer; the effectiveness of anti-estrogen therapy, the estrogen dependence of many human breast tumors, the positive association of breast cancer incidence with reproductive events (such as early menarche, late menopause and late first pregnancy, or nulliparity) and the dramatic effect of oophorectomy on lowering the incidence of breast cancer. High levels of plasma and urinary estrogens are related to human breast cancer, as shown in recent studies using improved analytical techniques. For example, Morreal et al. (1979), found elevated urinary estrogen in postmenopausal women with breast cancer and Moore et al. (1982), reported higher levels of total serum estradiol and non-protein found serum estradiol in postmenopausal patients with breast cancer. The non-protein bound estradiol was elevated in premenopausal breast cancer patients as well. Drafta et al. (1980), reported elevated serum estradiol concentrations in post menopausal women with breast cancer. MacMahon et al. (1983), found relative risks between 2.5 and 3.5 associated with the highest quartile of urinary estrogen values in premenopausal women. Elevated urinary estrogens have also been observed in the healthy daughters of women who have had breast cancer (Trichopoulos et al., 1981). In addition, Henderson et al. (1975), and Pike et al. (1977), found elevated serum and serum and urine estrogen in women at high risk by virtue of being the daughters of women with breast cancer.

Diet appears to influence the production, metabolism and excretion of estrogens and therefore may act to alter the incidence of breast cancer through this mechanism. Armstrong et al. (1981), studying American vegetarian and omnivores, found differences in serum prolactin and sex hormone binding globulin as well as urinary estrogens. In another study of plasma estrogen levels in vegetarian and non-vegetarian women, 14 premenopausal SDA women were compared with nine premenopausal omnivores (Shultz and Leklem, 1983). The vegetarian women consumed significantly less fat, especially saturated fat, than the omnivores. Plasma levels of estrone and estradiol were lower in the vegetarians. In a study from our laboratory involving omnivore and vegetarian women residing in Boston, the omnivores eating a "Western diet" had higher plasma and lower fecal estrogen levels than vegetarians (Goldin et al., 1982). Also, there was an inverse correlation between plasma estrogen levels and fecal estrogen excretion (Goldin et al., 1982). In a more recent investigation from our laboratory in which vegans (strict vegetarians), lacto-ovo-vegetarians and omnivores were studied, a positive correlation was observed between total fat intake and plasma estrogen concentration (unpublished results). We have also studied recent Oriental immigrants to Hawaii from Southeast Asia and compared their estrogen patterns to Caucasians residing in Boston. The Oriental pre- and post-menopausal subjects, who ate low fat diets (22 per cent fat) had lower plasma estrogen and higher fecal estrogen levels compared to the Boston omnivores. These studies suggest that dietary fat raises estrogen levels in the circulating blood by increasing absorption of estrogen from the intestine, thereby lowering fecal estrogen excretion. In this regard it should be noted that the metabolism of the sex steroid hormones involves an enterohepatic circulation which is dependent upon a biologically active excretion, bacterial deconjugation, and intestinal reabsorption similar to that of the bile acids. Approximately 60 per cent of circulating estrogens are conjugated in the form of glucuronides or sulfates and excreted in the bile (Ericksson and Gustafsson, 1971; Sandberg and Slaunwhite, 1957; Sandberg and Slaunwhite, 1965). Deconjugation, the preresquisite step of mucosal cell reabsorption, is catalyzed by the bacterial enzymes, β-glucuronidase and sulfatase, and it is nearly complete. Indeed, the small amount of estrogens excreted in the feces is 97 per cent in the deconjugated form, although virtually all of the estrogens in bile are conjugated.

Intravenous administration of radiolabelled estriol has demonstrated a two-step conjugation process in the liver (Emerson et al., 1967; Sandberg and Slaunwhite 1957; Sanberg and Slaunwhite, 1957). Initially, the 16-glucuronide is formed which is subsequently converted to estriol-3-sulfate-16-glucuronide and excreted in the bile. In the bowel, bacterial β-glucuronidase and sulfatase hydrolyze this double conjugated moiety to free estriol, most of which is reabsorbed by the mucosal cell. In the mucosal cell, free estriol is reconjugated to estriol-16-glucuronide (Floch et al., 1971). This compound returns to the liver where it is further conjugated to form estriol-3-sulfate-16-glucuronide which completes the enteroheptic cycle (Levitz and Katz, 1968). The mucosal cell can also reconjugate to estriol-3-glucoronide, a compound which is resistant to further conjugation (Floch et al., 1971). This moiety is not excreted in the bile and hence does not undergo an enterohepatic circulation; it is fated for rapid excretion in the urine. The presence of estriol-3-glucuronide in the urine can be used as an indicator of estrogen reabsorption in the lower gastrointestinal tract since the synthesis of this compound occurs only in colonic mucosal cells.

Dietary intake appears to have an effect on the intestinal metabolism of estrogens. There was a 3-fold increase in fecal excretion of estrogen among pre-menopausal vegetarian women when compared to omnivores (Goldin et al., 1982). Urinary excretion estriol-3-glucuronide was also reduced in vegetarians. These findings indicate a reduced enteroheptic circulation of estrogens in vegetarian women, which may be related to reduced intestinal bacterial enzymatic activity in this population.

Another indication that the microflora is involved in estrogen metabolism is the observation that oral antibiotics exert a profound effect on the enterohepatic circulation of estrogen. Studies have shown that there is decreased urinary estriol concentration following oral administration of ampicillin, penicillin or neomycin (Adlecreutz, 1975; Pulklinen and Willman, 1971; Pulkkinen and Willlman, 1973; Willman and Pulkkinen, 1971). The last antibiotic is of particular interest since it is poorly absorbed after oral administration, indicating that the observed effect is due to changes in the makeup of the intestinal flora and not to any systemic properties of the drug. When antibiotics were given, the urinary levels of total conjugated estriol and estriol-16-glucuronide were reduced, along with a 60-fold increase in the fecal excretion of conjugated estrogens and a 3-fold increase in unconjugated moieties (Adlercruetz et al., 1976). Ninety per cent of the observed reduction in urinary estrogen excretion following ampicillin administration could be accounted for by a decrease in the urinary excretion of the 3-glucuronide (Takkanen et al., 1973).

These findings confirmed the gastrointestinal origin of this effect since the synthesis of this conjugate occurs only in the intestinal mucosal cells. These results are most consistent with the postulate that the effect of antibiotics on the excretion of estriol is through suppression of the microflora with a consequent decrese in the bacterially-mediated deconjugation reaction.

FECAL MUTAGENS

Distribution in Different Populations

Bruce et al. (1977), first reported that organic extracts of human feces, contained material that was positive in the bacterial mutagenic test developed by Ames et al. (1975). Using a number of sepration techniques these investigators found that majority of mutagenic activity was associated with a single compound. During the course of these studies several groups investigated the occurrence and levels of fecal mutagens in populations at different risk for colon cancer. A study conducted in South Africa (Ehrich et al., 1979) in which fecal specimens were obtained from rural blacks a population with a very low risk of colon cancer and white South Africans in Johannesburg, who have a high rate of colon cancer, showed a significant difference in the frequency of mutagenic substrates found in the feces. Only 2 per cent of the fecal specimens obtained from the rural black population contained mutagens, in contrast, 15 per cent of the white population was positive. Reddy et al. (1980) measured fecal mutagenic actiity in three different populations: residents of New York City eating a typical "Western diet" and considered at high risk for colon cancer, and residents of the rural Finnish town of Kuopio a population at low risk for colon cancer. Fecal specimens were collected from the three groups and the specimens were freeze-dried, extracted, with ether, particularly purified by silica gel chromatography, and assayed with Salmonella tester strains TA98 and TA100 with and without a liver microsomal activating system. In this population at high risk for colon cancer 22 per cent of the fecal specimens were directly mutagenic on TA98, 11 per cent were directly active on TA100 and 6 per cent were active with S-9 activation on TA100, of the Kupio samples, 13 per cent were mutagenic on TA98, with microsomal activation required in all cases; no mutagenicity was observed on TA100, none of the Seventh-Day Adventists showed mutagenicity on any of the test strains. These data indicate a correlatin may exist between colon cancer incidence and the presence of mutagens in the fecal stream. In a subsequent study from the same laboratory (Reddy et al., 1980a) the presence of fecal comutagens were measured in two of the three populations discussed above, the residents from New York eating a "Western diet" and the Seventh Day Adventist.

Fecal specimens were selected on the basis of having no mutagenic activity in the previous study. Fecal extracts were prepared and tested for the ability to enhance the indirect-acting mutagen and carcinogen 2-acetylaminofluorene (2-AAF) and the direct acting mutagen N-methyl-N'-nitro-N-nitrosoguanine (MNNG). Dose related enhancment of 2-AAF on TA98 and TA100 was observed with the fecal extracts from both population groups, but the vegetarian group had significantly lower comutagenic activity on TA98. There was no difference between the groups in the comuntogenic activity toward MNNG.

Kuhnlein et al. (1981), observed significant differences in the mutagenicity of water extracts of feces collected from ovolactovegetarians. The mutagenic activity was tested with the fluctuation test as described by Green and Muriel (1976). Mutagenic activity was detected in as little as 1 mg/ml fecal supernatant, and its was shown that the vegetarians had significantly lower activity than nonvegetarians. There was, however, considerable variation among individuals. The subjects with the highest and lowest activity were both from the vegetarian group causing difficulty in interpreting results. Differences were noted in the mutagenic activity of the water extracts toward the tests strains indicating the presence of several different mutagens.

Ferguson et al. (1985), used a repair-proficient and repair-deficient mutant of E. coli, to investigate the DNA-damaging activity of ethanol-soluble fecal extracts. Feces from European colorectal cancer patients and age matched controls, Maore's, Samoans and European Seventh-Day Adventists who followed an ovo-lacto vegetarian diet were analyzed for DNA-modifying activity. Europeans had the highest activity regardless of whether or not they had cancer. The number of positive samples was less in the Polynesian groups, and there were no samples that could be unequivocably scored as positive in the Seventh-Day Adventist groups.

Isolation of a Ether Solbule Mutagen from Human Feces

Bruce first described the presence of mutagenic activity in an ether extract of freeze dried freeze (Bruce et al., 1979). The other extract demonstrated maximum activity when washed with acqueous sodium hydroxide and then neutralized prior to testing. The washed ether extract was subsequently dried and applied to benzene to silica gel column and was then eluated with benzene and ether. A single fraction contained most of the activity. This was the first evidence that the mutagenic activity in the ether fraction was associated with a single or similar class of compounds. The purification and ultraviolet spectra of the compound was then described by two different groups working in collaboration (Dion and Bruce, 1983; Wilkins et al., 1981). The compound has a ultraviolet spectrum 365 nm and an high extinction coefficient. The mutagen has a lime-green fluorescence when exposed to long wavelength UV light. The high absorbence allowed investigators (Wilkins et al., 1981) to devise a rapid HPLC method based on the area of optical density in column fractions which is ten fold more sensitive then the Ames test. The compound is very sensitive to oxidation and is inactivated by liver microsomal preparations normally added to bacterial mutagen assays for the purpose of activating compound by oxidation. The oxidation can be inhibited by inclusion of antioxidants, such as butylated hydroxytolene (BHT) in the organic solvents oxidation can be prevented completely by performing the purification under an atmosphere of argon in solvents containing BHT. The mutagen is very stable under strictly anaerobic conditions. When oxidation is allowed to proceed under controlled conditions, the three UV peaks shift to lower wavelength and the fluorescence disappears.

Bacterial Production of the Fecal Mutagen

The amount of mutagenic activity increases dramatically if a fecal specimen already containing mutagen is incubated anaerobically at 37°C for several days. This mutagen production is inhibited by oxygen, low temperature, autoclaving or radiation eliminates the production (Lederman et al., 1980).

It was not possible to generate a mutagen in vitro when fecal specimens were suspended in bacteriological media. This situation was reversed when bile was added to the media; this resulted in the production of mutagen (Van Tassall et al., 1982). It was then demonstrated that a precursor was present in the feces of individuals who produced mutagen. When this precursor was added to bacteriological media containing bile and innoculated with fresh feces and incubated anaerobically at 37°C mutagen was produced. Studies on pure cultures revealed that five strians of Bacteroides (B. fragilis, B. Ovatus, B. uniformis, B. thetaiotamicron and Bacteroides 3543A) produced the mutagen. These strains are commonly found in human feces. The in vitro production of mutagen was inhibited by fermentable carbohydrates, such as, glucose, starch or dextran. Some 40 other species of intestinal anaerobes have been tested for production of the mutagen and all have proved negative (Van Tassel et al., 1982a). The fact that the Bacteroides species is common in the human colon and only relatively small percentage of individuals produce the mutagen indicates the precursor is the determining factor in the mutagen production. This was confirmed by demonstrating that bacteria from feces of individuals who did not have mutagen were capable of producing mutagen in the presence of the precursor compound that is either a product of other bacteria in the colon, comes from the diet, or is a metabolite derived from the host is necessary in combination with Bacteroides for mutagen production. It has been subsequently demonstrated that cell free extracts of <u>Bacteroides</u> in the presence of bile could produce the mutagen. The bacterial enzyme system is not oxygen sensitive, however, the formation of product only occurs anaerobically (Wilkins et al., 1981).

Structure of the Fecal Mutagens

The structure of the fecal mutagen was first announced in 1982 (Hirai et al, 1982) and confirmed independently the following year (Grupta et al., 1983). The characteristic UV spectra and shift on oxidation implied the compound was a penetene. Chemical ionization mass spectrometry and NMR analysis elucidated the structure which is shown below.

$$CH_2O \ (CH = CH)_5 \ CH_2 \ CH_3$$

$$CHOH$$

$$CH_2OH$$

The chemical name of the compound is (S)-3-(1,3,5,7,9=dedecapenlaenyloxy)-1,2 propanediol. The compound is a vinyl ether and is a conjugated laurylglycerol. There are no known mutagens with similar structures. The mutagen has structural similarities to a group of ether linked lipids that are found in anaerobic bacteria and in small concentrations in some mammalian tissue (Wilkins et al., 1981).

ANIMAL TUMOR MODES

In previous sections information was presented indicating that the intestinal microflora can perform reactions that have the potential to produce carcinogens in situ in the large bowel. Evidence for the involvement of the intestinal microflora in the production of a mutagen which is present in the feces of humans has also been reviewed. All of the evidence is circumstantial and is derived either from in vitro metabolism, metabolic epidemiology (example: different levels of secondary bile acids in populations at different risk for colon cancer) or production of mutagenic which have not been shown to be colon carcinogens. There is one other line of evidence implicating bacteria in the etiology of colon cancer. This evidence is derived from animal models involving the chemical induction of colon tumors.

Dimethylhydrazine (DMH), an experimental carcinogen which is metabolized by the liver to methylazoxymethanol, is similar to cycasin in its structure and carcinogenic effects (Druckery et al., 1967). Rats on high beef diets were more susceptible to the carcinogenic effects of DMH. When DMH was fed to rats on high beef and grain diets, the rates of tumor production were 83 per cent and 31 per cent, respectively (Goldin and Gorbach, 1980).

When germ-free and convetional rats were challenged with 3,2'-dimethyl-4-aminobipehnyl (DMAB), there were significantly fewer colon tumors among germ-free animals (Reddy and Watunabe, 1978). The role of dietary fat in promoting colon carcinogensis was studied during challenge with DMAB in which more animals on high-fat diets had colon tumors than did animals receiving low-fat diet. Dietary fat had no effect on the incidence of tumors when germ-free animal were studied, further emphasizing the role of the microflora in this process.

The administration of oral antibiotics also influences the metabolic activity of the intestinal flora. Three groups of beef-fed rats were studied: a control group, a group receiving tetraycycline, and a group receiving erythromycin (Goldin and Gorbach, 1981). There was a striking reduction in the incidence of intestinal tumors in the antibiotic group after challenge with DMH. Colonic tumors developed in 74 per cent of control animals compared with 20 per cent in the tetracycline grop and 22 per cent in the erythromycin group. Fecal β-glucuronidase activity was also significantly reduced in the antibiotic treated animals. Similarly, administration of a β-glucuronidase inhibitor also decreased the formation of colon cancer in conventional animals treated with the experimental carcinogen azoxymethane (Takada et al., 1982).

In another study, beef-fed rats were given DMH to induce colon tumors, along with lactobacilli (Goldin and

Gorbach, 1980). There was significant reduction in colon cancers at the 20-week observation time, but no at 36 weeks. These findings suggest that dietary lactobacilli increase the latency or induction time for colon cancers, probably by influencing the metabolic activity of the colonic flora.

Although there is no direct evidence that the intestinal microflora increase the incidence of colon cancer in humans there is data which shows that the intestinal microflora are capable of performing reactions which can either generate carcinogens or tumors promoters in the large bowel.

REFERENCES

Adlecreutz H, Martin F, Pulkkinen M, Dencker H, Rimer U, et al. (1976). Intestinal metabolism of estrogens. J Clin Endocrinol Metab 43:497-505.
Adlecreutz H, Martin F, Tikanen MJ, Pulkkinen M (1975). Effect of ampicillin administration on the excretion of twelve oestrogens in pregnancy urine. Acta Endocrinologia 80:551-557.
Ames BN, McCann J, Yamasaki E (1975). Methods for detecting carcinogens and mutagens with the salmonella/mammalian-microsome mutagenicity test. Mutat Res 31:347-364.
Armstrong BK, Brown JB, Clarke HT, Crooke DK, Hahnel R, et al. (1981). Diet and reproduction hormones: A study of vegetarians and non-vegetarian postmenopausal women. J Natl Cancer Inst 67:761-767.
Bruce WR, Varghese AJ, Furrer R, Land PC (1977). A mutagen in the feces of normal humans. Cold Spring Harbor Conf Cell Profliferation 4:1641-1646.
Burkitt DP (1971). Epidemology of cancer of the colon and rectum. Cancer 28:3-13.
Chung KT (1983). The significance of azo-reduction in the mutagenesis and carcinogenesis of azo dyes. Mutation Res 114:269-281.
Chung KT, Fulk GE, Andrews AW (1978). The mutagenieity of methyl orange and metabolites produced by intestinal anaerobes. Mutation Res 58:375-379.
Chung KT, Fulk GE, Slein MW (1975). Tryptaphanase of fecal flora as a possibe factor in the etiology of colon cancer. J Natl Cancer Inst 54:1073-1078.

Carroll KK (1975). Experimental evidence of dietary factors and hormone dependence. Cancer Res 35:3374-3383.

Carroll KK, Gammal EB, Plunkett ER (1968). Dietary fat and mammary cancer. Cancer Med Assoc 98:590-594.

Dion P, Bruce WR (1983). Mutagenicity of different fractions of extracts of human feces. Mutation Res 119:151-160.

Doll R (1969). The geographical distribution of cancer. Br J Cancer 23:1-8.

Drasar BS, Hill MJ (1974). "Human Intestinal Flora." New York, Academic Press, p 263.

Drasar BS, Irving D (1973). Environmental facotrs and cancer of the colon and breast. Br J Cancer 27:167-172.

Drasar BS, Jenkins DJA, Cummings JH (1976). The influence of a diet rich in wheat fiber on the human fecal flora. J Med Microbiol 9:423-431.

Druckery H, Preussman R, Matzbies F, Ivantsovic S (1967). Selektive Erzengung Von Darmkrebs bei Ratten durch 1,2-dimethylhydrazin. Naturwissenschaften 54:285-286.

Dunn JE (1975). Cancer epidemology in populations of the United States with emphasis on Hawaii and California and Japan. Cancer Res 35:3240-3245.

Ehrich M, Aswell JE, Van Tassell RL, Wilkins TD (1979). Mutagens in the feces of 3 South African populations at different levels of risk for colon cancer. Mutat Res 64:231-240.

EL-Bayoumy K, Fharma C, Louis YM, Reddy B, Hecht SS (1983). The role of intestinal microflora in the metabolic reduction of 1-nitropyrene to 1-aminopyrene in conventional and germfree rats and in humans. Cancer Lett 19:311-316.

Emerman S, Twombly GH, Levitz M (1967). Biliary and urinary metabolites of estriol-15-^{3}H-3-sulfate-^{35}S in women. J Clin Endocrinol Metab 27:539-548.

Ender F, Ceh L (1968). Occurence of nitrosamines in foodstuffs for human and animal consumption. Food Cosmet Toxicol 6:569-571.

Eriksson H, Gustafsson JA (1971). Excretion of steroid hormones in adults: Steroids in feces from adults. Eur J Biochem 18:146-150.

Ferguson LR, Alley PG, Griffen BM (1985). DNA-damaging activity in ethanol-soluble fractions of feces from New Zealand Groups at varying risks of colorectal cancer. Nutr and Cancer J 7:93-103.

Finegold SM, Attebery HR, Sutter VL (1974). Effect of diet on human fecal flora: Comparison of Japanese and American diets. Amer J Clin Nutr 27:1456-469.

Finegold SM, Sutter VL, Sugihara PT, Elder HA, Lehmann SM, Phillips RL (1977). Fecal microbial flora in Seventh Day Adventist populations and control subjects. Am J Clin Nutr 30:1781-1792.

Fisher LJ, Millburn P, Smith RL (1966). The fat of 14C stilbesterol in the rat. Biochem J 100:69.

Floch MH, Gershengoren W, Elliott S, Apiro HM (1971). Bile acid inhibition of the intestinal microflora - a function for simple bile acids. Gastroenterology 61:228-233.

Goldin BR, Adlecreutz H, Gorbach SL, Warram JH, Dwyer JT, et al. (1982). Estrogen excretion patterns and plasma levels in vegetarian and omnivorous women. N Engl J Med 207:1542-1547.

Goldin BR, Gorbach SL (1976). The realtionship between diet and rat fecal bacterial enzymes implicated in colon cancer. J Natl Cancer Inst 57:371-375.

Goldin BR, Gorbach SL (1980). Effect of Lactobacillus acidophilus dietary supplements on 1,2-dimethylhydrazine dihydrochloride induced intestinal cancer in rats. J Natl Cancer Inst 64:263-265. J Natl Cancer Inst 64:263-265.

Goldin BR, Gorbach SL (1981). Effect of antibiotics on incidence of rat intestinal tumors induced by 1,2-dimethylhydrazine dihydrochloride. J Natl Cancer Inst 67:877-880.

Goldin BR, Swenson L, Dwyer J, Sexton M, Gorbach SL (1980). Effect of diet and Lactobaccilus supplements on human fecal bacterial enzymes. J Natl Cancer Inst 64:255-262. J Natl Cancer Int. 64:255-262.

Green MHL, Muriel WJ (1976). Mutagen testing using trp+ reversion in Escherichia coli. Mutat Res 38:3-32.

Gray GE, Pilse MC, Henderson BE (1979). Breast-cancer incidence and mortality rates in different countries in relation to known risk factors and dietary practices. Br J Cancer 39:1-7.

Gupta I, Baptista J, Bruce WE, Che CT, Furrer R, et al. (1983). Structures of fecapentaenes, the mutagens of bacterial origin isolated from human feces. Biochemistry 22:241-245.

Haenszel W, Berg JW, Segi M, Kurihara M, Locke FB (1973). Large bowel cancer in Hawaiian, Japanese. J Natl Cancer Inst 51:1765-1769.

Hartman CP, Falk CE, Andrews AW (1978). Azo reduction of trypan blue to a known carcinogen by a cell-free extract of a human intestinal anaerobe. Mutation Res 58:125-132.

Henderson BE, Gerkins V, Rosario I, Casagrande J, Pike MC (1975). Elevated serum levels of estrogn and prolactin in daughters of patients with breast cancer. N Engl J Med 293:790-795.

Hill MJ, Drasar BS, Aries VC, Crowther JS, Hawksworth GM, Williams REO (1971). Bacteria and etiology of cancer of large bowel. Lancet 1:95-99.

Hirai N, Kingston DGI, Van Tassell RL, Wilkins TD (1982). Structure elucidation of a potent mutagen from human feces. J Am Chem Soc 104:6149-6150.

Hirayama T (1978). Epidemiology of breast cancer with special reference to the rates of diet. Pre Med 7:173-195.

Howell MA (1976). The association between colorectal cancer and breast cancer. J Chron Dis 29:243-261.

Karpinsky GE, Rosenkranz HS (1980). The anaerobe-mediated mutagenicity of 2 nitroflurene and 2-aminofluroene for Salmonella Typirimurium. Environ Mutagen 2:353-358.

Kay RM (1981). Effects of diet on the fecal excretion and bacterial modification of acidic and neutral steroids, and implications for colon carcinogens. Cancer Res 42:3774-3777.

Kuhnlein V, Bergstrom D, Kuhnlein H (1981). Mutagens in feces from vegetarians and non-vegetarians. Mutat Res 85:1-12.

Laqueur GL, Spatz M (1975). Oncogenicity of cycasin and methylazoxymethanol. Gann Monogr Cancer Res 17:189-204.

Lederman M, Van Tassell RL, West SEH, Ehrich MF, Wilkins TD (1980). In vitro production of human fecal mutagen. Mutat Res 85:1-12.

Levitz M, Katz J (1968). Enterohepatic metabolism of estriol-3-sulfate-16-glucuronide in women. J Clin Endocrinol Metab 28:862-868.

Lindmark DG, Muller M (1976). Antitrichomanad action, mutagenicity and reduction of metronidazle and other nitromidazoles. Antimicrob Agents Chemother 10:476-482.

Lindop R, Tasman-Jones C, Thomsen LL, Lee SP (1985). Cellulose and pectin alter b-glucuronidase in the rat. Br J Nutr 54:21-26.

Lubin JH, Burns PE, Blot WJ, Ziegler RG, Lees AV, Frammeni JF (1981). Dietary factors and breast cancer risk. Int J Cancer 28:685-689.

MacDonald IA, Bussard RG, Hutchinson DM, Holderman LV (1984). Rutin-induced β-glucosidose activity in Strepcoccus faecium VGH-1 and Streptoccus SP. strain FRP-17 isolated from human feces: formation of the mutagen, quercetin from rutin. Appl Environ Micrscop 47:350-355.

MacDonald IA, Webb GR, Mahoney DC (1978). Fecal hydroxysteroid dehydrogenase activities in vegetarian Seventh-Day Adventist, control subjects and bowel cancer subjects. Am J Clin Nutr 31:5233-5238.

Mader JA, MacDonald IA (1985). Effect of bile acids on formation of the mutagen, quercetin, from two flavonol glycoside precursors by human gut bacterial preparations. Mutat Res 155:99-104.

Magee PH, Barnes JM (1956). The production of malignant primary hepatic tumors in the rat by feeding dimethylnitrosamine. Br J Cancer 10:114-122.

Maier BB, Flynn MA, Burton GG, Tsutakawa RK, Hentges DJ (1974). Effects of a high-beef diet on bowel flora: A preliminary report. Amer J Clin Nutr 27:1470-1474.

Mastromarino A, Reddy BS, Wynder EL (1976). Metabolic epidemiology of colon cancer: enzymatic activity of fecal flora. Am J Clin Nutr 29:1455-460.

Mastromarino A, Reddy BS, Wynder EL (1978). Fecal profiles of anaerobic microflora of large bowel cancer patients and patients with nonhereditary large bowel polyps. Cancer Res 38:4458-4462.

McCoy EC, Petrullo LA, Rosenkranz HS (1979). The demonstration of cooperative action of bacterial and intestinal mucosa enzymes in the activation of mutagens. Biochem Biophys Res Commun 89:859-862.

McCoy EC, Rosenkranz HS, Mermelstein R (1981). Evidence for the existence of a family of m-nitroreductases capable of activating nitrated polycyclics to mutagens. Environ Mutagen 3:421-427.

McCoy EC, Speck TS, Rosenkranz HS (1977). Activation of a procarcinogen to mutagen by cell-free extracts of anaerobic bacteria. Mutat Res 46:261-264.

Miller AB (1977). Role of nutrition in the etiology of breast cancer. Cancer 39:2704-2708.

Miller JA, Miller EC (1969). The metabolic activation of carcinogenic aromatic amines and amides. Prog Exp Tumor Res 11:273-301.

Moore WEC, Holderman LV (1974). Human fecal flora: The normal flora of 20 Japanese-Hawaiians. Appl Micro 27:961-979.

Moore WEC, Holderman LV (1975). Discussion of current bacteriological investigations of the relationships between intestinal flora, diet and colon cancer. Cancer Res 35:3418-20, 1975.

Morotomi M, Nanno M, Watanabe T, Sakurai T, Mutai M (1985). Mutagenic activation of biliary metabolites of 1-nitropyrene by intestinal microflora. Mut Res 149:171-178.

Morreal CE, Dao TL, Nemoto T, Lanegan PA (1970). Urinary excretion of estrone, estradiol, and estriol in postmenopausal women with primary breast cancer. J Natl Cancer Inst 63:1171-1174.

Mower HF, Ray RM, Shaff R, Stemmermann GN, Maura A, et al. (1979). Fecal bile acids in two Japanese populations with different colon cancer risks. Cancer Res 39:328-31, 1979.

Phillips RL (1975). Role of lifestyle and dietary habits in risk of cancer among Seventh Day Adventists. Cancer Res 35:3513-3522.

Pike MC, Casagrande JT, Brown JB, Gerkins V, Henderson BF (1977). Comparison of urinary and plasma hormone levels in daughters of breast cancer patients and controls. J Natl Cancer Inst 59:1351-1355.

Pulkkinen MO, Willman K (1971). Maternal estrogen levels during penicillin treatment. Br Med J 4:48.

Pulkkinen MO, WIllman K (1973). Reduction of maternal estrogen excretion by neomycin. Am J Obstet Gynecol 115:1153.

Reddy BS, Sharma C, Darby L, Losko K, Wynder EL (1980). Metabolic epidemology of large bowel cancer: fecal mutagens in high- and low-risk populations for colon cancer: A preliminary report. Mutat Res 72:511-519.

Reddy BS, Sharma C, Wynder EL (1980a). Fecal factors which modify the formation of fecal co-mutagens in high- and low-risk populations for colon cancer. Cancer Lett 10:123.

Reddy BS, Watanaboe K (1978). Effect of intestinal microflora on 3,2-dimethyl-4-aminobiphenyl-induced carcinogenesis in F344 rats. J Natl Cancer Inst 61:1269-271.

Reddy BS, Weisburger JH, Wynder EL (1974). Fecal bacterial beta-glucuronidase control by diet. Science 183:416-417.

Reddy BS, Wynder EL (1973). Large-bowel carcinogenesis: Fecal constituents of populations with diverse incidence rates of colon cancer. J Natl Cancer Inst 50:1437-442.

Reid TM, Morton KC, Wang CY, King CM (1983). Conversion of congo red and 2-azoxyfluorene to mutagens following in vitro reduction by whole-cell rat cecal bacteria. Mutation Res 117:105-112.

Sandberg AA, Slaunwhite Jr, WR (1957). Studies on phenolic steroids in human subjects. II. The metabolic fate and hepato-biliary-enteric circulation of ^{14}C-esterone and ^{14}C-estradiol in women. J Clin Invest 36:1266-1278.

Sandberg AA, Slaunwhite Jr, WR (1965). Studies on phenolic steroids in human subjects. VII. Metabolic fate of estriol and its glucuronide. J Clin Invest 44:694-702.

Schultz TD, Leklem JE (1983). Nutrient intake and hormonal status of premenopausal vegetarian Seventh-Day Adventists and premenopausal nonvegetarians. Nutr Cancer 4:247-259.

Takada H, Hirook T, Hiramatsu, Yamamato M (1982). Effect of β-glucuronidase inhibitor on azoxymethane-induced colonic carcinogenesis in rats. Cancer Res 42:331-334.

Tamura G, Gold C, Ferro-Luzzi A, Ames BN (1980). Fecalase: A model for activation of dietary glycosides to mutagens by intestinal flora. Proc Natl Acad Sci 77:4961-4965.

Tannenbaum SR, Sinsky AJ, Weisman M, Bishop W (1974). Nitrate in human saliva. Its possible relationship to nitrosamine formation. J Natl Cancer Inst 53:79-84.

Tikkanen MJ, Pulkkinen MO, Adlecreutz H (1973). Effect of ampicillin treatment on the urinary excretion of estriol conjugation in pregnancy. J Steroid Biochem 4:439-440.

Van Tassell RL, MacDonald DK, Wilkins TD (1982). Stimulation of mutagen production in human feces by bile and bile acids. Mutat Res 103:233-239.

Van Tassell RL, MacDonald DK, Wilkins TD (1982a). Production of a fecal mutagen by bacteriods Spp. Infect Immun 37:975-980.

Weisburger JH (1971). Colon carcinogens: their metabolism and mode of action. Cancer 28:60-70.

Weisburger JH, Grantham PH, Horton RE (1970). Metabolism of the carcinogen N-hydroxy-N-2-fluorenylacetamide in germ free rats. Biochem Pharmacol 19:151-162.

Weisburger JH, Weisburger EK (1966). Chemical as a cause of cancer. Chem Enz News 44:124-142.

Weisburger JH, Weisburger EK (1973). Biochemical formation and pharmacological, toxicological, and pathological properties of hydroxylamines and hydroxamic acid. Pharmacol Rev 25:1-66.

Wheeler LA, Soderberg FB, Goldman P (1975). The relationship between nitro group reduction and the intestinal microflora. J Pharmacol Exp Ther 194:135-144.

White BS, Lipsky RL, Fricke RJ, Hylemon PB (1980). Bile acid induction specificity of 7-α-dehydroxylase activity in an intestinal Eubacterium sp. Steroids 35:103-109.

Wilkins TD, Lederman M, Van Tassell RL (1981). Isolation of a mutagen produced in the human colon by bacterial action. Banburg Report 7:205-214.

Wilkins TD, Van Tassell RL (1983). "Human Intestinal Microlfora." Academic Press, New York, NY, pp 568.

Willman K, Pulkkinen MO (1971). Reduced maternal plasma and urinary estriol during ampicllin treatment. Am J Obstet Gynecol 109:893-896.

Wynder E, Shigimasu T (1967). Environmental factors of cancer of the colon and rectum. Cancer 20:1520-1561.

Dietary Fat and Cancer, pages 687–697

EICOSANOIDS AND CANCER

Rashida A. Karmali

Department of Nutrition, Rutgers University,
New Brunswick, New Jersey 08903 and
Memorial Sloan-Kettering Cancer Center,
New York, New York 10021

Investigations during the past decade suggest that
eicosanoids, a group of oxygenated arachidonic acid metabolites, which include prostaglandins (PGs), thromboxanes
(TXs), leukotrienes (LTs), and various hydroxy and hydroperoxy fatty acids, play an important role in cancer
development and progression. Prostaglandins are secreted
by a variety of animal and human tumors and current
evidence suggests that circulating prostaglandins may also
mediate a variety of paraneoplastic syndromes (Karmali,
1980, 1983; Metz et al. 1981).

This is not an all-inclusive literature review but an
attempt to examine critically the more recent evidence that
suggests that eicosanoid-mediated events may include tumor
initiation, neovascularisation, tissue invasiveness,
metastatic spread or subversion of immune surveillance. We
will also summarize our own work examining the possibility
of a role for eicosanoids in various steps in the complex
etiology of cancer.

An understanding of the biosynthetic pathways for the
eicosanoids and the interplay among substrates and products
may help in interpreting current evidence. The derivation
of eicosanoids from essential fatty acids is shown
schematically in Figure 1. Prostaglandins and thromboxanes
are produced from arachidonic acid ($C20:4\omega6$, the most
prevalent substrate in primates) via the cyclooxygenase
pathway, and the leukotrienes and hydroxy and hydroperoxy
acids are produced via the lipoxygenase pathways.
Dihomo-gamma-linolenic acid ($C20:3\omega6$) and eicosapentaenoic

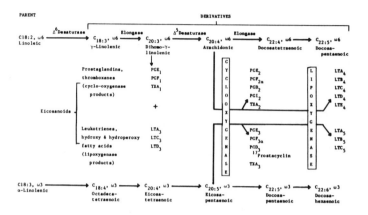

Figure 1. Derivation of eicosanoids from essential fatty acids.

acid are also used as substrates for eicosanoid synthesis by the cyclooxygenase and lipoxygenase enzymes. Eicosapentaenoic acid has been shown to competitively inhibit arachidonic acid metabolism by both enzymes and give rise to its own products, which have attenuated activity (Needleman et al., 1980; Lee et al. 1985). Modification in dietary intake of ω-3 and ω-6 polyunsaturated fatty acids affects availability of these substrates for eicosanoid biosynthesis.

Important discoveries have been made on the nature of the products of arachidonic acid metabolism. Thromboxane A_2 is a potent stimulus for platelet aggregation and constricts large blood vessels and has variable vasoconstrictor activity in the microcirculation (Hamberg et al., 1975). Prostacyclin, which is the main cyclooxygenase product of arachidonic acid in arteries, veins, and microcirculation (Goehlert et al., 1981), is a vasodilator, and the most potent naturally occurring inhibitor of platelet aggregation (Moncada and Vane, 1979). Prostaglandin E_2 has been shown to inhibit lymphocyte cytotoxicity in vitro (Goodwin and Webb, 1980) and exert immunosuppressive effects in tumor-bearing mice (Pelus and Strausser, 1976). The leukotrienes are of particular interest since LTB$_4$ has chemotactic activity (Palmer et al., 1980) and the sulfidopeptide leukotrienes comprise the activity previously recognized as slow reacting substance of anaphylaxis (Murphy et al, 1979) and are potent spasmogenic agents on nonvascular smooth muscle.

The cyclooxygenase enzyme is inhibited by nonsteroidal anti-inflammatory agents such as aspirin, indomethacin, ibuprofen, flurbiprofen, etc. Their effect on carcinogenesis and tumor growth is being tested in experimental tumor systems.

CHEMICAL CARCINOGENESIS

Chemical carcinogenesis in many experimental systems appears to be a multistage process in which the early phase may or may not require carcinogen metabolism followed by interaction with cells of the target tissue. The late phase encompasses the postcarcinogen period when a promoting agent may influence the development and growth of the tumor.

Recent studies have shown that cyclic hydrocarbons and other xenobiotics are cooxygenated to their carcinogenic forms during the oxidative metabolism of arachidonic acid (Marnett, 1981). Peroxidatic activation of procarcinogens, such as benzidine to electrophiles that covalently bind macromolecules, has been proposed as an additional pathway for initiation of chemical carcinogenesis (Zenser et al., 1980). Induction of mammary tumors with 7,12-dimethylbenz-(a)anthracene (DMBA) in rats was reported to be inhibited by indomethacin (McCormick et al., 1985). Similar results were reported in the 1,2-dimethyl-hydrazine hydrochloride-induced rat colon tumor model (Metzger et al., 1984).

In addition, eicosanoids may also act as tumor promoters since indomethacin was shown to inhibit the tumor-promoting effects of a high-fat (corn oil) diet in DMBA-induced mammary tumorigenesis (Carter et al., 1983). While some of the biological effects of the tumor promoter 12-0-tetradecanoyl phorbol-13-acetate are mediated by eicosanoid biosynthesis, their decisive role is unclear, since inhibition of eicosanoid synthesis both prevents and enhances promotion in the skin tumor model (Fischer and Slaga, 1982).

EICOSANOID PRODUCTION

Several types of malignant tissues in both humans and experimental animals have an enhanced ability to secrete eicosanoids into the tissue space. We have reported such studies of the R3230AC transplantable mammary adeno-carcinoma, the N-nitromethylurea-induced mammary tumors, Lewis lung carcinoma, human breast carcinoma, and head/neck cancer (Karmali et al., 1983, 1984, 1984). Although PGE_2 is quantitatively the major component, several studies in both rodent and human cancerous tissues indicate malignant tissues also contain other oxygenated metabolites of arachidonic acid, including other prostanoids, thromboxane, and hydroxy and hydroperoxy fatty acids.

Normal cells tend to produce a characteristic pattern of eicosanoids necessary for carrying out specific physio-logical functions. The rate of eicosanoid production is generally controlled in most normal cellular events, but it seems to reach exaggerated levels in some pathological conditions such as cancer. Some tumor cells have been shown to synthesize eicosanoids both in vivo and/or in vitro (Cohen and Karmali, 1984; Owen et al., 1980; Gebhardt et al., 1985). A significant portion of the eicosanoids associated with tumor tissues are derived from infiltrating cells such as macrophages and other inflammatory cells of the host. Thus factors such as cellular origin of tumor eicosanoids, tumor heterogeneity, and host-derived elements complicate interpretation of eicosanoid studies in solid tumors. Furthermore, design of methodology used to measure eicosanoids in tumor tissues should be based upon criteria that minimize procedural errors (Karmali et al., 1983).

Evidence that breast and lung carcinomas produced more PG-like material than normal tissue has been published by Bennett and associates (1977, 1979, 1982). Breast cancer tissues containing higher levels of PG-like material resulted in earlier death after surgery than those that produced lower levels (Bennett et al., 1979). In a series of 24 breast cancer patients, we found that steady-state tissue content of 5 compounds--PGE_1, PGE_2, $PGF_{2\alpha}$, 6-keto-$PGF_{1\alpha}$, and TXB_2--was higher in neoplastic tissue than in paired noncancerous breast tissue. Increased TXB_2 metabolism was related to tumor size, axillary lymph node metastases, and distant metastases (Karmali et al., 1983). Rolland et al. (1980) reported that increased synthesis of PGE_2 in vitro was associated with metastasis in a study involving 96 breast cancer patients. A study involving 11 ovarian cancer patients has documented that tumors of patients without response to chemotherapy contained more PGE_2, $PGF_{2\alpha}$, and 6-keto-$PGF_{1\alpha}$ than did tumors responding to chemotherapy (Bauknecht et al., 1985).

CONTROL OF CELL PROLIFERATION

The control of cell proliferation both in vivo and in vitro is a complex process, and to date the effect of a large number of eicosanoids or their analogue products have been tested (review, Karmali, 1983). Recent studies suggest that PGD_2 has growth inhibiting activity against several human leukemia cell lines and a variety of human malignant tumor cells, including melanoma, neuroblastoma, cervical cancer, rhabdomyosarcoma, osteosarcoma, breast cancer, and ovarian cancer. The dose of PGD_2 that was effective in inhibiting cell proliferation was equal to or greater than 5 µg/ml (Fukushima et al., 1982; Sakai and Yamaguchi, 1984). We have previously demonstrated in a lymphoid cell line that the effect of exogenous eicosanoids is most likely to be dose-related and concentrations above 1µg/ml are likely to result in inhibition of cell proliferation (Karmali et al., 1979). The significance of such in vitro data has to be evaluated in light of whether such high concentrations of eicosanoids can be administered in vivo in human subjects.

METASTASIS

The role of eicosanoids in metastatic spread and growth is not clearly defined, but indirect evidence supports the concept that there may be a net increase in TXA_2 (pro-aggregatory factor for platelets) and a decrease in PGI_2 (anti-aggregatory factor for platelets) activity. Hence, drugs that inhibit TXA_2 formation or increase PGI_2 activity would be antithrombotic and might be useful in the inhibition of tumor metastases. Honn and coworkers (1981, 1983) tested PGI_2 and Nafazatrom (a PGI_2-enhancing agent)

in the Lewis lung carcinoma and B16 melanoma tumor systems
in mice. They reported significant inhibition of
metastasis in these studies. Subsequent reports on the
effect of Nafazatrom suggest that the antimetastatic effect
of this drug is weak at best (Hass et al., 1985; Karmali et
al., 1986), and no clinically detectable biological
activity was observed in a Phase I trial of this drug in 48
cancer patients (Hortobaggi et al., 1985).

IMMUNE RESPONSES

Eicosanoids have profound effects on cellular and
humoral immune responses. Increased PGE_2 has been measured
in peripheral blood mononuclear cells in Hodgkin's disease
(Goodwin et al., 1977), melanoma (Murray and Kollmorgen,
1983), and head and neck cancer (Maca and Panje, 1982).
Regression of head and neck carcinoma was achieved with
indomethacin treatment (Panje, 1981). In Hodgkin's disease
attempts at reversing the defect in cell-mediated immunity
with indomethacin have been successful in part. Braun and
Harris (1984) studied solid tumor cancer patients and
reported that the immune function recovery in drug-treated
cancer patients is dependent, in part, on the effects of
chemotherapy on PGE synthesis by peripheral blood
mononuclear cells.

MODULATION OF ARACHIDONIC ACID METABOLISM IN EXPERIMENTAL TUMOR SYSTEMS IN OUR LABORATORY

Our own data would tend to reinforce the theory that
inhibition of arachidonic acid metabolism, specifically
PGE_2, can result in inhibition of tumor development and
growth. Pharmacological intervention with indomethacin,
ibuprofen, flurbiprofen, and specific immunotherapy against
PGE_2 resulted in inhibition of growth of the R3230AC
mammary tumors in rats maintained on rat chow (Karmali and
Marsh, 1985). However, indomethacin at the level of 0.004%
in a 20% corn oil diet was not found to inhibit tumor
growth, although plasma and tumor PGE_2 were reduced
(Feldman and Hilf, 1985). Differences are most likely
related to differences in the level of linoleic acid
between a rat chow diet and a 20% corn oil diet and the
dose of indomethacin used.

We have studied the effect of the tripeptide, reduced glutathione, on growth of the R3230AC mammary tumors. The data obtained suggest that tumor PGE_2 and growth were inhibited (Karmali, 1984).

A different approach was taken to modulate arachidonic acid metabolism with two dietary ω-3 fatty acids, eicosapentaenoic acid and docosahexaenoic acid. To date, we have found the fish oil rich in ω-3 fatty acids had antitumor effects in the R3230AC mammary adenocarcinoma (Karmali et al., 1984), DMBA-induced mammary tumors (Karmali, 1986), and the DU-145 prostatic tumor (Karmali et al., 1986). Results in these early studies suggest that the biochemical changes that accompany these effects on tumor development and/or growth involve inhibition of arachidonic acid metabolism in tumor tissues and in cultures of peritoneal macrophages and spleen leukocytes in vitro (Oza and Karmali, 1986). Data published by other investigators tend to reinforce these observations, for intervention with ω-3 fatty acids has resulted in inhibition of N-nitrosomethylurea- and DMBA-induced mammary tumors (Jurkowski and Cave, 1985; Carroll and Braden, 1985) and L-azaserine-induced preneoplastic pancreatic lesions (O'Connor et al., 1985). Since arachidonic acid metabolism may be amenable to safe nutritional alteration with ω-3 fatty acids, there is additional impetus to establish the optimum ratio of ω-3/ω-6 at which tumor protective effects will be achieved either with or without pharmacologic inhibition.

REFERENCES

Bauknecht T, Siegel A, Meerpohl HG, Zahradnik HP (1985). Formation of prostaglandins by ovarian carcinomas. Prostaglandins 29:665-672.
Bennett A, Berstock DA, Raja B, Stamford IF (1979). Survival time after surgery inversely related to the amounts of prostaglandins extracted from human breast cancers. Br J Pharmacol 66:451P.
Bennett, A, Carroll MA, Stamford IF, Whimster WF, Williams F (1982). Prostaglandins and human lung carcinomas. Br J Cancer 46:888-893.
Bennett A, Charlier EM, McDonald AM, Simpson JS, Stamford IF, Zebro T (1977). Prostaglandins and cancer. Lancet 2:624-626.

Braun DP, Harris JE (1984). Effect of combination chemotherapy on PGE-mediated immunoregulation in the peripheral blood mononuclear cells of solid tumor cancer patients. J Biol Response Modifiers 3:391-396.

Carroll KK, Braden LM (1985). Dietary fat and mammary carcinogenesis. Nutr Cancer 6:254-259.

Carter CA, Milholland RJ, Shea W, Ip MM (1983). Effect of prostaglandin synthetase inhibitor indomethacin on 7,12,dimethylbenz(a)anthracene-induced mammary tumorigenesis in rats fed different levels of fat. Cancer Res 43:3559-3562.

Cohen LA, Karmali RA (1984). Endogenous prostaglandin production by established cultures of neoplastic rat mammary epithelial cells. In Vitro 20:119-126.

Feldman JM, Hilf R (1985). Failure of indomethacin to inhibit growth of the R3230AC mammary tumor in rats. J Natl Cancer Inst 75:751-756.

Fischer SM, Slaga TJ (1982). Modulation of prostaglandin synthesis and tumor promotion. In Powles TJ, Bockman RS, Honn KV, Rainwell P (eds): "Prostaglandins and Cancer: First International Conference," New York: Alan R. Liss, pp 255-264.

Fukushima M, Kato T, Ueda R, Ota K. Narumiya S, Hayaishi O (1982). Prostaglandin D$_2$, a potential antineoplastic agent. Biochem Biophys Res Commun 105:956-964.

Gebhardt MC, Lippiello L, Bringhurst FR, Mankin HJ (1985). Prostaglandin E$_2$ synthesis by human primary and metastatic bone tumors in culture. Clin Orthopaed Rel Dis 196:300-305.

Goehlert UG, Ng Ying Kin NMK, Wolfe LS (1981). Biosynthesis of prostacyclin in rat cerebral microvessels and the choroid plexus. J Neurochem 36:1192-1201.

Goodwin JS, Messner RP, Bankhurst AD, Peake GT, Saiki JH, Williams RC. Prostaglandin-producing suppressor cells in Hodgkin's disease. N Engl J Med 297:963-967.

Goodwin JS, Webb DR (1980). Regulation of the immune response by prostaglandins. Clin Immunol Immunopathol 15:106-122.

Haas JS, Corbett TH, Haas CD (1985). Nafazatrom: lack of anti-metastatic effect. Proc Am Assoc Cancer Res 26:202.

Hamberg M, Svensson J, Samuelsson B (1975). Thromboxanes: a new group of biologically active compounds derived from prostaglandin endoperoxides. Proc Natl Acad Sci USA 72:2994-2998.

Honn KV, Buese WD, Sloane BF (1983). Prostacyclin and thromboxanes: implications for their role in tumor cell metastasis. Biochem Pharmacol 32:1-11.

Honn KV, Cicone B, Skeff A (1981). Prostacyclin: a potent antimetastatic agent. Science 212:1270-1272.

Hortobaggi G, Frye D, Papadoupoulas N, Buzdar A (1985). Phase I evaluation of Nafazatrom. Proc Am Assoc Cancer Res 26:687.

Jurkowski JJ, Cave WT Jr (1985). Dietary effects of menhaden oil on the growth and membrane lipid composition of rat mammary tumors. J Natl Cancer Inst 74:1145-1150.

Karmali RA (1984). Growth inhibition and prostaglandin metabolism in the R3230AC mammary adenocarcinoma by reduced glutathione. Cancer Biochem Biophys 7:147-154.

Karmali RA (1983). Prostaglandins and cancer. CA-A Cancer J for Clinicians 33:322-332.

Karmali RA (1980). Prostaglandins and cancer. Prostaglandins Leuk Med 5:11-28.

Karmali RA. Do tissue culture and animal model studies relate to human diet and cancer? Prog Lipid Res (in press).

Karmali RA, Otter G, Schmid F. Eicosanoids and metastasis: experimental aspects in Lewis lung carcinoma. Cancer Biochem Biophys (in press).

Karmali RA, Horrobin DR, Menezes J, Patel P (1979). The relationship between concentrations of prostaglandin A_1, E_1, E_2, and $F_{2\alpha}$ and rates of cell proliferation. Pharmacol Res Commun 11:69-75.

Karmali RA, Marsh J (1985). Antitumor activity in a rat mammary adenocarcinoma: the effect of cyclooxygenase inhibitors and immunization against prostaglandin E_2. Prostaglandins Leuk Med 20:283-286.

Karmali RA, Marsh J, Fuchs C (1984). Effect of omega-3 fatty acids on growth of a rat mammary tumor. J Natl Cancer Inst 73:457-461.

Karmali RA, Reichel P, Cohen LA (1986). Dietary effects of omega-3 fatty acids on the growth of the DU-145 prostatic tumor. Fed. Proc, St. Louis, Missouri.

Karmali RA, Thaler HT, Cohen LA (1983). Prostaglandin concentration and prostaglandin synthetase activity in N-nitrosomethylurea-induced rat mammary adenocarcinoma. Eur J Cancer Clin Oncol 19:817-823.

Karmali RA, Welt S, Thaler HT, Lefevre F (1983). Prostaglandins in breast cancer: relationship to disease stage and hormone status. Br J Cancer 48:689-696.

Karmali RA, Wustrow T, Thaler HT, Strong EW (1984). Prostaglandins in carcinomas of the head and neck. Cancer Lett 22:333-336.

Lee TH, Hoover RL, Williams JD, Sperling RI, Ravalese J III, Spur BW, Robinson DR, Corey EJ, Lewis RA, Austen KF (1985). Effect of dietary enrichment with eicosapentaenoic and docosahexaenoic acids on in vitro neutrophil and monocyte leukotriene generation and neutrophil function. N Engl J Med 312:1217-1224.

Maca RD, Panje WR (1982). Indomethacin sensitive suppressor cell activity in head and neck cancer patients pre and postirradiation therapy. Cancer 50:483-489.

Marnett LJ (1981). Polycyclic aromatic hydrocarbon oxidation during prostaglandin biosynthesis. Life Sci 29:531-546.

McCormick DL, Madigan MJ, Moon RC. Modulation of rat mammary carcinogenesis by indomethacin. Cancer Res 45:1803-1808.

Metz SA, McRae JR, Robertson RP (1981). Prostaglandins as mediators of paraneoplastic syndromes: review and update. Metabolism 30:299-316.

Metzger U, Meier J, Uhlschmid G., Weihe H (1984). Influence of various prostaglandin synthesis inhibitors on DMH-induced rat colon cancer. Dis Colon Rectum 27:366-369.

Moncada S, Vane JR (1978). Pharmacology and endogenous roles of prostaglandin endoperoxides, thromboxane A_2, and prostacyclin. Pharmacol Rev 30:293-331.

Murphy RC, Hammarstrom S, Samuelsson B (1979). Leukotriene C: a slow reacting substance from murine mastocytoma cells. Proc Natl Acad Sci USA 76:4275-4279.

Murray JL, Kollmorgen GM (1983). Inhibition of lymphocyte response by prostaglandin-producing suppressor cells in patients with melanoma. J Clin Immun 3:268-276.

Needleman P, Whitaker MO, Wyche A, Watters K, Sprecher H, Raz A (1980). Manipulation of platelet aggregation by prostaglandins and their fatty acid precursors. Pharmacological basis for a therapeutic approach. Prostaglandins 19:165-181.

O'Connor TP, Roebuck BD, Campbell TC (1985). Dietary intervention during the postdosing phase of L-azaserine-induced preneoplastic lesions. J Natl Cancer Inst 75:955-957.

Owen K, Gomolka D, Droller MJ (1980). Production of prostaglandin E_2 by tumor cells in vitro. Cancer Res 40:3167-3171.

Oza RP, Karmali RA (1986). Dietary effects of omega-3 fatty acids on the growth of the R3230AC mammary tumor. Fed Proc, St. Louis, Missouri.

Palmer RMJ, Stephey RJ, Higgs GA, Eakins KE (1980). Chemokinetic activity of arachidonic and lipoxygenase products on leukocytes of different species. Prostaglandins 20:411-414.

Panje WR (1981). Regression of head and neck carcinoma with a prostaglandin-synthesis inhibitor. Arch Otolaryngol 107:658-663.

Pelus LM, Strausser HR (1976). Indomethacin enhancement of spleen-cell responsiveness to mitogen stimulation in tumorous mice. Int J Cancer 18:653-660.

Rolland PH, Martin PM, Jacquemier J, Rolland AM, Toga M (1980). Prostaglandin in human breast cancer: evidence suggesting that an elevated prostaglandin production is a marker of high metastatic potential for neoplastic cells. J Natl Cancer Inst 64:1061-1070.

Sakai T, Yamaguchi N (1984). Prostaglandin D_2 inhibits the proliferation of human malignant tumor cells. Prostaglandins 27:17-26.

Zenser TV, Mattammal MB, Armbrecht HJ, Davis BB (1980). Benzidine binding to nucleic acids mediated by the peroxidative activity of prostaglandin endoperoxide synthetase. Cancer Res 40:2839-2845.

Dietary Fat and Cancer, pages 699–706
© 1986 Alan R. Liss, Inc.

FATTY ACID GROWTH REQUIREMENTS OF NORMAL AND NEOPLASTIC MAMMARY EPITHELIUM

William R. Kidwell

Laboratory of Tumor Immunology and Biology,
National Cancer Institute, Bethesda, Maryland
20892

INTRODUCTION

Although very strong correlations have been established between the incidence of human mammary cancer and the amount of lipid in the diet, cause-effect relationships between the two parameters have not yet been established in humans. In animals experimental manipulation of the diet clearly shows that both spontaneous and carcinogen-induced tumor development are enhanced by lipids indicating that lipids may be an etiological factor in human mammary cancer. Both direct and indirect effects of lipids on the mammary epithelium have been proposed as possible mechanisms by which lipids enhance the tumorigenic process. Proposed direct mechanisms include membrane lipid compositional changes that might alter peptide hormone receptors or their function or effect transport of nutrients and roles of lipids as substrates for prostaglandin synthesis or as modulators of C kinase. Indirect effects of lipids on mammary tumorigenesis that have been proposed include dietary lipid-induced changes in mammotrophic steroid and peptide hormone levels in blood or immunosuppression.

In examining the possible direct effects of lipids on mammary tumorigenesis we have combined approaches of in vitro culture of normal and neoplastic mammary epithelium and in vivo lipid compositional changes in growing or resting mammary glands and tumors. The results indicate that an intimate relationship exists between the mammary epithelial and adipose cells, the latter serving as a reservoir from which epithelial cells selectively draw needed unsaturated fatty acids in response to a proliferative stimulus.

RESULTS

Fatty acid effects on the growth of normal mammary cells are depicted in table 1. Ducts and alveoli were isolated from virgin, adult rats (Wicha et al, 1978) and incubated in delipidated serum-supplemened growth medium with or without hormones (hydrocortisone, prolactin and insulin) and fatty acids. Growth responses of rat mammary tumor cells are also given. As indicated, the normal and neoplastic cells were similar in that cell division was stimulated by linoleic acid and inhibited by stearic acid. Normal and tumor cells were different in their dependency on hormones for cell division. Some cell division was seen in the absence of hormones with tumor but not with normal cell cultures. These results are conistent with the fact that tumor cells produce growth factors that apparently autostimulate tumor cells whereas normal cells produce these agents in lesser amounts (Kidwell et al, 1984).

Table 1. Effect of hormone and fatty acid supplements on the growth of normal and neoplastic rat mammary cells in culture. Adapted from Wicha et al, 1978.

Medium additions	Cell doubling time (hrs)
A. Normal mammary cells	
None[a]	ND[b]
Hormones only	58 ± 5[c]
Linoleic acid only	ND
Linoleic acid + hormones	34 ± 4
Stearic acid + hormones	76 ± 8
B. Neoplastic mammary cells	
None	132 ± 12
Hormones only	89 ± 8
Linoleic acid + hormones	35 ± 5
Stearic acid + hormones	210 ± 40

[a]Growth medium plus 5% delipidated fetal calf serum.
[b]Cell division below detectable levels.
[c]Mean $\pm$ standard error.

Three observations suggests that the results given in table 1 are physiologically significant. First, following a proliferative stimulus to the mammary parenchyma in vivo, an enrichment of linoleic acid vs palmitic or stearic acids is seen in the mammary gland (Wicha et al, 1978). Second, in response to a growth stimulus in vivo there is an enrichment of epithelial cell membranes in unsaturated fatty acids (Kidwell et al, 1982). Third, in growing rat mammary tumors there is a depletion of unsaturated fatty acids in the adipose tissue immediately surrounding the tumor mass. These observations all suggest that mammary epithelium, wehether normal or neoplastic, recruits unsaturated fatty acids from adjacent adipocytes of the gland in support of the proliferation process. More importantly from a physiologic standpoint, the utilization of free fatty acids from the growth medium of cultured mammary cells is modulated by mammotrophic hormones such as prolactin (Kidwell et al, 1982). These results are depicted in tables 2-5.

Table 2. Enrichment of rat mammary gland in unsaturated fatty acids following a proliferative stimulus with perphenazine. Massive prolactin release was achieved by admnistering perphenazine at 16 and 4 hrs before sacrifice. Total fatty acids were quantitated by saponificatin followed by derivation with bromphenacylbromide and HPLC chromatography.

Mammary Gland Status[a]	Unsaturated:Saturated Fatty Acids	
	Experiment 1	Experiment 2
Non-proliferating	2.77	2.81
Proliferating	3.53	3.40

[a]Adapted from Wicha et al, 1978. Perphenazine treatment results in massive proliferation of the glandular elements as shown by histological examination (Wicha et al, 1980).

Table 3. Mammary cell membrane enrichment in linoleic acid following perphenazine treatment. Glandular proliferation was initiated as described in table 2. Sixteen hours later ducts and alveoli were isolated by collagenase digestion and Ficoll gradient sedimentation. Membranes were isolated by the method of Warren, 1974. Phospholipids were resolved by thin layer chromatography and saponified. Fatty acids were acylated and quantitated by gas chromatography on capillary columns. Adapted from Kidwell et al, 1982.

Experiment No.	% Linoleic Acid in Growing Cell Membranes / % Linoleic Acid in Resting Cell Membranes
1	3.4
2	1.8
3	1.3

Table 4. Ratio of unsaturated:saturated fatty acids in tissue adjacent to growing rat mammary tumors. Mammary tumors were located by palpitation. Tumors were excised along with surrounding fat tissue. Sections of fat tissue were taken at increasing distances from the tumor edge and these were analyzed for total tissue fatty acid contents by gas chromatography.

Animal No.	UFA:SFA Ratio	
	0 to 1 cm	1 to 2 cm
1	1.2	1.5
2	1.1	1.8
3	1.2	1.8
4	1.3	1.7

Table 5. Prolactin effects on the uptake of fatty acids from the growth medium of cultured rat mammary ducts and alveoli. Mammary cells were cultured for 24 hours at 37° C in the presence or absence of 100 ng prolactin/ml culture medium. Free fatty acids recovered from the growth medium using chloroform:methanol were acylated and quantitated on capillary columns by gas chromatography. Reproduced from Kidwell et al, 1982.

Fatty Acid	ug Fatty Acid Remaining in Medium	
	Minus Prolactin	Plus Prolactin
Palmitate	43.3	43.1
Stearate	17.6	16.0
Oleate	33.1	20.2
Linoleate	35.9	7.9

The effects on fatty acid uptake from culture medium in response to prolactin are quite remarkable. Following 24 hours stimulation the normal mammary cells consumed about 41 ug unsaturated fatty acids but only 2 ug of saturated fatty acids. This effect of prolactin could be dissociated from a growth response only because the mammary ducts and alveoli were cultured in suspension, a condition in which these cells do not divide (Wicha et al, 1979). Since the results shown in table 5 were obtained with pure mammary epithelium it is apparent that prolactin directly and selectively promotes unsaturated fatty acid metabolism by glandular epithelial cells. Prolactin also affects fatty acid metabolism in adipocytes of the mammary gland, albeit by an indirect mechanism. as shown in explant culture (Kidwell et al,1981). The ability of prolactin to effect a release of fatty acids from mammary tissue explants was found to be dependent on whether the explants contained glandular epithelium or not. Mammary tissue was cleared of glandular elements of 3 week old mice by cauterizing the nipple before the gland was developed. Other animals from the same group were taken as controls. At four months of age, the mammary glands were excised and cultured as explants to determine whether prolactin effected the release of free fatty acids. The results indicated that prolactin did not stimulate free fatty acid release into the culture medium unless the explanted tissue contained glandular epithelial elements. Since the epithelial cell component of the gland takes up rather than releasing free fatty acids in response to prolactin stimulation it seems very likely that prolactin acts on the mammary epithelium which in turn signals the adipocytes of the gland to release free fatty acids. The prolactin-stimulated epithelium then differentially takes up the unsaturated fatty acids from the free fatty acid pool as needed for proliferation.

Since the adipocytes and the epithelial cells are not in physical contact with each other it follows that a diffusing signal is transmitted somehow from epithelial to fat cell. In attempts to characterize such a signal we focused on agents reported to promote free fatty acid release from fat cells. One likely candidate is histamine, a compound present in very large amounts in mast cells, cells that are especially abundant in hormonally dependent mammary tumors (Strum et al, 1984). Histamine added at physiologic concentrations (10 ng/ml culture medium) doubled the amount of free fatty acids released by mammary explants after 24 hours incubation (680 vs 343 ug fatty acid/130 mg explant with and without histamine, respectively). However, we failed to find any effect of prolactin on the production of histamine by purified mammary epithelial cells. Thus if histamine is the agent responsible for free fatty acid release from fat cells it seems likely that it is derived from mast cells rather than mammary epithelial cells.

A model which encompasses our experimental results is presented in fig. 1. In response to a prolactin stimulus the glandular epithelium (which possesses most or all of the prolactin receptors of the gland) produces some signal as yet unidentified. The signal activates neighboring mast cells which release histamine. Histamine in turn activates lipases of nearby adipocytes which then release free fatty acids. The prolactin-activated glandular epithelium then differentially takes up the unsaturated fatty acids it needs for growth and inserts them into membrane phospholipids in place of the saturated acyl groups that were present before prolactin stimulation was manifest.

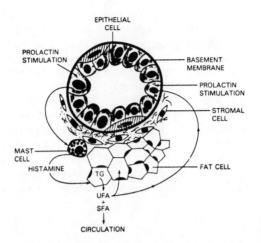

Figure 1. Model depicting the interactions between epithelial cells, mast cells and fat cells following prolactin stimulation. UFA, unsaturated fatty acid; SFA, saturated fatty acid; TG, triglyceride.

DISCUSSION

The model presented in fig. 1 outlines our current concepts of the physiologic interrelationships between cells in normal mammary glandular responses to hormonal stimulation. Based on limited experiments with cultured mammary tumor cells some aspects of this interrelationship between cells is maintained in the transformed state. Whether the results are etiologically important in explaining the role of dietary fat in mammary cancer remains to be seen. Epidemiological surveys suggest a strong correlation between total fat comsumption and breast cancer mortality rather than a correlation with polyunsaturated fat in the diet. As pointed out in table 1, unsaturated fatty acids are growth stimulatory while the opposite is true for the saturated fatty acids. The inhibition of the saturated fatty acids is, however, totally negated in culture by small amounts of unsaturated fatty acids. Consequently the following rationale may be formulated to explain the etiological findings. the adipocyte takes up efficiently almost all of the free fatty acids that are presented to the mammary gland. Unsaturated fatty acids then become rate lim-

iting for normal (or neoplastic) epithelial cell proliferation. The situation is reversed in response to hormonal
stimulation which indirectly activates the fat cells to
release fatty acids. Tumor cells, as a consequence of
transformation, make their own autostimulatory factors
but still retain the unsaturated fatty acid requirement.
If dietary fat consumption exceeds the buffering capacity
of the fat cells, free fatty acids are directly supplied
to the epithelium. As long as there is a small amount of
unsaturated fatty acid present in the free fatty acid pool
the epithelium can selectively utilize it and grow, even
if the unsaturated fatty acid is a small percent of the
total free fatty acid pool (Wicha et al, 1978).

REFERENCES

Kidwell WR, Knazek RA, Vonderhaar BK, Losonczy I (1982).
   Effects of unsaturated fatty acids on the development
   and proliferation of normal and neoplastic breast epi-
   thelium. In: Molecular Interrelations of Nutrition and
   Cancer, Arnott MS, van Eys J, Wang Y-M (eds), Raven Press,
   New York, pp 219-236.
Kidwell WR, Bano M, Salomon DS (1984). Growth of normal
   mammary epithelium on collagen in serum-free medium. In:
   Cell Culture Methods for Molecular and Cell Biology,
   Barnes DW, Sirbasku DA, Sato GH (eds), Alan R Liss, Inc.,
   New York, pp 105-125.
Kidwell WR, Shaffer J (1984). Growth stimulatory activity
   of unsaturated fatty acids for normal and neoplastic
   breast epithelium. J Amer Oil Chem Soc 61:1900-1905.
Strum J, Lewko WL, Kidwell WR (1981). Structural alterations within NMU-induced mammary tumors after in vivo
   treatment with cis-hydroxyproline. Lab Invest 45:347-
   354.
Warren L (1974). Isolation of plasma membranes from tissue
   culture L cells. Methods Enzymol 31:156-162.
Wicha M, Liotta LA, Kidwell WR (1978). Effects of unsaturated fatty acids on the growth of normal and neoplastic
   rat mammary epithelial cells. Cancer Res 39:426-435.
Wicha M, Liotta LA, Kidwell WR (1979). Basement membrane
   collagen requirements for attachment and growth of mammary
   epithelium. Exp Cell Res 124:181-190.
Wicha M, Liotta LA, Kidwell WR (1980). Effects of inhibition of basement membrane collagen deposition on rat mammary gland development. Dev Biol 80:253-266.

Dietary Fat and Cancer, pages 707–728
© 1986 Alan R. Liss, Inc.

FATTY ACID-INDUCED MODIFICATIONS OF MOUSE MAMMARY
EPITHELIUM AS STUDIED IN AN ORGAN AND CELL CULTURE SYSTEM

Nitin T. Telang

Surgical Oncology Research Laboratory, Department
of Surgery, Memorial Sloan-Kettering Cancer
Center, 1275 York Avenue, New York, NY 10021

INTRODUCTION

Laboratory investigations on animal models have not
only facilitated the understanding of etiology and
pathogenesis of mammary neoplasia, but have also provided
a facile experimental paradigm to examine the modulatory
influence of dietary components on the progression of
mammary tumors (Reddy et al., 1980; Abraham et al., 1984;
Bennett, 1984). Amongst the macronutrients, dietary fat
has been the most extensively studied component that
influences mammary tumorigenesis. In the animal models of
mammary cancer, high levels of dietary unsaturated fat
have been shown to enhance tumorigenesis (Chan and Cohen,
1975; Carrol and Khor, 1975; Hopkins et al., 1978;
Hillyard and Abraham, 1979). In contrast, maintenance of
animals on diet containing high levels of saturated fat
has been demonstrated to prolong the latent period of
tumor appearance and to inhibit the tumor incidence
(Hopkins et al., 1978; Tinsley et al., 1981; Abraham et
al., 1984; Bennett, 1984). However, little is known as
regards the exact mechanism of dietary fat in modulating
mammary tumorigenesis. Because of a well-defined
responsiveness of the mammary gland as well as mammary
tumors to steroid hormones it is tempting to speculate
that dietary fat may manifest its effect in vivo by
modulating the levels of ovarian steroid hormones and/or
by increasing the target tissue response to the hormonal
stimuli.

Mouse Model for Mammary Tumorigenesis

In contrast to the rat model, the mouse model has
been less extensively utilized to examine the dietary
modulation of mammary carcinogenesis. Several recent
investigations, however, have examined modulation of
spontaneous mammary tumorigenesis of mouse by dietary fat
or dietary calorie restriction (Tinsley et al., 1981;
Sarkar et al., 1982; Bennett, 1984). Inbred strains of
mice provide a useful experimental system because of a)
distinct strain-dependent difference in susceptibility to
murine mammary tumor virus (MTV)-induced mammary tumors,
b) susceptibility to chemical carcinogens, and c) the
existence of a distinct premalignant precursor lesion, the
hyperplastic alveolar nodule (HAN), that precedes the
emergence of mammary tumors. Indeed, MTV-expressing
strains of mice that have a high incidence of mammary
tumors exhibit an age-dependent increase in the premalignant HAN prior to the occurrence of mammary tumors
(Nandi and McGrath, 1973; Medina, 1973). It is the
presence of these precursor lesions in the mouse model
that makes it an attractive experimental system for
modulator studies on the pretumor phase(s) of cancer
progression. Recently, we and others have demonstrated
that calorie-restricted diet, low fat diet or administration of antineoplastic retinoids can inhibit the
development of HAN and the appearance of tumors (Sarkar et
al., 1982; Welsch, 1983; Abraham et al., 1984).

Organ Culture System for Mouse Mammary Tumorigenesis

In the presence of complex interacting influences of
systemic and humoral factors, it is difficult to understand how the target tissue responds at molecular and
cellular levels to selective dietary interventions in
vivo. Therefore, appropriate in vitro systems derived
from target organ and/or cell cultures provide a
potentially useful model wherein the limitations of whole
animal studies could be effectively circumnavigated.

Several investigators have made use of the tissue
culture techniques to develop the whole mammary gland
organ culture of immature mouse breast tissue, and have
examined multiple hormone interaction on the replication
and differentiation of mammary epithelium (Ichinose and

Nandi, 1966; Singh et al., 1970; Banerjee et al.,
1976,1980; Ono and Oka, 1980; Mehta et al., 1980). The
whole mammary gland organ culture system also has been
utilized to examine in vitro molecular and cellular
effects of a variety of nonviral carcinogens. At the
molecular level, mammary epithelium upon exposure to
radioactive 7,12-dimethylbenz(a)anthracene (DMBA) exhibits
covalent binding of the carcinogen to cellular DNA (Telang
et al., 1977,1978; Kundu et al., 1978). Exposure of the
mammary epithelium to other chemical carcinogens also has
been demonstrated to induce DNA repair and sister
chromatid exchange (Chatterjee and Banerjee, 1982;
Manoharan and Banerjee, 1985). These studies indicate
that mammary epithelium in organ culture is susceptible to
the DNA damaging effects of genotoxic chemical
carcinogens. At the cellular level, induction of
lactogenic hormone-independent lesions has been
demonstrated upon exposure of mammary epithelium to a
variety of chemical carcinogens (Banerjee et al., 1974;
Lin et al., 1976; Kundu et al., 1978; Tonnelli et al.,
1979; Dickens and Sorof, 1980). These lactogenic hormone-
independent alveolar lesions are also referred to as
nodule-like alveolar lesions (NLAL) which upon transplantation produce mammary adenocarcinoma (Telang et al.,
1979; Iyer and Banerjee, 1981). These alveolar lesions
are analogous to preneoplastic HAN found in vivo in MTV-
expressing mice or in MTV-nonexpressing mice that have
been exposed to chemical carcinogens and, therefore, serve
as the in vitro morphological markers of mammary
preneoplasia (Banerjee et al., 1980).

Based on the experience with immature mammary gland
organ cultures (Ichinose and Nandi, 1966; Singh et al.,
1970; Banerjee et al., 1976) and with the development of
an assay system for in vitro chemical carcinogenesis (Lin
et al., 1976; Kundu et al., 1978; Tonnelli et al., 1979;
Telang et al., 1979), an experimental system utilizing
mammary gland organ culture from adult mice has been
developed (Telang and Sarkar, 1983a,b; Telang et al.,
1984). It is observed that adult mammary gland organ
cultures from high breast cancer strains of mice,
especially RIII and GR, exhibit a high incidence of
lactogenic hormone-independent atypical alveolar lesions,
the mammary alveolar lesions (MAL). Since, similar to the
HAN, MAL are detectable in virgin mice and exhibit age-
dependent increased incidence prior to the appearance of

mammary tumors, these most likely are putative preneoplastic lesions of RIII and GR mice.

Cell Culture System for Mouse Mammary Cell Transformation

The entire mammary gland has a very heterogeneous
cellular composition. The epithelial component is
composed of three types of epithelial cells - ductal,
alveolar and myoepithelial, and the stromal component is
formed of the connective tissue cells, fibroblasts and
adipocytes. Thus, the in vitro system derived from the
whole mammary gland, although providing certain advantages
over the in vivo system, has certain limitations imposed
by the cellular heterogeneity. Recent evidence that
modulators such as fatty acids can effectively alter
growth of epithelial cells in vitro (Kidwell et al., 1978;
Wicha et al., 1979; Telang et al., 1984) provides evidence
that these modulators of mammary carcinogenesis also may
have a direct influence on the target cell. Attempts have
been made, therefore, to develop an epithelial cell
culture system from mouse mammary glands wherein the
genotypic and phenotypic modulations caused by selective
agents that initiate, promote and/or inhibit mammary
tumorigenesis can be examined (Telang and Sarkar,
1984). The unique advantage of this cell culture system
is that it facilitates analysis of modulator-induced
response of the specific target cell type in isolation
that upon transformation gives rise to mammary
carcinomas. An experimental system that combines the
organ culture and the cell culture approach provides an
insight into the interaction of various component cell
types of the breast as well as response of the target
epithelial cell in isolation to initiator as well as to
modulators of mammary carcinogenesis.

It is intended in this chapter to briefly review a)
the development of adult mouse mammary gland organ culture
from various strains of mice that differ in the risk of
developing spontaneous mammary tumors, and b) the
development of an in vitro model to examine molecular and
cellular effects of prototype initiators and their
modulation by diet-related agents such as fatty acids in
the mammary gland organ/cell culture system.

RESULTS

Effects of Hormones on the Genesis and Growth of MAL

It is known that under the influence of certain
ovarian steroid hormones the epithelium from immature
mouse mammary gland exhibits active growth and
multiplicity of ducts. If the culture medium is
supplemented with the combination of insulin + prolactin +
hydrocortisone, insulin + prolactin + aldosterone +
hydrocortisone or insulin + prolactin + hydrocortisone +
growth hormone, then the mammary epithelium exhibits
extensive lobuloalveolar development and evidence of
secretory activity (Ichinose and Nandi, 1966; Singh et
al., 1970; Banerjee et al., 1980; Ganguly et al., 1981).
It is also known that upon withdrawal of lactogenic
hormones the lobuloalveoli regress and the epithelial
component once again assumes a ductal morphology (Lin et
al., 1976; Dickens and Sorof, 1980; Banerjee et al.,
1980). These studies indicated that the immature mammary
epithelium is responsive in culture to mammotropic and
lactogenic stimuli from selected steroid and polypeptide
hormones, and that cyclic changes associated with
pregnancy, lactation and involution can be induced in
vitro by sequential exposure to hormones. It was of
interest, therefore, to examine whether or not the adult
mouse mammary epithelium is also responsive to the
selected lactogenic hormones.

For these studies the organ cultures were initially
maintained in lactogenic hormones for 8 days, and were
subsequently maintained for a further 14 days in
lactogenic hormone-free medium supplemented only with
insulin (Telang and Sarkar, 1983a,b; Telang et al.,
1984). Mammary gland organ cultures from strains of mice
differing in their risk for developing mammary cancer
showed comparable lobuloalveolar (LA) development, which
is strictly dependent on the presence of lactogenic
hormones in the medium. However, upon withdrawal of the
lactogenic hormones, most of the LA regressed, but
discrete areas of MAL were detectable, indicating the
lactogenic hormone-independent nature of these atypical
lesions. The incidence of MAL was higher in high risk
strains such as GR and RIII than in low risk strains such
as C57BL and BALB/c (Table 1).

TABLE 1. Effect of Select Polypeptide and Steroid Hormones on the Growth of MAL in Adult Mouse Mammary Glands Organ Cultures[a]

Duration in culture (days)	Hormone supplementation	Morphology of mammary glands							
		C57/BL		BALB/c		RIII		GR	
		LA[b]	MAL[c]	LA	MAL	LA	MAL	LA	MAL
0-1	I[d]	-	1.3[e] ±0.5	-	1.5 ±0.3	-	3.5 ±0.7	-	5.0 ±1.2
0-8	I[d]	-	1.5 ±0.3	-	1.2 ±0.2	-	3.8 ±0.5	-	4.5 ±1.0
0-8	IPAH[d]	+	ID[f]	+	ID	+	ID	+	ID
0-8 → 9-23	IPAH → I[g]	-	2.5 ±2.0		1.3 ±0.1	-	17.5 ±2.0	+	20.0 ±5.0

[a] Mammary gland organ cultures from adult mice were prepared as described (Telang and Sarkar, 1983a,b).
[b] Lobuloalveoli.
[c] Lactogenic hormone-independent mammary alveolar lesions.
[d] I: insulin 5 µg/ml; P: prolactin 5 µg/ml; A: aldosterone 1 µg/ml; H: hydrocortisone 5 µg/ml.
[e] Mean number of MAL/gland ± SD (n = 8-10).
[f] Indeterminate because of intense LA development.
[g] Sequential incubation with IPAH and I.

These data suggest that adult mouse mammary gland organ cultures respond to lactogenic hormones in a manner similar to that observed for immature mouse mammary glands in culture, indicating that the two-step culture model developed for immature mouse mammary gland organ cultures (Banerjee et al., 1980) is also effective in adult mouse mammary gland organ cultures, and that this model can be further extended for the study of MTV-induced or carcinogen-induced preneoplasia.

Effects of DMBA on MAL Incidence

The ability of DMBA to induce hormone-independent alveolar lesions has been repeatedly demonstrated in organ cultures from immature mice (Lin et al., 1976; Kundu et al., 1978; Tonnelli et al., 1979; Chatterjee and Banerjee, 1982). It has been also demonstrated recently that mammary gland organ cultures from mice fed a high fat diet exhibit increased cell proliferation when stimulated with estrogen and progesterone (Welsch et al., 1985). This diet-mediated modulation in the target tissue response to mammotropic hormones could conceivably render the epithelium more susceptible to carcinogenic insult. However, it is not known whether the target tissue from the adult mice is susceptible to carcinogens as is the immature epithelium, and whether dietary fat and/or selected hormones can modulate the response of the mature mammary epithelium to the carcinogenic insult. The ability of DMBA to induce lactogenic hormone-independent MAL was compared in organ cultures from 1-, 4-, 7-, and 16-month-old mice. The percent incidence of these lesions ranged from 80-90% in 1-, 4-, and 7-month-old mice and was reduced to 40% in the 16-month-old group. However, the frequency of MAL per gland was found to be 6.5±2, 3.8±0.36, 1.96±0.55 and 1.5±0.5, respectively (Table 2), indicating an age-dependent loss of susceptibility to DMBA. The high incidence and frequency of the atypical lesions in the 1-month-old group is consistent with the previous data (Lin et al., 1976; Kundu et al., 1978; Som et al., 1984). The carcinogen susceptibility of cultures from 4- and 7-month-old mice as observed in these experiments is conceivable since it is known that 4-month-old mice exposed in vivo to DMBA exhibit preneoplastic changes and mammary tumors appear in these mice at 7 months of age (Medina and Warner, 1976; Medina, 1979; Ethier and Ullrich, 1982,1984; Ethier et al., 1984).

Effects of Selected Fatty Acids on the MTV-induced MAL

The fat content of diet has been demonstrated to modulate the emergence of naturally occurring mammary cancer in high cancer risk strains of mice. Specifically, diet rich in unsaturated fatty acid enhances the appearance of tumors (Rao and Abraham, 1976; Hillyard and Abraham, 1979) whereas high levels of dietary saturated

TABLE 2. DMBA-induced MAL in Mammary Gland Organ Cultures from Adult Mice[a]

Age of mice at the time of culture (months)	Number of cultures with MAL/Total number of cultures examined (% incidence)	Frequency of MAL per gland (X ± SD)
1	16/20 (80)	6.5 ± 2.0^{b}
4	26/28 (92.8)	3.80 ± 0.36^{c}
7	11/12 (91.6)	1.96 ± 0.55^{d}
16	8/20 (40)	1.5 ± 0.50^{d}

[a] Mammary gland organ cultures from adult BALB/c mice were maintained in medium with IPAH for 9 days. Between the 3rd and 4th day of culture the glands were exposed to 7.8 μM/DMBA for 24 hr. Cultures were subsequently maintained in medium with I for an additional 14 days (Telang et al., 1979,1984).

[b-d] Values with dissimilar superscripts differed significantly ($p \leq 0.05$).

fat seem to retard tumor emergence (Tinsley et al., 1981; Bennett, 1984). It was, therefore, of interest to examine the influence of selected fatty acids on the growth and survival of premalignant lesions, MAL. The MAL frequency in the mammary gland organ cultures from 7-month-old RIII (high cancer risk) mice ranged from 13.7 ± 3.5 to 14.7 ± 2.4. In the presence of unsaturated fatty acid arachidonate the MAL frequency was increased to 24.0 ± 1.3 whereas the presence of saturated fatty acid stearate reduced MAL frequency to 4.0 ± 3.4 (Table 3). The potent inhibitor of prostaglandin synthesis, indomethacin, also had an inhibitory effect on the survival of MAL that was reversible by simultaneous exposure to indomethacin + arachidonate (Table 3). Since arachidonate is a precursor for prostaglandins and indomethacin inhibits their synthesis, it appears that prostaglandins may play a facilitative role in the survival of MAL. Indeed, the

TABLE 3. Effects of Fatty Acids and Indomethacin (IM) on the Survival of MAL in Mammary Gland Organ Cultures from RIII Mice [a]

Duration in culture (days)	Hormone supplementation to the medium [b]	Exposure [c]	Number of MAL per gland (X ± SD)
0-1	IPAH	None	13.7 ± 3.5 [d]
0-8	IPAH	None	ID [e]
0-8 → 9-23	IPAH → I	None	12.6 ± 2.5 [d]
0-8 → 9-23	IPAH → I	EtOH	14.7 ± 2.4 [d]
0-8 → 9-23	IPAH → I	ARA	24.0 ± 1.3 [f]
0-8 → 9-23	IPAH → I	STA	4.0 ± 3.4 [g]
0-8 → 9-23	IPAH → I	IM	5.0 ± 0.6 [g]
0-8 → 9-23	IPAH → I	IM + ARA	12.0 ± 3.1 [d]

[a] Mammary gland organ cultures were prepared as described (Telang et al., 1984). During the regression phase in I medium (days 9-23) cultures were exposed to the fatty acids, IM or ethanol (EtOH; solvent).

[b] Concentrations of hormones same as in TABLE 1.

[c] EtOH 0.1%, arachidonate (ARA) 10 µg/ml, stearate (STA) 10 µg/ml, IM 0.358 µg/ml.

[d,f,g] Mean values with dissimilar superscripts differed significantly ($p \leq 0.05$).

[e] ID indeterminate because of LA development.

modulation in MAL incidence by fatty acids and indomethacin could be correlated with the presence of prostaglandin E_2 in the culture medium (Telang et al., 1984). It should be pointed out that although the exposure to stearate resulted in suppression in the number

of MAL similar to that observed by indomethacin, this
fatty acid is not known to participate in the arachidonic
cascade, and thus is not a known precursor of prostaglandin
synthesis. It is, therefore, conceivable that modulation
in MAL incidence by saturated fatty acids may be operating
via a mechanism that is distinct from that for unsaturated
fatty acids.

Acute Effects of DMBA on Mammary Epithelial Cells

    The mammary gland is a complex organ exhibiting
extreme cellular heterogeneity. The mechanistic studies
aimed at understanding direct effects of initiators and
modulators of tumorigenesis will be, therefore, more
meaningful if carried out on the type of cell(s) that are
directly involved in tumor formation, namely, the
epithelial cells. We therefore undertook experiments
wherein the effect of the potent mammary carcinogen DMBA
was studied on the proliferative activity of nontransformed epithelial B/cMG Cl_1 cells. These cells were a
clonal derivative of the parental B/cMG(P) cell line that
was established by Lasfargues and Moore (1971). Since
this parental cell line was found to contain a mixed
population of elongated, fusiform cells and other cells
that had characteristic polygonal morphology, we cloned
the latter cell type. The B/cMG Cl_1 cells upon exposure
to various concentrations of DMBA exhibited dose-dependent
increase in the proliferative activity as evidenced by
increased mitotic index (Table 4). The DMBA-induced
increase in cell proliferative activity, 5 days after
carcinogen exposure, is qualitatively similar to our
earlier observations on colon epithelial cells in organ
culture (Telang and Williams, 1982; Reiss et al., 1983).

Effects of Selected Fatty Acid Modulators of Tumorigenesis
on DMBA-treated Mammary Epithelial Cells

    Since DMBA induces an increase in cell proliferative
activity it was of interest to examine whether or not
fatty acids and other agents that are known to modulate
mammary tumorigenesis in vivo can also modulate this acute
effect of mammary carcinogen. The modulatory effects of a
tumor promoter, tetradecanoyl phorbol acetate (TPA), the
unsaturated fatty acid, arachidonate (ARA), and the

TABLE 4. Effect of DMBA on Cell Proliferative Activity of B/cMG Cl_1 Mammary Epithelial Cells[a]

Concentration of DMBA (ng/ml)	Mitotic Index (MI) at 5 days after exposure[b] (%)
0 (DMSO)	0.45 ± 0.04[c]
5	0.64 ± 0.20[c]
10	1.97 ± 0.60[d]
20	2.08 ± 0.16[d]

[a] 1.0×10^4 B/cMG Cl_1 cells were seeded in 5 ml DMEM containing 0.24 IU/ml insulin and 10% serum. After 18-20 hr of attachment period, the cultures were exposed to different concentrations of DMBA or to 0.05% DMSO for 24 hr. The cultures were maintained in DMEM for 5 days. The cultures were then exposed to 4 μg/ml colchicine for 4 hr, incubated in 0.075 M KCl for 20 min at room temperature and fixed in Cornoy's fixative. Giemsa-stained cultures were taken for mitotic index determination.

[b] $MI = \dfrac{\text{Number of mitotic figures}}{\text{Total number of cells counted}} \times 100$

[c,d] Mean $\pm$ SD, values with dissimilar superscripts differed significantly ($p \leq 0.05$)

saturated fatty acid, stearate (STA), were evaluated by measuring the changes in the colony forming ability of B/cMG Cl_1 cells after exposure to DMBA. It was observed that ARA, similar to TPA, induced an increase in the number of colonies whereas STA exposure had no enhancing effect (Table 5). Malignant transformation of mammary epithelial cells upon exposure to DMBA or to NMU has been previously reported (Richards et al., 1980). Although, modulation in tumorigenicity of carcinogen-exposed mammary epithelial cells by the tumor promoter TPA is reported (Griener et al., 1983), little is known about the in vitro modulatory influence of other agents such as various fatty

TABLE 5. Effects of Selected Modulators of Mammary Tumorigenesis on DMBA-exposed Mammary Epithelial Cells[a]

Agent (concentration)	Cell Viability (%)[b]	Number of colonies (X ± SD)
None	95 ± 2	18.6 ± 2.0[c]
Ethanol (0.1%)	95 ± 3	16.0 ± 2.3[c]
TPA (20 ng/ml)	93 ± 2	26.8 ± 2.6[d]
ARA (20 ng/ml)	95 ± 2	24.0 ± 2.1[d]
STA (20 ng/ml)	92 ± 3	14.5 ± 1.1[c]

[a] Log phase cultures (>75% confluent) of B/cMG Cl$_1$ cells were exposed to 20 ng/ml DMBA for 24 hr. 1.0×10^4 cells were maintained in the presence of the test compounds for 5 days. On the fifth day 0.5×10^2 cells were seeded per T-25 flasks, and colonies that developed 10-14 days post-seeding were counted.
[b] Determined by trypan blue exclusion test prior to seeding for the clonal growth assay.
[c,d] Mean values (n = 6-8 flasks) with dissimilar superscripts differed significantly (p≤0.05).

---

acids that are known to modify tumorigenesis in mice or rats. Our observation that exposure of DMBA-treated cells to TPA and to ARA produced increased colony formation, whereas exposure to STA did not, suggests that unsaturated fatty acids like tumor promoter may favor replication in carcinogen-exposed epithelial cells. These results are in agreement with the observed modulatory effects of TPA as well as various fatty acids in vitro and in vivo (Kidwell et al., 1978; Wicha et al., 1979; Taketani and Oka, 1983;

Griener et al., 1983; Guzman et al., 1983; Abraham et al., 1984; Bennett, 1984).

Mutagenic Effect of DMBA and Its Modulation by Selected Fatty Acids

Many genotoxic carcinogens induce mutagenic changes in epithelial cells and thereby give rise to drug-resistant mutants (Gould, 1980; Moore et al., 1983,1984; Link et al., 1983; Tong and Williams, 1980; Tong et al., 1984). B/cMG Cl_1 cells upon exposure to DMBA gave rise to a high incidence of mutant colonies that were resistant to the cytotoxic effects of the purine antimetabolite 6-thioguanine (TG). The incidence of TG^r colonies could be further enhanced by the exposure of DMBA-treated cells to the tumor promoter TPA (Telang and Sarkar, 1984). The cells from DMBA-induced TG^r colonies were clonally expanded and were analyzed for persistence of TG-resistance and for the levels of the purine salvage pathway enzyme hypoxanthine-guanine phosphoribosyl transferase (HGPRT). The mutant cells were found to be persistently resistant to TG for at least 20 passages, and exhibited about 90-96% inhibition in HGPRT levels. It is known that HGPRT is required for the formation of the cytotoxic metabolite of TG. It is, therefore, conceivable that TG-resistance in the mutant cells is at least in part due to the deficiency of HGPRT.

An assay system based on cell-mediated mutagenesis has been developed to examine the biological effects of several epigenetic type modulators of tumorigenesis (Trosko et al., 1980; Williams et al., 1980,1981; Yotti et al., 1979). This assay measures the modulation in a specific type of membrane-mediated intercellular communication, the metabolic cooperation. The process of metabolic cooperation is implied to be important in the transport of low molecular weight metabolites between contiguous cells via membrane-associated gap junctions. We have sought to develop a metabolic cooperation assay for mouse mammary epithelial cells whereby the effects of modulators of mammary tumorigenesis could be evaluated.

For evaluating the effects of TPA and various fatty acids on metabolic cooperation in mammary epithelial cells, the cloned TG-resistant (TG^r, HGPRT$^-$) mutant cell line, B/cDTG^r Cl$_1$, was cocultivated with the wild type TG-sensitive (TG^S, HGPRT$^+$) mammary epithelial cells, B/cMG Cl$_1$, and the modulation in the survival of TG^r mutant colonies was evaluated after the cultures were exposed to the modulating agents, TPA, ARA and STA (Table 6). The wild type TG^S cells did not grow in the selective medium containing TG, whereas the TG^r mutants exhibited normal growth, indicating a selective toxicity of TG towards the TG^S phenotype. However, when cocultures of TG^S and TG^r cells were maintained in selective medium, a significant decrease in the recovery of TG^r phenotype was observed. Mechanistically, it is possible that TG^S (HGPRT$^+$) cells incorporate TG, metabolize it to the toxic phosphorylated derivative, and pass the metabolite through membrane-associated gap junctional complexes to the adjacent TG^r (HGPRT$^-$) cells, thereby killing the TG^r phenotype. The decrease in the recovery of TG^r cells appears, at least in large part due to active metabolic cooperation between the two phenotypes. A similar metabolic cooperation has been demonstrated to occur between epithelial cells from rat liver (Williams et al., 1981), mouse mammary tumor cells, a variety of nontransformed mouse cells (Miller et al., 1983), as well as hamster fibroblasts (Yotti et al., 1979; Trosko et al., 1981; Aylsworth et al., 1984). The exposure of the cocultures to TPA and ARA appeared to rescue TG^r cells as evidenced by the enhancement of mutant recovery, while exposure to STA did not result in increased recovery of mutants. These findings are in agreement with a similar study on Chinese hamster V79 cells (Aylsworth et al., 1984).

A mechanism that could fully explain the fatty acid-induced modulation of mammary tumorigenesis has not been established. Indirect, endocrine-related mechanisms for their action have been implied in the modulatory response (Cohen, 1981; Welsch and Aylsworth, 1982,1983). The observations that fatty acids modulate the growth of normal and neoplastic rat mammary epithelial cells (Kidwell et al., 1978; Wicha et al., 1979), and of MAL in organ culture (Telang et al., 1984) or modulate inter-cellular communication between V79 cells (Aylsworth et al., 1984) are perhaps the most direct evidence of a cause and effect of these agents on the cells. More imporantly, studies examining the modulation in intercellular communication by fatty acids may be considered particularly relevant to the in vivo condition where

TABLE 6. Effects of Selected Modulators of Mammary Tumorigenesis on Intercellular Communication in Mammary Epithelial Cells[a]

Number of cells per flask				
TG^r cells (HGPRT$^-$)	TG^s cells (HGPRT$^+$)	Agent (concentration)	Number of TG^r mutant colonies (X ± SD)	% Recovery of TG^r mutant colonies[b]
0	5.0 x 10^5	None	0	0
100	0	None	73.7 ± 4.0[c]	100
100	0	Ethanol (0.1%)	70.0 ± 5.0[c]	95.5
100	5.0 x 10^5	Ethanol (0.1%)	4.7 ± 2.1[d]	6.7
100	5.0 x 10^5	TPA (20 ng/ml)	22.7 ± 1.7[e]	32.4
100	5.0 x 10^5	ARA (20 ng/ml)	19.7 ± 2.2[e]	20.1
100	5.0 x 10^5	STA (20 ng/ml)	5.5 ± 2.0[d]	7.8

[a] The thioguanine-resistant mutants (TG^r) and thioguanine-sensitive (wild type, TG^s) cells were cocultivated. After an attachment period of 18-20 hr the cultures were exposed continuously for 4 days to the test agents or to ethanol (solvent). The medium was aspirated and the cultures were maintained in the selective medium (20 µg/ml TG) for 10-14 days. The colony counts were determined from Giemsa-stained fixed cultures.

[b] % recovery relative to TG^r cells cultured in the absence of TG^s cells and maintained in the presence of 0.1% ethanol.

[c-e] Mean values (n = 6-8 flasks) with dissimilar superscripts differed significantly (p≤0.05).

putative tumorigenic cells are known to be present in close association with normal cells. Conceivably, epigenetic modulators like fatty acids may exert their biological effects by altering membrane-mediated gap junctional contacts between adjacent cells that are important in transfer of low molecular weight regulatory substances.

SUMMARY AND CONCLUSIONS

The results obtained from the experiments described in this article may be summarized as follows:

1. Mammary glands from adult mice of various strains can be maintained in a chemically defined medium for at least 23 days. The mammary epithelium in this _in vitro_ system responds to selected steroid and polypeptide hormones in a manner similar to that observed in the explant cultures of immature mice.

2. The incidence of spontaneous or carcinogen-induced lactogenic hormone-independent, putative preneoplastic MAL has a strong correlation with the age of mouse and the risk of developing mammary cancer.

3. Selected fatty acids that are known to modulate mammary tumor incidence are also able to alter MAL incidence in mammary gland organ cultures from a high cancer incidence strain of mouse.

4. Nontransformed mammary epithelial cells in culture respond to the potent mammary carcinogen DMBA by exhibiting increased proliferation and specific mutation that renders the cells resistant to cytotoxic TG. Selected fatty acids modulate DMBA-induced changes, at least in part, by modulating the process of metabolic cooperation between normal and mutant phenotypes.

5. The present _in vitro_ assays could be valuable to evaluate the direct effects of agents that initiate, promote and/or inhibit neoplastic transformation in mammary epithelium.

Acknowledgment

I wish to express my appreciation to Drs. Nurul H. Sarkar, Richard S. Bockman and Mukund J. Modak for helpful discussions that led to the writing of this Chapter. Special thanks are due to Patricia Z. Higgins for excellent secretarial assistance. This Chapter is dedicated to Dr. Mihir R. Banerjee who introduced me to the field of in vitro mammary carcinogenesis and has been a constant source of encouragement.

REFERENCES

Abraham S, Faulkin LJ, Hillyard LA, Mitchell DJ (1984). Effect of dietary fat on tumorigenesis in the mouse mammary gland. J Natl Cancer Inst 72: 1421-1429.
Aylsworth CF, Jone C, Trosko JE, Meites J, Welsch CW (1984). Promotion of 7,12-dimethylbenz(a)anthracene-induced mammary tumorigenesis by high dietary fat in the rat: possible role of intercellular communication. J Natl Cancer Inst 72: 637-645.
Banerjee MR, Wood BG, Washburn LL (1974). Chemical carcinogen-induced alveolar nodules in organ cultures of mouse mammary gland. J Natl Cancer Inst 53: 1387-1393.
Banerjee MR, Wood BG, Lin FK, Crump LR (1976). Organ culture of the whole mammary gland of the mouse. Tissue Cult Assoc Manual 2: 457-462.
Banerjee MR, Ganguly N, Mehta NM, Iyer AP, Ganguly R (1980). Functional differentiation and neoplastic transformation in an isolated whole mammary organ in vitro. In McGrath CM, Brennan MJ, Rich MA (eds): "Cell Biology of Breast Cancer," New York: Academic Press, pp 485-516.
Bennett AS (1984). Effect of dietary stearic acid on the genesis of spontaneous mammary adenocarcinomas in strain A/ST mice. Int J Cancer 34: 529-533.
Carrol KK, Khor HT (1975). Dietary fat in relation to tumorigenesis. Prog Biochem Pharmacol 10: 308-353.
Chan PC, Cohen LA (1975). Dietary fat and growth promotion of rat mammary tumors. Cancer Res 35: 3384-3386.
Chatterjee M, Banerjee MR (1982). N-Nitrosodiethylamine-induced nodule-like alveolar lesion and its prevention by a retinoid in BALB/c mouse mammary gland in whole organ culture. Carcinogenesis 3: 801-804.

Cohen LA (1981). Mechanisms by which dietary fat may stimulate mammary carcinogenesis in experimental animals. Cancer Res 41: 3808-3810.

Dickens MS, Sorof S (1980). Retinoid prevents transformation of cultured mammary glands by procarcinogens but not by many activated carcinogens. Nature (Lond) 285: 581-584.

Ethier SP, Ullrich RL (1982). Induction of mammary tumors in virgin female BALB/c mice by single low dose of 7,12-dimethylbenz(a)anthracene. J Natl Cancer Inst 69: 1199-1203.

Ethier SP, Ullrich RL (1984). Factors influencing expression of mammary ductal displasia in cell dissociation derived mammary outgrowths. Cancer Res 44: 4523-4527.

Ganguly N, Ganguly R, Mehta NM, Crump LR, Banerjee MR (1981). Simultaneous occurrence of pregnancy like lobuloalveolar morphogenesis and casein gene expression in a culture of the whole mammary gland. In Vitro 17: 55-60.

Gould MN (1980). Mammary gland cell mediated mutagenesis of mammalian cells by organ specific carcinogens. Cancer Res 40: 1836-1841.

Griener JW, DiPaolo JA, Evans CH (1983). Carcinogen induced phenotypic alterations in mammary epithelial cells accompanying the development of neoplastic transformation. Cancer Res 43: 273-278.

Guzman RC, Osborn RC, Richards JE, Nandi S (1983). Effects of phorbol esters on normal and tumorous mouse mammary epithelial cells embedded in collagen gels. J Natl Cancer Inst 71: 69-73.

Hillyard LA, Abraham S (1979). Effect of dietary polyunsaturated fatty acids on growth of mammary adenocarcinoma in mice and rats. Cancer Res 39: 4430-4437.

Hopkins GJ, Hard GC, West CE (1978). Carcinogenesis induced by 7,12-dimethylbenz(a)anthracene in C3H-A^{vy}fB mice: incluence of different dietary fats. J Natl Cancer Inst 60: 849-853.

Ichinose RR, Nandi S (1966). Influence of hormones on lobuloalveolar differentiation of mouse mammary glands in vitro. J Endocrinol 35: 331-340.

Iyer AP, Banerjee MR (1981). Sequential expression of preneoplastic and neoplastic characteristics of mouse mammary epithelial cells transformed in organ culture. J Natl Cancer Inst 66: 893-505.

Kidwell WR, Monaco ME, Wicha MS, Smith GS (1978).
Unsaturated fatty acid requirements for growth and
survival of a rat mammary tumor cell line. Cancer Res
38: 4091-4100.
Kundu AB, Telang NT, Banerjee MR (1978). Binding of 7,12-
dimethylbenz(a)anthracene to BALB/c mouse mammary gland
DNA in organ culture. J Natl Cancer Inst 61: 465-469.
Lasfargues EY, Moore DH (1971). A method of continuous
cultivation of mammary epithelium. In Vitro 7: 21-25.
Lin FK, Banerjee MR, Crump LR (1976). Cell cycle related
hormone carcinogen interaction during chemical
carcinogen induction of nodule like alveolar lesions in
mammary gland organ culture. Cancer Res 36: 1607-1614.
Link KH, Heidelberger C, Landolph JR (1983). Induction of
oubain resistant mutants by chemical carcinogens in rat
epithelial cells. Environ Mutagen 5: 33-48.
Manoharan K, Banerjee MR (1985). Measurements of chemical
carcinogen-induced sister chromatid exchanges in a whole
organ in vitro. Mutat Res 147: 165-169.
Medina D (1973). Preneoplastic lesions in mouse mammary
tumorigenesis. Meth Cancer Res 7: 3-53.
Medina D (1976). Preneoplastic lesions in murine mammary
cancer. Cancer Res 36: 3584-3595.
Medina D (1979). Serial transplantation of chemical
carcinogen induced mouse mammary ductal displasias. J
Natl Cancer Inst 62: 397-405.
Medina D, Warner MR (1976). Mammary tumorigenesis in
chemical carcinogen treated mice. IV. Induction of
mammary ductal hyperplasias. J Natl Cancer Inst 57:
331-337.
Mehta NM, Ganguly N, Ganguly R, Banerjee MR (1980).
Hormonal modulation of casein gene expression in a
mammogenesis-lactogenesis culture model of the whole
mammary gland of the mouse. J Biol Chem 255: 4430-4434.
Miller BE, Roi LD, Howard LM, Miller FR (1983).
Quantitative selectivity of contact mediated
intercellular communication in a metastatic mouse
mammary tumor line. Cancer Res 43: 4102-4107.
Moore CJ, Gould MN (1984). Differences in mediated
mutagenesis and polycyclic hydrocarbon metabolism in
mammary cells from pregnant and virgin rats.
Carcinogenesis 5: 103-108.

Moore CJ, Bachuber AJ, Gould MN (1983). Relationship of mammary tumor susceptibility, mammary cell mediated mutagenesis and metabolism of polycyclic aromatic hydrocarbons in four types of rats. J Natl Cancer Inst 70: 777-784.

Nandi S, McGrath CM (1973). Mammary neoplasia in mice. Adv Cancer Res 17: 354-414.

Ono M, Oka T (1980). The differential actions of cortisol on the accumulation of α-lactalbumin and casein in mid pregnant mouse mammary gland in culture. Cell 19: 473-480.

Rao AR, Abraham S (1976). Enhanced growth rate of transplanted mammary adenocarcinoma induced in C3H mice by dietary linoleate. J Natl Cancer Inst 56: 431-432.

Reddy BS, Cohen LA, McCoy GD, Hill P, Weisburger JH, Wynder EL (1980). Nutrition and its relationship to cancer. Adv Cancer Res 32: 237-345.

Reiss B, Telang NT, Williams GM (1983). The application of organ culture to the study of colon carcinogenesis. In Autrup H, Williams GM (eds): "Experimental Colon Carcinogenesis," Florida: CRC Press Inc, pp 83-94.

Richards J, Guzman R, Yang J, Nandi S, Konrad M (1980). Chemical carcinogenesis of mammary epithelium in cell culture. In McGrath CM, Brennan MJ, Rich MA (eds): "Cell Biology of Breast Cancer," New York: Academic Press, pp 467-484.

Sarkar NH, Fernandes G, Telang NT, Kourides IA, Good RA (1982). Low calorie diet prevents the development of mammary tumors in C3H mice, reduces circulating prolactin levels, murine mammary tumor virus expression and proliferation of mammary alveolar cells. Proc Natl Acad Sci USA 79: 7758-7762.

Singh DV, DeOme KB, Bern HA (1970). Strain differences in response of mouse mammary glands to hormones in vitro. J Natl Cancer Inst 45: 657-675.

Som S, Chatterjee M, Banerjee MR (1984). β-Carotene inhibition of DMBA-induced transformation of murine mammary cells in vitro. Carcinogenesis 5: 937-940.

Taketani Y, Oka T (1983). Tumor promoter 12-0-tetradecanoylphorbol acetate, like epidermal growth factor, stimulates cell proliferation and inhibits differentiation of mouse mammary epithelial cells in culture. Proc Natl Acad Sci USA 80: 1646-1649.

Telang NT, Sarkar NH (1983a). In vitro regression of naturally occurring alveolar lesions of mouse mammary glands induced by vitamin A. In Meyskens FL, Prasad KN (eds): "Modulation and Mediation of Cancer by Vitamins." New York: S. Karger, pp 67-77.

Telang NT, Sarkar NH (1983b). Long term survival of adult mouse mammary glands in culture and their response to a retinoid. Cancer Res 43: 4891-4900.

Telang NT, Sarkar NH (1984). A cell mediated mutagenesis assay for mouse mammary epithelial cells: Effects of an initiator and a promoter. In Vitro 20: 247

Telang NT, Williams GM (1982). Carcinogen induced DNA damage and cellular alterations in rat colon organ cultures. J Natl Cancer Inst 68: 1015-1052.

Telang NT, Kundu AB, Crump LR, Banerjee MR (1977). Nodule-like alveolar lesions (NLAL) induced by DMBA and hormonal influence of its binding to mammary DNA in organ culture. Proc Am Assoc Cancer Res 18: 116.

Telang NT, Kundu AB, Banerjee MR (1978). Arylhydrocarbon hydroxylase (AHH) activity induced by 7,12-dimethyl-benz(a)anthracene (DMBA) and its binding to DNA of mammary cells in organ culture. In Vitro 14: 337.

Telang NT, Banerjee MR, Iyer AP, Kundu AB (1979). Neoplastic transformation of epithelial cells in whole mammary in vitro. Proc Natl Acad Sci USA 76: 5886-5890.

Telang NT, Bockman RS, Sarkar NH (1984). Fatty acid induced modifications of mouse mammary alveolar lesions in organ culture. Carcinogenesis 5: 1123-1127.

Tinsley JJ, Schmitz JA, Pierce DA (1981). Influence of dietary fatty acids on the incidence of mammary tumors in the C3H mouse. Cancer Res 41: 1460-1465.

Tong C, Williams GM (1980). Definition of conditions for the detection of genotoxic chemicals in the adult rat liver epithelial cell/hypoxanthine-guanine phosphoribosyl transferase (ARL/HGPRT) mutagenesis assay. Mutat Res 74: 1-9.

Tong C, Telang S, Williams GM (1984). Differences in the responses of 4 adult rat liver epithelial cell lines to a spectrum of chemical mutagens. Mutat Res 130: 53-61.

Tonnelli QJ, Custer RP, Sorof S (1979). Transformation of cultured mouse mammary glands by aromatic amines and amides and their derivatives. Cancer Res 39: 1784-1792.

Trosko JE, Aylsworth C, Chang CC (1985). Possible involvement of arachidonate products in tumor promoter inhibition of cell-cell communication. In Fischer SM, Slaga TJ (eds): "Arachidonic Acid Metabolism and Tumor Promotion," Boston: Martin Nijhoff Publishing, pp 170-197.

Trosko JE, Yotti LP, Dawson B, Chang CC (1981). In vitro assay for tumor promoters. In Stich H, San RHC (eds): "Short Term Tests for Chemical Carcinogens," New York: Springer Verlag, pp 420-427.

Welsch CW, Aylsworth CF (1982). The interrelationship between dietary lipids, endocrine activity, and the development of mammary tumors in experimental animals. In Perkins EG, Visek WJ (eds): "Dietary Fat and Health," Monograph #10, Champagne, IL: Am Oil Chemists Soc, pp 212-240.

Welsch CW, Aylsworth CF (1983). Guest Editorial: Enhancement of murine mammary tumorigenesis by feeding high levels of dietary fat: A hormonal mechanism? J Natl Cancer Inst 70: 215-221.

Welsch CW, DeHoog JV, Moon RC (1983). Inhibition of mammary tumorigenesis in nulliparous C3H mice by chronic feeding of the synthetic retinoid, N-(4-hydroxyphenyl) retinamide. Carcinogenesis 4: 1185-1187.

Welsch CW, DeHoog JV, O'Connor DH, Sheffield LG (1985). Influence of dietary fat levels on development and hormone responsiveness of mouse mammary gland. Cancer Res 45: 6147-6154.

Wicha MS, Liotta LA, Kidwell WR (1979). Effects of free fatty acids on the growth of normal and neoplastic rat mammary epithelial cells. Cancer Res 39: 426-435.

Williams GM (1980). Classification of genotoxic and epigenetic hepatocarcinogens using liver culture assays. Ann NY Acad Sci 349: 273-282.

Williams GM, Telang S, Tong C (1981). Inhibition of intercellular communication between liver cells by the liver tumor promoter 1,1,1-trichloro-2,2-bis(p-chlorophenyl) ethane. Cancer Lett 11: 339-344.

Yotti LP, Chang CC, Trosko JE (1979). Elimination of metabolic cooperation in Chinese hamster cells by a tumor promoter. Science (Wash) 206: 1089-1091.

VI. Potential Responses to and Impacts of Epidemiological and Experimental Data on Dietary Fat and Cancer

Dietary Fat and Cancer, pages 731–771
© 1986 Alan R. Liss, Inc.

DIETARY GUIDELINES

Thomas P. O'Connor, Ph.D. and
T. Colin Campbell, Ph.D.
Division of Nutritional Sciences,
Cornell University,
Ithaca, NY 14853

INTRODUCTION:

This chapter will review the numerous sets of dietary guidelines proposed by Government Agencies, Private Organizations and individual scientists both in the United States and elsewhere. This topic has been reviewed previously in two brief reviews (McNutt 1980, Palmer 1983).

Dietary guidelines have been proposed as preventive measures against the major chronic diseases which account for the bulk of mortality in Western countries. It is generally accepted that these diseases are multifactorial in nature. Diet is recognized as a very important etiological factor. It is also generally acknowledged that adherence to these dietary guidelines will not eliminate the incidence of these chronic diseases -- coronary heart disease, cancer, obesity, hypertension and adult onset diabetes -- but adherence will significantly decrease the probability of their occurrence or delay their onset. While most dietary guidelines have been formulated to aid in prevention of coronary heart disease, the dietary modifications proposed in these guidelines are similar to dietary modifications proposed in guidelines specifically pertaining to cancer.

A number of scientists and industry groups have criticized some of the dietary guidelines.(Harper 1978; Olson 1979; Pariza 1984; CAST 1977). These scientists believe that sufficient evidence is not available, at this time, to make general recommendations to the public with respect to dietary modification and prevention of chronic diseases.

This issue will be discussed in the Summary section of the chapter.

The data base relating diet to chronic disease is obviously incomplete -- there is no absolute proof of this relationship. However, the consistency of evidence in epidemiological studies, clinical studies, animal studies and the biological plausibility of the relationships are impressive and, in our opinion, provide overwhelming support for guidelines such as those of the McGovern Committee (Select Committee on Nutrition 1977 a, b). Opponents of the dietary guidelines suggest that the current United States diet containing about 40% of calories from fat, 20% for sugar, 500-700 mg/day cholesterol and 8-10 g salt daily is the best diet that can be recommended to Americans. As Hegsted (Hegsted 1978) has observed, it is "inconceivable that anyone familiar with the literature can arrive at (this) conclusion."

Almost 70% of the U.S. population dies from either atherosclerotic disease or cancer (Surgeon General 1979). In our view, it is irresponsible to withhold dietary advice from the public and demand further research before reaching any conclusions. The data are imperfect and further research is required to refine our understanding of them. However, the data are more that sufficient to propose rational dietary guidelines to the public that are consistent with good nutritional practices and are very likely to decrease the probability and delay the onset of chronic disease. The public, which ultimately supports biomedical research, has a right to this information. As Grobstein has elegantly stated: " In fundamental science we properly demand incontrovertible evidence, else we would be building on shifting sands. In applied science, however, aggressive application often begins before the requirements for full certainty are satisfied. We would be remiss to withhold what can be useful because it is not perfect." (Grobstein 1983)

HISTORICAL PERSPECTIVES

Dietary advice to the public has been propagated for centuries. Li (Li 1982) quotes Yan's (Yan) advice: "One should eat and drink in moderation (not in excess, not at a rapid rate, foods not too hot and not overly hard), maintain an even temperament, eat a good diet and Ye Ge will not develop." Ye Ge was the old Chinese term for what is now called esophageal cancer.

Dr. William Lambe (Lambe 1815) in 1815, in a paper considering cancer and other chronic diseases, argued strongly for moderation and warned against excesses in food consumption, particularly meat and other protein products. Dr. John Hughes Bennett (Bennett 1865), in 1865, suggested that nutrition was an important parameter in the etiology of cancer.

Dr. John Shaw (Shaw 1907), a member of the Royal College of Surgeons, England, in 1907 listed some of the conditions tending to promote cancer as:
1. Deficiency of vegetable foods.
2. Excess of animal foods.
3. The abuse of alcohol, tea, tobacco and drugs.

Dr. W. Roger Williams (Williams 1908), published a massive treatise in 1908 on the Natural History of Cancer in which he stated: "Probably no single factor is more potent in determining the outbreak of cancer in the predisposed, than excessive feeding."

In 1921, Dr. L. Duncan Bulkley (Bulkley 1921) stated that: "Candid and thoughtful men must recognize that deranged, disturbed, perverted nutrition is the bottom fact of all erroneous growth, whether it be obesity, rickets or cancer." Fallscheer-Zurcher, in 1930, (19) in a paper on Cancer and Diet, recommended a number of dietary steps to prevent cancer:
1. More uncooked than cooked food.
2. Mainly vegetarian food.
3. Less food of any kind.
4. Only 2, or at most 3, meals a day.
5. Food to prepared as simply as possible.
6. Food not to be eaten hot.
7. Food to be well chewed.
8. No alcohol, nicotine or coffee; no preserves.
9. Three or four fast days in every month.

Dr. E. Brown Thompson (Thompson 1932), in 1932, published a treatise called "Cancer: Is it preventable?", and advocated a diet high in fruit and vegetables especially those rich in cellulose. He advised moderation in the consumption of meat, especially pickled and salted meat. He also favored the use of wholemeal bread over white bread and pastries.

Hoffman (Hoffman 1937), in a major review of Diet and Cancer concluded that "cancer, unquestionably, in its causative factors and progress towards a fatal termination, is profoundly affected by dietary and nutritional factors" and that "excessive nutrition" is either the "chief cause " of cancer or "at least a contributory factor of the first importance."

MODERN DIETARY GUIDELINES

United States:

Basic Four:

Dietary advice to the public has traditionally been based upon the 1957 report "Essentials of an Adequate Diet" from the U.S. Department of Agriculture which emphasized choosing a wide variety of food from the four "basic" food groups. (Page and Phipard 1957) These groups are:
1. Milk group -- 2 or more servings daily.
2. Meat group (including legumes and nuts) -- 2 or more servings daily.
3. Vegetable/fruit group -- 4 or more servings daily.
4. Bread/cereal group -- 4 or more servings daily.

It was stated that the minimum number of servings listed above
formed the foundation for a good diet. Meals could be rounded out and appetite satisfied by using more of these foods and other foods not specified; eg. butter, margarine, other fats, oils, sugars and unenriched refined grain products.

Nutrition educators sought to educate the public to use this plan to consume a "balanced" diet. However, these efforts may not have been very successful, as knowledge of nutrition even among physicians and medical students is generally poor (Podell et al 1975). An updated version of the "Basic 4", including a fifth group for fats, oils, sugar, and alcohol was published in 1979 (USDA 1979) and a similar type plan was published by the Canadian Government (Dept National Health and Welfare 1979) in 1979. While no one quarrels with the idea of eating a varied diet, a major problem with the Basic 4 approach is that it does not caution about the risk associated with overconsumption in any group.

It became increasingly apparent, however, that the very high incidence of chronic disease in the United States -- coronary heart disease, cancer, obesity, hypertension -- was causally related to several environmental parameters, one of which was diet. Thus, since the 1957 U.S.D.A report (Page and Phipard 1957), numerous reports from both Federal Agencies and Private Organizations have suggested dietary modification as a means to aid prevention of these chronic diseases.

American Heart Association (A.H.A.):

In 1957, the A.H.A. prepared a report on Atherosclerosis and the Fat Content of the Diet (Page et al 1957). No specific dietary recommendations were made but the report suggested that:
1. Diet may play an important role in the pathogenesis of atherosclerosis.
2. The fat content and total calories in the diet are probably important factors.
3. The ratio between saturated and unsaturated fat may be the basic determinant.
4. A wide variety of other factors beside fat, both dietary and non-dietary may be important.

In 1961, a second A.H.A. Committee prepared a new report on the relationship of fat intake to heart attacks and strokes (Page et al 1961). Two of the authors of the 1961 report were also involved in the preparation of the 1957 report. The 1961 report recommended:
1. Maintenance of correct body weight.
2. Moderate exercise, e.g. walking, to aid in weight reduction.
3. Reduced intake of total fat, saturated fat and cholesterol. Increased intake of polyunsaturated fat.
4. Men with a strong family history of atherosclerosis should pay particular attention to diet modification.
5. Dietary changes should be carried out under medical supervision.

Since 1961, the A.H.A. has issued several updated statements on diet and coronary heart disease. (A.H.A. 1965, 1968, 1973, 1978, 1980) The 1965 statement (A.H.A. 1965) recommended:

1. Caloric restriction to achieve desirable weight.
2. Substitution of polyunsaturated fats for saturated fats where possible.
3. Reduction in cholesterol intake.
4. Inclusion of the whole family in dietary changes.

The 1968 statement (A.H.A. 1968) made similar recommendations. In 1973, a new statement was published (A.H.A. 1973) that attempted to quantify desirable intakes of specific nutrients. The dietary recommendations were:
1. A caloric intake adjusted to achieve and maintain ideal body weight.
2. A reduction from the usual 40-45% of total calories from fat to no more than 35%.
3. Less than 10% of total calories should come from saturated fatty acids and up to 10% from poly-unsaturated fatty acids.
4. A cholesterol intake not greater than 300 mg/day.
5. Increased consumption of foods containing natural complex carbohydrates such as fruits, vegetables and cereals.
6. Avoid excessive salt intake.

Essentially, similar recommendations were made in two subsequent A.H.A. statements in 1978 and 1980. (A.H.A. 1978,1980).

The most recent recommendations from the A.H.A., published in 1982 (A.H.A. 1982), suggest that no more than 30% of total calories come from fat, with not more than 10% from saturated fat and not more than 10% from polyunsaturated fat. The remaining recommendations are similar to the 1973 recommendations listed above.

Dietary Goals for the United States:

In January of 1977, the Senate Select Committee on Nutrition and Human Needs chaired by Senator George McGovern, released a report entitled "Dietary Goals for the United States." (Select Committee on Nutrition 1977 a) Senator McGovern noted that this report was the first comprehensive statement by any branch of the Federal Government on risk factors in the American diet.

The report noted that "...during this century, the composition of the average diet in the United States has changed radically. Complex carbohydrates -- fruit, vegetables and grain products -- which were the mainstay of diet, now play a minority role. At the same time, fat and sugar consumption have risen to the point where these two dietary elements alone now comprise at least 60% of total calorie intake."

Moreover, the report stated that : "Given the wide impact on health that has been traced to the dietary trends outlined, it is imperative, as a matter of public health policy, that consumers be provided with authoritative dietary guidelines or goals that will encourage the most healthful selection of foods."

The dietary goals outlined were:

1. Increase carbohydrate consumption to account for approximately 55 to 60% of energy intake.
2. Reduce overall fat consumption from approximately 40% to 30% of energy intake.
3. Reduce saturated fat consumption to account for about 10% of total energy intake; and balance that with polyunsaturated and monosaturated fats, which should account for 10% of energy intake each.
4. Reduce cholesterol consumption to about 300 mg/day.
5. Reduce sugar consumption by about 40% to account for about 15% of total energy intake.
6. Reduce salt consumption by about 50 to 85% to about 3 g/day.

The report indicated that the goals suggest changes in food selection and preparation.

1. Increase consumption of fruits and vegetables and whole grains.
2. Decrease consumption of meat and increase consumption of poultry and fish.
3. Decrease consumption of foods high in fat and partially substitute polyunsaturated fat for saturated fat.
4. Substitute non-fat milk for whole milk.
5. Decrease consumption of butterfat, eggs and other high cholesterol sources.
6. Decrease consumption of sugar and foods high in sugar content.
7. Decrease consumption of salt and foods high in salt content.

The Dietary Goals generated a tremendous amount of debate, interest and controversy among scientists, consumers and the Food Industry.

Many of these supplemental views were published in a second publication called "Dietary Goals for the United States -- Supplemental views." (Select Committee on Nutrition 1977 c). In an Editorial on the Dietary Goals, the Lancet (Editorial 1977) noted that: "Nutrition education of the public is poor. The seven (or four) basic food groups are out of date; they were not designed to meet current nutritional problems... The American goals will be welcomed by people who have thought seriously about the diet of modern Western man."

The American Medical Association (Senate Select Committee on Nutrition 1977 c) believed that it would be inappropriate at the present time to adopt the Dietary Goals. The National Dairy Council questioned the belief that adherence to the Dietary Goals would decrease the incidence of chronic diseases. (Senate Select Committee on Nutrition 1977 c). The Council for Agricultural Science and Technology prepared a report on the Goals. (CAST 1977). This report acknowledged that the Goals had merit for subgroups of the population at risk but as a whole the Goals were "not appropriate for application to the general public."

In December 1977, the Select Committee on Nutrition and Human Needs published a Second Edition (Senate Select Committee on Nutrition 1977 b) which reflected some of the supplemental views expressed since the publication of the first edition. The revised Dietary Goals were:

1. To avoid overweight, consume only as much energy (calories) as is expended; if overweight, decrease energy intake and increase energy expenditure.
2. Increase the consumption of complex carbohydrates and naturally occurring sugars from about 28% of energy intake to about 48% of energy intake.
3. Reduce the consumption of refined and processed sugars by about 45% to account for about 10% of total energy intake.
4. Reduce overall fat consumption from approximately 40% to about 30% of energy intake.
5. Reduce saturated fat consumption to account for about 10% of total energy intake; and balance that with polyunsaturated and monosaturated fats, which should account for about 10% of energy intake each.

6. Reduce cholesterol consumption to about 300 mg/day.
7. Limit the intake of sodium by reducing.. the intake of salt to about 5 g/day.

The following changes in food selection and preparation were also recommended:

1. Increase consumption of fruits and vegetables and whole grains.
2. Decrease consumption of refined and other processed sugars and foods high in such sugars.
3. Decrease consumption of foods high in total fat, and partially replace saturated fats, whether obtained from animal or vegetable sources, with polyunsaturated fats.
4. Decrease consumption of animal fat, and choose meats, poultry and fish which will reduce saturated fat intake.
5. Except for young children, substitute low-fat and non-fat milk for whole milk, and low-fat dairy products.
6. Decrease consumption of butterfat, eggs and other high cholesterol sources. Some consideration should be given to easing the cholesterol goal for pre-menopausal women, young children and the elderly in order to obtain the nutritional benefits of eggs in the diet.
7. Decrease consumption of salt and foods high in salt.

The report states that individuals "...should recognize that these dietary recommendations do not guarantee improved protection from the killer diseases. They do, however, increase the probability of improved protection."

Surgeon-General's Report:

In 1979, the Surgeon-General's Report on Health Promotion and Disease Prevention entitled "Healthy People" made a number of dietary recommendations to the American people. (Surgeon General 1979). While acknowledging the overall health of Americans was excellent, the Surgeon-General believed that Americans would probably be healthier if they consumed:

1. Only sufficient calories to meet body needs and maintain desirable weight (fewer calories if overweight).

2. Less saturated fat and cholesterol.
3. Less salt.
4. Less sugar.
5. Relatively more complex carbohydrates such as whole grains, cereals, fruits and vegetables.
6. Relatively more fish, poultry, legumes and less red meat.

United States Department of Agriculture/ United States Department of Health, Education and Welfare (Health and Human Service)

The USDA/USDHEW (USDHSS) published Dietary Guidelines for Americans in 1980 and a more recent edition in 1985 (USDA 1980,1985). The guidelines are designed for healthy Americans. The publication notes that: "Food alone cannot make you healthy. But food eating habits based on moderation and variety can keep you healthy and even improve your health."
The dietary guidelines are:
1. Eat a variety of foods.
2. Maintain desirable weight.
3. Avoid too much fat, saturated fat and cholesterol.
4. Eat foods with adequate starch and fiber.
5. Avoid too much sugar.
6. Avoid too much sodium.
7. If you drink alcohol, do so in moderation.

Inter-Society Commission for Heart Disease Resources:

In 1984, the Inter-Society Commission for Heart Disease Resources (Inter-Society Commission 1984) suggested that "the entire family should be involved in a program involving the following aspects of atherosclerotic disease prevention." The dietary recommendations made by the Commission were:
1. Control of obesity.
2. Calories derived from fat should not exceed 30% of total energy intake, of which no more than 10% should be derived from polyunsaturated and 8% from saturated fats.
3. Cholesterol intake should be less than 250 mg/day.
4. Salt intake should be less than 4 g/day.
5. Any calorie deficit should be made up with unrefined carbohydrates including fruits, vegetables, whole grains and legumes.

Consensus Conference on Lowering Blood Cholesterol to
Prevent Heart Disease:

The National Heart, Lung and Blood Institute (NHLBI)
and the National Institutes of Health Office of Medical
Applications of Research organized a Consensus Development
Conference on Lowering Blood Cholesterol to Prevent Heart
Disease from December 10-12, 1984. The Expert Panel's
conclusions were published in 1985 (Consensus Conference
1985).

The Panel concluded that "Elevation of blood
cholesterol levels is a major cause of coronary artery
disease. It has been established beyond a reasonable doubt
that lowering definitely elevated blood cholesterol levels
(specifically, blood levels of low-density lipoprotein
cholesterol) will reduce the risk of heart disease... we are
persuaded that the blood cholesterol levels of most
Americans are undesirably high, in large part because of our
high dietary intake of calories, saturated fat and
cholesterol."

The Consensus Panel also stated that "there is no
doubt that appropriate changes in our diet will reduce blood
cholesterol levels." The dietary recommendations proposed
by the Panel for all Americans (except for children younger
than 2 years of age) are:
1. Reduce total dietary fat intake from the current
    level of about 40% of total calories to 30% of
    total calories.
2. Reduce saturated fat intake to less than 10% of
    calories.
3. Increase polyunsaturated fat intake to no more
    than 10% of total calories.
4. Reduce daily cholesterol intake to 250-300 mg or
    less.
5. Intake of total calories should be reduced, if
    necessary, to maintain ideal body weight.
    Regular moderate-level exercise is helpful in
    this regard.

The Panel noted that these dietary changes can be
readily made while intake of protein, vitamins and minerals
is maintained to satisfy the Recommended Dietary Allowances
of the Food and Nutrition Board of the National Research
Council. (Food and Nutrition Board 1980 a). Moreover, they

stated that it is desirable to begin dietary protective measures in childhood because patterns of lifestyle are developed in childhood.

The Panel recommended intensive dietary treatment under the guidance of a physician for individuals with blood cholesterol levels above the 75th percentile. Appropriate drugs should be added to the dietary treatment regimen, if the response to diet is inadequate.

Food and Nutrition Board/ National Academy of Sciences (FNB/NAS):

A report called The Role of Dietary Fat in Human Health was first published in 1958 by the FNB/NAS (Food and Nutrition Board 1958). In 1966, a revised version of this report was published under the title Dietary Fat and Human Health (Food and Nutrition Board 1966).

At that time, the report stated "...Sufficient data for firm recommendations for radical dietary changes" were not available. However, the FNB considered that "... for many Americans, moderate reduction in total fat intake and some substitution of polyunsaturated fat for saturated fat may be indicated. The degree to which this is done must be judged on an individual basis and, in adjustment of the diet, other changes in caloric and nutrient intake must be taken into consideration."

In 1980, the 9th edition of the Recommended Dietary Allowances (RDA's) was published by the FNB/NAS. (Food and Nutrition Board 1980 a). The Committee made recommendations on desirable amounts and proportions of dietary fat and carbohydrate. While recognizing the multifactorial nature of chronic disease, the Committee believed that "... there is sufficient evidence to support some recommendations for dietary changes that would be consonant with better health." The Committee recommended controlling caloric intake and increasing physical activity to maintain desirable body weight. However, the Committee did not believe that it was desirable to make blanket recommendations for dietary change for the entire population, however, for individuals suspected or known to be at high risk for certain diseases, the Committee recommended:
      1. Total fat intake should not comprise more than 35% of dietary energy.

2. There should be a greater reduction in saturated fats, such as from animal sources, than in vegetable fats containing predominantly unsaturated fatty acids.
3. An upper limit of 10% of dietary energy for polyunsaturated fats is advisable.
4. Intake of refined sugar should be reduced and complex carbohydrates maintained or even increased.
5. Decrease alcohol consumption.

In 1980, the FNB/NAS also published a brief report titled "Towards Healthful Diets" (Food and Nutrition Board 1980 b). The FNB made the following recommendations to adult Americans:

1. Select a nutritionally adequate diet from the foods available, by consuming each day appropriate servings of dairy products, meats or legumes, vegetables and fruits and cereals and breads.
2. Select as wide a variety of foods in each of the major food groups as is practicable in order to ensure a high probability of consuming adequate quantities of all essential nutrients.
3. Adjust dietary energy intake and energy expenditure so as to maintain appropriate weight for height; if overweight, achieve appropriate weight reduction by decreasing total food and fat intake and by increasing physical activity.
4. If the requirement for energy is low (e.g. reducing diet), reduce consumption of food such as alcohol, sugars, fats and oils, which provide calories but few other essential nutrients.
5. Use salt in moderation; adequate but safe intakes are considered to range between 3 and 8 g of sodium chloride daily.

The Board considered it "...scientifically unsound to make single, all-inclusive recommendations to the public regarding intakes of energy, protein, fat, cholesterol, carbohydrates, fiber and sodium." with respect to prevention of chronic diseases such as coronary heart disease and cancer. However, they proceeded to make an "all-inclusive recommendation" with respect to sodium and failed to do so for fat even though the evidence with respect to fat and health is considerably stronger than that relating salt to health.

This report was extremely controversial and gave rise to heated debate in the scientific world and in the media. This will be discussed further below.

American Medical Association (A.M.A.)

In 1972, the A.M.A Council on Foods and Nutrition published a joint statement on Diet and Coronary Heart Disease with the Food and Nutrition Board (American Medical Association 1972). The statement acknowledged that "there is abundant evidence that the risk of developing CHD is positively correlated with the level of cholesterol in the plasma."

It also stated that "the average level of plasma lipids in most American men and women is undesirably elevated" (emphasis ours). The statement also acknowledged that "there is extensive evidence that the level of cholesterol in the plasma of most people can be lowered by appropriate dietary modification. Generally, such lowering can be achieved most practically by partial replacement of the dietary sources of saturated fat with sources of unsaturated fat, especially those rich in polyunsaturated fatty acids, and by a reduction in the consumption of foods rich in cholesterol."

The Council recommended early intervention with these dietary modifications: "As would be expected in dealing with a chronic disease of this kind, early intervention appears to be more effective than intervention after the disease is evident." The Council stressed maintenance of desirable weight by appropriate combination of physical activity and calorie intake.

In 1979, the A.M.A Council on Scientific Affairs published a report entitled "American Medical Association Concepts of Nutrition and Health." (American Medical Association 1979). The Council supported the idea of consuming a widely varied diet drawn from the four basic food groups outlined in the USDA guide. (Page and Phipard 1957). The report also noted that "... perhaps the most overlooked aspect are the number and size of servings in the meat group. Note that only 57-86 g (2 to 3 oz.) is considered a serving.:" The Basic 4 plan calls for 2 or more servings from the meat group (including legumes) daily.

The Council recommended that "Full-term, newborn infants should be breast fed, unless there are specific contraindications or breast feeding is unsuccessful." For older children, the Council noted that "... immoderate habits learned early in life may be difficult to change later on."

The Council recommended to the American public achievement and maintenance of the most desirable body weight through a combination of dietary control and exercise. It recommended to the healthy population to restrict dietary salt intake to less than 12 g/day.

For individuals falling into risk categories for coronary heart disease on the basis of their plasma lipid profile, the Council recommended achievement and maintenance of desirable body weight and individualized dietary advice based on the type of hyperlipidemia diagnosed. Reduction in plasma cholesterol levels can be achieved by regulation of the amount of dietary cholesterol and saturated fatty acids, as well as total calorie intake. The Council also noted that for healthy people, moderation in fat intake should become the rule of thumb.

American Health Foundation:

In 1972, the American Health Foundation published a Position Statement on Diet and Coronary Heart Disease that made several dietary recommendations to the American population (American Health Foundation 1972):
1. Adjust total caloric intake to avoid obesity.
2. Decrease total dietary fat intake to approximately 35% of calories daily.
3. Change the dietary fat from predominantly saturated to approximately isocaloric amounts of saturated, monounsaturated and polyunsaturated.
4. Decrease dietary cholesterol to about 300 mg/day.
5. Adjust carbohydrate intake so complex types will predominate.
6. Reduce salt intake to approximately 5 g/day.

American Academy of Pediatrics and Canadian Pediatric Society:

The American Academy of Pediatrics Committee on Nutrition released a statement "Towards a Prudent Diet for

Children" in 1983 (American Academy of Pediatrics 1983). The Committee took the position that "... the safety of diets designed to decrease caloric intake, increase consumption of complex carbohydrates, decrease intake of refined sugars, decrease consumption of fat and cholesterol, and limit sodium intake has not been established in growing children."

However, the Nutrition Committee of the Canadian Pediatric Society (Canadian Pediatric Society 1981) believes that "... there is no indication that a decreased intake of cholesterol and saturated fats compromises growth and brain development." The Canadian Committee made a number of dietary recommendations for children 2 years of age and older on the basis that, (a) dietary habits are formed in childhood and can be modified only with difficulty later in life and (b) the assumption that improved plasma lipid profile in childhood may slow the progression of athersclerosis. The recommendations were:

1. Energy intake adjusted to achieve and maintain ideal weight.
2. Reduction in dietary fat to 35% of total energy intake. A source of linoleic acid should be included.
3. Increased consumption of whole grain products, fruits and vegetables, with reduced consumption of salt and refined sugars.
4. Increased physical activity.

DIETARY GUIDELINES WITH REPSPECT TO REDUCING THE RISK OF CANCER

There is a vast body of literature on the relationship between diet, nutrition and cancer. It is generally recognized that diet is a very important factor in the etiology of cancer. Various estimates have been made as to the exact contributions of diet to cancer incidence. Wynder and Gori (Wynder and Gori 1977) suggested that diet was an important factor in the etiology of 60% of cancers in women and 40% of cancers in men. Doll and Peto (Doll and Peto 1981) suggested that diet was a causal factor in between 10 and 70% of all cancers with their best estimate being 35%. In 1979, Dr. Arthur Upton, Director of the National Cancer Institute, submitted a statement on Diet, Nutrition and

Cancer to the Senate Committee on Agriculture, Nutrition and Forestry. (Upton 1979). Dr. Upton suggested reduction in dietary fat intake, moderation in alcohol consumption and an increase in dietary fiber intake as dietary principles significant in cancer prevention.

National Academy of Sciences/ National Research Council:

In 1982, the National Academy of Sciences/National Research Council Committee on Diet, Nutrition and Cancer published a landmark report entitled "Diet, Nutrition and Cancer" (National Academy of Sciences 1982). The Committee reviewed the vast literature on this subject. The Committee did not attempt to estimate the exact percentage of cancers causally related to diet, but stated instead that "...cancers of most major sites are influenced by dietary patterns... the data are not sufficient to quantitate the contribution of diet to the overall cancer risk or to determine the percent reduction in risk that might be achieved by dietary modifications."

On the basis of the available evidence the Committee made a number of Interim Dietary Guidelines to decrease cancer risk:
1. Reduce total fat intake, both saturated and unsaturated from the current level of 40% to approximately 30% of total calories. Indeed, the data could be used to justify an even greater reduction.
2. Include fruits, vegetables and whole grain cereals in the daily diet.
3. Reduce consumption of smoked, pickled and salt-cured foods.
4. Consume alcohol only in moderation.

The Committee noted that "It is not now possible and may never be possible, to specify a diet that would protect everyone against all forms of cancer." Nevertheless, the Committee believed that the above guidelines are both consistent with good nutritional practices and likely to reduce the risk of cancer.

The findings of this Expert Committee of the National Academy of Sciences on Diet, Nutrition and Cancer did not agree with the earlier brief report "Towards Healthful Diets" published by the Food and Nutrition Board of the

National Academy of Sciences (Food and Nutrition Board 1980 b) which concluded that no sound scientific basis existed for recommending dietary changes to reduce cancer risk.

In 1984, the United States Government Accounting Office addressed this discrepancy in findings between the two reports (U.S. General Accounting Office 1984). The GAO suggested that "... different scientists' philosophies about what scientific evidence is necessary as a basis for providing the public with dietary advice to reduce the risk of cancer are a major factor in the reports' different conclusions and recommendations."

It is important to note also that the Committee on Diet, Nutrition and Cancer spent over two years reviewing the vast literature in this area before coming to their carefully considered conclusions on diet and cancer and proposing Interim Dietary Guidelines. Diet, Nutrition and Cancer is a 460 page comprehensive scientific document. (U.S. General Accounting Office 1984). On the other hand, Towards Healthful Diets is a 24 page position statement and the GAO noted that it did not fully document the methodology used to arrive at its conclusions about diet's relationship to chronic diseases. It devoted 1 1/2 pages to cancer (U.S. General Accounting Office 1984) and listed only 6 references on this topic.

American Institute for Cancer Research (A.I.C.R.):

In 1983, the American Institute for Cancer Research published "Dietary Guidelines to Lower Cancer Risk." (American Institute for Cancer Research 1983). These guidelines were essentially similar to the Interim Dietary Guidelines recommended by the Committee on Diet, Nutrition and Cancer (National Academy of Sciences 1982). The A.I.C.R. Guidelines noted, however, that the guideline to consume less salt-cured, smoked and charcoal broiled foods is intended for those consuming excessive quantities of these products. There is little evidence that there are many Americans in this category.

American Cancer Society (A.C.S):

In 1984, the American Cancer Society published a number of dietary guidelines to reduce cancer risk. (American Cancer Society 1984)
1. Avoid obesity.
2. Cut down on total fat intake.
3. Eat more high fiber foods such as whole grain cereals, fruits and vegetables.
4. Include food rich in vitamins A and C in the daily diet.
5. Include cruciferous vegetables, such as cabbage, broccoli, Brussels Sprouts, kohlrabi and cauliflower in the diet.
6. Be moderate in consumption of alcoholic beverages.
7. Be moderate in consumption of salt-cured, smoked and nitrite-cured foods.

National Cancer Institute (N.C.I.):

In 1984, the National Cancer Institute published cancer tips including some dietary recommendations (National Cancer Institute 1984):
1. If you drink alcoholic beverages, do so only in moderation.
2. Eat foods low in fat.
3. Include fresh fruits, vegetables, and whole grain cereals in your daily diet.

DIETARY GUIDELINES IN OTHER COUNTRIES

Britain:

In 1974, the Advisory Panel of the Committee on Medical Aspects of Food Policy (Nutrition) on Diet in relation to Cardiovascular and Cerebrovascular Disease published a report on Diet and Coronary Heart Disease. (DHSS 1974). The Committee noted the multifactorial nature of the disease and pointed out that "simple dietary changes alone cannot solve a problem of such complexity." Nevertheless, on the basis of the available evidence the Panel proposed a number of dietary changes to decrease the risk of coronary heart disease. The changes were recommended for adults but the Panel stated that they may safely apply to children as well.

The recommendations were:
1. Obesity should be avoided both in the child and the adult.
2. The majority of the members of the Panel recommend that the amount of fat in the United Kingdom diet, especially saturated fat from both animal and plant sources, should be reduced.
3. The Panel unanimously agree that they cannot recommend an increase in the intake of ' polyunsaturated fatty acids in the diet as a measure intended to reduce the risk of the development of ischaemic heart disease. In their opinion, the available evidence that such a dietary alteration would reduce the risk in the United Kingdom at the present time is not convincing.
4. The Panel recommends that the consumption of sucrose, as such or in foods and drinks, should be reduced, if only to diminish the risk of obesity and its possible sequelae.
5. The Panel recommends that any proposals for softening the water supply in any part of the country should be considered in the light of knowledge about the observed positive relationship between the death rate from ischaemic heart disease and the softness of the local water supply.

In 1976, a Joint Working Party of the Royal College of Physicians of London and the British Cardiac Society (Royal College of Physicians 1976) made a number of dietary recommendations to reduce the incidence of coronary heart disease.
1. Avoid obesity.
2. Reduce consumption of saturated fats.
3. Reduce total fat consumption towards 35% of total calories.
4. Increase the intake of polyunsaturated fats.
5. Eat less meat and egg yolks, eat more poultry and fish. Choose lean meat.
6. Reduce sugar and alcohol consumption to help in avoiding obesity.
7. Increase vegetable and fruit consumption.

In 1978, the Department of Health and Social Security published a series of dietary recommendations entitled "Eating for Health" (DHSS 1978). A balanced diet is stressed. A reduction in the consumption of total fat, protein, salt, alcohol and sucrose and an increased consumption of fruits, vegetables and bread is recommended. Obesity should be avoided and breast feeding of babies is encouraged. It is pointed out that dietary habits are formed in childhood and thus the recommendations are important for children as well as adults.

Dr. J.I. Mann (Mann 1979) proposed a prudent diet for Britain in 1979 as a preventative measure in the etiology of coronary heart disease, maturity-onset diabetes, diverticular disease and dental caries. Dr. Mann's recommendations were:
1. To maintain ideal body weight.
2. To increase the consumption of complex carbohydrates such as whole grain cereals and unprocessed fruits and vegetables at the expense of fats, simple sugars and refined carbohydrates.
3. To decrease total fat intake from 40% of total calories to 30% of total calories.
4. To substitute polyunsaturated fat for saturated fat as much as possible.

The author admitted that this last recommendation is controversial. However, he believed that, while conclusive scientific evidence for these recommendations was lacking, circumstantial evidence is extremely strong and that they could not be in any way harmful.

In 1979, also, three other eminent British nutritionists Passmore, Hollinsworth and Robertson gave a prescription for a better British diet (Passmore et al 1979). They proposed modest (15%) reductions in the intake of fat, sugar, meat, and a 25% reduction in the intake of alcohol, and 15% increases in the consumption of potatoes, vegetables, fruit and grain products. Intake of dairy products (except butter), eggs, fish, pulses and nuts were to remain unchanged. Passmore, et al, state that "the suggested changes in the national diet are large enough to be meaningful, yet would not disrupt agricultural or trade policies if implemented over the next decade."

A stronger set of recommendations for the prevention of CHD was proposed in 1982 by an ad hoc working group of 23 experts in the field (Ad hoc Working Group 1982). The dietary recommendation advocated were:

1. Obesity should be avoided.
2. Total fat intake should be reduced to provide 30% of total energy intake.
3. Saturated fat should provide no more than 10% of total energy.
4. Increased consumption of foods rich in complex carbohydrates particularly bread, vegetables, potatoes and fruit. This would also increase dietary fiber intake.

The ad hoc committee agreed that special attention should be directed to children since dietary habits are often established early in life.

The National Advisory Committee on Nutrition Education (NACNE), in September 1983, published a report entitled "Proposals for nutritional guidelines for health education in Britain." (NACNE 1983) The specific guidelines were:

1. Total fat should be reduced from the present level of 38% of total energy (including alcohol) to 34% of total energy in the 1980's and to 30% of total energy in the long term.
2. Sucrose should be reduced from the present 38 kg per head per year (104g per day) to 34 kg (93g) in the 1980's and to 20 kg (55g) in the long term, of which not more than half should be in drinks and snacks before meals.
3. Dietary fiber should be increased from the present 20g to 25g in the 1980's and 30g in the long term; both cereal fiber and fruit and vegetable fiber should be increased.
4. Alcohol should be reduced from 6% of total energy to 5% in the 1980's and 4% in the long term.
5. Energy levels should be maintained because more exercise throughout the population is to be encouraged.

The Committee stated its recommendations apply to all age groups "although a few additional recommendations for babies, the elderly and ethnic minorities may be necessary."

Ten years after its previous report (DHSS 1974) on diet and coronary heart disease, the Committee on Medical Aspects of Food Policy published a new report on the same topic in 1984. (DHSS 1984) The report recommended for the general population:

1. A reduction in total fat intake to 35% of food energy.
2. A reduction in saturated fat intake to 15% of food energy.
3. An increase in consumption of complex carbohydrate-rich foods.
4. A decrease in salt consumption.
5. Avoidance of obesity.

The Committee stated that their recommendations applied to children above the age of 5 as well as adults. For groups at high risk of CHD, the report recommended a reduction in total fat intake to 30% of caloric intake, saturated fat to 10% of caloric intake, cholesterol to 100mg/1000kcal and an increase in dietary fiber intake to 30g/day.

Ireland

The Health Advisory Committee of An Foras Taluntais (An Foras Taluntais 1977) made a number of recommendations to reduce the risk of CHD.

1. A reduction in caloric intake to a level compatible with normal energy expenditure.
2. A decrease in consumption of total fats and refined carbohydrate as a major element in decreasing caloric intake.
3. An increase in caloric expenditure.
4. An increase in the consumption of fibrous foods demonstrating hypocholesterolaemic effects. e.g. apples, carrots, beans, peas, oats.

The most recent guidelines from the Health Advisory Committee (1984) recommend consuming a varied diet, maintenance of ideal body weight, reduction in total fat intake to 35% of calories, reduction in saturated fat intake, increase in dietary fiber intake to 22-35 g/day, moderation in salt, sugar and alcohol consumption and a reduction in protein intake to 1 g/kg body weight/day with a greater emphasis on vegetable sources of protein.

Canada

Quebec's Nutritional Goals have been reported by Molitor (Molitor 1979). The goals are:
1. To cut sugar intake by half.
2. To cut fat intake by 25% by eating less meat, fried foods and by using low fat milk, yogurt and cheeses.
3. To be moderate in intake of alcohol.
4. To increase the intake of starchy foods and fiber.
5. To conserve nutritive values by using proper refrigerated storage and avoiding overcooking.
6. To eat a wide variety of food to ensure a well balanced diet.
7. To exercise regularly.

In 1979, the Nutrition Recommendations for Canadians were reviewed and amended (Murray and Ral 1979). The new recommendations were:
1. Consumption of a nutritionally adequate diet as outlined in Canada's Food Guide (Dept of National Health and Welfare).
2. A reduction in fat intake to 35% of total calories. A source of linoleic acid should be included in the diet.
3. Emphasize whole grain cereals, fruits and vegetables and minimize alcohol, salt and refined sugars in the diet.
4. Polyunsaturated fats should be substituted for saturated fats as much as possible.

Norway

In 1975, the Royal Norwegian Ministry of Agriculture made the following recommendations to the Storting: (Royal Norwegian Ministry of Agriculture 1975)
1. Total dietary fat intake should be reduced from the 1973 level of 42% of calories to 35% of calories.
2. Intake of starchy foods should be increased.
3. Sugar intake should be decreased.
4. Polyunsaturated fats should be substituted for saturated fats as much as possible.

Earlier recommendations had been made in 1968 by the combined Medical Boards of Finland, Norway and Sweden aimed at reducing the prevalence of obesity and coronary heart disease (Keys 1968). These recommendations were:

1. The supply of calories in the diet should in many cases be reduced to avoid overweight.
2. Total fat intake should be reduced from 40% to between 25% and 35% of total calories.
3. The consumption of saturated fats should be reduced and the consumption of polyunsaturated fats be increased simultaneously.
4. The consumption of sugar should be decreased.
5. The consumption of vegetables, fruit, potatoes, skimmed milk, fish, lean meat and cereal products should be increased.
6. Regular exercise should be emphasized.

Sweden

Two sets of dietary recommendations have been published in Sweden (Molitor 1979; National Board of Health and Welfare 1972; Swedish National Food Administration 1981). Basically similar recommendations are contained in both reports.

1. Reduce calories to avoid obesity.
2. Reduce total fat intake to 25-35% of calories.
3. Reduce saturated fat intake and increase the intake of polyunsaturated fats.
4. Cholesterol consumption should be decreased.
5. Reduce intake of simple sugars by 25%.
6. Reduce alcohol intake.
7. Regular exercise should be stressed.
8. Increase complex carbohydrate intake to 50-60% of calories.

This final goal was contained in the second report. (Swedish National Food Administration 1981)

Australia

The Committee on Diet and Heart Disease of the National Heart Foundation of Australia (National Heart Foundation of Australia 1974), in 1974, suggested a number of dietary recommendations to reduce the risk of coronary heart disease.

1. Total fat intake should be limited to 30-35% of calories.
2. Cholesterol intake should be less than 300 mg/day.
3. Achieve a P:S ratio of 1.5.
4. Decrease alcohol consumption.

The Committee believed these dietary modifications to be safe and beneficial. The Committee suggested that these recommendations be followed by the over one-third of the middle aged population whose serum cholesterol level exceeded 250 mg/day. The Committee noted, however, that since the development of athersclerosis and coronary artery disease occurs over many years and may begin in the first two decades of life, a trend in the national diet away from the present high intakes of calories and fat was desirable.

A Food and Nutrition Policy, including Dietary Goals, was proposed in Australia in 1979 by the Commonwealth Department of Health. (Langsford 1979). The goals were:
1. Increase breast feeding.
2. Provide nutrition education on a balanced diet for all Australians.
3. Reduce the incidence of obesity.
4. Decrease total fat consumption.
5. Decrease refined sugar consumption.
6. Increase consumption of complex carbohydrates and dietary fiber; i.e. wholegrain cereals, vegetables and fruits.
7. Decrease consumption of alcohol.
8. Decrease consumption of salt.

World Health Organization (W.H.O.)

A W.H.O. Expert Committee issued a report on "Prevention of Coronary Heart Disease" in 1982 which contained dietary recommendations. (WHO 1982). The Committee recommended:
1. Reduce total fat intake to 20-30% of total energy intake.
2. Reduce saturated fat intake to less than 10% of total energy intake. Polyunsaturated fat intake should be no more than 10% of total calories.
3. Reduce cholesterol intake to below 100mg/1000kcal.
4. Avoid obesity.

5. Increase complex carbohydrate consumption.
6. Salt consumption should be less than 5g/day.

As a means of achieving these goals, the Committee suggested:
1. Emphasis on foods of plant origin -- beans, cereal grains, vegetables and fruit.
2. Fish, poultry and lean meats, used in small portions and eaten less often as the main dish.
3. Low-fat dairy products for adults.
4. Less oils and fats in food preparation and in spreads.
5. Less high-fat meats from domestic breeds as the principal protein source.
6. Less high-fat dairy products.
7. Less whole eggs, unless a major source of protein.
8. Less commercially baked products.
9. Less alcoholic beverages.

Food and Agriculture Organization/ World Health Organization

In 1977, a joint FAO/WHO expert consultation group produced a report on Dietary Fats and Oils in Human Nutrition (FAO/WHO 1977). For population groups with a high incidence of atherosclerosis, obesity and maturity-onset diabetes, the recommended composition of a diet adequate to maintain ideal body weight is 10-15% of calories as protein and 30-35% of calories as fat. The latter should have a reduced saturated fat content and a linoleic acid content of at least one third of total fat calories. The diet should be low in sugar and alcohol and contain less than 300mg/day of cholesterol.

New Zealand

A Committee of the National Heart Foundation of New Zealand, in 1971, made a number of recommendations to reduce the risk of coronary heart disease in the general population (National Heart Foundation of New Zealand 1971).
1. Maintain optimum weight.
2. Reduce consumption of saturated fatty acids. This should be done in childhood rather than later life.

3. Cholesterol intake should be curtailed to prudent levels (i.e. between 300-600 mg/day). In general terms this means reducing egg consumption to about one egg per day.

For those identified at higher risk from coronary disease the Committee recommended greater modification of diet.

1. Maintain optimum weight.
2. Total fat consumption should be restricted to 35% of total calories.
3. There should be a more rigorous restriction of saturated animal fats and cholesterol-containing foods. i.e. egg consumption being kept to one every other day.
4. Substitute certain polyunsaturated vegetable oils for saturated fat in the diet.
5. Sugar consumption should be restricted when excessive weight or diabetes are present.
6. Limitation of alcohol is indicated for weight reduction.

The Netherlands

The Netherlands Nutrition Council made recommendations on the amount and nature of dietary fats in relation to atherosclerosis in 1973. (Netherlands Nutrition Council 1973; Vergroesen and Gottenbos 1975).

1. The total caloric intake should be regulated individually to achieve and maintain "normal" body weight.
2. Dietary fat intake should account for about one third of total calories. Saturated fat should be restricted.
3. Polyunsaturated fatty acids should account for 10-13% of total caloric intake.
4. Protein should account for 10-12% of total calories and about 30-50% of this should be animal protein.
5. The remaining calories will be supplied by carbohydrate, preferably whole grain cereals and pulses and as little as possible from sugar.
6. Cholesterol intake should not exceed 250-300mg per day.

SUMMARY

The majority of dietary guidelines discussed above suggest a reduction in the % of dietary calories derived from fat. Currently, approximately 40% of calories in Western countries come from fat. Some of the more recent guidelines call for a reduction in fat intake to 30% of calories. Indeed, the Committee on Diet, Nutrition and Cancer (National Academy of Sciences 1982) and the World Health Organization Report on Prevention of Coronary Heart Disease (WHO 1982) suggested that the evidence warranted an even lower fat intake, but 30% of calories is a moderate and practical target.

Diets containing 30% of calories as fat are undoubtedly safe for the general population. During and immediately after the Second World War in Britain, dietary fat intake was at or about this level and no deleterious effects in the population were noted. (Greaves and Hollingsworth 1966). Indeed, the overall state of health of the population seemed improved. Futhermore, most of the world population exists and has existed on a primarily plant based diet, low in fat content, with no apparent ill effects and lower rates of chronic disease.(Mintz 1985).

Most dietary guidelines recommend a reduction in saturated fat intake. The more recent guidelines suggest saturated fat should be restricted to less than 10% of total calories.

While some of the earlier guidelines suggested an increase in polyunsaturated fat intake, more recent guidelines stress that polyunsaturated fat intake should not exceed 10% of calories. Thus, the focus of more recent guidelines appears to be to decrease total fat intake.

Essentially all guidelines stress avoidance of obesity by avoiding excess caloric intake and increasing caloric expenditure. Diets low in total fat content are beneficial in this regard, a fact acknowledged in the Food and Nutrition Board's report "Towards Healthful Diets." (Food and Nutrition Board 1980 b)

Most guidelines advise a decrease in calories derived from processed sugars and a concomitant increase in complex carbohydrate intake. This is best achieved by stressing whole grain cereals, fruits and vegetables in the diet.

More recent recommendations advise moderation in the use of alcohol. Moderation in salt use is also a common theme. It is our belief that guidelines should be general in nature and not identify specific nutrients, e.g. vitamin A and C in foods, or specific foods themselves, e.g. cabbage, as conferring special benefits. The available data base does not support such specific claims. However, available data does support strongly more general guidelines relating to classes of foods, e.g. increased consumption of whole grains, vegetables and fruits and decreased consumption of animal products.

Furthermore, guidelines relating to foods should not be extended to supplements of individual nutrients found in those foods, e.g. vitamin A, C, E, selenium, etc. Epidemiological data pertain to foods containing these nutrients and a multitude of other constituents both nutrient and non-nutrient. Thus, one should not extrapolate epidemiological data indicating a protective effect of a class of foods, e.g. vegetables, to the use of a vitamin supplement. Epidemiological data on foods give one no information on intake (dose) of a vitamin and, say, cancer risk. Because of the complex composition of foods, very many nutrient and non-nutrient interactions may occur that influence cancer risk. A further concern relating to supplement use is that supplements may confer a false sense of security in the user. Thus the user may believe he or she need not alter other aspects of his/her lifestyle (such as smoking or diet) to reduce cancer risk.

Hegsted has discussed the progress of nutrition research in the United States from its early years through the era of discovery of vitamins and then the era of studying nutritional deficiency diseases (Hegsted 1985). Traditionally, nutrition research has focused on better defining nutrition requirements. By the end of the Second World War, nutritional deficiency disease had all but disappeared from the U.S. and Western countries. A new era of nutrition research began to focus on the effects of diet on the incidence of chronic diseases. With the elimination of deficiency diseases and the great reduction in infectious diseases due to improvements in medical treatment and in antibiotics, it become apparent that significant improvement in the health status of Americans depended on controlling the incidence of chronic diseases (Hegsted 1985).

This fact has also been noted by the Office of Technology Assessment: (Office of Technology Assessment 1978)   "...the Federal Government has failed to adjust the emphasis of its human nutrition research activities to deal with the changing health problems of the United States. The consequence of continuing to pursue the present preoccupation with nutritional deficiency diseases will seriously affect the quality of life of present and future generations into the 21st century."

"...The role of nutrition must be given priority in the prevention and improved management of today's major health problems. Nutritional factors deserve particular attention for two reasons. First, it is possible to change diets while some of the other factors that influence disease development cannot be altered. Second, nutrition is basic to health and deserves attention as one of the many factors that influence health and disease."

Some opponents of dietary guidelines argue against them on the basis that the proposed changes are not safe and may affect the availability of essential nutrients.(Harper 1978; Olson 1979) However, as noted above, no deleterious effects were observed in Britain during the war and most of the world population exists on diets that readily meet the goals of dietary recommendations. There is no requirement for 40% of calories as fat in the diet or for high levels of saturated fat and no benefits have been claimed for intakes at this level. Consumption of some animal products high in both total fat and saturated fat would decrease but would not be eliminated from the diet. Furthermore, low-fat animal products are readily available. Achievement of the dietary guidelines would mean a shift from a diet emphasizing animal products to a diet emphasizing more plant-derived foods. Apart from the potential health benefits of this type of diet, there are economic and ecological benefits. A diet emphasizing plant-derived foods with the bulk of calories coming from grains, legumes, fruits and vegetables is cheaper and more ecologically sound than the current American diet which emphasizes animal-derived foods. (Connor 1979)

Critics of dietary guideline accept current Western diets as if they had been scientifically developed on the basis of good evidence. In reality, current Western diets are more a product of economic influences which have increased the intake of fat, sugar, salt, etc. and decreased the intake of plant foods and low-fat wild animals on which humans evolved and subsisted on for eons (Blackburn 1979).

Rose (Rose 1981) has distinguished between two types of mass preventive measures. The first consists of removal of an unnatural factor and restoration of "biological normality" e.g. a substantial reduction in saturated fat intake, avoidance of obesity, avoidance of physical inactivity and avoidance of cigarettes. Such measures may be presumed to be safe and should be advocated on the basis of a reasonable presumption of benefit. The second type of mass preventive measure involves addition of some other unnatural factor in the hope of conferring protection, e.g. a high intake of polyunsaturated fat or long-term medication. These types of preventive measures require a much greater level of evidence of efficacy and, especially, safety before they can be advocated.

While the vast majority of the dietary guidelines discussed above are directed to the general population, some authorities believe such guidelines (decreased intake of fat, saturated fat, sugar, salt and cholesterol, etc.) should be given only to those individuals at "high-risk" for these chronic diseases. (Food and Nutrition Board 1980 b; AMA 1979). As approximately 70% of the U.S. population dies from either atherosclerotic diseases or cancer, we would submit that most of the population is in a "high-risk" category.

Furthermore, identification of "high-risk" individuals is likely to be enormously expensive (Bloom and Soper 1986). This strategy will do very little for those for whom the first indication of risk is death from a heart attack.

This should not be interpreted as an argument against efforts to identify and treat "high-risk" individuals. Such efforts are to be commended, however, the relative societal benefits are likely to be small. A public health campaign emphasizing dietary guidelines such as those of the McGovern Committee (Select Committee on Nutrition 1977 b) should be actively pursued in parallel with efforts to identify high risk individuals.

In the case of coronary heart disease, the largest number of coronary attacks occur in individuals below the

90th percentile for plasma cholesterol level, although the relative risk is greatest above this level i.e. in high-risk individuals. (Kannel and Gordon 1970) Thus the potential impact of a public health campaign to educate the entire public on dietary guidelines is much greater (Rose 1981). A 1% decrease in plasma cholesterol levels can decrease the risk of coronary heart disease by 2% (Lipid Research Clinics Program 1984) or by 1.6-2%. (R. Peto, personal communication.)

As Connor (Connor 1979), has noted: "...it is recognized that deficiency diseases are best prevented on a mass population basis." Indeed, that is the rationale behind the RDA's. We fortify foods with vitamin D for all in order to protect the very few who might still be susceptible to rickets. This concept of advice to the general population for the benefit of the few pervades all aspects of society, e.g. all are advised to wear seat belts even though very few of us will ever be involved in an accident. This concept derives from the recognition that prevention is easier, cheaper and involves less suffering than injury or illness and subsequent treatment.

A further argument against exclusive use of the identification of "high-risk" individuals approach is that by the time those individuals are identified, potentially irreversible damage has been done to their health. Giving dietary advice to these individuals, while commendable, is, in our opinion, a classic example of bolting the stable door long after the horse has gone. Chronic diseases, such as coronary heart disease and cancer, have a long latency period and maximal potential benefit of dietary intervention will be achieved only if these dietary modifications are made early in life, preferably in childhood. It is generally recognized that eating habits and preferences are developed in childhood and intensive efforts should be made to educate children on the importance of consuming a diet that meets recommended dietary guidelines.

Critics of dietary guidelines also argue that they are "draconian" and "unrealistic" and cannot be achieved (Marr and Morris 1982; Oliver 1983). However, recent USDA data suggests that total fat intake in the United States is beginning to decrease (Rizek et al 1986). People's food habits can and do change and will respond to an aggressive public health policy of education on how to implement dietary guidelines. This education process should be initiated in childhood. Restaurants, school lunch programs and Government food programs should provide meals that meet dietary recommendations. The Food Industry should intensify efforts to develop more low-fat, low-sugar products. That low-fat, high-complex carbohydrate type diets are palatable is testified by the popularity of Asian, Mexican and Mediterranean type cuisine. As Hegsted has noted, the only risk in this process is to the well-being of certain segments of the Food Industry, and while "...these industries deserve some consideration, their interests cannot supersede the health interests of the population they must feed." (Hegsted 1975).

Another argument against dietary guidelines is that there is no scientific "proof" that adherence to these guidelines will decrease the incidence and /or delay the onset of chronic diseases. Similar arguments are used by tobacco interests with respect to tobacco consumption and lung cancer.

Proof of this nature may be impossible to obtain. It would involve following thousands of subjects for 30, 40, 50 years or so. More limited trials, such as the Multiple Risk Factor Intervention Trial (MRFIT) (MRFIT 1982), involving dietary intervention for a limited time period in middle-aged men may not be an adequate test of the dietary hypothesis. Atherosclerosis develops slowly over many years. The much cited studies (Enos et al 1955) in young U.S. victims of the Korean War who exhibited a significant degree of atherosclerosis in their 20's even though heart attacks are not a serious public health problem until the 40's and later are testimony to this fact. In the absence of definitive proof that would be provided by a lifetime clinical trial, scientists and public policy makers must base policy on existing evidence. Existing evidence, both epidemiological, clinical and animal, and the biological plausibility of this evidence, supports strongly the rationale of dietary guidelines such as the U.S. Dietary Goals (Senate Select Committee on Nutrition 1977 a,b).

The evidence supporting dietary guidelines is as strong or stronger than the evidence for many of the Recommended Dietary Allowances (Food and Nutrition Board 1980 a). The RDA's are essentially guidelines to prevent deficiency diseases. The RDA's are the best estimates that can be made based upon limited epidemiological, clinical and animal evidence. More evidence is always desirable but RDA's have to be set based upon the evidence at hand. A similar situation exists with respect to dietary guidelines -- they are the best advice that we can give based upon available evidence.

It will be difficult to make major changes in the United States' diet but the effort is worthwhile as the potential benefits are great. However as Trowell et al have noted (Trowell et al 1985) : "Minimal changes will achieve only minimal results. Enlightened individuals have already made major changes in their own diet."

ACKNOWLEDGEMENTS

This work was supported by NIH Grant No. CA 33638 and CA 34205.

REFERENCES

Ad hoc Working Group on Coronary Prevention. (1982) Prevention of Coronary Heart Disease in the United Kingdom. Lancet i: 846-847.
American Academy of Pediatrics Committee on Nutrition. (1983) Towards a prudent diet for children. Pediatrics 71: 78-80.
American Cancer Society. (1984) Nutrition and Cancer: Cause and Prevention. Special Report New York, American Cancer Society.
American Health Foundation. (1972) Position Statement on Diet and Coronary Heart Disease. Preventive Med 1: 255-286.
American Heart Association. (1965) Diet and Heart Disease. Dallas, American Heart Association.
American Heart Association. (1968) Diet and Heart Disease. Dallas, American Heart Association.
American Heart Association. (1973) Diet and Coronary Heart Disease. Dallas, American Heart Association.
American Heart Association. (1978) Diet and Coronary Heart Disease. Dallas, American Heart Association.
American Heart Association. (1980) Risk Factors and Coronary Disease. Circulation 62: 449A-445A.

American Heart Association. (1982) Rationale of the Diet-Heart Statement of the American Heart Association. Circulation. 65: 839A-854A.

American Institute for Cancer Research. (1983) Dietary Guidelines to Lower Cancer Risk. Falls Church, VA. American Institute for Cancer Research.

American Medical Association Council on Foods and Nutrition and Food and Nutrition Board/National Research Council. (1972) Diet and Coronary Heart Disease. J Am Med Assoc 222: 1647.

American Medical Association Council on Scientific Affairs. (1979) American Medical Association Concepts on Nutrition and Health. J Am Med Assoc 242: 2335-2338.

Bennett, J H, (1865) Clinical Lectures on the Principals and Practice of Medicine. 4th edition Adam and Charles Black, Edinburgh.

Blackburn, H, (1979) Diet and mass hyperlipidemia: a public health view. In Levy, R, Rifkin, B, Dennis, B, Ernst, N (eds) Nutrition, Lipids and Coronary Disease New York, Raven Press, pp. 309-347.

Bloom, B S and Soper, K A (1986) Diagnostic testing for coronary artery disease in a large population. Am J Prev Med 2: 35-41.

Bulkley, L D (1921) Cancer and its Non-Surgical Treatment. W Wood and Co., New York.

Canadian Pediatric Society Nutrition Committee (1981) Children's diets and atherosclerosis. Can Med Assoc J 124: 1545-1548.

Connor, W E (1979) Too little or too much: the case for preventive nutrition. Am J Clin Nutr 32: 1975-1978.

Connor, W E (1981) U.S. Dietary Goals. A Pro View, with Special Emphasis upon the Etiological Relationships of Dietary Factors to Coronary Heart Disease. In P J Garry (ed) Human Nutrition -- Clinical and Biochemical Aspects. Am Assoc Clin Chem Washington, D.C. pp. 44-80

Consensus Conference (1985) Lowering blood cholesterol to prevent heart disease J Am Med Assoc 253: 2080-2086.

Council for Agricultural Science and Technology (CAST) (1977) Dietary Goals for the United States -- A commentary. Report No 71.

Department of Health, Education and Welfare (1979) Healthy People: The Surgeon General's Report on Health Promotion and Disease Prevention. DHEW (Public Health Service) Publication No 79-55071 Washington, D.C. Printing Office.

Department of Health and Social Security (1974) Report on Health and Social Subjects, No 7 Diet and Coronary Heart Disease. London, Her Majesty's Stationary Office.

Department of Health and Social Security (1978) Eating for Health. London, Her Majesty's Stationary Office.

Department of Health and Social Security (1984) Report on Health and Social Subjects No 28 Diet and Cardiovascular Disease. London, Her Majesty's Stationary Office.

Department of National Health and Welfare (1979) Canada's Food Guide Ottawa.

Doll, R and Peto, R (1981) The causes of cancer: quantitative estimates of avoidable risks of cancer in the United States today. J Natl Cancer Inst 66: 1191-1308.

Editorial (1977) Review of the Dietary Goals of the United States Lancet i: 887-888.

Enos, W F Jr, Beyer, J C and Holmes, R H (1955) Pathogenesis of coronary disease in American soldiers killed in Korea. J Am Med Assoc 158: 912-916.

Fallscheer-Zurcher, J (1930) Cancer and Diet. Cancer Review 5(1).

Food and Agriculture Organization of the United Nations and World Health Organization (1977) Dietary fats and oils in human nutrition. FAO Food and Nutrition Paper No 3 Rome.

Food and Nutrition Board/National Research Council (1958) The Role of Dietary Fat in Human Health. NAS-NRC Publication No 575 National Academy of Sciences. Washington, D.C.

Food and Nutrition Board/National Research Council (1966) Dietary Fat and Human Health. NAS-NRC Publication No 1147. National Academy of Sciences Washington, D.C.

Food and Nutrition Board Committee on Dietary Allowances (1980 a) National Research Council. Recommended Dietary Allowances -- Ninth Edition. National Academy of Sciences Washington, D.C.

Food and Nutrition Board/National Research Council (1980 b) Towards Healthful Diets. National Academy of Sciences Washington, D.C.

Greaves, J P and Hollingsworth, D F (1966) Trends in food consumption in the United Kingdom. World Rev Nutr Diet 6: 34-89.

Grobstein, D (1983) Should imperfect data be used to guide public policy? Science 83: 4910) 18.

Harper, A E (1978) Dietary Goals -- a Skeptical view. Am J Clin Nutr 31: 310-321.

Health Advisory Committee (1977) An Foras Taluntais (Agricultural Institute) Prevention of Coronary Heart Disease -- Diet and the Food Supply, Dublin.

Hegsted, D M (1978) Dietary Goal -- a progressive view. Am J Clin Nutr 31: 1504-1509.

Hegsted, D M (1978) Nutrition: The changing Scene. Nutr Rev 43: 357-367.

Hoffman, F L (1937) Cancer and Diet -- with facts and observations on related subjects. The Williams and Wilkins Co. Baltimore.

Inter-State Commission for Heart Disease Resources (1984) Optimal resources for primary prevention of atherosclerotic diseases. Circulation 70: 153A-205A.

Kannel, W B, Gordon, T, (eds.) (1970) Section 26 Some characteristics related to the incidence of cardiovascular disease and death: Framingham Study, 16 year follow-up. Washington, D.C. U.S. Government Printing Office.

Keys, A (1968) Official collective recommendations on diet in the Scandanavian countries. Nutr Rev 26: 259-263.

Lambe, W (1815) Additional Reports on the Effects of a peculiar Regimen in cases of Cancer, Scrofulus, Consumption, Asthma and other Chronic Diseases. London.

Langsford, W A (1979) A food and nutrition policy. Food Nutr Notes Rev 36: 100-103.

Li, J Y (1982) Epidemiology of esophageal cancer in China. Natl Cancer Inst Monogr 62: 113-120.

Lipid Research Clinics Program: The Lipid Research Clinics Coronary Primary Prevention Trial Results (1984) I Reduction in incidence of coronary heart disease. J Am Med Nutr 33: 57-63.

Mann, J I (1979) A prudent diet for the nation. J Human Nutr 33: 57-63.

Marr, J and Morris, J N (1982) Changing the national diet to reduce coronary heart disease. Lancet i: 217-218.

McNutt, K (1980) Dietary advice to the public: 1957-1980 Nutr Rev 38: 353-360.

Mintz, S W (1985) Sweetness and Power -- The Place of Sugar in Modern History. Viking Press, New York.

Molitor, G T (1979) National nutrition goals -- How far have we come? In: M Chou and D P Harmon (eds) Critical Food issues of the Eighties pp 134-141. New York Pergamon Press.

Multiple Risk Factor Intervention Trial (MRFIT) (1982) J Am Med Assoc 248: 1465-1468.

Murray, T K and Rae, J (1979) Nutrition recommendations for Canadians. Can Med Assoc J 120: 1241-1242.

NACNE (1983): A discussion paper on proposals for nutritional guidelines for health education in Britain. Prepared for the National Advisory Committee on Nutrition Education by an ad-hoc working party under the chairmanship of Professor W P T James. London, Health Education Council.

National Academy of Sciences (1982) Committee on Diet, Nutrition and Cancer. Diet, Nutrition and Cancer, Washington D.C. Nation Academy Press.

National Board of Health and Welfare (1972) Diet and Exercise. Report from the National Board of Health and Welfare. Stockholm.

National Cancer Institute (1984) Cancer Prevention. NIH Publication No 84-2671 U.S. Department of Health and Human Services. Public Health Service. National Institutes of Health.

National Heart Foundation of Australia Committee on Diet and Heart Disease (1974) Dietary fat and coronary heart disease -- a review 1: 575-579, 616-620,663-668.

National Heart Foundation of New Zealand (1971) Coronary heart disease -- a New Zealand Report. National Heart Foundation.

Netherlands Nutrition Council (1973) Recommendation on amount and nature of dietary fats. Voeding 34: 552-557 (in Dutch)

Office of Technology Assessment (1978) "The Role of Diet in the Prevention of Chronic Disease and Obesity" Nutrition Research Alternatives. OTA-D-74 U.S. Congress, Washington, D.C.

Oliver, R E (1979) Should we not forget about mass control of risk factors? Lancet ii: 37-38.

Olson, R E (1979) The U.S. Quandary: Can we formulate a rational nutrition policy? in: M Chou and D P Harmon (eds) Critical Foods Issues of the Eighties. pp. 119-133 New York, Pergamon Press.

Page, I H, Stare, F J, Corcoran, A C, Pollack, H and Wilkinson, C F (1957) Atherosclerosis and the fat content of the diet. Circulation 16: 163-178.

Page, I H, Allen, E B, Chamberlain, F L, Keys, A, Stamler, J and Stare, F J (1961) Dietary fat and its relation to heart attacks and strokes. Circulation 23: 133-136.

Page, L and Phipard, E H (1957) Essentials for an Adequate Diet. Home Economics Research Report No 3. Agriculture Research Service. U.S. department of Agriculture. Washington, D.C. Government Printing Office.

Palmer, S (1983) Diet, Nutrition and Cancer: The Future of Dietary Policy. Cancer Res 43: 2509s-2514s.

Pariza, M W (1984) A perspective on Diet, Nutrition and Cancer. J Am Med Assoc 251: 1455-1458.

Passmore, R, Hollingsworth, D and Robertson, J (1979) Presrciption for a better British diet. Br Med J 1: 527-531.

Podell, R N, Gary, L R and Keller, K (1975) A profile of clinical nutrition knowledge among physicians and medical students. J Med Educ 50: 888-892.

Rizek, R, Riddick, H and Trippett, K (1986) U.S. Department of Agriculture. Food and Nutrient intake of women and children. Fed Proc 45(4) Abstract No 1876.

Rose, G (1981) Strategy of prevention: lessons from cardiovascular disease. Br Med J 282: 1847-1851.

Royal College of Physicians of London and British Cardiac Society (1976) Prevention of Coronary Heart Disease. Report of a Joint Working Party. J R Coll Physic Lond 10:213-275.

Royal Norwegian Ministry of Agriculture 1976 on Norwegian Food and Nutrition Policy. Report No 32 (1975-1976) to the Storting.

Select Committee on Nutrition and Human Needs, United States Senate (1977a) Dietary Goals for the United States. Stock No 052-070-03913-2 Washington, D.C. Government Printing Office.

Select Committee on Nutrition and Human Needs, United States Senate (1977b) Dietary Goals for the Untied States -- Second Edition. Stock No 052-070-04376-8 Washington, D.C. Government Printing Office.

Select Committee on Nutrition and Human Needs, United States Senate (1977c) Dietary Goals for the United States -- Supplemental Views. Washington, D.C. Government Printing Office.

Shaw, J (1907) The Cure of Cancer: and How Surgery Blacks the Way. London.

Swedish National Food Administration (1981) Swedish Nutrition Recommendations. Uppsala, Sweden. The National Food Administration.

Thompson, E B (1932) Cancer: Is it preventible? London.

Trowell, H, Burkitt, D and Heaton, K (1985) Summaries. In: H Trowell, D Burkitt and K Heaton (eds) Dietary Fiber, Fiber-Depleted Foods and Disease. Academic Press. London. pp. 419-427.

United States Department of Agriculture, Science and Education Administration (1979) Food. Home and Garden Bulletin No 228, USDA. Washington, D.C.

United States Department of Agriculture and United States Department of Health, Education and Welfare (1980) Nutrition and Your Health: Dietary Guidelines for Americans. Home and Garden Bulletin No 232. Washington, D.C. Government Printing Office.

United States Department of Agriculture and United States
  Department of Health and Human Service (1985) Nutrition
  and Your Health: Dietary Guidelines for Americans --
  Second Edition. Home and Garden Bulletin No 232.
  Washington, D.C. Government Printing Office.
United States General Accounting Office (1984) National
  Academy of Sciences' Reports on Diet and Health -- Are
  they Credible and Consistent? Gaithersburg, MD. U.S.
  General Accounting Office.
Upton, A C (1979) Statement on Diet, Nutrition and Cancer.
  Hearings of the Subcommittee on Nutrition and Forestry.
Vergroesen, A J and Gottenbos, J J (1975) The Role of fats
  in human nutrition -- an Introduction. in: Vergroesen, A J
  (ed) The Role of Fats in Human Nutrition. Academic Press
  London, pp. 1-41.
Williams, W R (1908) The Natural History of Cancer with
  Special Reference to its Causation and Prevention.
  William Heineman, Publisher. London.
World Health Organization (1982) Prevention of Coronary
  Heart Disease, Geneva. World Health Organization.
  Technical Report Series: No 678.
Wynder, E L and Gori, G B (1977) Contribution of the
  environment to cancer incidence: and epidemiological
  exercise. J Natl Cancer Inst 58: 825-833.
Yan, Y H : Ji Sheng Fang. In: Medical Book of the Song
  Dynasty, (in Chinese)

Dietary Fat and Cancer, pages 773–788
© 1986 Alan R. Liss, Inc.

THE DIET AND CANCER BRANCH, NCI: CURRENT PROJECTS AND
FUTURE RESEARCH DIRECTIONS

Ritva R. Butrum, Elaine Lanza, and Carolyn
K. Clifford
Diet and Cancer Branch, Division of Cancer
Prevention and Control, National Cancer Institute,
Silver Spring, Maryland

INTRODUCTION

The Diet and Cancer Branch (DCB) has the lead responsibility within the Prevention Program of the Division of
Cancer Prevention and Control (DCPC), National Cancer
Institute (NCI), for encouraging and supporting research on
the role of diet and nutrition in cancer control. The
primary goal of the Branch's programs is the reduction of
cancer incidence through dietary modification. In view of
the existing gaps in our knowledge regarding the type of
dietary modification to reduce cancer incidence, the Diet
and Cancer Branch is organized to: develop, plan, direct,
and coordinate a research program in diet, nutrition, and
cancer as it relates to cancer prevention; develop, refine,
and test hypotheses of diet and the etiology and prevention
of cancer; develop quantitative methods to monitor nutritional
intake in large populations and to facilitate accurate
conversion of diet into nutrient content; study baseline
dietary data on populations participating in controlled
clinical trials, assess strategies for altering diet in
relation to cancer risks, assess scientific knowledge and
the impact of such strategies, and conduct applied research
on dietary modification and cancer; and oversee diet,
nutrition, and cancer activities in other divisions of the
NCI, other National Institutes of Health (NIH) programs,
and other research and health agencies.

The specific objectives for immediate implementation
relate to the first three cancer control research phases of
NCI: hypothesis testing, methods development, and controlled

clinical trials. With the newly planned projects outlined below, the DCB will seek to: identify areas for applied and basic research on specific dietary factors that serve as inhibitors or promoters of carcinogenesis; develop and refine dietary and nutritional assessment methodologies, including refining of nutrient data banks, to permit reliable and valid measurement of specific dietary factors; develop methods for enabling desirable changes in eating behavior and for measuring such changes; and provide, through support of risk reduction clinical trials, scientifically-based information on the preventive role of dietary factors in carcinogenesis and prevention. Particular emphasis is on diet in relation to cancer development and progression. As the knowledge base of the role of nutritional factors in the development and progression of cancer continues to expand, the opportunity exists to develop and evaluate dietary modifications that potentially can prevent as much as 35 percent of all human cancer (Doll and Peto, 1981).

Current efforts in the diet and cancer research area include: expansion of the knowledge base of the metabolism of nutrients and their role in cancer causation and prevention, the interaction of nutrients and their role in cancer causation and prevention, the interaction of genetic-nutrient-environmental factors in cancer initiation or progression, and the influence of nutritional factors on cancer treatment and patient recovery. Basic research is required on the nutrient content of various foods, the effects of processing on food, retail practices, identification of determinants of dietary practices, and development of methods to change such practices within defined populations.

DIRECTIONS OF DIET AND CANCER RESEARCH

In order to fulfill the needs of the Diet and Cancer Program, DCB staff members are involved with numerous extramural and intramural activities. The extramural needs are met through the development, implementation, and success-ful administration of appropriate projects performed under the mechanisms of contracts, cooperative agreements, grants, and interagency agreements. It should be understood that a clear distinction is made between the DCB program and the chemoprevention program conducted by the Chemoprevention Branch (CB) of DCPC. The DCB program focuses on research and clinical trials that assess the role of specific foods or food groups in the prevention of cancer. Within this framework, intervention trials may be expressed as dietary guidelines or recommendations. In contrast, the chemoprevention program focuses its efforts on human studies related to the intake of specific chemicals, nutrient analogues, or nutrients.

As the knowledge base regarding the role of nutritional factors in the development and progression of cancer continues to expand, the opportunity exists to develop and evaluate dietary modifications which have the potential for preventing a significant percentage of human cancer. This expansion of knowledge regarding human nutrition and the identification of effective cancer preventive diets offer a cancer prevention approach which can be widely adopted by the general public.

The DCB has conceptualized the diet and cancer research program in a convergence plan framework which provides a rational structure for testing and evaluating solid research leads in terms of pre-established criteria to determine their efficacy in reducing the cancer incidence in human populations. This convergence plan has three basic components: Laboratory Studies, Epidemiological Studies and Human Intervention Studies (see Figure 1). Each of the three components is subdivided into stages or phases which are separated by decision points. Progress from one research stage or phase to the next requires the satisfactory fulfillment of criteria at each decision point. The Board of Scientific Counselors and the NCI staff of DCPC determine that the criteria at each decision point in the process have been satisfied sufficiently to warrant proceeding to the next research stage or phase.

For example, the first step in conducting laboratory studies is the evaluation of literature to identify possible leads that warrant further study. Initial investigations of efficacy are then conducted in animal models and in other types of laboratory studies to determine which dietary factors may have the greater cancer prevention potential. If the initial studies prove to be positive, the research lead is introduced to a decision process that selects the more favorable leads for subsequent comparative studies. This process is designed to identify and promote the dietary factors that have the greatest potential for cancer preven-

Figure 1

DCB Research Convergence Plan

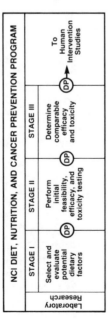

LABORATORY RESEARCH STAGES

NCI DIET, NUTRITION, AND CANCER PREVENTION PROGRAM

	STAGE I	STAGE II	STAGE III	
Laboratory Research	Select and evaluate potential dietary factors	Perform initial feasibility, and efficacy, and toxicity testing	Determine comparable efficacy and toxicity	To Human Intervention Studies

HUMAN INTERVENTION STUDIES PHASES

NCI DIET, NUTRITION, AND CANCER PREVENTION PROGRAM

PHASE I	PHASE II	PHASE III	PHASE IV	PHASE V
Evaluate clinical, laboratory, and epidemiologic findings	Establish dose level methods studies	Prevention trials	Defined population studies	Demonstration and implementation studies

EPIDEMIOLOGIC RESEARCH STAGES

NCI DIET, NUTRITION, AND CANCER PREVENTION PROGRAM

STAGE I	STAGE II	
Descriptive Studies	Analytic Studies	To Human Intervention Studies

DP = Decision Point

EP = Evaluation Point

tion and that can be safely and effectively moved into human intervention studies. To move from the laboratory or epidemiological study phase to the human intervention phase, a lead must not only meet the criteria established at each of the appropriate decision points but also must be identified as a priority research topic which has a significant potential for reducing cancer in human populations.

The Laboratory Research component of the convergence planning framework has three stages: 1) the selection and evaluation of potential cancer prevention dietary factors; 2) the performance of initial feasibility, efficacy and toxicity tests, and 3) the evaluation of the comparable efficacy and toxicity of the test factor. To be selected for introduction into human intervention studies, a research lead must fulfill these requirements: the laboratory results are relevant for consideration in human clinical trials, there are no adverse interactions with other dietary factors or drugs, all necessary long-term toxicity and survival studies have been initiated or completed, and the model being tested is relevant to human situations and metabolism.

Similarly, within the Epidemiological Research component, the decision process is divided into two stages. The first stage identifies the dietary factors with a high potential for impacting the incidence of cancer in human populations which, therefore, warrant additional study. This first stage also identifies populations for further study, e.g., populations which have unique diets and/or patterns of cancer. Previous "natural" experimental studies, e.g. wartime changes in food supplies, which may provide important research leads are identified at this stage. Based upon positive scientific assessment, the promising research leads are moved on to the next stage of higher level analytical and refined epidemiologic studies, e.g., case-control and cohort studies. The purpose of these more sophisticated studies is to further define the preventive potential of a dietary strategy. These studies are usually analytic in nature, providing the basis for human intervention studies. The key criteria to be satisfied before proceeding to human intervention trials are: 1) establishing evidence of a causal association between the proposed dietary strategy and cancer incidence and 2) determining that an appropriate target population can be identified.

The final testing ground of any hypothesis or lead from laboratory or epidemiological studies is its application to human intervention studies (see Figure 1). The initial study process is the evaluatation of the information from laboratory and/or epidemiological studies (Phase I). Once positively evaluated in Phase I, initial feasibility studies are conducted to determine the level of acceptance of the proposed dietary intervention by the study population(s), the degree of change needed to gain acceptability, and safety of the intervention since certain dietary factors in excess can be toxic (Phase II). The next step is the conduct of controlled studies which involve randomized clinical trials, e.g. the comparison group receiving its usual diet and the study group receiving the "experimental" diet (Phase III).

If these initial clinical trials are successful, the intervention will be brought into ever widening circles of study populations (Phases IV). The final phase is the introduction of a dietary intervention to the general population (Phase V).

Given this cohesive research planning structure as a basis, the DCB has initiated a number of important dietary studies to clarify the roles various nutrients play in the causation and reduction of cancer incidence. The current program is concentrated in three research areas: 1) dietary f ?) dietary fiber, and 3) vitamin A and carotenoids. The rationale for these foci is based on the current status of diet-related cancer research. The program also encompasses related piojects with a broader nutrition focus which supports diet and cancer research.

DIETARY FAT

A substantial body of epidemiological evidence supports a direct relationship between dietary fat and the incidence of cancer of the breast and colon (Armstrong and Doll, 1975; Gray et al., 1979; Correa, 1981; Carroll and Khor, 1975). Other cancers, including rectal, ovarian, endometrial, and prostate, have also been associated with dietary fat. These epidemiological observations have been supported by laboratory research using a variety of carcinogens in several animal models (Carroll et al., 1968). Overall, a significant number of laboratory and epidemiological studies suggest a link between dietary fat and cancer incidence, sufficiently strong to warrant human clinical trials.

The DCB is sponsoring two human clinical trials to determine whether a reduced fat diet will reduce the incidence and recurrence of breast cancer. Specifically, the two trials, both in the feasibility study stage, are designed to test whether low fat diets can reduce the cancer incidence in high-risk women and reduce cancer recurrence in women diagnosed as having stage II breast cancer. Both trials are studying the effects of a diet in which no more than 20% of all calories is obtained from fat intake.

The Women's Health Trial (WHT) will test the hypothesis that intake of 20-25% of calories from fat is better than the customary intake of fat in the American diet in reducing the incidence of breast cancer in women at increased risk. The feasibility study is now underway for the WHT and three clinical sites will recruit 100 subjects each. Overall goals of the feasibility study are to provide opportunities to: 1) demonstrate that women at increased risk of breast cancer can be recruited to undertake a rather stringent dietary regimen; 2) prove that a dietary intervention can reduce substantially the level of fat intake in women over a six-month period; and 3) develop and test forms, procedures, organization and methods that will be needed if the full-scale trial is subsequently undertaken. The primary study endpoint is the occurrence of histologically-diagnosed breast cancer in women free of this condition. Secondary study endpoints include occurrence of cancer in a primary site, other than the breast or nonmelanotic skin cancer, and death from any cause.

The Nutrition Adjuvant Study (NAS) focuses on increasing the cancer-free interval and overall survival of women with Stage II breast cancer. The thrust for initiating the study was generated from the hypothesis that the research data pointing to fat as a cause of human breast cancer also suggest that fat plays a major role in the progression of the disease. Evidence for this hypothesis came from data on breast cancer patients in Japan where survival rates are significantly more favorable than in the U.S. population. These survival rate differences were more marked in post-menopausal populations than in pre-menopausal populations. The present feasibility phase of the Nutrition Adjuvant Study will test the overall research design in a small number of

breast cancer patients. The full scale trial will include
approximately 2,000 women with stage II surgically treated
breast cancer.

DIETARY FIBER

An expanding body of research findings suggests that
foods known to be high in fiber content have a significant
cancer prevention effect, especially with regard to colon
cancer (Bingham et al., 1979; Reddy, 1982). In a recent
literature review, 17 of 20 epidemiological studies showed
an inverse correlation between dietary fiber intake and
large bowel cancer (Greenwald and Lanza, 1985). The overall
data support the hypothesis that a high fiber diet has a
protective effect against colon cancer development.

Sufficient qualitative and quantitative information on
the content of total dietary fiber and its components in the
U.S. food supply is not available. The DCB is sponsoring
two major investigations in dietary fiber. One focuses on
improved methodology and analytical procedures to measure
total fiber and fiber components in foods. Subsequently,
these procedures will be used to analyze foods in the U.S.
food supply. The research will provide a reliable database
which will serve as an important research tool for dietary
assessment and intervention trials.

The other investigation focuses on the physiological
effects of dietary fiber in humans. The goal of this study
is to elucidate the role of dietary fiber in human carcinogenesis. Foci of investigation include the effects of
dietary fiber on: fecal mutagenic activity, fecal content
of bile salts and bile acids, fecal pH and oxidation/reduction
status, and colonic cell kinetics, morphology and physiology.
The data from these investigations are required for human
intervention trials.

VITAMIN A (RETINOIDS) AND CAROTENOIDS

Overall evidence to date is very strong in support of the
hypothesis that foods containing vitamin A, especially
those high in total carotenoids, may protect against some

cancers. The protective effect of these micronutrients appears to be most pronounced within a broad spectrum of epithelial cancers. Epidemiological studies have linked the intake of foods containing carotenoids and/or vitamin A with protection against lung cancer (Shekelle et al., 1981; Kvale et al., 1983; Palgi, 1984; Ziegler et al., 1981). Biochemical epidemiological studies of vitamin A and beta-carotene have also shown inverse relationships with cancer risk in some (Wald et al., 1980; Salonen et al., 1985) but not all instances (Wald et al., 1984; Willett et al., 1984). Also animal studies focused on vitamin A, retinol and retinoids have shown a cancer preventive effect over a wide spectrum of cancer sites (Kummet et al., 1983).

The homeostatic and metabolic controls of carotenoids and retinol in the human body are incompletely understood, and knowledge about the carotenoid and retinoid composition of foods is lacking. Based upon these research needs, the DCB has initiated two major studies.

One focuses on the methodology and analysis of retinoids and carotenoids in selected foods. The goal of this study is to aid in the development of sensitive analytical procedures to measure retinoids and carotenoids in food. Using these enhanced procedures, foods which are the major contributors of these components in the U.S. food supply will be analyzed. The resulting data will provide a database for calculation of dietary intake of these compounds in clinical trials, dietary interventions, dietary assessment studies and nutrition counseling.

The second study focuses on the metabolism and physio--logy of retinoids and carotenoids in humans. The goal of this study is to enhance the present level of understanding of the absorption, metabolism and physiological functions of dietary carotenoids and retinoids in humans. Specific study foci include: absorption of dietary retinoids and carotenoids, cleavage of these compounds in the intestinal mucosa, fate of the cleavage products and the regulatory mechanism controlling the rate of these events; extra-intestinal metabolism of various compounds of vitamin A and their significance and/or specificity on target tissues; organ and tissue concentrations and homeostatic control mechanisms; and effects of other dietary constituents on the absorption and utilization of retinoids and carotenoids.

In addition to the above two carotenoid/retinoid studies, DCB staff are also involved in the design, implementation and analysis of a study evaluating plasma carotenoid response to a single dose and long-term ingestion of beta-carotene and selected vegetables. The DCB staff are planning a project to analyze the metabolism of carotenoids and retinoids in humans using stable isotopes.

OTHER PROJECTS

The development of the International Food Composition Data System (INFOODS) project will provide a complete, reliable and comprehensive database on the nutrient and nonnutrient composition of foods, beverages and their ingredients (Butrum and Young, 1984). The objectives of this project are to: 1) develop a network between nutritional databases, professional workers and interested organizations; 2) establish standards and guidelines relating to nutritional data gathering, storage, interchange and usage; 3) maintain a secretariat (organization) to handle information collection, dissemination, coordination, need identification and resource allocation; and 4) establish an international journal devoted to food composition studies. The System's data will greatly enhance comprehensive studies of intakes of nutrients and other components of foodstuffs, including contaminants, toxic substances and non-nutritive chemicals and will support a variety of biomedical studies. Current diet and disease studies require data on the human requirements for essential nutrients and data on the ability of the food supply to provide these factors. In addition, information on other chemical components of food that represent protection for, or risk to, good health is needed. Such a comprehensive data system will be helpful in providing criteria for formulating public policy on diet-related health issues. To date, seven regional centers have been established: EUROFOODS (Western Europe), NORFOODS (Scandinavia), NOAFOODS (North America), LATINFOODS, (Latin America), MEDIFOODS (Mediterranean Countries), ASIAFOODS (Asia), AFRICAFOODS (North Africa and Middle East), and OCEANIAFOODS (Pacific Islands). Early plans are underway to promote regional groups covering Australia, New Zealand, and the Soviet Union and Eastern European nations.

Finally, DCB this year will fund a project titled the Modification of Eating Behaviors in Support of Future Clinical Trials. The rationale for the project lies in the fact that important behavior changes will have to be adopted by the community in order to maximally benefit from the findings of cancer research, e.g., eating and diet patterns may require alteration in order to come into accord with recommended cancer prevention dietary guidelines. The adoption of a recommended diet will not be easy for most people because eating habits are deeply ingrained. The Modification of Eating Behavior Project is designed to aid NCI researchers draw valid conclusions regarding the most effective and efficient sequence of intervention activities, the likely duration, and the level of effort required to achieve dietary interventions on an individual and group basis. The research will result in the development of validated methods and protocols for implementing dietary changes and serve as an important research tool for NCI in conducting future clinical intervention trials. The overall objective of the project is to develop new methodologies or perfect existing methodologies for the design, implementation, evaluation and standardization of dietary behavior modification procedures which will result in reduction of dietary fat intake from current U.S. levels ($> 40\%$) to $< 30\%$ of calories, and the approximate doubling of dietary fiber levels from the current average of $+ 11$ grams to 20-25 grams daily. The study will focus on both short and long term adherence to the recommended dietary fat and fiber intakes as well as monitor compliance through the use of biological markers.

The DCB supports three Clinical Nutrition Research Units (CNRU's), one each in Alabama, New York and California (Combs et al., 1984). These centers are part of a larger network of seven CNRUs; the remaining four centers are funded by the National Institute of Arthritis, Diabetes, Digestive and Kidney Diseases. The objectives of the CNRUs are to: 1) create and strengthen biochemical research within institutions for the purpose of developing new knowledge about specific nutrients in health, human development, and the prevention and treatment of disease, 2) to strengthen training environments in order to improve the education of medical students, medical staffs, practicing physicians and

paramedic personnel involved in clinical nutrition, and 3)
to enhance patient care and promote good health by focusing
attention on clinical nutrition and generating nutrition
information for the public.

FUTURE PROGRAM DIRECTIONS

As stated previously, the primary goal of the DCB's
program is to reduce the incidence of cancer through dietary
modification. The most compelling need presently is to
conduct large-scale human intervention trials which incorporate multiple dietary changes, including reduced fat,
increased fiber, and increased micronutrients. Studies of
this type have the potential for decreasing the risk of
cancer of many sites, including breast, colon, prostate,
endometrium, and lung, and thereby significantly reducing
the overall incidence of cancer. To address this need the
DCB will continue to fund its current programs and expand
initiatives in the following study areas: 1) etiologic
factors, 2) methodologic issues and behavioral modification,
and 3) human clinical trials.

Etiologic Factors

Etiological studies will be conducted to help select
and evaluate potential dietary factors in order to develop,
refine and test hypotheses of diet and cancer prevention.
Etiological study efforts currently planned or underway
include: 1) the analysis of dietary components of data obtained from national surveys, such as the National
Health and Nutrition Examination Surveys, to ascertain
correlations between diet and site-specific cancer incidence
and the cancer risk of defined racial and sex groups; 2)
the analysis of the effects of diet manipulation on the proliferation characteristics of colonic mucosa, and 3) the cond
of research to investigate the relationship of folic acid
intake and cancer incidence, specifically in relation to
cervical dysplasia.

The role of folic acid in cancer prevention will be an
added focus of research for DCB. The literature has suggeste
that this nutrient may have anti-carcinogenic characteristics
in humans. The thrust of DCB's efforts will be to evaluate

the folic acid status and requirements in man and conduct
epidemiological studies on folic acid and cancer.

Methodology for Diet and Cancer Research

Measurement tools are essential to dietary intervention
trials in humans. The DCB plans to support development
methods for collecting and automating dietary assessment
data for application in clinical trials. The goal of
dietary assessment is to find methods that accurately reflect
current and past food intake and which verify the biochemical
and anthropometric measures of the nutritional status of
study subjects. Accurate measurement of dietary compliance
is necessary for obtaining reliable data from clinical
intervention trials. The DCB gives priority to development and
improvement of dietary assessment methodologies and development of sensitive biological markers for measuring dietary
compliance.

Human Intervention Studies

Etiological and methodological studies are necessary
groundwork to the implementation of human intervention
studies in which dietary guidelines are tested as to their
efficiency in reducing the incidence of cancer in high risk
groups and the general population. Human intervention
trials planned by DCB in the near future include: 1) feasibility studies on colon and gastric cancer 2) dietary
interventions for high-risk occupation groups, and 3) pilot
testing a model community-based dietary intervention strategy
focusing on reducing intake of dietary fat and increasing
dietary fiber and vitamins A and C, through the selection
of specific types of food products.

A feasibility study is being developed to assess the
effects of diet on colon cancer incidence. The hypothesis to
be tested is that decreased fat and increased fiber and calcium intake will reduce the risk and incidence of colon
cancer. The study will include: 1) dietary modification and
monitoring compliance, and 2) evaluation of intermediate
endpoints to demonstrate the efficacy of dietary changes in
reducing the potential risk of cancer. If the feasibility
study proves positive, a full-scale controlled intervention
trial will be initiated.

A feasibility study on gastric cancer will test the hypothesis that precursor lesions (atrophic gastritis) which precede gastric cancer are influenced by diet. A pilot intervention which will also collect data on current and past dietary patterns, migrant status, occupation and other demographic data is being planned.

SUMMARY

Diet, perhaps more than any other environmental factor, has a significant potential for reducing the incidence of cancer. It has been projected that as much as 35 percent of all human cancer can be prevented through effective dietary modification strategies.

The comprehensive research program of the DCB significantly directs diet and cancer research toward the ultimate cancer prevention goal of modifying dietary habits of the general population for optimal health.

The DCB is currently supporting projects along the entire continuum from laboratory research to human intervention trials: basic research projects in food composition, encompassing dietary fiber, vitamin A and carotenoids and development of INFOODS; physiologic studies establishing safe and effective levels of dietary fiber and carotenoids; modification of eating behavior; human intervention trials of low fat diets in prevention of breast cancer; and clinical nutrition research units.

REFERENCES

Armstrong B, Doll R (1975). Environmental factors and cancer incidence and mortality in different countries, with special reference to dietary practices. Int J Cancer 15:617-631.

Bingham S, Williams DRR, Cole TJ, James WPT (1979). Dietary fiber and regional large-bowel cancer mortality in Britain. Rb J Cancer 40: 456-463.

Butrum R, Young VR (1984). Development of a nutrient data system for international use: INFOODS (International Network of Food Data Systems). JNCI, 73 (6): 1409-1413.

Carroll KK, Gammal EB, Plunkett ER (1968). Dietary fat and mammary cancer. Canadian Medical Association Journal 98: 590-591.

Carroll KK, Khor HT (1975). Dietary fat in relation to tumorigenesis. Prog Biochem Pharmacol 10: 308-353.

Combs GR, Suld ME, Gardner L, DeWys WD (1984). Report on clinical nutrition research units. American Journal of Clinical Nutrition 40: 855-864.

Correa P (1981). Epidemiological correlations between diet and cancer frequency. Cancer Res 41: 3685-3689.

Doll R, Peto R (1981). The causes of cancer: Quantitative estimates of avoidable risks of cancer in the United States today. JNCI 66: 1192-1308.

Gray GE, Pike MC, Henderson BE (1979). Breast cancer incidence and mortality rates in different countries in relation to known risk factors and dietary practices. Br J Cancer 39: 1-7, 1979.

Greenwald P, Lanza E (1985). Role of Dietary Fiber in the Prevention of Cancer. In: V. DeVita and S. Rosenberg (eds) Important Advances in Oncology New York, Lippincott

Kvale G, Bjelke E, Gart JJ (198). Dietary habits and lung cancer risk. Int. J. Cancer 3:397-405.

Kummet T, Moon TE, Meyskens Jr, FL (1983). Vitamin A: Evidence for its protective role in human cancer. Nutrition and Cancer 5(2):96-106, 1983.

Palgi A (1984). Vitamin A and lung cancer: A prospective. Nutrition and Cancer 6(2):105-120.

Reddy BS (1982). Dietary fiber and colon carcinogenesis: A critical review. In: Vahouny GV and Kritihesky D, (eds). Dietary Fiber in Health and Disease. New York: Plenum Press, 1982.

Salonen JT, Salonen R, Lappetelainer-Maenpaa PH, Alfthan G, Puska P (1985). Risk of cancer in relation to serum concentrations of selinium and vitamins A and E: Matched case-control anaylsis of prospective data. British Medical Journal, 290:417-420.

Shekelle RB, Liu S, Raynor Jr, WJ, Lepper M, Maliza C, Rossof AH (1981). Dietary vitamin A and risk of cancer in the Western Electric Study. Lancet:1185-1190.

Wald N, Idle M, Boreham J (1980). Low serum-vitamin-A and subsequent risk of cancer, Preliminary results of a prospective study. Lancet:813-815.

Wald NJ, Boreham J, Hayward JL, Bulbrook RD (1984). Plasma retinol, B-carotene and vitamin E levels in relation to the future risk of breast cancer. Br J Cancer 49: 321-324.

Willett WC, Polk BF, Underwood BA, Stampfer MJ, Pressel S, Rosner B, Taylor JO, Schneider K, Hames CG (1984). Relation of serum vitamins A and E and carotenoids to the risk of cancer. N Engl J Med 310:430-434.

Ziegler RG, Morris LE, Blot WJ, Pottern LM, Fraumeni Jr JF (1981). Esophageal cancer among black men in Washington, D.C. II. Role of nutrition. JNCI 67(6):1199-1206.

Dietary Fat and Cancer, pages 789–799
© 1986 Alan R. Liss, Inc.

CANCER AND DIET INTERACTIONS

Mark A. Bieber

Best Foods Research and Engineering Center,
CPC International, Union, NJ 07083

INTRODUCTION

Numerous recommendations have been proposed to lower
fat and to increase fiber, certain vitamins and minerals in
the hopes of reducing the risks from certain types of
cancer. The chapter by Campbell in this volume has outlined
these recommended changes and given a rationale for their
validity. This chapter shows that while moderate dietary
change is feasible, great care must be taken to ensure that
the best potential benefits are derived from the selected
changes and to caution against radical or severe dietary
changes which can be problematic.

FOOD PATTERNS

Food Selection. Diet modification must be undertaken
with care. The simple but often forgotten fact is that when
one component is decreased, another must be increased in
order to maintain a desired caloric intake. If fat intake
is to be lowered (and fiber intake increased), then it might
seem simple to ask people to eat less high fat foods, such
as oils, butter, margarine, high fat dairy and meat products
and more whole grains, legumes, beans, fruits and
vegetables. However, total food intake must increase
significantly to maintain caloric balance. The nutrient
density of foods replacing the higher fat, more nutrient
dense foods, is low. For the 34 million Americans who are
overweight (or overfat) (NIH, 1985) a caloric deficit could
occur with modest fat reduction; this could only be

beneficial for this population. However, in those persons
at desirable weight, further loss should not be encouraged.
Making appropriate food choices can actually be more
difficult than many people realize. Adequate nutrient
intakes must be maintained. In this regard, iron, zinc and
Vitamin B_{12} are especially important (Peterkin et al.,
1979); levels of these nutrients are very high in animal
foods which might be selected less frequently.
"Anti-nutritional factors" such as oxalates and phytates are
present in recommended foods which are high in fiber. As
well, proteinase inhibitors, chlorogenic acid, cyanogenetic
glycosides and other toxins are present in legumes and dark
leafy vegetables. There are no reliable data to indicate
that in a well nourished population any of these
anti-nutritionals have a significant impact on overall
health, growth or development. However, in less well
nourished populations where scarcity of and a lack of
variety in food sources exists, serious deficiencies have
been observed, such as zinc deficiency in Egypt (Prasad,
1985) or selenium deficiency in China (Guang-lu et al.
1985). Therefore, potential does exist for nutritional
problems in selected populations if food selection is poor.
The accepted way to guard against potential nutrient
imbalances is to select from the widest variety of foods
possible (USDA, 1979). The theme of balance, variety and
moderation has been repeated consistently and constantly in
all dietary recommendations.

Dietary Patterns. Peterkin et al. (1981) proposed
several eating patterns that would satisfy nutrient and
dietary guideline recommendations. Table 1 presents their
calculations. The usual pattern was determined from
analysis of the 1977-78 USDA Household Food Consumption
Survey. The patterns formulated were based on the premise
that new patterns should resemble current ones as closely as
possible with the following criteria: 1980 RDA for energy,
9 vitamins and 5 minerals; 30% of calories from fat; 10% of
calories each from saturated fat and sweeteners; and 300 mg
of cholesterol per day. A second diet, with all standards
relaxed by 15% was also derived. The major change is a
significant increase in bread consumption with a decrease in
fats and oils and eggs. Of course, many different dietary
patterns can be derived to fulfill any number of criteria.
However, this scheme, based on current patterns, is reasonable in that the overall impact on agriculture and the food
industry, except for eggs, is quite minimal. Walker (1983)

TABLE 1. A Day's Food, as Served, in Consumption Patterns and Diets that Meet Standards (from Peterkin et al., 1981)[a]

Food[b]	Unit	Number of Units per Day					
		Man 20-50 years			Women 20-50 years		
		Usual Pattern	Diet 1	Diet 2	Usual Pattern	Diet 1	Diet 2
vegetables, fruit	1/2 c	5.2	6.1	5.7	4.7	5.4	5.1
cereal, pasta, dry	1 oz[c]	1.5	3.1	2.6	1.2	2.6	2.1
bread[d]	1 sl	4.4	8.7	7.2	2.8	5.0	4.6
bakery products[d]	1 sl	1.4	1.7	1.9	1.0	1.0	1.2
milk, yogurt	1 c	1.2	1.3[e]	1.3[e]	0.8	0.9[e]	0.9[e]
cheese	1 oz	1.0	0.3	1.0	1.0	0.5	1.1
meat, poultry, fish, boned[f]	1 oz	7.3	7.1[g]	7.9[g]	4.8	7.6[g]	6.0[g]
eggs (per week)	no.	6.2	2.0	2.6	4.3	2.2	4.0
dry beans, peas, cooked; nuts	1/2 c	0.3	0.6[h]	0.4[h]	0.2	0.4[h]	0.3[h]
fats, oils	1 T	3.4	2.3[h]	2.4[h]	2.8	0.9[h]	1.7[h]
sugar, sweets	1 T	2.6	1.9	3.2	2.2	1.1	2.0
soft drinks, punches, ades	1 c	1.8	0.9	0.9	1.6	0.8	0.8

[a]Diet 1 meets standards drawn from 1980 RDAs and Dietary Goals; Diet 2 meets standards used for Diet 1 relaxed by 15 percent. Usual patterns are derived from the USDA 1977-78 National Food Consumption survey.
[b]Excludes commercially prepared mixtures except bakery products.
[c]1 oz. of dry cereal and pasta is about 1 serving.
[d]Bread is commercially prepared bread and bread assumed to have been made at home from flour and meal and some milk, fat, and sugar, in terms of food as purchased. Ingredients used in homemade bakery products in excess of those required to make bread are included in the groups of the ingredients. Bakery products shown are only commercially prepared types.
[e]Low-fat types.
[f]Includes bacon, sausage, and lunch meat.
[g]Only lean meat and poultry flesh are consumed.
[h]Primarily soft margarine and vegetable oils.

and Jollans (1984) both calculated the impact and feasibility of dietary change and concluded that modest change is achievable and would have minor disruptive impact on agriculture and the food industry.

DIETARY CHANGE

Dietary Fat Reduction. In reducing fat content the quality of the fat used should be monitored carefully. Results from experimental animal studies show that the requirement for essential fatty acids (EFA), although nominally placed at about 2% of calories, is quite variable (FAO, 1977). Animals eating diets high in fat, saturated fat (SFA), trans fatty acids or sugar seem to require more EFA to maintain their EFA status as indicated by triene/tetraene ratios (Holman, 1971; Holman, 1978) as well as cholesterol balance (Dupont et al., 1985) and maximal ex vivo prostaglandin synthesis (Mathias and Dupont, 1985). In much of past animal experimentation, the EFA level has been below that shown to produce maximal induced tumor growth and development. In a high fat diet, Ip et al. (1985) have shown that about 4% EFA by weight or about 8% of calories are needed for maximal tumor growth. Therefore, much of the past data indicating that polyunsaturated fatty acids (PUFA) are strong promoters of induced tumor growth compared to SFA are artifacts of the experiment due to a relative EFA deficiency in the high SFA diets. This also helps explain the observation that in high fat diets, some fats such as lard and olive oil promoted equally as well as corn or other high PUFA oils since enough EFA was supplied (Carroll and Khor, 1975; Dayton et al., 1977). In low fat diets, lard and olive oil acted more like SFA oils. If these animal models do have any relationship to the human experience, then a reduction in total fat, not PUFA might be called for; however, the ability to extrapolate from animal model data to the human situation has been seriously challenged (Wands and Visek, 1986). A balanced, varied diet of common foods contains significant PUFA levels (Goor, 1985).

Adequate PUFA Intake. Maintaining adequate PUFA intake is an important consideration in view of the wide body of research that shows that PUFA helps lower while SFA elevates serum cholesterol levels (McGandy and Hegsted, 1975). Numerous human studies have shown that at a high fat intake (>35% fat calories) PUFA has a significant effect on cholesterol levels (Schaefer et al., 1981; Gustafsson et al., 1985). At a low fat intake (<23% of fat calories) the effect is not as strong (Kuusi et al., 1985) and at very low fat intakes (<12% fat calories, Schaefer, et al., 1981) data seem to indicate that the quality of the fat is less important. The gray area is obviously then between the tested points of 35% and 23%, the target area for fat reduction to fall to. In long-term monkey feeding studies, Nicolosi et al. (1984) showed that in monkeys eating diets with 42 or 30 percent of calories from fat at P/S ratios of 0.45 or 1.0, the level of polyunsaturates was more important than reduction of fat intake to lower blood cholesterol levels. Therefore, without data, it seems essential to maintain adequate PUFA intake for maintenance of lowered serum cholesterol levels. As fat is reduced, if PUFA rich foods were preferentially deleted from the diet, a change in the national average P/S ratio could result leading to higher average serum cholesterol levels. Stamler (1985) has pointed to the radical decline in coronary heart disease observed over the past 15 years. He strongly cautions against any changes which would be counterproductive to this twenty-year trend.

As well as sustaining a lower blood cholesterol level, a fat-modified diet with adequate PUFA can result in lowered blood pressure and decreased platelet aggregation (Iacono and Dougherty, 1983) and better control of the diabetic (Houtsmuller, 1975). Therefore, not only might the risks of some cancers be decreased by use of a fat-modified diet, but that of heart disease as well. Peto et al. (1985) summarized results of 17 studies (involving 36,000 subjects) of cholesterol-lowering trials by diet and drugs to assess the impact on overall mortality. They concluded that the benefits of cholesterol-lowering were significantly stronger than any proposed risk of excess mortality from non-cardiovascular diseases.

Special Food Products. Food product standards could be formulated and implemented when knowledge of optimal nutrient intake to reduce disease risk becomes more definitive. This approach would circumvent the problems of slow and less effective mass nutrition education programs. In the meantime, dietary guidelines and nutrition education are the only viable courses of action. In order to effect dietary changes, the need for modified products has been

assessed. A conference held at the American Health
Foundation (Livingston et al., 1982) concluded that
modifying products was feasible and could be readily
accomplished if consumer demand were present to make these
products economically viable. Many fat-modified products
are currently available, e.g., low fat milk, egg
substitutes, filled cheeses, "no-oil" salad dressings. Some
of these products have been very successful; many have
failed. The food industry is capable of producing a myriad
of new products if consumer demand were high enough to
warrant it. However, it was also noted at the Conference
that the wide choice and variety of food currently available
in a typical supermarket provides the consumer with all the
foods necessary to follow diet recommendations. As well,
nutrition information is available for most foods in the
marketplace either through a nutrition information panel on
the label, point of purchase material in the supermarket
(which is growing in popularity), or directly from the food
manufacturer. The U.S. food supply is the largest and
safest in the world; if appropriate food choices are made
special products are not required.

ANIMAL AND EPIDEMIOLOGY DATA PERSPECTIVE

Data Presentation. Presentation format of data can
confuse or clarify the results. Many factors can confound
data interpretation. Tumor incidence or number of tumors
per tumor-bearing animal alone can be misleading under some
experimental conditions. For example, DMBA-induced mammary
tumors increase in number and size as dietary fat intake
increases but caloric restriction reduces tumor number and
size even at high fat intakes. However, since the total
number of animals with tumors may remain the same, it is
essential therefore to report tumor weight. Kritchevsky et
al. (1985) reported total tumor burden (tumor weight times
number per tumor-bearing animal) to give a clearer
indication of the impact of graded fat intake and caloric
restriction. Comparison of human nutrient and fiber intakes
on cancer incidence without correcting for caloric intake
can give totally opposite results (Willet and MacMahon,
1984).

Animal Diet. In interpreting data, especially from
induced tumor animal model experiments, attention must be
paid to diet variables. Comparison of dietary fats at

different intakes and with different levels of EFA appears
to have produced great confusion in the animal tumor model
literature. Most investigators have formulated diets with a
linoleic acid requirement based on a biochemical definition,
not to maximize tumor burden (Ip et al., 1985). Protein
content and type may influence the potential tumor yield.
Hawrylewicz (1983) has shown that a high protein diet leads
to greater tumor yield. However, experimental data of Visek
and Clinton (1983) do not support these conclusions. More
work obviously is needed. The National Research Council
Committees on Nutrient Requirements of Laboratory Animals
(1978) recommends a protein level of 12% for growth and 4.2%
for maintenance, while most natural ingredient or purified
diets contain about 20%. Nutter et al. (1983) showed that
in DMH-induced colon cancer, rats fed casein, whether at
high or low fat levels in the diet, developed significantly
more tumors than rats fed beef protein, especially when high
protein levels were fed.

Caloric Intake. Potentially more important than any
single dietary constituent may be total caloric intake or
the ad libitum pattern of feeding (O'Connor, 1985).
Although it has been widely believed that rats balance
caloric intake with expenditure, as rats age they definitely
gain excess weight, even in strains like the Fischer 344
which have been thought to be somewhat obesity resistant
(Solleveld et al., 1984). The recent experiments of
Kritchevsky et al. (1984, 1985), Ip et al. (1985) and
Pollard and Luckert (1985) all show that excess calories may
be the most significant determinant of eventual induced
tumor burden. Changing an ad libitum animal to any form of
caloric restriction, for example, allowing access to food
for a limited time, seems to reduce the eventual tumor load
(Ip, personal communication 1986). The idea that caloric
intake must be carefully considered is strengthened by a
reappraisal of past epidemiological cancer studies by Willet
and MacMahon (1984). This group recalculated nutrient
intakes per 1000 Kcals and found no relationships existed
between specific nutrient intakes and breast cancer.
However, a relationship between dietary fiber and colon
cancer emerged. The chapter by deWaard in this volume shows
that a correlation of breast cancer incidence to excess body
weight, and by inference increased caloric intake exists.
As well, Phillips and Snowdon (1985) and Nomura et al.
(1985) showed a strong relationship between body mass index
and colon cancer.

CONCLUSIONS

The promises of dietary change for reducing the risks of certain cancers have yet to be fulfilled in the way they have been for coronary heart disease risk reduction. Consumer education is desperately needed in food composition and selection so that a balanced and varied diet which meets nutrient requirements is chosen, and that the resultant dietary patterns have the potential to help reduce risk of all nutrition related degenerative diseases.

ACKNOWLEDGMENTS

I would like to thank Drs. R.E. Landers, M.J. Norvell and P.R. Wells for critical reading of the manuscript.

REFERENCES

Carroll KK, Khor HT (1975). Dietary fat in relation to tumorigenesis. Progr Biochem Pharmacol 10:308-353.
Dayton S, Hashimoto S, Wollman J (1975). Effect of high-oleic and high-linoleic safflower oils on mammary tumors induced in rats by 7,12-dimethylbenz(a)anthracene. J Nutr 107:1353-1360.
Dupont J, Ewens-Luby S, Mathias MM (1985). Cholesterol metabolism in relation to aging and dietary fat in rats and humans. Lipids 20:825-833.
Food and Agriculture Organization/World Health Organization (1977). Dietary fats and oils in human nutrition: Report of an expert consultation. FAO Food and Nutrition Paper No. 3, Rome.
Goor R, Hosking JD, Dennis BH, Graves KL, Waldman GT (1985). Nutrient intakes among selected North American populations in the Lipid Research Clinics Prevalence Study: Composition of fat intake. Am J Clin Nutr 41:299-311.
Guang-lu X, Shan-yang H, Hong-bin S, Jung-kui X (1985). Keshan disease and selenium deficiency. Nutr Res 5(I):S-187-S-192.
Gustafsson I-B, Vessby B, Karlstrom B, Boberg J, Boberg M, Lithell H (1985). Effects on the serum lipoprotein concentrations by lipid-lowering diets with different fatty acid compositions. J Am Coll Nutr 4:241-248.

Hawrylewicz EJ, Huang HH, Kissane JQ, Drab EA (1982). Enhancement of 7,12-dimethylbenz(a)anthracene (DMBA) mammary tumorigenesis by high dietary protein in rats. Nutr Rep Intl 26:793-806.

Holman RT (1971). Biological activities of and requirements for polyunsaturated acids. Progr Chem Fats Other Lipids 9:611-682.

Holman RT (1978). How essential are essential fatty acids? J Am Oil Chem Soc 55:774A-81A.

Houtsmuller AJ (1975). The role of fat in the treatment of diabetes mellitus. In Vergroesen AJ (ed): "The Role of Fats in Human Nutrition," New York: Academic Press, pp 231-302.

Iacono JM, Dougherty RM (1983). The role of dietary polyunsaturated fatty acids and prostaglandins in reducing blood pressure and improving thrombogenic indices. Prev Med 12:60-69.

Ip C, Carter CA, Ip MM, (1985). Requirement of essential fatty acid for mammary tumorigenesis in the rat. Cancer Res 45:1997-2001.

Jollans JL (1984). Implementing the NACNE report: An agricultural viewpoint. Lancet 1:382-384.

Kritchevsky D, Weber MM, Klurfeld DM (1984). Dietary fat versus caloric content in initiation and promotion of 7,12-dimethylbenz(a)anthracene-induced mammary tumorigenesis in rats. Cancer Res 44:3174-3177.

Kritchevsky D, Weber MM, Klurfeld DM (1985). Calories, fat and cancer. Fed Proc 44:411.

Kuusi T, Enholm C, Huttunen JK, Kostiainen E, Pietinen P, Leino U, Uusitalo U, Nikkari T, Iacono JM, Puska P (1985). Concentration and composition of serum lipoproteins during a low-fat diet at two levels of polyunsaturated fat. J Lipid Res 26:360-367.

Livingston GE, Moshy RJ, Chang CM (1982). "The Role of Food Product Development in Implementing Dietary Guidelines." Westport, CT: Food & Nutrition Press.

Mathias MM, Dupont J (1985). Quantitative relationships between dietary linoleate and prostaglandin (eicosanoid) biosynthesis. Lipids 20:791-801.

McGandy RB, Hegsted DM (1975). Quantitative effects of dietary fat and cholesterol on serum cholesterol in man. In Vergroesen AJ (ed): "The Role of Fats in Human Nutrition." New York: Academic Press, pp 221-230.

National Institutes of Health (1985). Health implications of obesity. Consensus Development Conference Statement 5:No. 9.

National Research Council (1978). Nutrient Requirements of Laboratory Animals, 3rd revised edition. Washington, DC: National Academy Press.

Nicolosi RJ, Hegsted DM, Hartley LH (1984). Lipoprotein levels with the American Heart Association (AHA) recommended diet. Circulation 70(II):291.

Nomura A, Heilbrun LK, Stemmermann GN (1985). Body mass index as a predictor of cancer in man. J Natl Cancer Inst 74: 319-323.

Nutter RL, Gridley DS, Kettering JD, Goude AG, Slater JM (1983). BALB/c mice fed milk or beef protein: Differences in response to 1,2-dimethylhydrazine carcinogenesis. J Natl Cancer Inst 71:867-874.

O'Connor TP (1985). Dietary fat, calories and cancer. Contemp Nutr 10:No. 7.

Peterkin BB, Shore CJ, Kerr RL (1979). Some diets that meet the dietary goals for the United States. J Am Diet Assoc 74:423-430.

Peterkin BB, Patterson PC, Blum AJ, Kerr RL (1981). Changes in dietary patterns: One approach to meeting standards. J Am Diet Assoc 78:453-459.

Peto R, Yusuf S, Collins R (1985). Cholesterol-lowering trial results in their epidemiologic context. Circulation 72(II):451.

Phillips RL, Snowdon DA (1985). Dietary relatioships with fatal colorectal cancer among Seventh-Day Adventists. J Natl Cancer Inst 74:307-317.

Pollard M, Luckert PH (1985). Tumorigenic effects of direct- and indirect-acting chemical carcinogens in rats on a restricted diet. J Natl Cancer Inst 74:1347-1349.

Prasad AS (1985). Clinical and biochemical manifestations of zinc deficiency in human subjects. J Am Coll Nutr 4:65-72.

Schaefer EJ, Levy RI, Ernst ND, VanSant FD, Brewer HB (1981). The effects of low cholesterol, high polyunsaturated fat, and low fat diets on plasma lipid and lipoprotein cholesterol levels in normal and hypercholesterolemic subjects. Am J Clin Nutr 34:1758-1763.

Solleveld HA, Haseman JK and McConnell EE (1984). Natural history of body weight gain, survival, and neoplasia in the F-344 rat. J Natl Cancer Inst 72:929-940.

Stamler J (1985). Coronary heart disease: Doing the "right things". N Engl J Med 312:1053-1055.

U.S. Dept Agriculture (1979). "Food." Sience and Education
   Administration, Home & Garden Bulletin No. 228.
Visek WJ, Clinton SK (1983). Dietary fat and breast cancer.
   In Perkins EG, Visek WJ (eds): "Dietary Fats and Health,"
   Champaign, IL: American Oil Chemists' Society,
   pp 721-740.
Walker CJ (1983). Implementing the NACNE report. Lancet
   2:1351-1356.
Wands RC, Visek WJ (1986). "Symposium on the Biological
   Bases for Interspecies Extrapolation of Carcinogenicity
   Data." Bethesda, MD: Life Science Research Office, FASEB.
Willett WC, MacMahon B (1984). Diet and cancer -- an
   overview. N Engl J Med 310:697-703.

Dietary Fat and Cancer, pages 801–814
© 1986 Alan R. Liss, Inc.

DIETARY FAT AND CANCER: A PERSPECTIVE FROM THE LIVESTOCK AND MEAT INDUSTRY

Donald M. Kinsman, Department of Animal Sciences, University of Connecticut, Storrs, CT 06268

George D. Wilson, American Meat Institute, Washington, DC 20007

Introduction

The current concern about dietary fat and its influence on human health is a major factor in the food consumption trends in the U.S.A. These concerns were initiated first by calories and weight control, then the cholesterol impact, followed by atherosclerosis and hypertension, each of which was considered closely associated with fat intake. Most recently, the correlation with various cancers has given added impetus to studies of the effects of dietary fat.

It is generally recognized that one should maintain a reasonable weight for one's height, body type and age. This necessitates consuming no more calories or energy than one expends physically. Many factors are involved in this balance of intake-output including age, exercise, life-style, stress, eating habits, sources of nutrients and dietary balance. It is also generally conceded that the types of fat may play an important role in health. A balance of saturated and unsaturated fats is important as is the relationship of plant and animal fats toward maintaining a proper equilibrium in health. The most recent U.S. dietary recommendations (1985) suggest a reduction of approximately 10% in fat intake; that not over 30% of our caloric intake come from dietary fat and that saturated fat provide no more than 10% of these total calories. In addition, a daily dietary limit of 300mg of cholesterol is recommended.

The second edition of "Dietary Guidelines for Americans," commissioned by the National Academy of Sciences and released in September 1985, reflects the latest thinking of a panel of nine distinguished nutrition scientists. One part of the report expresses concerns about the link between diet and some forms of cancer, but does not express a definitive cause and effect relationship between the two nor does it point to any one element, such as dietary fat in any of these associations. In an attempt to provide a first line of defense against certain chronic diseases, the panel recommends:

*Eat a variety of foods
*Maintain desirable weight
*Avoid too much fat, saturated fat and cholesterol.
*Eat foods adequate in starch and fiber.
*Avoid too much sugar.
*Avoid too much salt.
*If you drink alchoholic beverages, do so in moderation.

When one considers the leading causes of death in the U.S.A., it is of great interest to note the changing patterns in this century alone and to ponder the causes for this shift in rank in conjunction with the many factors that have changed during that 80-year period. Is diet a major consideration in the two conditions that have elevated so dramatically, heart disease (41.6% points) and cancer (17.2% points)? Do our national nutritional habits account for these changes in part or in whole?

Animal Products Trends

Ever since the domestication of animals, man has attempted to mold their attributes to his needs for food, fiber and draft purposes as well as companionship. With food-producing animals, there is a natural tendency to store fat in and on the body for reserve requirements. The sequence of fat deposition which is nature's way of providing reserve energy for the animal is internally, around the kidneys and heart and in the pelvic region; intermuscularly as "seam" fat; externally or subcutaneously over the carcass; and intramuscularly, between the muscle bundles and muscle fibers as marbling.

Through improved selection, genetics, nutrition and management practices, livestock producers have succeeded in reducing the fat content of U.S. meat animals. Consequently, there is a lesser degree of fat at any of the aforementioned locations, and that fact is reflected in the U.S.D.A. meat grading standards that now require less marbling and external fat for a given quality and yield grade. Furthermore, meat animals are marketed at a much younger age and therefore have less fat deposited and consequently becomes less highly-saturated in that abbreviated time. It is estimated that in the most recent 30 years alone (1950-1980) muscle or lean meat production per head has increased some 6% in beef and lamb, and 30% in pork with corresponding reductions in fat or adipose tissue without sacrificing palatability or quality of product. Although the consumption of fat increased approximately 25% (125g per capita to 159g) in the period of 1909 -1978, fat from animal sources declined from 104g to 91g per capita during that same period of time. Thus, the increases in fat consumption in the U.S.A. are entirely attributable to vegetable sources. (Figure 1).

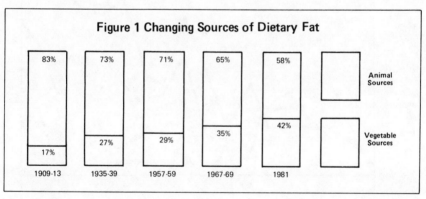

Figure 1 Changing Sources of Dietary Fat

Source: AMI compilation of data from U.S.D.A. and R. Marston and S. Welsh, "Nutrient Content of the U.S. Food Supply, 1981," National Food Review, NFR-21, 1983

In general, our sources of energy in U.S.A. diets are approximately 16% from protein, 40% from carbohydrates and 44% from fats of all kinds. The dietary fats are derived, on the average, from:

1)	meat, poultry, fish	–	40%
2)	milk products	–	15%
3)	eggs	–	15%
4)	fats and oils	–	15%
5)	grains and legumes	–	8%
6)	fruits and vegetables	–	7%

One should recognize that these figures vary by age group.

The 1985 U.S.D.A. Agriculture Handbook #652 depicting the trends in food consumption, portrays a definite increase in ingestion of all foods during the past 20 years, with crop products distinctly out-distancing animal products 10.6% vs. 4% respectively. (Figure 2).

Figure 2 Per Capita Consumption of Foods

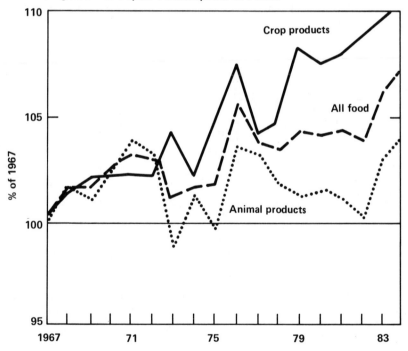

When one studies the U.S. per capita consumption of selected animal products, it is obvious that poultry is up markedly (49%), egg consumption is down (19% less today than in 1967), red meat is down slightly (-3%), dairy (mainly cheese) has risen 5% and fish is up approximately 25%. (Figure 3).

Figure 3 Per Capita Consumption of Selected Animal Products

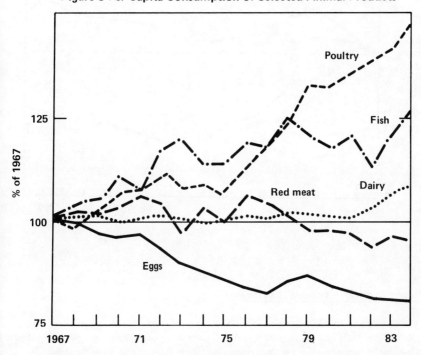

Therefore, the foods containing the more unsaturated fat (crop products, poultry and fish) have made noticeable increases, and the more saturated fat carrying foods (red meats and dairy products) have decreased or increased only modestly. More significantly, the per capita consumption of total fats and oils has increased 14% which is the net effect of a 40% increase in vegetable oils and a 20% decrease in animal fats since 1967. (Figure 4).

Figure 4 Per Capita Consumption of Fats and Oils

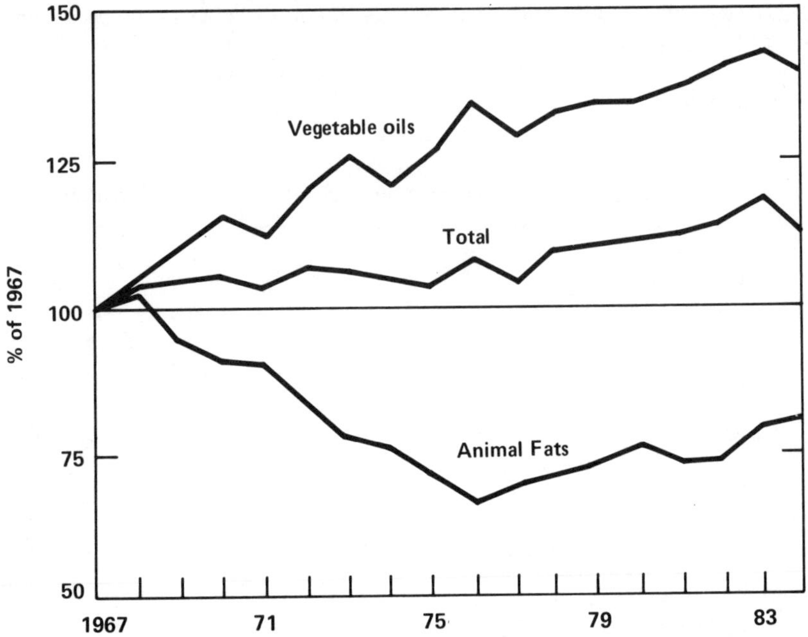

Animal fats include butter.

Meat Consumption Patterns

U.S. health care officials and health organizations recommend daily consumption of 4 to 6 ounces per person from the meat group. The recommendation is based on actual ingested product excluding fat and bone. Often food and meat consumption figures are quoted on a basis of national raw material produced divided by population. (Figure 5). Thus, the total production of red meat animal carcass weight is approximately 170 pounds of red meat consumed per person annually (7.5 ozs/day). However, when one realizes that carcass weight includes trimmable fat, bone and connective tissue representing approximately 35% inedible tissue, the 170 pounds total is reduced to a more realistic 110 pounds edible raw meat. Cooking losses average approximately 25% due to fat drippings and moisture loss, thus reducing the actual annual consumption of red meat in the U.S. to approximately 85 pounds, assuming that no other losses occur from slaughter to consumption and what is served is consumed. This annual consumption of 85 pounds is 3.73 ounces of red meat per day. (Figure 6).

Figure 5 Per Capita Disappearance of Red Meat, Carcass & Retail Weight Basis, 1960 - 84

	BEEF		VEAL		PORK		LAMB & MUTTON		TOTAL RED MEAT	
	Carcass	Retail	Carcass	Retail	Carcass	Retail	Carcass	Retail	Carcass	Retail
1960	85.1	64.2	6.1	5.2	64.9	60.3	4.8	4.3	160.9	134.0
1961	87.8	65.8	5.6	4.7	62.0	57.7	5.1	4.5	160.5	132.7
1962	88.9	66.2	5.5	4.6	63.5	59.1	5.2	4.6	163.1	134.5
1963	94.4	69.9	4.9	4.1	65.4	61.0	4.9	4.4	169.6	139.4
1964	99.9	73.9	5.2	4.3	65.4	61.0	4.2	3.7	174.7	142.9
1965	99.5	73.6	5.2	4.3	58.7	54.7	3.7	3.3	167.1	135.9
1966	104.1	77.0	4.6	3.8	58.1	54.4	4.0	3.6	170.8	138.8
1967	106.5	78.8	3.8	3.2	64.1	60.0	3.9	3.5	178.3	145.5
1968	109.7	81.2	3.6	3.0	66.2	61.4	3.7	3.3	183.2	148.9
1969	110.8	82.0	3.3	2.7	65.0	60.5	3.5	3.1	182.6	148.3
1970	113.5	84.0	2.9	2.4	66.4	62.3	3.2	2.9	186.0	151.6
1971	112.7	83.4	2.7	2.2	73.0	68.3	3.2	2.8	191.5	156.7
1972	115.5	85.4	2.2	1.9	67.4	62.9	3.3	2.9	188.4	153.1
1973	108.8	80.5	1.8	1.5	61.6	57.3	2.6	2.4	174.8	141.7
1974	115.7	85.6	2.3	1.9	66.6	61.8	2.3	2.0	186.9	151.3
1975	118.8	87.9	4.1	3.4	54.8	50.7	2.0	1.8	179.7	143.7
1976	127.5	94.4	4.0	3.3	58.2	53.7	1.8	1.6	191.5	153.0
1977	124.0	91.8	3.8	3.2	60.5	55.8	1.7	1.5	190.0	152.3
1978	117.9	87.2	2.9	2.4	60.3	55.9	1.6	1.4	182.7	146.9
1979	105.5	78.0	2.0	1.7	68.8	63.8	1.5	1.3	177.8	144.8
1980	103.4	76.5	1.8	1.5	73.5	68.3	1.5	1.4	180.2	147.7
1981	104.2	77.1	1.9	1.6	69.9	65.0	1.6	1.4	177.6	145.1
1982	104.3	77.2	2.0	1.6	62.7	59.0	1.7	1.5	170.6	139.3
1983	106.4	78.7	2.0	1.6	66.2	62.2	1.7	1.5	176.2	144.1
1984	106.2	78.6	2.2	1.8	65.7	61.7	1.7	1.5	175.7	143.7

Source: U.S. Department of Agriculture

For reasons attributable to animal characteristics, traditional consumer tastes, technological capability and economics the fat content of meat products ranges from 5 to 50% but an estimate by product class shows they average less than 24%. With increased emphasis on reducing the fat on meat, the average percentage of fat is probably less. However, if the average is as high as 24%, 3.73 ounces of cooked meat contains 25.4 gms of fat. The above estimates are in good agreement with National Live Stock and Meat Board (NLSMB) 1985 calculations of 3.9 ounces of total meat and 23.7 grams of fat per day. However, using the larger of the estimates the total contribution of animal fat is less than 11.4% of a 2000 kcal diet. The saturated fat contribution is

Figure 6 Per Capita Disappearance and Actual Consumption of Red Meat

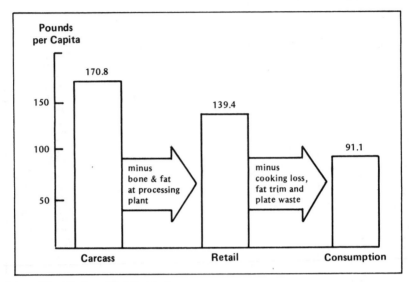

Source: "Contribution of Red Meat to the
U.S. Diet," National Live Stock and Meat
Board

Note: Figures are for 1982

about 11.4 grams and represent 5.1% of a 2000 kcal diet. These estimates clearly indicate that average red meat consumption is not excessive and are well within the recommended dietary guidelines for fat and saturated fat intake from red meat sources. (Figure 7).

Today's consumer is increasingly aware of the association of diet and health. According to a report entitled, "The Consumer Climate for Red Meat," conducted by Yankelovich, Skelly and White (1985), there has been a significant shift in terms of increased support for diet and health factors relative to the purchase and consumption of red meat. Concerns about diet and health were evident among 2 out of 3 consumers. Those consumers classified as adhering to an "active lifestyle" who were regular meat consumers increased from 16% in 1983 to 26% in 1985; and those who were "health-oriented" increased from 17% to 24% during the last two years. About 90% of those interviewed reported

Figure 7
Per Capita Disappearance of Red Meat,
Poultry & Fish, Retail Weight Basis, 1960 - 84

	TOTAL RED MEAT	VARIETY MEATS	POULTRY	FISH	TOTAL RED MEAT, POULTRY AND FISH
			Pounds		
1960	134.0	10.9	34.0	10.3	189.2
1961	132.7	10.7	37.3	10.7	191.4
1962	134.5	10.7	36.8	10.6.	192.6
1963	139.4	10.1	37.6	10.7	197.8
1964	142.9	11.1	38.5	10.5	203.0
1965	135.9	10.4	40.7	10.8	197.8
1966	138.8	10.6	43.4	10.9	203.7
1967	145.5	11.1	44.9	10.6	212.1
1968	148.9	11.2	44.6	11.0	215.7
1969	148.3	11.0	46.7	11.2	217.2
1970	151.6	11.2	48.4	11.8	223.0
1971	156.7	11.3	48.5	11.5	228.0
1972	153.1	10.8	50.7	12.5	227.1
1973	141.7	9.8	48.9	12.8	213.2
1974	151.3	10.7	49.5	12.1	223.6
1975	143.7	10.2	48.6	12.2	214.6
1976	153.0	10.6	51.8	12.9	228.3
1977	152.3	10.4	53.2	12.7	228.6
1978	146.9	9.5	55.9	13.4	225.7
1979	144.8	10.4	60.5	13.0	228.7
1980	147.7	9.5	60.6	12.8	230.6
1981	145.1	9.4	62.4	12.9	229.8
1982	139.3	8.7	63.9	12.3	224.2
1983	144.1	9.1	65.1	13.1	231.4
1984	143.7	9.1	67.1	13.6	233.5

Source: U.S. Department of Agriculture

Meat Consumption Shares

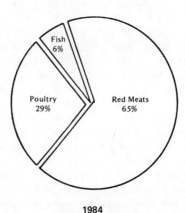

1984
Includes variety meats

exercising care with respect to fat intake. A high level of consumer responsiveness to the concept of leaner, calorie-reduced meat products was obvious. It was also evident that their concern was principally <u>amount</u> of fat intake rather than type or source of fat.

Animal Fats in the Future

A desire and demand on the part of consumers for reduced fatness of animal products - red meat, poultry and dairy products has been noted and heeded by the livestock and meat industry. There has been a reduction in the production of animal fats and a reduction in the amount of fat in both fresh and processed products. The accompanying diagram, based on NLSMB (1984) data, demonstrates the current red meat:fat:calorie:diet relationship which appears to have a proper balance and is within the recommendations (Figure 8).

Some genetic variation exists in livestock and can and is being utilized to change the fat composition of animals and their products. Additionally, carcass composition is primarily a function of body weight and/or maturity. Thus, feeding the ration that produces the most economical gains and marketing the animals at reduced body weights will limit carcass fat.

The livestock and meat industry is interested in providing the most wholesome and healthful products possible to the consuming public. The meat industry currently provides lean meat products ranging from closely-trimmed, lean, primal cuts to almost completely fat-free cold cuts and other processed meats. It should be recognized, however, that some fat in these products is a necessary component which contributes very significantly to the flavor and other sensory qualities of these highly-nutritious products contributing proteins, vitamins, minerals, essential fatty acids and energy as well as satiety to a complete and balanced diet.

The development of many "Lite" (meat) products with a 25% reduction in fat from the existing standards is commonplace today. This reduction in fat represents a 20% reduction in calories on the average. "Lean" and "Extra Lean" hams and other prepared meat with 10% and 5% fat respectively are also a growing market segment. Undoubtedly,

Figure 8 Fat and Calories from Average Daily Meat Consumption

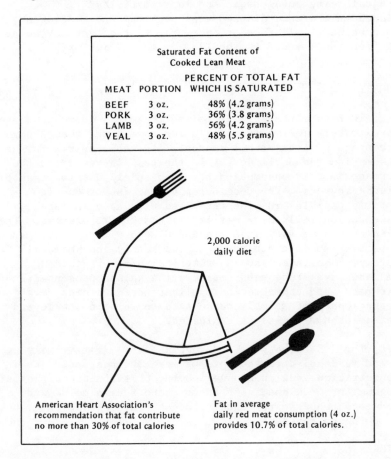

Saturated Fat Content of Cooked Lean Meat		
MEAT	PORTION	PERCENT OF TOTAL FAT WHICH IS SATURATED
BEEF	3 oz.	48% (4.2 grams)
PORK	3 oz.	36% (3.8 grams)
LAMB	3 oz.	56% (4.2 grams)
VEAL	3 oz.	48% (5.5 grams)

2,000 calorie daily diet

American Heart Association's recommendation that fat contribute no more than 30% of total calories

Fat in average daily red meat consumption (4 oz.) provides 10.7% of total calories.

the present trend toward a reduction in the production and consumption of fats of animal origin will continue and efforts will continue to modify fats to meet the nutritional requirements of the U.S. consumer. As research findings uncover new knowledge, the meat industry will adjust its action accordingly. The recent discovery of the anticarcinogenic activity of fried ground beef which resulted in up to 44% reduction in tumors in mice is noteworthy and may well lead to other investigations concerning the relationship of diet and especially dietary fats and red meat to cancer (Pariza and Hargraves, 1984). Can it be that those foods which have been identified as containing mutagens also have balancing mutagenesis modulator activity? If so, balanced diets and balanced meal patterns and moderation in consumption of all food products may be the best advice as has been recommended by the 1985 Dietary Guidelines for Americans.

SUMMARY

It has been a popular belief that U.S. consumers ingest approximately 40% of their calories as fat and that a high percentage is from animal sources. In fact, animal fat consumption has declined 23% in the past 20 years and the increase in fat consumption has been solely due to vegetable (plant) sources. The decline in animal fat production probably explains why the estimates discussed in this presentation fall below earlier literature references. The validity of the estimates presented here will be determined as part of an in depth study undertaken by the National Academy of Sciences' Board of Agriculture. If this comprehensive study substantiates the values presented in this paper and other recent publications, a reconsideration of the impact of animal source fats on caloric intake and diet related diseases is indicated.

The U.S. livestock and meat industry is extremely aware of and responsive to the role of meat and meat products in the nutrition, health and well-being of the nation. Research programs are designed with these factors as a guide and producers continue to adjust product characteristics to meet the changing needs.

REFERENCES

American Meat Institute. 1985. Meatfacts: a statistical summary about America's largest food industry. Washington, DC.

Breidenstein, B.C. 1984. Food and Nutrition News. National Live Stock and Meat Board. Chicago, IL.

Breidenstein, B.C. 1985. Red meat: nutrient composition and actual consumption. National Live Stock and Meat Board. Chicago, IL.

Council for Agricultural Science and Technology. 1980. Food
    from animals. CAST Report No. 82. Ames, IA.

Hoover, S. R. 1973. Research into foods from animal
    sources: I. Controlling level and type of fat; II.
    Developments in beef and dairy products. Pre. Med. 2:(I)
    346-360; 2:(II) 361-365.

Leveille, G. A. 1974. Issues in human nutrition and their
    probable impact on foods of animal origin. J. Anim.
    Sci. 41(2):723.

National Research Council, National Academy of
    Sciences, Food and Nutrition Board. 1976.
    Fat content and composition of animal
    products. Symposium Proceedings.
    Washington, DC.

National Research Council, National Academy of Sciences, Food
    and Nutrition Council. 1980. Toward healthful diets.
    Washington, D.C.

National Research Council, National Academy of Sciences,
    Committee on Diet, Nutrition and Cancer. 1982. Diet,
    nutrition and cancer. National Academy Press.
    Washington, D.C.

Pariza, M. W. and W. A. Hargraves. 1985. A beef-derived
    mutagenesis modulator inhibits initiation of mouse
    epidermal tumors by 7,12-dimethylbenz(a)anthracene.
    Carcinogenesis 6: 591-593.

National Research Council, National Academy of Sciences,
    1985 Committee on Technical Options to Improve
    Nutritional Attributes of Animal Products.
    Washington, DC. (Completion date, 1986)

Paul, D.L. and Foget, K.S. 1983. Leaner products in the
    meat industry. Proc. Meat Industry Research Conf. pps.
    23-37. Washington, D.C.

Reiser, R. 1973. Saturated fat in the diet and serum
    cholesterol concentration: a critical examination of the
    literature. Am. Jnl. Clinical Nutr. 26(5):524-555.

USDA 1984/85. Handbook No. 8 Composition of foods.
Washington, D.C.

USDA and U.S. Dept. of Health and Human Services. 1985.
Nutrition and your health: Dietary Guidelines for
Americans. Second edition. Washington, D.C.

USDA 1985. Agricultural Chartbook, Agricultural Handbook No.
652. Washington, D.C.

Yankelovich, Skelly and White. 1985. The consumer climate
for red meat. Executive summary prepared for American
Meat Institute. Washington, D.C.

Dietary Fat and Cancer, pages 815–861
© 1986 Alan R. Liss, Inc.

CHANGING PATTERNS IN THE DAIRY INDUSTRY

Lois D. McBean, Emerita N. Alcantara, and
Elwood W. Speckmann

National Dairy Council
Rosemont, Illinois 60018

INTRODUCTION

As the second leading cause of death in the United
States, cancer is projected to be responsible for an
estimated 472,000 deaths in 1986 (American Cancer Society,
1986). For this same year, the American Cancer Society
(1986) estimates that 930,000 new cases of cancer will be
diagnosed. Despite these alarming statistics, age-adjusted
cancer death rates for nearly all forms of cancer have
remained stable and, in some cases (e.g., stomach and uterine
cancer), actually have declined over the past five decades
(American Cancer Society, 1986; Figure 1). An exception is
the increase in lung cancer which is attributed to tobacco
smoking. The specific cause of most other cancers remains
unknown (Doll and Peto, 1981).

While heredity undoubtedly influences cancer risk,
epidemiological findings of worldwide differences in cancer
incidence and changes in incidence with migration suggest
that environmental factors may be more important than genetic
factors in cancer causation (Armstrong and Doll, 1975; Doll
and Peto, 1981; Committee on Diet, Nutrition and Cancer
1982). On the basis of epidemiologic data, Wynder and Gori
(1977) estimated that 80 to 84% of human cancer incidence is
caused by environmental, life-style, and occupational
factors. Tobacco smoking, alcohol, occupational hazards,
viruses, environmental pollutants, medicines (e.g.,
estrogens), and dietary deficiencies and excesses are among
the various environmental factors incriminated in cancer
causation (Doll and Peto, 1981).

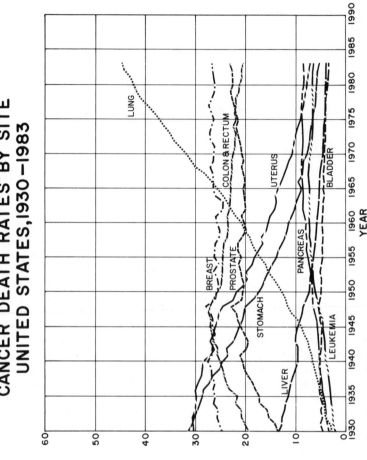

CANCER DEATH RATES* BY SITE
UNITED STATES, 1930–1983

RATE PER 100,000 POPULATION

YEAR

EPIDEMIOLOGY & STATISTICS DEPT.
AMERICAN CANCER SOCIETY, 2-86

FIGURE 1

* Rate for the population standardized for age on the 1970 U.S. population
  Sources of Data: National Center for Health Statistics and
  Bureau of the Census, United States.

Note: Rates are for both sexes combined except breast and uterus female population only
  and prostate male population only.

While findings from experimental studies conducted more than 40 years ago reveal an association between diet and cancer (Tannenbaum, 1942), only recently has the importance of diet and nutrition as determinants of the risk of developing certain types of cancer received considerable attention (Committee on Diet, Nutrition and Cancer, 1982; Lowenthal, 1983; National Cancer Institute, 1985). However, the extent to which diet contributes to cancer incidence and mortality is controversial (Brown, 1983). The Committee on Diet, Nutrition and Cancer (1982), after a comprehensive assessment of the evidence linking diet and nutrition to cancer, was unable to quantitate the contribution of diet to overall cancer risk.

With respect to diet, fat intake has been singled out as one of the most prominent factors responsible for differences in incidence rates of various cancers particularly those of the breast, colon, and prostate. (Armstrong and Doll, 1975; Doll and Peto, 1981; Committee on Diet, Nutrition and Cancer, 1982). Although the relationship between dietary fat and cancer has yet to be precisely defined, dietary recommen-dations have been issued to the American public to reduce total fat intake and some fat-containing foods including certain dairy products to decrease the risk of this disease (Committee on Diet, Nutrition and Cancer, 1982; American Cancer Society, 1984; National Cancer Institute, 1984). This raises questions regarding how much fat in our diet comes from dairy products and what adjustments consumers have made in their intake of foods in this food group.

This chapter reviews changes in dairy product consump-tion and the dairy industry's response to changes in consumer demands for their products. In addition, data on dietary fat and cancer in relation to dairy products will be addressed. The evidence presented below shows that not only is the link between dietary fat in general and fat in dairy products in particular inconsistent, but other nutrients and components in dairy foods (e.g., calcium, bacterial cultures in cultured dairy foods) may protect against specific types of cancer.

CHANGES IN DAIRY PRODUCT CONSUMPTION

During this century there have been significant changes in the consumption of dairy products and dietary fat, as well as the contribution of dairy products to total fat intake (Rizek et al., 1983). While total fat available in the nation's food supply has increased since the beginning of the century, most of this increase is explained by the greater availability of vegetable sources of fat. Overall consumption of dairy foods has declined with foods in this group providing a smaller percentage of fat available in the 1980s than in the early 1900s. Moreover, dairy foods supply a much smaller percentage of fat available (i.e., 11.4%) than either fats and oils (44.7%) or meat, poultry, and fish (34.1%). Actual food intake data from national surveys support these findings. Within the dairy group, there has been a shift in preferences for specific dairy foods. For example, per capita consumption of fluid whole milk and buttermilk has declined whereas that of lowfat milk, yogurt, and most types of cheeses has increased. This means that within the dairy group, fluid whole milk is providing a smaller share of fat than in earlier years and that the contribution of fat from lowfat milk and cheeses is greater than in earlier years. Compared to 1909-13, cholesterol in the food supply and the percentage contributed by dairy foods (i.e., 15%) are about the same in the 1980s.

Availability of Dairy Foods

Most of the information on food intake is obtained indirectly by per capita "disappearance" data or sales figures. This information reveals the amount of food available or sold and not actual intake. Nevertheless, such data are useful for tracking trends in food consumption (Rados, 1985).

Dairy foods traditionally have been an important part of the American diet, accounting for almost 22% of the 1,423 lbs of food used per capita in 1983 (Bunch, 1985a). However, over the past two decades, there has been a significant and steady decline in the overall consumption of dairy foods (Bunch, 1985a). For example, in 1983 the average American used 307 lbs of dairy foods which is 49 lbs less than 20 years earlier (i.e., 356 lbs) (Bunch, 1985a). Several reasons are given for this downward shift in total intake of

dairy foods. Among these are changes in life-styles,
demographics, including an increase in the aged and in the
black populations, competition from other beverages,
particularly soft drinks, and consumer concerns about fat and
energy (calories) (Bunch, 1985a; Rados, 1985).

While total consumption of dairy products has decreased
compared with 20 years ago, intake of some dairy foods has
increased whereas that of others has declined (Bunch, 1985a).
As shown in Tables 1 and 2 and Figure 2, consumption of
several dairy products such as yogurt, lowfat milk, sour
cream and dips, American and most other cheeses, flavored
milk and drinks, and eggnog has increased over the past 10 to
20 years, whereas use of whole milk, butter, and buttermilk
has declined. Between 1964 and 1984, per capita consumption
of whole milk (3.5% fat) fell 116 lbs (Bunch, 1985a).
Expressed in terms of total fluid milk products, per capita
use of whole milk declined from 85% in 1964 to 51% in 1984.
In contrast, increasing consumer concerns about health and
nutrition led to a greater intake of several other dairy
foods (Bunch, 1985a). Consumption of lowfat milk (1-2% fat),
for example, increased over 1000% during these years
(Table 1). And while per capita intake of yogurt (i.e., a
966% increase) and flavored milks (i.e., a 28% increase) also
rose, per capita consumption of creams (light cream, heavy
cream, half and half and buttermilk fell (Table 1).

Table 1. Per Capita Consumption of Fluid Milk Products Shifts (Bunch, 1985a)

Year	Plain whole milk	Low-fat milk	Skim milk	Flavored milk and drinks	Butter-milk	Yogurt	Eggnog	Half-and-half	Light cream	Heavy cream	Sour cream	Total Consumption
							Pounds					
1960	250.9	2.3	10.7	7.0	6.7	0.3	0.25	4.6	1.46	1.04	.9	286.1
1961	243.2	3.4	11.3	7.3	6.2	.3	.26	4.6	1.32	.97	.9	279.8
1962	240.8	4.7	11.6	7.5	6.5	.2	.28	4.4	1.23	.97	1.0	279.3
1963	240.4	6.4	12.2	8.2	6.4	.3	.27	4.2	1.06	.92	1.0	281.5
1964	238.6	8.7	12.6	8.5	6.3	.3	.25	4.1	.94	.88	0.9	282.0
1965	236.5	10.9	12.6	8.8	6.1	.3	.26	4.0	.86	.84	1.0	282.2
1966	234.1	14.5	11.0	9.0	6.0	.4	.27	3.8	.75	.78	1.0	281.7
1967	223.7	18.4	10.7	8.6	5.9	.5	.26	3.6	.65	.72	.9	273.9
1968	218.6	22.7	11.3	9.0	5.8	.6	.30	3.4	.52	.65	1.0	273.8
1969	212.1	27.3	11.7	8.8	5.8	.8	.29	3.2	.46	.57	1.0	272.1
1970	206.9	30.7	11.9	8.8	5.7	.8	.31	3.0	.38	.56	1.1	270.2
1971	199.3	35.8	11.5	9.2	5.6	1.2	.41	2.8	.33	.55	1.2	267.9
1972	195.0	40.1	12.6	9.7	5.6	1.4	.47	2.7	.28	.57	1.3	269.8
1973	186.2	44.0	14.1	9.8	5.2	1.5	.44	2.7	.39	.58	1.3	266.2
1974	175.2	46.4	14.1	9.9	4.8	1.6	.45	2.5	.40	.56	1.5	257.4
1975	173.2	54.9	11.9	10.0	4.8	2.1	.38	2.5	.42	.57	1.7	262.5
1976	165.5	58.6	11.9	11.0	4.8	2.2	.40	2.5	.36	.61	1.6	259.5
1977	157.4	62.3	12.1	11.6	4.7	2.4	.43	2.5	.31	.59	1.7	256.0
1978	152.6	65.6	11.7	11.3	4.5	2.6	.43	2.5	.32	.56	1.7	253.8
1979	146.9	68.3	11.8	10.7	4.3	2.5	.42	2.5	.30	.63	1.8	250.1
1980	140.6	71.8	11.8	10.2	4.2	2.6	.42	2.5	.24	.66	1.8	246.8
1981	135.0	74.1	11.5	10.1	3.9	2.6	.44	2.5	.24	.68	1.9	242.8
1982	130.5	75.6	11.0	9.5	4.1	2.7	.46	2.6	.27	.71	2.0	239.5
1983	127.2	77.7	11.0	10.1	4.3	3.2	.49	2.7	.29	.80	2.1	239.9
1984	122.6	80.7	11.9	10.9	4.3	3.6	.49	2.9	.31	.90	2.3	240.9

1/ Per capita U.S. sales. Data based primarily on information from Government-regulated State and Federal fluid milk markets. Excludes milk produced and consumed on farms. Per capita figures are based on estimated population using fluid products from purchased sources.

TABLE 2. Trends in Per Capita Consumption of Other Milk Products, 1963-1983 (National Economics Division, 1984)

Year	Butter	CHEESE Whole and Part Whole-milk Cheese American	Other	Cottage	CONDENSED AND EVAPORATED MILK Canned Whole Milk	Canned and Bulk Skim Milk	Bulk Whole Milk	FROZEN DAIRY PRODUCTS Ice Cream	Sherbert	Ice Milk	Other Frozen Products	DRY MILK PRODUCTS Nonfat Milk	Whole Milk	Butter-milk	Other Dry Products
1963	6.9	6.1	3.1	4.6	9.5	4.5	2.1	18.0	1.5	6.0	0.2	5.8	0.3	0.4	0.5
1964	6.9	6.2	3.2	4.7	9.2	4.8	2.2	18.3	1.5	6.3	.2	5.9	.3	.4	.6
1965	6.4	6.2	3.4	4.7	8.6	5.0	2.0	18.5	1.5	6.6	.2	5.6	.3	.4	.7
1966	5.7	6.2	3.6	4.6	7.9	5.4	1.9	18.2	1.6	6.8	.2	5.9	.3	.3	.8
1967	5.5	6.4	3.7	4.5	7.3	5.0	1.7	17.8	1.5	7.0	.2	5.6	.3	.3	1.0
1968	5.7	6.6	4.0	4.6	7.1	4.8	1.8	18.4	1.6	7.2	.2	5.8	.2	.3	1.2
1969	5.4	6.7	4.2	4.8	6.4	5.0	1.5	18.0	1.7	7.6	.2	5.8	.2	.3	1.3
1970	5.3	7.1	4.4	5.2	5.9	5.0	1.2	17.6	1.6	7.8	.2	5.3	.2	.2	1.6
1971	5.1	7.4	4.7	5.4	5.7	5.1	1.1	17.5	1.6	7.7	.2	5.3	.2	.3	1.7
1972	4.9	7.8	5.3	5.5	5.1	4.7	1.2	17.3	1.6	7.7	.3	4.6	.1	.2	1.9
1973	4.8	7.9	5.7	5.3	4.8	4.3	1.1	17.3	1.6	7.6	.3	5.3	.1	.2	1.9
1974	4.5	8.6	6.0	4.7	4.4	3.5	1.2	17.4	1.5	7.7	.3	4.2	.1	.2	2.3
1975	4.7	8.2	6.1	4.7	3.9	3.6	1.4	18.5	1.5	7.7	.3	3.3	.1	.2	2.3
1976	4.3	9.0	6.7	4.7	3.7	3.6	1.3	17.9	1.5	7.3	.3	3.5	.2	.2	2.5
1977	4.3	9.3	6.8	4.7	3.2	3.9	1.1	17.5	1.5	7.8	.4	3.3	.2	.3	2.5
1978	4.4	9.6	7.4	4.7	3.1	3.5	1.1	17.4	1.4	7.7	.4	3.1	.3	.2	2.6
1979	4.5	9.6	7.6	4.5	3.0	3.4	1.1	17.1	1.3	7.3	.3	3.3	.3	.2	2.8
1980	4.5	9.7	7.9	4.5	2.8	3.3	1.0	17.4	1.3	7.2	.3	3.0	.3	.2	2.7
1981	4.3	10.3	8.1	4.4	2.9	3.2	1.2	17.2	1.3	7.0	.6	2.7	.2	.2	2.8
1982	4.6	11.5	8.6	4.2	2.8	3.0	1.3	17.5	1.3	6.7	.7	2.7	.1	.2	2.9
1983	5.1	11.6	9.0	4.2	2.7	3.2	1.2	17.9	1.3	7.0	.6	3.1	.2	.2	3.0

*   All per capita consumption figures use civilian population.

**   Includes quantities used in other dairy products.

*** Excludes pot and baker's cheese.

**** Includes dried whey and, until 1979, malted milk.

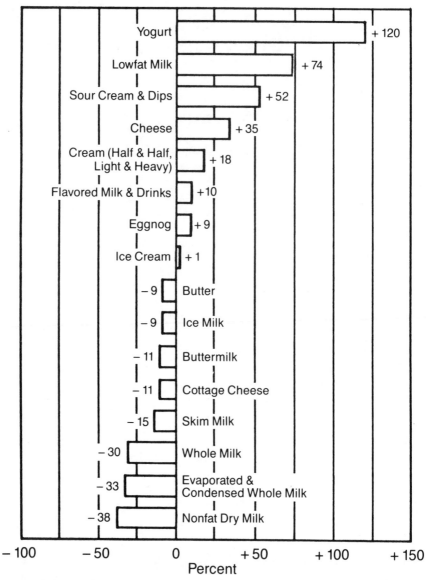

FIGURE 2. PERCENT CHANGE IN PER CAPITA SALES OF DAIRY FOODS, 1974-1984 (MILK INDUSTRY FOUNDATION, 1985).

Per capita consumption of all types of cheeses, with the exception of cottage cheese which has remained relatively stable, has risen over 100% between 1963 and 1983 (Table 2). In contrast, per capita consumption of butter decreased by 26% (Table 2). Likewise, per capita consumption of dry milk products such as nonfat milks, whole milk, buttermilk, and other dry products, decreased 7% during these years (Table 2).

Despite the overall decline in total consumption of dairy foods and the shift in preferences, consumption of total fluid milk products was 1.4% higher in 1983 than in the previous year, representing the first gain in eight years (Bunch, 1985b; Rados, 1985). As shown in Table 3, per capita consumption of all dairy products increased from 301.4 lbs. in 1982 to 306.7 lbs. in 1983 to an estimated 309 lbs. in 1984 (Bunch, 1985b). Over 60% of this gain in dairy product consumption was accounted for by lowfat milk, with yogurt, cheese, and frozen desserts providing the remainder (Bunch, 1985b). While intake of whole milk continued to decline in 1983, it was the smallest decrease in over twenty years (Bunch, 1985b).

TABLE 3. Per Capita Consumption of Selected Dairy Foods and Fats and Oils (including butter)* (Bunch, 1985b).

FOOD	1960-63	1970-73	1982	1983	1984**
			pounds		
All dairy products (product weight)	358.6	333.4	301.4	306.7	309.0
Fluid milk products	292.8	274.5	241.7	245.1	245.4
Cheese	8.8	12.6	20.1	20.6	22.4
Butter	7.3	5.0	4.6	5.1	5.4
Ice Cream	18.0	17.4	17.5	17.9	17.7
Fats and Oils (including butter)	48.7	55.9	61.4	62.7	66.7
Animal fats	19.6	14.4	12.5	13.0	13.9
Vegetable Oils	29.2	41.6	48.9	49.7	52.8

* Retail weight equivalent

** Preliminary

According to Bunch (1985b), some of the same factors that have led to the decrease in consumption of whole milk and some other dairy foods now are turning in favor of these foods. The population, for example, is becoming more sophisticated in its knowledge of nutrition. Despite consumer concerns about fat and energy intake, awareness of the nutritional value of milk, especially lowfat milk, has increased (Bunch, 1985a). Data collected by the United States Department of Agriculture reveal that milk and other dairy foods contribute significant proportions of many nutrients to the U.S. food supply (Marston and Raper, 1985; Table 4). In 1984, milk, cheese, yogurt, and other dairy foods (excluding butter) contributed 75.8% of the calcium, 35.8% of the phosphorus, 34.7% of the riboflavin, 20.9% of the protein, 20.1% of the vitamin B_{12}, 19.1% of the magnesium, and a substantial percentage of several other vitamins and minerals, while contributing only 10.3% of the food energy (calories) and only 11.7% of the fat in the food supply (Marston and Raper, 1986; Table 4).

TABLE 4. Contribution of Dairy Foods (excluding butter) to Nutrient Supplies Available for Civilian Consumption, USA (Marston and Raper, 1986)

NUTRIENT	1984
	% of total nutrients available for consumption
Calcium	75.8
Phosphorus	35.8
Riboflavin	34.7
Protein	20.9
Vitamin B_{12}	20.1
Magnesium	19.1
Vitamin A value	11.6
Fat	11.7
Vitamin B_6	11.5
Food energy (calories)	10.3
Thiamin	8.9
Carbohydrate	6.0
Ascorbic Acid	3.1
Iron	2.3
Niacin	1.6

Because of the public's increased awareness of the importance of calcium in milk and other dairy foods in relation to diseases such as osteoporosis and hypertension, it is expected that the upward turn in the use of total fluid milk products will continue (Bunch, 1985a). Recent research findings suggest that an adequate intake of calcium may help protect against osteoporosis (Heaney et. al., 1982; The American Society for Bone and Mineral Research, 1982; Consensus Development Panel, 1984; Avioli, 1984; Recker and Heaney, 1985; Sandler et al., 1985) and hypertension (McCarron, 1984; Resnick, 1985; McCarron and Morris, 1985; McCarron, 1985; Henry et al., 1985). Osteoporosis, an age-related disorder in which bone mass decreases and susceptibility to fractures increases, affects as many as 15 to 20 million persons in the U.S., mostly postmenopausal women (Consensus Development Panel, 1984). Inadequate calcium intake is thought to be one of the primary causes of this potentially debilitating disease (Consensus Development Panel, 1984; Avioli, 1984). Evidence also is accumulating that increasing calcium consumption lowers blood pressure in some individuals (Parrott-Garcia and McCarron, 1984; Resnick, 1985; McCarron and Morris, 1985; Henry et al., 1985).

The availability of milk and other dairy foods with variable amounts of fat and energy (Table 5) has provided consumers with a variety of choices within the milk group (Bunch, 1985a). The dairy industry continually is pursuing product development using the latest advances in dairy science and technology to further expand consumers' choices. Consumer demand for reduced fat products has led to the development of lower fat milk, cheese, cream, ice cream, frozen dessert, and sour cream.

Table 5.   Fat and Energy Content of Selected Dairy
Products (Agricultural Research Service, 1976)

Dairy Product	% Fat g/100g	Fat g/serving	Energy kcal/serving
Skim milk, 1 cup	0.18	0.44	86
Evaporated skim milk, 1/2 cup	0.20	0.26	99
Cottage cheese, dry curd, 1/2 cup	0.42	0.48	96
Buttermilk, cultured, 1 cup	0.88	2.16	99
Lowfat (1%) chocolate milk, 1 cup	1.00	2.50	158
Lowfat (1%) milk, 1 cup	1.06	2.59	102
Yogurt, plain lowfat, 8 fl. oz.	1.55	3.52	144
Lowfat (2%) milk, 1 cup	1.92	4.68	121
Sherbet, orange, 1 cup	1.98	3.82	270
Lowfat (2%) chocolate milk, 1 cup	2.00	5.00	179
Yogurt, plain, whole milk, 8 fl. oz.	3.25	7.38	139
Whole milk, 1 cup	3.3	8.15	150
Chocolate milk, 1 cup	3.4	8.48	208
Ice milk, vanilla, 1 cup	4.3	5.63	184
Cottage cheese, creamed, 1/2 cup	4.5	5.10	117
Eggnog, 1 cup	7.48	19.00	342
Evaporated whole milk, 1/2 cup	7.56	9.53	169
Ricotta cheese made with part skim milk, 1/2 cup	7.9	9.81	171
Sweetened condensed whole milk, 1 fl. oz.	8.7	3.32	123
Ice cream, vanilla, 1 cup	10.77	14.32	269
Half-and-half, 1 tablespoon	11.5	1.72	20
Ricotta cheese, whole milk, 1/2 cup	13	16.10	216
Mozzarella cheese, part skim, 1 oz.	16	4.51	72
Light cream, 1 tablespoon	19.3	2.90	29
Sour cream, 1 tablespoon	21	2.52	26
American cheese spread, 1 oz.	21.2	6.02	82
Mozzarella cheese, 1 oz.	21.6	6.12	80
American cheese food, 1 oz.	24.5	6.93	94
Medium cream, 25% fat, 1 tablespoon	25	3.75	37
Jetost cheese, 1 oz.	29.5	8.37	132
Light whipping cream, 1 tablespoon unwhipped	30.9	4.64	44
Cheddar cheese, 1 oz.	33.1	9.40	114
Cream cheese, 1 oz.	34.9	9.89	99
Heavy whipping cream, 1 tablespoon unwhipped	37	5.55	52
Butter, 1 pat	81	4.06	36

Changes in the Availability and Intake of Dietary Fat and the
Contribution of Dairy Products to Fat Availability

Since the beginning of the century, total fat as well as
per capita consumption in the nation's food supply has
increased almost 31%, from 124g per capita per day in 1909-13
to 162g per capita per day in 1982 (Marston and Welsh, 1984).
Expressed as a percentage of energy available, fat provided
32% in 1909 compared with 43% in 1982 (Rizek et al., 1983;
Marston and Welsh, 1984).

Not only has the quantity of fat in the nation's food
supply increased, but the sources of fat have changed. (Risek
et al., 1983; Marston and Welsh, 1984; Figure 3). The
increase in the total amount of fat in the food supply is
explained largely by the sharp increase in fat available from
vegetable sources which provided 17% of the fat in 1909-13
compared with 43% in 1982 (Rizek et al., 1983; Marston and
Welsh, 1984). During this same period, the contribution of
fat provided by animal sources fell from 83% in 1909-13 to
57% in 1982 (Rizek et al., 1983; Bunch and Hazera, 1984;
Marston and Welsh, 1984).

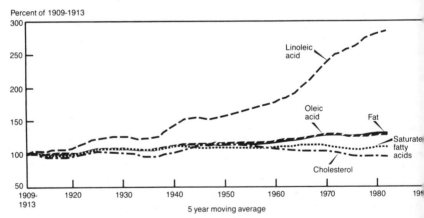

FIGURE 3. FAT, FATTY ACIDS, AND CHOLESTEROL CHANGES IN THE
U.S. FOOD SUPPLY 1909-13 TO 1982 (MARSTON AND
WELSH, 1984).

With respect to food sources of fat, three food groups--fats and oils; meat, poultry, fish; and dairy products--have provided about 90% of the total fat in the nation's food supply since the beginning of the century (Rizek et al., 1983). However, the proportion of fat provided by each of these groups has changed over the years. As shown in Figure 4 (Marston and Welsh, 1984; Marston and Raper, 1986), fats and oils provided 44.0% of fat available in the food supply in 1984 (Marston and Raper, 1986), an increase from 37.1% in 1909-13 (Marston and Welsh, 1984). In contrast, the amount of fat contributed by meat, poultry and fish declined from 37.3% in 1909-13 to 34.2% in 1984. Likewise, dairy products provided only 11.7% of the fat available in 1984 compared with 14.7% in 1909-13 (Figure 4).

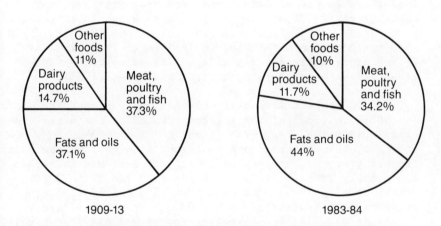

1909-13   1983-84

FIGURE 4. CHANGES IN PROPORTIONATE CONTRIBUTIONS BY MAJOR FOOD GROUPS TO TOTAL FAT BETWEEN 1909-13 AND 1983 (MARSTON AND WELSH, 1984; MARSTON AND RAPER, 1986).

Within the fats and oils group, butter and margarine have reversed their position as sources of fat since the beginning of the century (Rizek et al., 1983; Bunch and

Hazera, 1984). Between 1909-13 and 1980, the proportion of fat in this group contributed by butter declined from 38% to 6% at the expense of margarines made with vegetable oils (Rizek et al, 1983; Bunch and Hazera, 1984). Compared with its peak consumption of 18.5 lbs per person in the early 1930s, use of butter decreased to 4.5 lbs in 1982 (Bunch and Hazera, 1984). Expressed as a percentage of total fat available in the food supply, butter contributed 12% in 1940 compared with 3% in 1982 (Bunch and Hazera, 1984).

With respect to dairy products, this food group provided about the same amount of fat early in the century (18.6g per capita/day) as in 1980 (19.9g per capita/day) (Rizek et al., 1983). However, between 1909-13 and 1984 the proportion of fat in the food supply contributed by dairy products declined from 14.7% to 11.7%, respectively (Rizek et al., 1983; Marston and Welsh, 1984; Marston and Raper, 1986). In 1947-49, when use of dairy foods was near its peak, these foods provided 17% of the fat in the food supply (Rizek et al., 1983). Thereafter, fat from this group fell to 14% in 1960 to 12% in both 1970 and in 1982 to 11.7% in 1984 as shifts occurred in the use of specific dairy foods in this group (Rizek et al., 1984, Marston and Raper, 1986).

Fluid whole milk contributed a smaller proportion of fat in 1980 (i.e., 36% of the fat contributed by the dairy group) than in 1909-13 (i.e., 67%) (Rizek et al., 1983). In contrast, the proportionate contribution of fat in the dairy product group by cheeses and frozen desserts has increased appreciably from 9% early in the century to 31% in 1980 (Rizek et al., 1983). Between 1909-13 and 1980, fat from cheese almost quadrupled from 1.6 to 6.1g per capita/day (Rizek et al., 1983). Likewise, fat from fluid lowfat milk, despite its low fat content, has more than quadrupled since 1909-13, accounting for 9% of all the fat from dairy products in 1980 (Rizek et al., 1983). And fat from ice cream and other frozen desserts has risen from 2% in 1909-13 to 15% of the fat contributed by dairy products in 1980 (Rizek et al., 1983). On the other hand, fat from processed milks (e.g., evaporated, condensed, dry) has remained about the same between 1909-13 and 1980, while fat from fluid cream has decreased sharply (Rizek et al., 1983). In 1980, cream supplied 1.1g fat per capita/day, about one-third as much as in 1909-13 (Rizek et al., 1983).

In contrast to total fat in the food supply which has risen since the beginning of the century, cholesterol has remained about the same (i.e., 507 and 479 mg per capita/day in 1909-13 and 1982, respectively) (Marston and Welsh, 1984). However, in between these years, cholesterol in the food supply has fluctuated considerably, reaching 575 mg per capita/day in 1947-49 (Rizek et al., 1983; Marston and Welsh, 1984). Similarly, the percentage of cholesterol in the U.S. food supply contributed by dairy products was about the same in 1982 as in 1909-13 (i.e., 15%), however, this also has fluctuated over the years (Marston and Welsh, 1984; Figure 5). For example, the contribution of cholesterol from dairy products was greater in 1947-49 when use of fluid whole milk and cream was high than in later years (Rizek et al., 1983). Fluid whole milk, cheese, fluid lowfat milk, and frozen dairy products are the main contributors to cholesterol in the dairy group, although the proportions from each have varied (Rizek et al., 1983). For example, the decreased contribution of cholesterol from fluid whole milk and cream in recent years has been offset by the increased cholesterol from cheese, lowfat milk, and frozen desserts (Rizek et al., 1983).

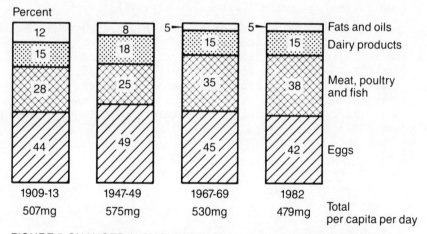

FIGURE 5. CHANGES IN CHOLESTEROL IN THE U.S. FOOD SUPPLY BY FOOD GROUP BETWEEN 1909-13 AND 1982 (MARSTON AND WELSH, 1984).

The above data reveal fat and cholesterol available in the nation's food supply or that which "disappears" into civilian consumption. This information, while useful, overestimates actual intake by individuals (Rizek et al., 1983). Data collected as part of national surveys such as the 1977-78 Nationwide Food Consumption Survey (NFCS) and the Second National Health and Nutrition Examination Survey, 1976-1980 (NHANES-II) provide a more realistic indication of what individuals consume (Rizek et al., 1983). Data from the 1977-78 NFCS show that the average person ingested 83g fat/day, an amount much lower than the 161g fat per capita/day in 1977 based on food supply data (Rizek et al., 1983). The difference is explained by food waste and how the data are compiled (Rizek et al., 1983). In contrast, the proportion of food energy contributed by fat consumed by individuals in the 1977-78 NFCS was about the same (i.e., 42%) as that calculated from the national food supply (i.e., 43%) (Rizek et al., 1983).

According to data from NHANES-II (1976-1980), mean fat intake for males six months to 74 years of age is 98g/day, while that for females of the same age range is 64g/day (Carroll et al., 1983). For both sexes, this level of fat intake represents 37% of energy intake. The mean dietary intake of cholesterol is 405 and 266 mg for males and females, respectively (Carroll et al., 1983).

In terms of the percentage of fat consumed from various categories of food, data from NHANES-II (1976-1980) reveal the following: meat 31.5%; "others" (e.g., fats, sweets, alcohol)--30.5%; milk and other dairy foods--19.2%; grains--7.8%; combination foods (soups, gravies, mixed protein dishes)--7.6%; and fruits and vegetables--5.4% (National Health and Nutrition Examination Survey (NHANES-II) 1976-1980; Figure 6).

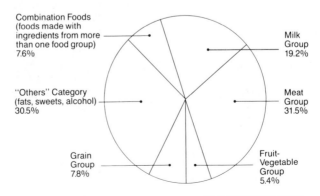

FIGURE 6. PERCENTAGE OF FAT INTAKE PROVIDED BY VARIOUS CATEGORIES OF FOOD (NATIONAL HEALTH AND NUTRITION EXAMINATION SURVEY, NHANES II, 1976-80).

Within the dairy group some of the sources of fat such as butter or ice cream actually provide a much smaller proportion of total fat intake than one would expect, according to dietary data from 11,658 adults in the NHANES-II, 1976-80 (Block et al., 1985). As shown in Table 6, for example, butter and ice cream provided only 2.39% and 2.05% of total fat intake, respectively (Block et al., 1985).

Table 6.   Contribution of Dairy Products to Fat and Cholesterol in the U.S. Diet: Data from the NHANES II Survey, 1976-1980 (Block et al., 1985)

Dairy Product	% of Total Fat	% of Total Saturated Fat	% of Total Cholesterol
Whole milk, whole milk beverages	5.98	9.11	5.41
Cheeses, excluding cottage cheese	4.54	7.28	3.05
Butter	2.39	3.67	1.70
Ice cream, frozen desserts	2.05	3.11	1.71
2% milk	1.37	2.48	0.79
Skim milk, buttermilk	-*	-	0.22
Cream, half and half	0.44	0.68	0.37
Sour cream, dips	-	0.25	-
Yogurt	-	0.22	0.08

* dashes denote lack of data.

DIETARY FAT AND CANCER IN RELATION TO DAIRY PRODUCTS

Evidence linking dietary fat in general and fat in animal foods such as milk and dairy products to cancer is inconsistent. The difficulties in singling out a sole nutrient such as fat in cancer causation are many. Not only is the contribution of diet to cancer risk unknown, but there is no reliable evidence that dietary changes will be of major importance in preventing this disease or decreasing overall mortality (Pariza, 1984; Sherwin, 1985).

Evidence Linking Dietary Fat to Cancer

One of the most studied, yet controversial relationships between diet and cancer is that between dietary fat and cancer (Doll and Peto, 1981; Committee on Diet, Nutrition and Cancer, 1982). Most of the data supporting a role for fat in carcinogenesis comes from epidemiological surveys of human populations and experimental animal studies (Armstrong and Doll, 1975; Doll and Peto, 1981; Carroll, 1982; Committee on Diet, Nutrition and Cancer, 1982; Jensen, 1983; Kolonel et al., 1983; Shamberger, 1984; Willett and MacMahon, 1984; Creasey, 1985; Miller, 1985). Many of these types of investigations have shown an association between dietary fat and the occurrence of, or mortality from, cancer at several sites, especially the breast, colon, and prostate, the second, third, and fourth most common cancers, respectively, in the U.S.

With respect to breast cancer, several international correlation studies have shown a positive association between per capita fat intake and age-adjusted incidence of or mortality from this type of cancer (Armstrong and Doll, 1975; Committee on Diet, Nutrition and Cancer, 1982; Willett and MacMahon, 1984; Mettlin, 1984; Carroll, 1985; Kakar and Henderson, 1985; Simpopoulos, 1985). For example, countries such as Japan with a low per capita intake of fat (i.e., about 10% of energy intake) have a reduced incidence of and mortality from breast cancer compared with that in countries such as the U.S. with a higher per capita fat level (i.e., 40% of energy intake) (Committee on Diet, Nutrition and Cancer, 1982; Brown, 1983; Rose, 1983; Visek and Clinton, 1983; Creasey, 1985).

Some intra-country studies also support the above findings (Gaskill et al., 1979; Visek and Clinton, 1983; Kolonel et al., 1983). Within the U.S., age-adjusted breast cancer mortality was found to be positively associated with per capita intake of animal foods (Gaskill et al., 1979). An association between dietary fat and cancer of the breast also is supported by studies of migrants who, upon moving from a country with a low per capita fat intake to one with a higher per capita fat intake, experience an increased incidence of this type of cancer similar to that of their adopted country (Committee on Diet, Nutrition and Cancer, 1982).

In case-control studies such as the one in northern Italy, for example, involving 368 women with breast cancer and 373 age-matched controls, more frequent consumption of animal foods was associated with increased risk of breast cancer (Talamini et al., 1984). In addition, studies of human populations that follow a unique lifestyle support an association between fat intake and breast cancer (Visek and Clinton, 1983; Shamberger, 1984). Seventh-Day Adventists, for example, who consume a lowfat lacto-ovo-vegetarian diet have a lower incidence of breast cancer than the average U.S. population (Visek and Clinton, 1983). For individuals with breast cancer, increased fat consumption has been related to poorer survival time following diagnosis, according to an historical prospective study of 953 women with this disease (Gregorio et al., 1985).

Similar to epidemiological studies, a number of experimental animal investigations of spontaneous, chemically induced, transplantable, and radiation-induced tumors, reveal that high fat diets are associated with the development of breast cancers (Committee on Diet, Nutrition and Cancer, 1982; Welsch and Aylsworth, 1983; Kakar and Henderson, 1985). Unlike most human epidemiological studies, however, experimental animal studies show that under some circumstances, breast tumor incidence varies with both the quantity and the type of fat consumed (Committee on Diet, Nutrition and Cancer, 1982; Carroll, 1985). When fat intake is low (i.e., 5%), polyunsaturated fatty acids stimulate mammary tumor growth in experimental animals to a greater extent than saturated fatty acids (Committee on Diet, Nutrition and Cancer, 1982; Carroll, 1983; Carroll, 1985). However, when fat intake is increased (i.e., 20%) and the need for essential fatty acids is met, the type of fat (saturated vs. polyunsaturated) appears to be less important in carcinogenesis (Carroll, 1985). In general, intake of a high fat diet increases breast tumorigenesis in experimental animals when fed _after_ a carcinogen is administered, not during or before tumor initiation. This suggests that dietary fat exerts a promoting effect on mammary tumorigenesis, as opposed to initiating or causing the disease (Committee on Diet, Nutrition and Cancer, 1982; Visek and Clinton, 1983; Carroll, 1983; Mettlin, 1984; Carroll, 1985).

Similar to breast cancer, several epidemiological studies reveal a positive association between total fat intake and colon carcinogenesis (Armstrong and Doll, 1975; Carroll and Khor, 1975; Jain et al, 1980; Carroll, 1980; Reddy, 1981; Jensen, 1983; Reddy, 1984; Willett and MacMahon, 1984; Weisburger, 1985). Correlations of international incidence and mortality rates for colon cancer in relation to various dietary components suggest a strong association with total dietary fat (Armstrong and Doll, 1975; Jensen, 1983; Willett and MacMahon, 1984). In addition, some studies of population groups within countries and some case-control studies point to a positive association between fat intake and colon cancer incidence (Carroll and Khor, 1975; Jain et al, 1980; Reddy, 1981; Reddy, 1983). Fat from animal sources such as beef, pork, eggs, and milk also has been correlated with increased mortality from colon cancer (Correa, 1981).

Experimental animal studies reveal that raising dietary fat intake from 5 to 20% increases the incidence of colon cancer induced by a variety of carcinogens (Reddy, 1983; Sakaguchi et al, 1984; Willett and MacMahon, 1984; MacLennan, 1985). Similar to mammary tumorigenesis, a promoting effect of dietary fat is suggested (Willett and MacMahon, 1984; MacLennan, 1985). In addition, there is some suggestion from experimental animal studies that unsaturated fats may be more important in increasing colon cancer risk than saturated fats (Reddy, 1983; Willett and MacMahon, 1984).

Prostate cancer also has been associated epidemiologically with fat intake, although the evidence is less convincing than that for either breast or colon cancer (Committee on Diet, Nutrition and Cancer, 1982). A comparison of per capita fat intake with prostate cancer in a number of countries suggests an association between high fat intake and increased incidence of and mortality from this type of cancer (Armstrong and Doll, 1975; Committee on Diet, Nutrition and Cancer, 1982). Some studies within countries also support this association (Blair and Fraumeni, 1978; Kolonel et al., 1983; Shamberger, 1984). Furthermore, findings from a few case-control studies suggest that fat in general and animal fats specifically increase the risk of prostate cancer (Rotkin, 1977; Meikel et al., 1982; Graham et al., 1983; Snowdon et al., 1984; Heshmat et al., 1985). In the case-control studies carried out both by Graham et al. (1983) and Kolonel et al. (1983), increased fat intake was associated with greater risk of developing prostate cancer in men 70 years of age and older, but not in younger men.

Inconsistencies/Discrepancies in the Dietary Fat-Cancer Hypothesis

Several authors have pointed out inconsistencies in the epidemiological correlations between fat intake and the above types of cancer (Doll and Peto, 1981; Enstrom, 1981; Committee on Diet, Nutrition and Cancer, 1982,; Higginson, 1983; Jensen, 1983; Kolonel et al., 1983; Mendeloff, 1983; Mettlin, 1984; Willett and MacMahon, 1984; Nair, 1984; Shamberger, 1984; Simopoulos, 1985; MacLennan, 1985). Reasons given for the discrepancies include the difficulty in obtaining reliable dietary data for individuals and the long latency period (e.g., 20 to 30 years) between the initiation and diagnosis of cancer (Simopoulos, 1985). As pointed out by Simopoulos (1985), national per capita food intake or food "disappearance" data may be an inaccurate measure of food consumed by an individual. Moreover, it is difficult if not impossible to obtain reliable information regarding what individuals ate 20 years previously (Simopoulos, 1985).

With respect to breast cancer, many surveys within countries have failed to support a positive association between this type of cancer and dietary fat (Gaskill et al., 1979; Doll and Peto, 1981; Simopoulos, 1985). For example, when other factors known to influence breast cancer risk such as age at time of first pregnancy were taken into account, the apparently direct correlation between breast cancer mortality and fat intake within the U.S. by state disappeared (Gaskill et al., 1979). Also within the U.S., the trend since the beginning of the century has been toward increased total fat consumption and in particular, increased use of polyunsaturated fatty acids, yet breast cancer incidence in the U.S. has changed very little (Mettlin, 1984; Figure 1). A number of case-control studies also have shown either a weak or no association between dietary fat and breast cancer (Graham et al., 1982; Kolonel et al., 1983; Willett and MacMahon, 1984; Mettlin, 1984; Carroll, 1985). In a case-control study carried out by Kolonel et al. (1983), the correlation between dietary fat and breast cancer was much weaker than reported associations of other risk factors (e.g., family history of breast cancer, age at first pregnancy) for this cancer. And in a case-control study in Buffalo, New York involving over 2000 women with breast cancer and almost 1500 women without this disease, no association between dietary fat and breast cancer was observed (Graham et al., 1982).

Similar to breast cancer, numerous inconsistencies in the epidemiological evidence relating dietary fat to colon cancer have been reported (Lyon and Sorenson, 1978; Bingham et al., 1979; Doll and Peto, 1981, Enstrom, 1981; Jensen et al., 1982; Mendeloff, 1983, Jensen, 1983; Kolonel et al., 1983; Nair, 1984; Willett and Mac Mahon, 1984; Shamberger, 1984; Smith et al., 1985). A comparison of two Scandinavian populations with different risks for colon cancer showed no difference in fat intake between the high-risk Danes in Copenhagen and the low-risk Finns in Kuopio (i.e., rural Finland) (Report from the IARC Intestinal Microecology Group, 1977; Shamberger, 1984). Also, when dietary fat intake of a population in New York with a high risk for colon cancer was compared with that of low-risk Finns, no differences in total fat intake were evident (Reddy et al., 1978). Likewise, surveys within countries such as Britain (Bingham et al., 1979) and the U.S. (Lyon and Sorenson, 1978) have failed to show any correlation between fat intake and incidence of colon cancer. Also, colon (and breast) cancer mortality and incidence) are the same among Mormons as Seventh-Day Adventists in the U.S. even though the amount of fat consumed by Mormons is far greater than that consumed by the Seventh-Day Adventists (Enstrom, 1975; Jensen, 1983; Nair, 1984). Likewise, Smith et al. (1985) reported no difference in fat consumption between Maori and Non-Maori New Zealanders despite the higher incidence of colon cancer in the latter.

With respect to prostate cancer, MacLennan (1985) in a review of epidemiological evidence for and against relating dietary fat to human gastrointestinal and prostate cancers, points out the inconsistencies in the data implicating dietary fat to this type of cancer. Armstrong and Doll (1975), for example, found a positive correlation between per capita fat intake and mortality from but not incidence of prostate cancer.

In contrast to epidemiological findings of a positive association between the availability of animal foods and cancer risk, other investigations have revealed either no clear relationship or a lower risk of cancer (Mettlin and Graham, 1979; Jensen et al., 1982; McKeown-Eyssen and Bright-See, 1984; Phillips and Snowdon, 1985). Phillips and Snowdown (1985), for example, observed no association between colon cancer mortality and frequent use of meat, cheese, milk, or eggs in a 21-year follow-up study of over 25,000 California Seventh Day Adventists. And Mettlin and Graham (1979) reported a negative association between intake of milk and bladder cancer. Likewise, other investigators (Jensen et al., 1982; McKeown-Eyssen and Bright-See, 1984) have shown an inverse relationship between the availability of milk and milk products and colon cancer. Although the low risk of colon cancer in Finns who are high consumers of dairy products has been suggested to be due to their fiber-rich diet which may protect against cancer (Report from the IARC Intestinal Microecology Group, 1977; Shamberger, 1984), dairy foods, as discussed below, are an excellent source of calcium which possibly may protect against colon cancer.

Since the beginning of the century, extensive changes have taken place in the U.S. in total fat intake, the contribution of fat to total energy intake, and sources of dietary fat, including dairy products. In contrast, overall U.S. cancer rates at most sites other than the lung and stomach have remained relatively stable for several decades (American Cancer Society, 1986). As reviewed above, animal fat intake has remained relatively constant or even decreased slightly during this century and ingestion of common animal fats such as butter and whole milk has decreased while intake of vegetable fats has increased steadily. This suggests that fat's effect on cancer is minimal or non-existent, or that dietary changes have occurred too recently to be influential, or that some dietary changes have had a positive and others a negative effect on cancer incidence and mortality (Committee on Diet, Nutrition and Cancer, 1982).

It is apparent that the interpretation of both human epidemiological studies and experimental animal investigations is very complex, rendering clear-cut conclusions regarding fat intake and cancer risk difficult. Although an association between fat intake and some forms of cancer has been found, the findings are by no means consistent. Moreover, associations do not necessarily imply causation and results of animal studies may not be relevant to cancer in humans (Committee on Diet, Nutrition and Cancer, 1982).

In addition to the inconsistencies in epidemiological and experimental animal studies implicating dietary fat intake in cancer causation, the mechanism(s) by which dietary fat enhances tumorigenesis is unknown (Committee on Diet, Nutrition and Cancer, 1982). However, most experimental studies suggest that dietary fat acts as a promoter, as opposed to an initiator of carcinogenesis, although the latter cannot be excluded (Committee on Diet, Nutrition and Cancer, 1982; Carroll, 1983; Reddy, 1983; Welsch and Aylsworth, 1983; Kakar and Henderson, 1985; Carroll, 1985). The mechanisms by which dietary fat influences carcinogenesis are thought to be complex, multifactorial, and specific to different cancers (Carroll, 1983; Creasey, 1985). With respect to breast cancer, dietary fat has been suggested to promote this type of cancer by altering the immune response or hormonal or endocrine status (e.g., estrogen, prolactin) of the individual or by influencing the synthesis of prostaglandins or the composition and physical characteristics of cell membranes and hence their fluidity and transport process (Vitale and Broitman, 1981; Welsch and Aylsworth, 1983; Visek and Clinton, 1983; Rose, 1983).

Dietary fat may affect colon cancer by increasing the excretion of certain bile sterols and bile acids, some of which may be tumor promoters (Carroll, 1982). Several studies suggest that fecal bile acids and cholesterol metabolites possess co-carcinogenic properties (Committee on Diet, Nutrition and Cancer, 1982; Reddy, 1983). Also, in individuals at high-risk for colon cancer and in experimental animals fed high fat diets, excretion of fecal neutral steroids and bile acids is increased (Willett and MacMahon, 1984). However, to-date no active carcinogen derived from bile acids has been isolated from human or animal feces (Carroll, 1982). Dietary fat also may affect colon carcinogenesis by altering the metabolic activity of the intestinal flora which may convert fecal steroids into compounds with carcinogenic or cocarcinogenic potential (Committee on Diet, Nutrition and Cancer, 1982; Reddy, 1983). Fat-induced changes in the hormonal milieu (i.e., the effective levels and balance between androgens and estrogens) may promote the development of prostate cancer (Creasey, 1985; Heshmat et al., 1985).

Not only is the mechanism by which dietary fat influences carcinogenesis unknown, but questions have been raised regarding the effect of different types of dietary fats on the development of cancer (Sherwin, 1985). On the basis of epidemiological data, total fat intake and to a lesser extent animal fat intake have been associated most frequently with carcinogenesis. In contrast, in experimental animal studies, dietary polyunsaturated fatty acids appear to stimulate mammary and colon tumorigenesis to a greater extent than saturated fatty acids, at least when fat intake is low (Carroll and Khor, 1975; Carroll and Hopkins, 1979; Carroll, 1980, Carroll, 1982; Carroll, 1983; Visek and Clinton, 1983, Sakaguchi et al., 1984, Sakaguchi et al., 1986). According to studies carried out by Carroll and Hopkins (1979) and Carroll (1982, 1983), polyunsaturated fatty acids apparently are required to provide a source of essential fatty acids during tumor promotion. Ip et al (1985) found that about 4% of essential fatty acids (linoleate) was required for maximal expression of mammary tumorigenesis in carcinogen-induced laboratory rats. Once the requirement for essential fatty acids is met, additional tumor development appears to depend on the amount rather than on the source of dietary fat (Carroll, 1983; Visek and Clinton, 1983; Carroll, 1985).

How polyunsaturated fatty acids enhance tumorigenesis is not yet established, but diets high in polyunsaturated fatty acids in relation to saturated fatty acids are suggested to be more immunosuppressive and better promoters of tumorigenesis (Vitale and Broitman, 1981). Other possible mechanisms of unsaturated fatty acids involve increased excretion of bile acids (Sakaguchi et al., 1986) and enhanced formation of active oxidation products of fatty acids (e.g., the carcinogen, fatty acid hydroperoxide) (Ip and Sinha, 1981; Carroll, 1985). While the data in experimental animal studies reveal that both the quantity and type of fat consumed are important in tumorigenesis, dietary data in human subjects do not permit a clear distinction to be made among the effects of different components of fat (saturated, monounsaturated, polyunsaturated) or between different sources (animal or vegetable).

Dietary cholesterol is another dietary component which has been associated with a small-to-medium increase in risk of mammary and colon cancers in epidemiological studies (McMichael et al., 1984; Sherwin, 1985) . However, the close association between dietary cholesterol and other fats and nutrients precludes a causal inference between cholesterol and cancer (McMichael et al., 1984; Sherwin, 1985). While dietary cholesterol has been reported to enhance the yield of dimethylhydrazine-induced colon cancers in some experimental animal studies (Sherwin, 1985), the opposite effect (i.e., an inhibitory action on colon cancer) also has been found (Cohen

et al., 1982). Of related interest is the observation that
individuals with low blood cholesterol levels (185 mg/100
ml) have a higher mortality from cancer, particularly colon
cancer in males (Sidney and Farguhar, 1983; McMichael et al.,
1984; Salmond et al., 1985; Sherwin, 1985). In a review of
20 studies, each initiated to investigate the relationship
between blood cholesterol levels and coronary heart disease,
an inverse association between blood cholesterol and overall
cancer risk was found in 12 of the studies (McMichael et al.,
1984). The association was most marked for colon cancer in
men (McMichael et al., 1984). There is recent evidence
suggesting that in some cases low blood cholesterol is a
result of or a metabolic response to preclinical cancer
(McMichael et al., 1984; Sherwin, 1985). This is supported
by findings of a study reviewed by Sherwin (1985) in which
361,662 middle aged American men who were screened as
potential participants in the Multiple Risk Factor
Intervention Trial (MRFIT) were followed for six-to-eight
years. In this study, there was no relationship between
serum cholesterol and death from cancer occurring more than
five years after measurement of blood cholesterol (Sherwin,
1985).

Some of the discrepancies or inconsistencies in the
epidemiological findings relating dietary fat to cancer may
be explained by the difficulties in determining an
independent effect of dietary fat (Visek and Clinton, 1983).
Fat in the diet does not exist alone, but rather in
combination with other nutrients (e.g., protein) and food
components (e.g., fiber) which may interact with fat either
synergistically or antagonistically. Animal protein intake,
for example, is highly correlated with fat intake in many
studies (Kolonel et al., 1983). Also, because fat (9 kcal/g)
provides more than twice the metabolizable energy of either
carbohydrate or protein (4 kcal/g), and because fat calories
are used more efficiently by the body than calories from
other energy sources (Donato and Hegsted 1985; Boissonneault
et al. 1986; Donato, 1986) it has been suggested that the
enhancing effect of fat on carcinogenesis may be mediated via
increased energy availability. (Kritchevsky et al., 1984;
Kritchevsky 1985; Kritchevsky and Klurfeld, 1986; Kritchevsky
et al., 1986; Boutwell and Pariza, 1986; Boissonn Cault et
al., 1986). The subject of calories and energy expenditure
in cancer recently was addressed at a symposium in
Washington, DC (International Life Sciences Institute-
Nutrition Foundation, 1986).

As reviewed by Boutewll and Pariza (1986) and Kritchevsky and Klurfeld (1986), the effect of energy intake on tumor growth has been recognized for more than 75 years. In the early 1900s several studies showed less growth of spontaneous, transplanted, or carcinogen-induced tumors in underfed experimental animals. A reduction in food intake was shown not only to decrease the incidence of carcinogen-induced or spontaneous tumors but also to increase the lifespan of the experimental animals (MacCay et al., 1939). These early observations subsequently were supported in the 1940s by more systematic studies which showed that energy restriction inhibited the growth of spontaneous or carcinogen-induced tumors in laboratory animals. Further-more, it was demonstrated that low energy-high fat diets resulted in fewer tumors than high energy-low fat diets.

This interest in the importance of energy intake, especially in relation to fat enhancement of cancer, recently has been renewed. Results of epidemiological investigations suggest that energy restriction inhibits tumor development or conversely that overweight (e.g., by 40%) increases the risk of some forms of cancer (Armstrong and Doll, 1975; Lew and Garfinkel, 1979; Talamini et al., 1984; Willett and Mac Mahon, 1984; Garfinkel, 1985; Simopoulos, 1985; Phillips and Snowdon, 1985). For example, in a prospective study conducted by the American Cancer Society of 750,000 men and women followed for 12 years, men who were 40% overweight exhibited significantly high mortality for colorectal and prostate cancers whereas women who were 40% overweight had higher rates for cancers of the endometrium, gallbladder, ovary, and breast than normal weight individuals (Lew and Garfinkel, 1979; Garfinkel, 1985). While obesity may increase risk of breast cancer in older women, the reverse may be true among premenopausal women (Willett et al., 1985).

Findings from some recent experimental animal studies suggest that energy intake may be a more critical determinant of some types of cancer than dietary fat (Kritchevsky, 1985, 1986; Kritchevsky and Klurfeld, 1986; Kritchevsky et al., 1984, 1986; Boissonneault et al., 1986). When carcinogen-treated laboratory rats were fed an energy restricted (by 40%) diet, the incidence and yield of mammary (Kritchevsky et al., 1984, 1986) and colon (Kritchevsky et al., 1986) tumors were significantly lower than in control ad libitum fed animals despite twice the amount of fat consumed by the energy restricted rats.

Additional investigations were carried out to determine the effects of the degree of energy restriction on tumor incidence and growth (Kritchevsky and Klurfeld, 1986; Kritchevsky et al; 1986). Rats were fed either a lowfat (5% corn oil) diet ad libitum (i.e., control diet) or a diet, restricted in energy by 10, 20, 30, or 40% (Kritchevsky and Klurfeld, 1986). When energy intake was restricted by 10%, tumor incidence was not affected, but the number of tumors per tumor-bearing rat and the tumor burden were reduced compared to the control group. When energy intake was restricted 20 and 30%, tumor incidence, frequency, and size were further decreased and only one tumor was observed in the 40% energy restricted group (Kritchevsky and Klurfeld, 1986).

Because the diets used in the above studies were relatively low in fat, the effect of moderate energy restriction (by 25%) and increased levels of fat were examined (Kritchevsky and Klurfeld, 1986; Kritchevsky et al., 1986). Carcinogen-induced rats were fed ad libitum diets containing 5, 15, or 20% corn oil or a diet moderately restriced in energy (by 25%) providing 20 or 26.7% fat (i.e., equivalent to the ad libitum groups fed 15 or 20% fat (Kritchevsky and Klurfeld, 1986; Kritchevsky et al., 1986). Mammary tumor incidence and size increased sharply when fat was raised from 5 to 15 to 20%. But when energy intake was restricted by 25%, tumor incidence, frequency and size were significantly lower than in rats fed ad libitum a diet containing one-third to one-quarter as much fat. These findings suggest that energy restriction significantly reduces tumor growth even in the presence of a high fat intake (Kritchevsky and Klurfeld, 1986; Kritchevsky et al., 1986).

Studies with growing animals have shown that fat provides about 11 kcal/g or 124% of the expected 9 kcal/g (Donato and Hegsted, 1985; Donato, 1986). This increased efficiency of fat calories as compared to calories from other energy sources is related in part to the inefficient process of synthesizing fat from dietary carbohydrate and protein when low fat diets are consumed (Boissonneault et al., 1986; Boutwell and Pariza, 1986). To determine whether the enhancing effect of fat on tumorigenesis is due to the increased efficiency of utilization of fat calories, carcinogen-induced rats were fed ad libitum either a lowfat (5% corn oil) or a high fat (30% corn oil) diet, or a high fat (30% corn oil) diet slightly restricted to provide a level of usable energy equivalent to the low fat group (Boissonneault et al., 1986). After 24 weeks on the above diets, the incidence of mammary tumors was 73% in the high fat ad libitum fed animals, 43% in the low fat ad libitum fed rats, and 7% in the animals fed the high fat diet at a restricted level. That is, rats consuming a high fat diet developed fewer tumors than those fed a low fat diet when net energy was restricted (38). The findings of this study led the authors to conclude that tumor incidence is independent of the percent of dietary fat per se or the amount of fat consumed. Instead, mammary tumor development appears to depend on a complex interaction involving energy intake, energy retention within the body (body fat versus lean body mass), and ultimate body size (Boissonneault et al., 1986).

The means by which energy intake affects tumorigenesis is unknown (Kritchevsky et al., 1984), although the obesity-related increase in the production of hormones is implicated in the development of cancers of the breast and endometrium (Simopoulos, 1985; Boutwell and Pariza, 1986). The precise relationship between energy intake per se and cancer incidence in humans is difficult to define because the energy content of the diet and the efficiency of utilization of energy can be affected by differences in various energy sources. Moreover, obesity or overweight can result not only from excess energy intake but also from low energy expenditure.

Dietary Recommendations Regarding Fat Intake and Cancer

Many inconsistencies and unknowns surround the dietary fat-cancer hypothesis including the mechanism(s) of action and the amount and type of fat necessary to increase tumorigenesis. Furthermore, fat in the diet does not exist alone but in combination with many other nutrients and food components which may modulate carcinogenesis. Yet in spite of the lack of evidence of a causal relationship between fat intake and cancer, dietary recommendations have been made to the general public aimed at reducing the risk of cancer (Committee on Diet, Nutrition and Cancer, 1982; American Cancer Society, 1984; National Cancer Institute, 1984).

In 1982, the Committee on Diet, Nutrition and Cancer of the National Research Council/National Academy of Sciences (NRC/NAS) issued a series of interim dietary recommendations including the recommendation to reduce total fat intake from the present level of about 40% of total energy intake to 30%. This recommendation to lower fat intake subsequently was supported by other groups such as the American Cancer Society (1984) and the National Cancer Institute (1984).

These dietary recommendations to reduce cancer risk are not universally accepted. Many scientists, professional organizations, and government agencies claim that available scientific data are inadequate to support any specific dietary recommendations to reduce cancer (American Medical Association Council on Scientific Affairs, 1979; Doll and Peto, 1981; Enstrom, 1981; Council for Agricultural Science and Technology, 1982; Mendeloff, 1983; Pariza, 1984; Willett and MacMahon, 1984; U.S. Department of Agriculture, 1984; Sherwin, 1985).

It is unknown what fraction of cancer could be reduced by modifications in diet in general and in dietary fat in particular (Committee on Diet, Nutrition and Cancer, 1982; Visek and Clinton, 1983). Moreover, there is no conclusive evidence that lowering dietary fat intake is beneficial in terms of reducing overall mortality in humans (Enstrom, 1981; Pariza, 1984; Sherwin, 1985). In a number of coronary heart disease intervention studies employing a fat modified diet, the decrease in coronary heart disease mortality was offset by a corresponding increase in deaths from cancer or other causes such that total mortality in the population remained unchanged (Multiple Risk Factor Intervention Trial Research Group, 1982; McNamara, 1982; Sherwin, 1985). Furthermore, a recent analysis of data from the Honolulu Heart Program revealed that men consuming low fat diets had a higher mortality rate, particularly from cancer and stroke, than those whose fat intake was greater (McGee et al., 1985).

The long-term consequences of a diet low in fat, saturated fatty acids, and cholesterol and high in polyunsaturated fatty acids are unknown (McNamara, 1982; Sherwin, 1985). The safety of high intakes of polyunsaturated fatty acids is questioned, particularly in relation to gallstone formation, cancer incidence and alterations in cell membrane composition and fluidity (Sturdevant et al., 1973; McNamara, 1982; Sherwin, 1985). As reviewed above, not only have polyunsaturated fatty acids been shown to promote the growth of certain experimentally induced tumors (Carroll and Khor, 1971; Carroll and Hopkins,

1979; Carroll, 1980; Carroll, 1982; Carroll, 1985), but they are thought to be more immunosuppressive than saturated fatty acids (Vitale and Broitman, 1981; Kakar and Henderson, 1985). Furthermore, unsaturated fatty acids and cholesterol are more susceptible than saturated fatty acids to oxidation and free radical formation (Ames, 1983). Free radicals can damage membranes and cellular DNA and are involved in several pathologic processes including carcinogenesis (Kakar and Henderson, 1985). A diet high in polyunsaturated fatty acids may increase the requirement for protective antioxidants such as vitamin E (tocopherol), B-carotene, selenium, and ascorbic acid (Ames, 1983; Kakar and Henderson, 1985).

Lowering intake of fat or limiting foods such as dairy products, meat, or eggs because of their fat content to reduce cancer risk not only is unlikely to change mortality but potentially could lead to nutrient deficiencies (Council for Agricultural Science and Technology, 1982; Pariza, 1984). This in turn could lead to increased risk of other diseases. Moreover, as discussed below, cutting back on dairy foods possibly may increase the risk of cancer. In making dietary recommendations for the general population, it is important to consider not only the possible benefits but also how the changes may influence other diseases and the general health and well-being of the population (Carroll, 1985).

Milk And Milk Products As Potential Inhibitors Of Carcinogenesis

Findings from some epidemiological studies have suggested that increased consumption of milk protects against cancers of the bladder (Mettlin and Graham, 1979), stomach (Hirayama, 1967; Hirayama, 1977; Hirayama, 1984), and colon (Phillips, 1975; MacLennan et al., 1978; Jensen et al., 1982; McKeown-Eyssen and Bright-See, 1984; Garland et al., 1985). For example, Hirayama (1967) reported an inverse association between daily consumption of milk and stomach cancer in a case-control study in Japan. This finding was supported ten years later in a prospective cohort study involving over 260,000 persons (Hirayama, 1977). In this study, consumption of two glasses of milk/day was associated with a lower incidence of gastric cancer (Hirayama, 1977). The mechanism by which milk protects against stomach cancer is unknown, although it has been suggested that milk reduces the stomach's production of nitrosamines, a potent carcinogen in laboratory animals (Kurechi and Kikugawa, 1979; Rooma and Uibu, 1983). In an in vitro study carried out in the USSR, milk products with a fat content of 0.6 to 3.2% decreased the level of nitrites available for nitrosamine formation by 20 to 60% (Rooma and Uiby, 1983).

Of considerable recent interest is the suggestion that milk and dairy products, due to their calcium content, possibly may protect against colon cancer (Wargovich et al., 1983; Wargovich et al., 1984; Newmark et al., 1984; Garland et al., 1985; Anonymous, 1985; Lipkin and Newmark, 1985; Bresalier and Kim, 1985). In a 19-year prospective investigation of 1954 middle-aged men who completed a 28-day dietary history between 1957 and 1959, it was found that risk of colorectal cancer was inversely associated with dietary vitamin D and calcium (Garland et al., 1985). The association remained significant after adjusting for confounding factors such as age, cigarette smoking, body mass index, alcohol intake, and percentage of calories from fat (Garland et al., 1985; Anonymous, 1985). This finding supports the previously reported association between high milk intake and low cancer incidence in Finland as compared to Denmark (Report from the IARC Intestinal Microecology Group, 1977; MacLennan et al., 1978; Anonymous, 1985). A suggested confounding factor, however, is the higher consumption of dietary fiber by the Finnish population as compared to the Danish (Report from the IARC Intestinal Microecology Group, 1977; MacLennan et al., 1978; Anonymous, 1985). However, there is no conclusive evidence that dietary fiber protects against colon-rectum cancer in humans (Committee on Diet, Nutrition and Cancer, 1982).

Increasing calcium intake by 1.5 times the Recommended Dietary Allowance for this mineral recently has been shown to decrease cell growth in colonic epithelial cells in ten asymptomatic subjects at high risk for this type of cancer (Lipkin and Newmark, 1985; Bresalier and Kim, 1985). After two to three months of dietary supplementation with calcium (1250 mg/day), the profile of proliferating epithelial cells in the colonic crypts of subjects at high risk for colonic cancer was characteristic of that in individuals at low risk (Lipkin and Newmark, 1985). The mechanism by which calcium protects against colon cancer is unknown. As discussed above, dietary fat may promote colon cancer by increasing colonic levels of free ionized fatty acids and bile acids which may possess co-carcinogenic properties (Committee on

Diet, Nutrition and Cancer, 1982). Experimental animal studies reveal that calcium reduces the effects of fatty acids and bile acids on the colon epithelium or blocks the reported cell-damaging activity of these agents by forming biologically inert calcium soaps (Wargovich et al., 1983; Wargovich et al., 1984; Newmark et al., 1984). However, as neither bile acids nor calcium complexes were measured in the human subjects participating in Lipkin and Newmark's study (1985), it is unknown whether this mechanism or any other mechanism explains calcium's protective effect against colon cancer. The findings that risk of colon cancer is lower in some populations known to be high consumers of dairy products and that the cancer promoting effect of fat may be modulated by calcium merit further investigation. This is particularly important considering that cancer of the colon and rectum (colorectal cancer) affects about 6% of the U.S. population and is estimated to be responsible for 60,000 deaths in 1986 (American Cancer Society 1986; Bresalier and Kim, 1985).

A number of investigations carried out over the past decade suggest that intake of cultured and culture-containing dairy foods may inhibit the growth or formation of tumor cells. In 1973, Reddy et al. observed a 28% reduction in Ehrlich ascites tumor cell proliferation in male Swiss mice fed yogurt ad libitum for several days. Similar findings later were reported by Friend et al. (1982) and Reddy et al. (1983). Moreover, fecal bacterial enzymes associated with risk of bowel cancer were reduced by the intake of lactic cultures (Goldin and Gorbach, 1976; Goldin and Gorbach, 1977; Goldin et al., 1980; Ayebo et al., 1981; Gorbach, 1982; Goldin and Gorbach, 1984).

In humans consuming an omnivorous "Western-type" diet, fecal activities of enzymes associated with the conversion of chemical procarcinogens to proximal carcinogens in the large bowel were greater than those in vegetarians (Goldin et al., 1982). When viable Lactobacillus acidophilus organisms were added to the diet of omnivores, activities of fecal bacterial enzymes associated with colon cancer decreased (Goldin et al., 1982). Also, in human subjects fed Lactobacillus acidophilus milk or oral supplements of viable Lactobacillus acidophilus, activities of these fecal enzymes were significantly reduced (Ayebo et al., 1981; Goldin and Gorbach, 1984). Once the lactobacilli feeding was discontinued, however, fecal enzyme activities returned to baseline levels (Ayebo et al., 1981; Goldin and Gorbach,

1984). In addition, lactic cultures have been reported to reduce the incidence of tumors in laboratory animals receiving a chemical carcinogen (Goldin and Gorbach, 1980; Gorbach, 1982; Shackelford et al., 1983).

Although the evidence to-date is suggestive, it remains to be determined whether lactic bacteria in cultured and culture-containing dairy foods reduce the risk of large bowel cancer in humans (Gorbach, 1982; Goldin and Gorbach, 1984). The carcinogen in colon cancer has yet to be identified and the significance in terms of carcinogenesis of lowered bacterial enzyme activity induced by lactic cultures is unknown (Goldin and Gorbach, 1977; Goldin and Gorbach, 1984).

The above findings that calcium in milk and other dairy foods and Lactobacilli cultures in cultured dairy foods may protect against cancer are not conclusive. Nevertheless, they do raise questions concerning the advisability of reducing intake of foods such as milk and other dairy products as sources of fat in an effort to decrease the risk of cancer.

CONCLUSION

While total fat available in the nation's food supply has increased since the beginning of the century, most of this increase is explained by the greater availability of vegetable rather than animal sources of fat. Overall consumption of dairy foods has declined despite the recent upswing in total fluid milk consumption with foods in the dairy group providing a smaller percentage of fat available in the 1980s than in the early 1900s. Moreover, dairy foods contribute a much smaller percentage of fat available (only 11%) than other food groups such as fats and oils (44.7%).

While some nutrients or food components have been suggested to promote cancer, others may be protective (Doll and Peto, 1981; Committee on Diet, Nutrition and Cancer, 1982; Jensen, 1983; Willett and MacMahon, 1984). Also, different nutrients may exert different effects on specific types of cancer (Committee on Diet, Nutrition and Cancer, 1982). Consequently, limiting certain foods in our diet in an effort to prevent cancer may in fact increase the risk of this disease. For example, restricting the intake of dairy foods because of their fat content could lead to a deficiency of calcium, a nutrient suggested to possibly protect against colon cancer as well as other major chronic diseases such as osteoporosis and hypertension. For individuals who need or wish to reduce their intake of fat, a variety of milk products is available with different fat and energy levels.

With the exception of lung cancer, which is attributed to tobacco smoking, there is no convincing evidence that most other cancers in the U.S. have increased over the past several decades (Ames, 1983). Moreover, life expectancy in this country is steadily increasing (Ames, 1983). Until more is known about the cause(s) of cancer and in particular the association between diet and this disease, "a nutritious diet providing adequate amounts of all nutrients and the proper energy content to achieve desirable weight is important for general health and for vigorous defense mechanisms against cancer as well as other diseases," according to the Food and Nutrition Board (1980).

REFERENCES

Agricultural Research Service, US Department of Agriculture (1976). "Composition of Foods, Dairy and Egg Products, Raw, Processed, Prepared." Agriculture Handbook No. 8-1. Washington DC: US Government Printing Office.

American Cancer Society (1984). "Nutrition and Cancer: Cause and Prevention." Special Report. New York: Am Cancer Society.

American Cancer Society (1986). "1986 Cancer Facts & Figures." New York: American Cancer Society.

American Medical Association Council on Scientific Affairs (1979). Concepts of Nutrition and Health. JAMA 242:2335-2338.

Ames BN (1983). Dietary carcinogens and anticarcinogens. Science 221:1256-1264.

Anonymous (1985). Calcium and vitamin D intakes influence the risk of bowel cancer in men. Nutr Rev 43:170-172.

Armstrong BK, Doll R (1975). Environmental factors and cancer incidence and mortality in different countries with special reference to dietary practices. Int J Cancer 15: 617-631.

Avioli LV (1984). Calcium and osteoporosis. Ann Rev Nutr 4:471-491.

Ayebo AD, Shahani KM, Dam R (1981). Antitumor component(s) of yogurt: fractionation. J Dairy Sci 64:2318-2323.

Bingham S, Williams DRR, Cole TJ, James WPT (1979). Dietary fibre and regional large-bowel cancer mortality in Britain. Br J Cancer 40:456-463.

Blair A, Fraumeni JF Jr (1978). Geographic patterns of prostate cancer in the United States. J Natl Cancer Inst 61:1374-1384.

Block G, Dresser CM, Hartman AM, Carroll MD (1985). Nutrient sources in the American diet: quantitative data from the NHANES II Survey. II Macronutrients and fats. Am J Epidemiol 122:27-40.

Boissonneault GA, Elson CE, Pariza MW (1986). Net energy effects of dietary fat on chemically induced mammary carcinogenesis in F344 rats. J Natl Cancer Inst 76: 335-338.

Boutwell RK, Pariza MW (1986). Historical perspective: calories and energy expenditure in carcinogenesis. AM J Clin Nutr. In press.

Bresalier RS, Kim YS (1985). Diet and colon cancer. N Engl J Med 313:1413-1414.

Brown RR (1983). The role of diet in cancer causation. Food Technol 37:49-56.

Bull AW, Soulier BK, Wilson PS, Hayden MT, Nigro ND (1979). Promotion of azoxymethane-induced intestinal cancer by high fat in rats. Cancer Res 39:4956-4959.

Bunch K (1985a). Whole milk is no longer the beverage of choice. Natl Food Rev 29:21-24.

Bunch K (1985b). US food consumption on the rise. National Food Rev 29:1-4.

Bunch K, Hazera J (1984). Fats and oils: consumers use more but different kinds. National Food Rev 26:18-21.

Carroll KK (1975). Experimental evidence of dietary factors and hormone-dependent cancers. Cancer Res 35:3374-3383.

Carroll KK (1980). Lipid and carcinogenesis. J Envir Path Toxicol 3:253-271.

Carroll KK (1982). Dietary fat and its relationship to human cancer. In Stich HF (ed): "Carcinogens and Mutagens in the Environment," Vol 1. Food Products. Boca Raton Fla: CRC Press, Inc., pp 31-38.

Carroll KK (1983). The role of dietary fat in carcinogenesis. In Perkins EG, Visek WJ (eds): "Dietary Fats and Health," Champaign IL: American Oil Chemists' Society, pp 710-720.

Carroll KK (1985). Dietary fat and breast cancer. Nutrition Update 2:29-47.

Carroll KK, Hopkins GJ (1979). Dietary polyunsaturated fat versus saturated fat in relation to mammary carcinogenesis Lipids 14: 155-158.

Carroll KK, Khor HT (1975). Dietary fat in relation to tumorigenesis. Prog Biochem Pharmacol 10:308-353.

Carroll MD, Abraham S, Dresser CM (1983). "Dietary Intake Source Data: United States 1976-80." Vital and Health Statistics, Series II, No 231, DHHS Pub No (PHS) 83-1681. National Center for Health Statistics, Public Health Service, Washington DC: US Government Printing Office.

Cohen BI, Raicht RF, Razzini E (1982). Reduction of N-methyl-N-nitrosourea-induced colon tumors in the rat by cholesterol. Cancer Res 42:5050-5052.

Committee on Diet, Nutrition and Cancer, Assembly of Life Sciences. National Research Council (1982). "Diet, Nutrition and Cancer." Washington DC: National Academy Press.

Consensus Development Panel, Office of Medical Applications of Research, National Institutes of Health (1984). Osteoporosis. JAMA 252:799-802.

Correa P (1981). Epidemiological correlations between diet and cancer frequency. Cancer Res 41:3685-3690.

Council for Agricultural Science and Technology (1982). "Diet, Nutrition and Cancer: A Critique". Special publication 13. Ames, Iowa: Council for Agricultural Science and Technology.

Creasey WA (1985). "Diet and Cancer." Philadelphia: Lea & Febiger, pp 83-107.

Donato K, Hegsted DM (1985). Efficiency of utilization of various sources of energy for growth. Proc Natl Acad Sci USA 82:4866-4870.

Donato KA (1986). Efficiency and utilization of various energy sources for growth. Paper presented at the International Life Sciences Institute-Nutrition Foundation symposium on "Calories and Energy Expenditure in Carcinogenesis," February 24 & 25.

Doll R, Peto R (1981). The causes of cancer: quantitative estimates of avoidable risks of cancer in the United States today. J Natl Cancer Inst 66:1191-1308.

Enstrom JE (1975). Cancer mortality among Mormons. Cancer 36:825-841.

Enstrom JE (1981). Reassessment of the role of dietary fat in cancer etiology. Cancer Res 41:3722-3723.

Food and Nutrition Board, Division of Biological Sciences, Assembly of Life Sciences, The National Research Council (1980) "Toward Healthful Diets," Washington DC: National Academy Press.

Friend BA, Farmer RE, Shahani KM (1982). Effect of feeding and intraperitoneal implantation of yoghurt culture cells on Ehrlich ascites tumor. Milchwissenschaft 37:708-710.

Garfinkel L (1985). Overweight and cancer. Ann Intern Med 103:1034-1036.

Garland C, Shekelle RB, Barrett-Connor E, Criqui MH, Rossof AH, Paul O (1985). Dietary vitamin D and calcium and risk of colorectal cancer: A 19-year prospective study in men. The Lancet 1:307-309.

Gaskill SP, McGuire WL, Osborne CK, Stern MP (1979). Breast cancer mortality and diet in the United States. Cancer Res 39:3628-3637.

Goldin BR, Gorbach SL (1976). The relationship between diet and rat fecal bacterial enzymes implicated in colon cancer. J Natl Cancer Inst 57:371-375.

Goldin B, Gorbach SL (1977). Alterations in fecal microflora enzymes related to diet, age, lactobacillus supplements, and dimethylhydrazine. Cancer 40:2421-2426.

Goldin BR, Gorbach SL (1980). Effect of Lactobacillus acidophilus dietary supplements on 1,2-dimethylhydrazine dihydrochloride-induced intestinal cancer in rats. J Natl Cancer Inst 64:263-265.

Goldin BR, Gorbach SL (1984). The effect of milk and lactobacillus feeding on human intestinal bacterial enzyme activity. Am J Clin Nutr 39:756-761.

Goldin BR, Swenson L, Dwyer J, Sexton M, Gorbach SL (1980). Effect of diet and Lactobacillus acidophilus supplements on human fecal bacterial enzymes. J Natl Cancer Inst 64:255-261.

Gorbach SL (1982). The intestinal microflora and its colon cancer connection. Infection 10:379-384.

Graham S, Haughey B, Marshall J, Priore R, Byers T, Rzepka T, Mettlin C, Pontes JE (1983). Diet in the epidemiology of carcinoma of the prostate gland. J Natl Cancer Inst 70:687-692.

Graham S, Marshall J, Mettlin C, Rzepka T, Nemoto T, Byers T (1982). Diet in the epidemiology of breast cancer. Am J Epidemiol 116:68-75.

Gregorio DI, Emrich LJ, Graham S, Marshall JR, Nemoto T (1985). Dietary fat consumption and survival among women with breast cancer. J Natl Cancer Inst 75:37-41.

Heaney RP, Gallagher JC, Johnston CC, Neer R, Parfitt AM, Whedon GD (1982). Calcium nutrition and bone health in the elderly. Am J Clin Nutr 36(supp):986-1013.

Henry HJ, McCarron DA, Morris CD, Parrott-Garcia M (1985). Increasing calcium intake lowers blood pressure: the literature reviewed. J Am Diet Assoc 85:182-185.

Heshmat, MY, Kaul L, Kovi J, Jackson MA, Jackson AG, Jones GW, Edson M, Enterline JP, Worrell RG, Perry SL (1985). Nutrition and prostate cancer: a case-control study. The Prostate 6:7-17.

Higginson J (1983). Summary: nutrition and cancer. Cancer Res (suppl) 43:2515-2518.

Hirayama T (1967). The epidemiology of cancer of the stomach in Japan with special reference to the role of diet. In Harris RJC (ed): "Proceedings of the 9th International Cancer Congress," UICC Monograph Series Volume 10. New York: Springer-Verlog, pp 37-48.

Hirayama T (1977). Changing patterns of cancer in Japan with special reference to the decrease in stomach cancer mortality. In Hiatt HH, Watson JD, Winsten JA (eds): "Origins of Human Cancer. Book A, Incidence of Cancer in Humans," Cold Spring Harbor New York: Cold Spring Harbor Laboratory, pp 55-75.

Hirayama T (1984). Epidemiology of stomach cancer in Japan. With special reference to the strategy for the primary prevention. Jpn J Clin Oncol 14:159-168.

International Life Sciences Institute, Nutrition Foundation, American Medical Association, American Dietetic Association, Agricultural and Food Chemistry Division, American Chemical Society, US Department of Agriculture (1986). "Calories and Energy Expenditure in Carcinogenesis." Washington DC: February 24 and 25.

Ip C, Carter CA, Ip MM (1985). Requirement of essential fatty acid for mammary tumorigenesis in the rat. Cancer Res 45:1997-2001.

Ip C, Sinha DK (1981). Enhancement of mammary tumorigenesis by dietary selenium deficiency in rats with a high polyunsaturated fat intake. Cancer Res 41:31-34.

Jain M, Cook GM, Davis FG, Grace MG, Howe GR, Miller AB (1980). A case-control study of diet and colo-rectal cancer. Int J Cancer 26:757-768.

Jensen OM (1983). Epidemiological evidence associating lipids with cancer causation. In Perkins EG, Visek WJ (eds): "Dietary Fats and Health," Champaign IL: American Oil Chemists' Society, pp 698-709.

Jensen OM, MacLennan R, Wahrendorf J (1982). Diet, bowel function, fecal characteristics, and large bowel cancer in Denmark and Finland. Nutr Cancer 4:5-19.

Kakar F, Henderson M (1985). Diet and breast cancer. Clin Nutr 4:119-130.

Kolonel LN, Nomura AMY, Hinds MW, Hirohata T, Hankin JH, Lee J (1983). Role of diet in cancer incidence in Hawaii. Cancer Res (suppl) 43:2397-2402.

Kritchevsky D (1983). Lipids and carcinogenesis session: summary of discussion. Cancer Res (suppl) 43:2508.

Kritchevsky D (1985). Calories and chemically induced tumors in rodents. Comprehensive Ther 11:35-39.

Kritchevsky D, Klurfeld DM (1986). Caloric effects in experimental mammary tumorigenesis. Paper presented at the International Life Sciences Institute-Nutrition Foundation symposium on "Calories and Energy Expenditure in Carcinogenesis." Washington DC: February 24 and 25.

Kritchevsky D, Weber MM, Klurfeld DM (1984). Dietary fat versus caloric content in initiation and promotion of 7,12-dimethylbenzanthracene-induced mammary tumorigenesis in rats. Cancer Res 44:3174-3177.

Kritchevsky D, Weber MM, Buck CL, Klurfeld, DM (1986). Calories, fat and cancer. Lipids. In press.

Kutechi T, Kikugawa K (1979). Nitrite-lipid reaction in aqueous system: inhibitory effects on nitrosamine formation. J Food Science 44:1263-1266, 1971.

Lew EA, Garfinkel L (1979). Variations in mortality by weight among 750,000 men and women. J Chron Dis 32:563-576.

Lipkin M, Newmark H (1985). Effect of added dietary calcium on colonic epithelial-cell proliferation in subjects at high risk for familial colonic cancer. N Engl J Med 313:1381-1384.

Lowenthal JP (ed) (1983). "Proceedings of the Workshop Conference on Nutrition in Cancer Causation and Prevention," held in Fort Lauderdale Florida, 18-20 October 1982. Sponsored by the American Cancer Society. Cancer Res (suppl) 43:2386.

Lyon JL, Sorenson AW (1978). Colon cancer in a low risk population. Am J Clin Nutr 31:227-230.

MacCay CM, Ellis GH, Barnes LL, Smith CAH, Sperling G (1939). Chemical and pathological changes in aging and after retarded growth. J Nutr 18:15-25.

MacLennan R (1985). Fat intake and cancer of the gastrointestinal tract and prostate. Med Oncol & Tumor Pharmacother 2:137-142.

MacLennan R, Jensen OM, Mosbech J, Vuori H (1978). Diet, transit-time, stool weight and colon cancer in two Scandinavian populations. Am J Clin Nutr 31:S239-S242.

Marston RM, Raper NR (1986). The nutrient content of the food supply. Natl Food Rev 32:   .

Marston RM, Welsh SO (1984). Nutrient content of the US food supply, 1982. Natl Food Rev 25:7-13.

McCarron DA (1985). Is calcium more important than sodium in the pathogenesis of essential hypertension? Hypertension 7:607-627.

McCarron DA, Morris CD (1985). Blood pressure response to oral calcium in persons with mild to moderate hypertension. Ann Intern Med 103:825-831.

McGee D, Reed D, Stemmerman G, Rhoads G, Yano K, Feinleib M (1985). The relationship of dietary fat and cholesterol to mortality in 10 years: the Honolulu Heart Program. Int J Epidemiol 14:97-105.

McKeown-Eyssen GE, Bright-See E (1984). Dietary factors in colon cancer: international relationships. Nutr & Cancer 6:160-170.

McMichael AJ, Jensen OM, Parkin DM, Zaridze DG (1984). Dietary and endogenous cholesterol and human cancer. Epidemiol Rev 6:192-216.

Meikel A, Stanish W, West D (1982). Risk factors for prostate cancer. Abstracts of the American Public Health Association Meeting. Montreal Canada. November 14-18, p 30.

Mendeloff, AI (1983). Appraisal of "Diet, Nutrition, and Cancer." Am J Clin Nutr 37:495-498.

Mettlin C (1984). Diet and the epidemiology of human breast cancer. Cancer 53:605-611.

Mettlin C, Graham S (1979). Dietary risk factors in human bladder cancer. Am J Epidemiol 110:255-263.

Milk Industry Foundation (1985). "Milk Facts." Washington DC: Milk Industry Foundation, p 20.

Miller AB (1985). Diet, nutrition and cancer. An epidemiological overview. J Nutr Growth and Cancer 2:159-171.

Multiple Risk Factor Intervention Trial Research Group (1982). Multiple Risk Factor Intervention Trial: risk factor changes and mortality results. JAMA 248:1465-1477.

Nair PP (1984). Diet, nutrition intake, and metabolism in populations at high and low risk for colon cancer. Am J Clin Nutr 40:880-886.

National Cancer Institute, US Department of Health and Human Services, Public Health Service, National Institutes of Health (1984). "Cancer Prevention." NIH Publication No. 84-2671.

National Cancer Institute, Division of Cancer Etiology and the Division of Cancer Prevention and Control (1985). Symposium on the "Role of Nutrients in Carcinogenesis," held at the National Institutes of Health, Bethesda MD, 30 January -1 February.

National Economics Division, Economic Research Service, US Department of Agriculture (1984). "Food Consumption, Prices, and Expenditures, 1963-83." Statistical Bulletin Number 713.

National Health and Nutrition Examination Survey (HANES II), 1976-80. Unpublished data. Values represent a weighted mean of the raw data which were presented as means for various age groups.

Nauss KM, Locniskar M, Newberne PM (1983). Effect of alterations in the quality and quantity of dietary fat on 1,2-dimethylhydrazine-induced colon tumorigenesis in rats. Cancer Res 43:4083-4090.

Newmark HL, Wargovich MJ, Bruce WR (1984). Colon cancer and dietary fat, phosphate, and calcium: a hypothesis. J Natl Cancer Inst 72:1323-1325.

Pariza MW (1984). A perspective on diet, nutrition, and cancer. JAMA 251:1455-1458.

Parrott-Garcia M, McCarron DA (1984). Calcium and hypertension. Nutr Rev 42:205-213.

Phillips RL (1975). Role of life-style and dietary habits in risk of cancer among Seventh Day Adventists. Cancer Res 35:3513-3522.

Phillips RL, Snowdon DA (1985). Dietary relationships with fatal colorectal cancer among Seventh-Day Adventists. J Natl Cancer Inst 74:307-317.

Rados B (1985). Eggs and dairy foods: dietary mainstays in decline. FDA Consumer 19:11-17.

Recker RR, Heaney RP (1985). The effect of milk supplements on calcium metabolism, bone metabolism and calcium balance. Am J Clin Nutr 41:254-263.

Reddy BS (1981). Dietary fat and its relationship to large bowel cancer. Cancer Res 41:3700-3705.

Reddy BS (1983). Experimental research on dietary lipids and colon cancer. In Perkins EG, Visek WJ (eds): "Dietary Fats and Health, " Champaign IL: American Oil Chemists' Society, pp 741-760.

Reddy GV, Friend BA, Shahani KM, Farmer RE (1983). Antitumor activity of yogurt components. J Food Protection 46:8–11.

Reddy BS, Hedges AR, Laakso K, Wynder EL (1978). Metabolic epidemiology of large bowel cancer: fecal bulk and constituents of high-risk North American and low-risk Finnish populations. Cancer 42:2832–2838.

Reddy GV, Shahani KM, Banerjee MR (1973). Inhibitory effect of yogurt on Ehrlich ascites tumor cell proliferation. J Natl Cancer Inst 50:815–817.

Report from the IARC (International Agency for Research on Cancer) Intestinal Microecology Group (1977). Dietary fibre, transit-time, fecal bacteria, steroids, and colon cancer in two Scandinavian populations. Lancet 2:207–211.

Resnick LM (1985). Calcium and hypertension: the emerging connection. Ann Intern Med 103:944–947.

Rizek RL, Welsh SO, Marston RM, Jackson EM (1983). Levels and sources of fat in the US food supply and in diets of individuals. In Perkins EG, Visek WJ (eds): "Dietary Fats and Health," Champaign IL: American Oil Chemists' Society, pp 13–43.

Rooma M, Uibu J (1983). Influence of various milk products on the concentration of nitrite and the formation of nitrosodimethylamine in vitro. Nutr Cancer 4:171–175.

Rose DP (1983). Diet, hormones, and cancer. Food Technol 37:58–67.

Rotkin ID (1977). Studies in the epidemiology of prostate cancer: expanded sampling. Cancer Treat Rep 61:173–180.

Sakaguchi M, Hiramatsu Y, Takada H, Yamamura M, Hioki K, Saito K, Yamamoto M (1984). Effect of dietary unsaturated and saturated fats on azoxymethane-induced colon carcinogenesis in rats. Cancer Res 44:1472–1477.

Sakaguchi M, Minoura T, Hiramatsu Y, Takada H, Yamamura M, Hioki K, Yamamoto M (1986). Effects of dietary saturated and unsaturated fatty acids on fecal bile acids and colon carcinogenesis induced by azoxymethane in rats. Cancer Res 46:61–65.

Salmond CE, Beaglehole R, Prior IAM (1985). Are low cholesterol values associated with excess mortality? Br Med J 290:422–424.

Sandler RB, Slemenda CW, LaPorte RE, Cauley JA, Schramm MM, Barresi ML, Kriska AM (1985). Postmenopausal bone density and milk consumption in childhood and adolescence. Am J Clin Nutr 42:270–274.

Shackelford LA, Rao DR, Chawan CB, Pulusani SR (1983). Effect of feeding fermented milk on the incidence of chemically induced colon tumors in rats. Nutr Cancer 5:159–164.

Shamberger RJ (1984). "Nutrition and Cancer." New York: Plenum Press, pp 53-70.

Sherwin R (1985). Nutrition, cancer, cardiovascular disease, and mortality. Clin Nutr 4:143-146.

Sidney S, Farquhar JW (1983). Cholesterol, cancer, and public health policy. Am J Med 75:494-508.

Simopoulos AP (1985). Fat intake, obesity, and cancer of the breast and endometrium. Med Oncol & Tumor Pharmacother 2:125-135.

Smith, AH, Pearce NE, Joseph JG (1985). Major colorectal cancer aetiological hypotheses do not explain mortality trends among Maori and non-Maori New Zealanders. Int J Epidemiol 14:79-85.

Snowdon, DA, Phillips RL, Choi W (1984). Diet, obesity, and risk of fatal prostate cancer. Am J Epidemiol 120:244-250.

Stemmermann GN, Nomura AMY, Heilbrun LK (1984). Dietary fat and risk of colorectal cancer. Cancer Res 44:4633-4637.

Sturdevant RAL, Pearce ML, Dayton S (1973). Increased prevalence of cholelithiasis in man ingesting a serum-cholesterol-lowering diet. N Engl J Med 288:24-27.

Talamini R, LaVecchia C, Decarli A, Franceschi S, Grattoni E, Grigoletto E, Liberati A, Tognoni G (1984). Social factors, diet and breast cancer in a northern Italian population. Br J Cancer 49:723-729.

Tannenbaum A (1942) The genesis and growth of tumors III. Effects of a high-fat diet. Cancer Res 2:468-475.

The American Society for Bone and Mineral Research (1982). "Osteoporosis," Kelseyville, California.

U.S. Department of Agriculture (1983). Response to the report "Diet, Nutrition and Cancer" of the Committee on Diet, Nutrition and Cancer, Assembly of Life Sciences, National Research Council, 1982.

Visek WJ, Clinton SK (1983). Dietary fat and breast cancer. In Perkins EG, Visek WJ (eds): "Dietary Fats and Health," Champaign IL: American Oil Chemists' Society, pp 721-740.

Vitale JJ, Broitman SA (1981). Lipids and immune function. Cancer Res 41:3706-3710.

Wargovich MJ, Eng VWS, Newmark HL (1984). Calcium inhibits the damaging and compensatory proliferative effects of fatty acids on mouse colon epithelium. Cancer Letters 23:253-258.

Wargovich MJ, Eng VWS, Newmark HL, Bruce WR (1983). Calcium ameliorates the toxic effect of deoxycholic acid on colonic epithelium. Carcinogenesis 4:1205-1207.

Welsch CW, Aylsworth CF (1983). Enhancement of murine mammary tumorigenesis by feeding high levels of dietary fat: a hormonal mechanism? J Natl Cancer Inst 70:215-221.

Willett WC, Browne ML, Bain C, Lipnick RJ, Stampfer MJ, Rosner B, Colditz GA, Hennekens CH, Speizer FE (1985). Relative weight and risk of breast cancer among premenopausal women. Am J Epidemiol 122:731-740.

Willett WC, MacMahon B (1984). Diet and cancer - an overview. N Engl J Med 310:697-703.

Index

AAF
  liver cancer, dietary fat and carcinogen metabolism, 463, 475
  metabolic activation, 599–600
Acinar cells, atypical nodules, pancreas, 336, 338–339, 346–350
Adaptation. *See* Fatty acid oxidation and triglyceride synthesis, adaptation to high-fat diet; Glucose metabolism adaptation to high-fat diet; *under* Cholesterol
Adenocarcinoma, pancreatic, enhancement by dietary fat, 343–345
Adenoma, pancreatic, enhancement by dietary fat, 343, 345
Adipocytes, breast epithelium cultures, fatty acid effects, 703–706
Adipose tissue, glucose metabolism adaptation to high-fat diet, 533, 535, 540
Ad libitum feeding, 368, 387, 388
  cf. calorie-restricted diet, 499–504
    DMBA breast tumorigenesis, mice, 517, 520–524
  see also Calorie-restricted diet *entries*
  carcinogenesis testing, 368
  dairy products, 843–845
Adrenocorticoids, calorie-restricted diet, and DMBA breast tumorigenesis, mice, 519
Aflatoxin
  liver cancer, 463–464, 466, 468
  metabolic activation, 598–599
Age and breast cancer
  chemically induced, rats, 266
  at menarche, 20, 21
AHH, metabolic activation, 589, 593, 595, 596, 598, 600
AIN-76 diet, 342, 344, 345, 378
Albumin, free fatty acid transport, 541, 542
Alcohol

dietary guidelines for heart disease and cancer reduction, 760
  fatty, 156
Aldosterone, breast epithelium cultures, fatty acid effects, 711–715
American Academy of Pediatrics, 745–746
American Cancer Society, 749
American Health Foundation, 745
American Heart Association, 735–736
American Institute for Cancer Research, 748
American Medical Association, 738, 744–745
Ames test, 199, 588, 599
  and intestinal microflora, 658, 660–662, 673
Anaerobic bacteria, intestinal, 656, 657
Androstenedione, aromatization into estrone, prostate carcinoma, 49–50, 58
Animal fat
  breast tumorigenesis, endocrine-dietary fat interaction, 624–625
  and colon cancer, 70, 71, 313–314
  cf. vegetable fats, U.S. food supply data, since 1910, 132, 148
  see also Dairy products *entries*; Livestock and meat industry perspective; specific fats
Animal models
  breast cancer prevention, low-fat-diet clinical trials, 100, 102–103
  dietary modification and cancer
    caloric intakes, 794
    tumor data interpretation, 794–795
  intestinal microflora, dietary fat, and cancer, 676–678
  see also Epidemiologic data, dietary fat and cancer, relation to experimental data
Animal protein and colon cancer, 71–72, 78
Antibiotics, oral, and intestinal microflora, 671–672, 677

Antigens
    H-2, 557, 562–564
    lymphocytes, 557–559, 575
Anti-inflammatory agents, nonsteroidal, 689,
    692
    indomethacin, 714–716
AOMand colon carcinogenesis, 389, 390,
    392
Arachidonic acid
    breast epithelium cultures, 714–721
    carcinogens, metabolic activation, 590,
        591, 596
    cascade, fish oil perturbation, 289–290
    and essential polyunsaturated fatty acids,
        211–212, 214, 222, 225
    immune function and dietary fat, 572–
        574, 579
    metabolism, eicosanoids, 687, 692–693
    see also Eicosanoids and cancer;
        Prostaglandins
ATP, glucose metabolism adaptation to high-
    fat diet, 535, 536
Australia, dietary guidelines, 755–756
Azaserine. See under Pancreatic cancer, en-
    hancement by dietary fat
Azoreductase, intestinal microflora, dietary
    fat, and cancer, 660, 667
Azoxymethane-induced colon cancer, 296,
    299–304
    colon cancer, dietary fat and, variable an-
        imal results, 315
    trans fatty acids, 287–288

Bacteria, colonic. See Intestinal microflora
Bacteroides, intestinal, 656, 657, 662–664,
    675–676
Basic Four Food Groups, 734–735, 738
B cells. See under Immune response, dietary
    fatty acid modulation
Beef cf. pork, food supply data, U.S. since
    1910, 137–138, 143, 145–149
Beef fat (tallow)
    and colon cancer, animal studies, 299,
        305
    dietary calcium, 490–492
    variable results, 315, 317–319
    food supply data, U.S. since 1910, 136,
        143, 148, 152

liver cancer, dietary fat and carcinogen
    metabolism, 466, 468
Benign prostatic hypertrophy, 51, 53, 56–58
Benzo(a)pyrene
    calorie-restricted diets and cancer, 495,
        497, 502
    fats, heated and oxidized, 195–196
    metabolic activation, 588–591, 593,
        595–599
Benzyl acetate, carcinogenesis-toxicity test-
    ing, corn oil gavage test, rodents,
    357, 369
BHA, BHT, 273, 275–276, 599–600
Bifidobacterium, intestinal, 656, 657, 664,
    665
Bile acids
    cholesterol metabolism adaptation, high-
        fat diets, 545, 546
    fecal, and colon cancer, 72, 77–81,
        305–306
        and dietary fiber, 507, 508
        and intestinal microflora, 666, 676
        metabolism into mutagens/carcino-
            gens, 82–84
        relation between dietary and serum
            cholesterol, 449, 453–454
        see also under Calcium
Blastogenesis, immune function, and dietary
    fat, 568
Bleaching in fat and oil processing, 167
Body weight, 368, 387, 388
    breast cancer, fat-protein interaction, de-
        fined two-generation studies,
        408–411
    calorie-restricted diets and cancer,
        502–504
        DMBA breast tumorigenesis, mice,
            518, 522, 524, 525
    carcinogenesis-toxicity testing, corn oil
        gavage test, rodent, 362–364,
        366–369
    colon cancer, dietary fat and, variable an-
        imal results, 320–322
    pancreatic carcinogenesis, enhancement
        by dietary fat, 340
BOP-induced pancreatic carcinogenesis, en-
    hancement by dietary fat, 331–342,
    349-350

Brain carcinogenesis, animal, and neutral fats and fatty acids, 250
Breast cancer
  calorie-restricted diets and cancer, 499–504
  carcinogenesis-toxicity testing, corn oil gavage test, rodent, 363–365
  cf. colon cancer, 834–835, 837–838, 843, 845
  dairy products, 834–835, 837–838, 843, 845
  eicosanoid production, 690, 691
  enterohepatic circulation of estrogens, intestinal microflora, 668–672
  fats, heated and oxidized, mutagens, 194, 197, 199
  cf. prostate carcinoma, 44, 45, 49–50
  see also Estrogens and breast cancer; Gap junction-mediated intercellular communication (metabolic cooperation), breast tumor promotion; Mammary; Prolactin and breast cancer
Breast cancer, DMBA-induced, 342
  calorie-restricted diet, mouse, 517–526
  dietary fat, 379–384
    fish oil, 290, 291
    immune system, 382–383
    ovarian hormones, 381–382
    prolactin, 382
    saturated cf. unsaturated, 384
    soybean oil, 382, 383
    trans fatty acids and tumorigenesis, 284–288
  dietary protein, 384–387
  energy intake, 387–389
    ad libitum, 387, 388
    underfeeding/calorie-restricted diets, 388
  initiation cf. promotion, 381, 386
  role of macronutrients, 377–389
Breast cancer epidemiology, dietary fat and, 7, 10, 17–28
  age at menarche, 20, 21
  breast fluid cholesterol, 21
    cholesterol epoxide, 21–22
  Canada, 22–24, 26, 27
  case control studies, 22–24, 26, 27, 33

dietary changes recommended, 25–26
cf. experimental data, 231, 232, 234–236, 238, 239, 241, 242
intervention studies, 27–28
Israel, 18, 24
Japan, 18, 19, 24–25, 38–39
Japan-Hawaii Cancer Study, 24, 39
methodologic issues, 7, 10
mortality rates, 19
selenium deficiency, 20
Seventh Day Adventists, 18, 22
U.S., 18, 19
Breast cancer, fat–protein interaction, defined two-generation studies, 403–431
  and breast development, 415, 421, 422, 423, 428
    terminal end buds, 421–423
  casein, 403–405, 407, 417, 420
  diets, composition, 407
  DMBA, 405, 414, 415, 420, 427–429, 431
  epidemiologic data, 403
  experimental data, summary, 403–404
  and food consumption and weight gain, 408–411
  and hormone regulation, 411–420
    dopamine, 411, 415, 416
    estrogen, 415, 420
    progesterone, 415
    prolactin, 411, 413–415, 417–419
    sexual maturation and estrous cycle, 408, 411–412, 418–420, 424
  NMU, 408, 418, 419, 430, 431
  and ^{3}H-thymidine incorporation, DNA, 421, 424–426
  tumor incidence, 424, 427–430
Breast cancer, obesity and, 21, 27, 33–39
  estrogen, extra-ovarian production, 33–36
  estrogen-receptor status, 35, 37, 38
  as growth enhancer, late in carcinogenic process, 35
  and height, 20, 21, 34, 38
  intervention, weight reduction, 37
  post-menopausal, 35, 37, 39
  public health impact, 38–39
Breast cancer prevention, low-fat-diet phase III clinical trials, NCI, 93–111, 779–780

epidemiologic and experimental back-
    ground, 99–103
  animal studies, 100, 102–103
  Nutrition Adjuvant Study, stage II breast
    cancer patients, 93, 107–111,
    779–780
  objectives and scope of feasibility studies,
    103–104
  trial development process, 95–99
    management structure, 96
  Women's Health Trial, women at risk,
    93, 104–107, 779
Breast dysplasia, dietary-fat reduction, clini-
    cal trials, Canada, 117–124
  assessment of outcome, 122
    dietary practices after study, 122–123
  compliance, 120–122
  feasibility, 118–119
  maintenance of patients after entry,
    119–120
    drop-outs, 119, 120
  patients, 118
  randomization, 120
  screening, 119–120
Breast epithelium cultures, fatty acid effects,
    rodents, 699–706, 707–722
  and adipocytes, 703–706
  DMBA, 709, 713, 714, 716–722
    mitotic index, 716, 717
  hyperplastic alveolar nodule, 708, 709
  linoleic acid, 700–703, 705–706
  mammary alveolar lesions, 709, 711–716,
    720
  mast cells, histamine release, 704–705
  membranes, 701, 702
  MTV, 708, 712
  organ cultures, 708–710, 714–715
  perphenazine, 701
  prolactin, 701, 703–705
  TG-resistant, HGPRT$^-$, 719–721
  TPA, 716–721
  unsaturated fatty acids, 713–716
    arachidonic acid, 714–721
    prostaglandins, 714–716
    /saturated ratio, 701, 702
    cf. stearic acid, 717–718, 720–721
Breast tumor, chemically induced, dietary fat
    modulation, rats, 255–276

borderline/pre-malignant, 270
  coconut oil, 270, 272
  coffee/caffeine, 275
  corn oil, 267–270, 272–274
    and dietary protein, 274
  DMBA, 256–263, 266–268, 270–272,
    274, 275
  essential fatty acids, 267, 272
  hormone-dependence, 257, 274
  lard, 270, 271, 273, 274
  linoleic acid, 270, 272
  mechanisms, 272–273
  MNU, 261–267, 269, 270, 272, 274, 275
    age-dependence, 266
    Ha-ras-1 oncogene, 266
  natural cf. purified diet, 257–259, 263–
    265, 271
  PUFA, 267, 272, 274
  retinoids, 275
  selenium, 274, 275
  terminal duct lobular units, 260, 273
    DNA synthesis, 273
  terminal end buds, 260
  timing and duration, 273
  vitamin E, 274
Breast tumorigenesis, endocrine–dietary fat
    interaction, 623–641
  animal fats, 624–625
  Ca^{2+}, 638, 639
  cell proliferation enhancement, 638
  diacylglycerol, 638–641
  DMBA, 628–630, 633–635
  EFA status, 633, 636
  estrogen receptors, 635
  estrogens, 628–629, 632–634, 636
  estrous cycle, 631, 632
  experimental results, summary, 623–624
  glucocorticoids, 629–630, 634–635
  growth hormone, 627–628, 631–632
  hormone responsiveness (receptors),
    635–637
  initiation vs. promotion, 625
  insulin, 630, 631
  ovaries, 625, 632, 634, 635
  phospholipids, 638–639
  pituitary, 625, 634, 635
  progesterone, 629, 632, 636
  prolactin, 626–627, 632–634

fibroadenomas, 627
  receptors, 636
protein kinase C, 638–641
thyroid hormones, 630–631, 634–635
unsaturated, 624–625, 638
  long-chain (fish oil), 624
Britain, dietary guidelines, 749–753
  World War II, low-fat diet, 759, 761
Butter, 181–182, 824, 829, 830, 833
  food supply data, U.S. since 1910, 134,
    143, 145, 148, 152
Butters, cocoa/hard, 180–181

Caffeine and chemically induced breast tu-
    mor, rats, 275
Calcium, 214
  -activated protein kinase C, 618, 638–641
  breast tumorigenesis, endocrine–dietary
    fat interaction, 638, 639
  and colon cancer, 76, 82, 83
  dairy products, 825, 826
  effect on bile acid and fat, colonic crypt
    epithelium, mice, 487–492
    beef fat, 490–492
    cholic acid, 489, 492
    corn oil, 490–492
    free fatty acids, 487
    inhibition of carcinogenesis, 848, 849
    membrane damage, 487
    proliferation, 489, 490, 492
  influx, immune function and dietary fat,
    576
Calorie intake
  and colon carcinogenesis, 394
    dietary fat and, variable animal re-
      sults, 323
  dairy products, 843–845
  and DMBA-induced breast carcinogene-
    sis, 387–389
  overnutrition, carcinogenesis testing with
    corn oil gavage test, 362–364,
    366–369
  pancreatic carcinogenesis, enhancement
    by dietary fat, 341
  percent from fat
    epidemiologic data, relation to experi-
      mental, 235–236
    food supply data, since 1910, U.S.,
      131, 141–142

see also Ad libitum feeding
Calorie-restricted diet, 388, 496–504
  cf. ad libitum diet, 499, 501–504
  benzo(a)pyrene, 495, 497, 502
  body weight, 502–504
  colon, 495–496, 499–500
  dairy products, 843, 844
  DMBA, 495, 499–502
    with essential nutrient underfeeding, 498
  fat, low cf. medium, 498–500
  graded calorie restriction, 501, 502
  mammary, 499–504
  MCA, 495, 498, 499
  cf. other weight loss modalities, 502
  fiber, 508
Calorie-restricted diet, acute, and DMBA-
    breast tumorigenesis, mouse, 517–526
  cf. ad libitum feeding, 517, 520–522, 524
  adrenocorticoids, 519
  body weight, 518, 522, 524, 525
  estrogen, 519–522, 524
  estrous cycles, 519, 523, 524
  growth hormone, 520, 521
  immunology, 525–526
    cf. other chronic diseases, 525–526
    thymus, 525–526
  pituitary insufficiency, 518–519
  prolactin, 519–522, 524
  timing, 519–520, 523
Canada
  breast cancer, 22–24, 26, 27
  breast dysplasia, dietary-fat reduction,
    clinical trials, 117–124
  dietary guidelines, 746, 753
Canadian Pediatrics Society, 745–746
Cancer reduction, U.S. See Dietary modifi-
    cation and cancer, overview; Guide-
    lines, dietary entries
Candicidin and colon cancer, 450
Carbohydrates, percent of calories from, epi-
    demiologic cf. experimental data,
    235–236
Carcinogenesis inhibition, dairy products,
    847–850
Carcinogenesis-toxicity testing, corn oil gav-
    age test-compound effects (NTP), ro-
    dents, 357–370
  alternatives (microencapsulation), 369

benzyl acetate, 357, 369
breast, 363–365
carbon tetrachloride, 358–360
chloroform, 358–360
chronic bioassays, 360–366
  extrapolation of carcinogenesis data,
    365–366
  untreated control vs. vehicle control
    tumors, 361–365
leukemia, 363, 364, 366
methylene chloride, 357, 369
overnutrition, 362–364, 366–369
  ad libitum feeding, 368
  diet composition, 366–368
  lack of exercise, 368
  tumor growth modulation mechanism,
    368–369
pancreatic, 361–363, 369, 370
prechronic studies, 358–360
  maximum tolerated dose, 358–360
  pharmacokinetics, 360
teratogenicty, 360, 369
Carcinogens, metabolic activation, overview,
    587–601
AAF mutagenicity, 599–600
aflatoxin, 598–599
AHH, 589, 593, 595, 596, 598, 600
benzo(a)pyrene, 588–591, 593, 595–599
BHT, 599–600
dietary fat and, 591–601
  colon cancer, 297, 299, 300
  corn oil, 593–595, 597–600
  essential fatty acid deficiency, 593
  fish oil, 594, 595, 598, 601
  polyenoic acids, 592
  polyunsaturated, 592, 596, 597
DMN, 593–595, 599, 600
DNA binding, 588–591, 597–599
epoxides, 588–590, 593, 598, 599
glutathione-S-transferase, 591, 596,
    599–601
3-methylcholanthrene, 593, 594, 598
MFO, liver microsomal, 587–593, 596,
    600
  cytochromes P-450, 587, 589, 592,
    594–596, 600
  phenobarbital, 588, 592, 594–596,
    599

PAH, 588
  bay regions, 589
  prostaglandin endoperoxide synthase,
    590–591, 593, 596
  arachidonic acid, 590, 591, 596
  tumorigenicity, 600–601
  see also Liver cancer, dietary fat and car-
    cinogen metabolism
Carnitine palmitoyl transferase, adaptation to
    high-fat diet, 542
Carotenoids, 156–157
β-carotene, 198
  NCI (U.S.), 780–782
Casein and breast cancer, 403–405, 407, 417,
    420
Causality, epidemiologic criteria, 100
Cell proliferation
  breast tumorigenesis, endocrine–dietary
    fat interaction, 638
  DMBA, breast epithelium cultures, fatty
    acid effects, 716–717
  eicosanoids and, 691
Cervical dysplasia, 784
Charcoal broiling, mutagens, 185, 195–196
  PAH, 185, 190–191, 195–197, 199
Cheese, 818–819, 821–823, 825, 827, 830,
    831
  food supply data, U.S. since 1910, 140,
    143, 147, 149
Chemoprevention, NCI (U.S.), 774
Chlorophyll, 156–157
Cholesterol
  blood, dairy products, 842
  breast-fluid, and breast cancer, 21
    cholesterol epoxide, 21–22
  dietary, dairy products, 831, 832,
    841–842
  food supply data, U.S. since 1910,
    146–149
    eggs, 147, 149, 152
  metabolism adaptation, high-fat diets,
    545–547
  see also Colon cancer, relation between
    dietary and serum cholesterol;
    Guidelines, dietary entries
Cholesterol dehydrogenase and intestinal mi-
    croflora, 666
Cholestyramine

colon cancer, relation between dietary
    and serum cholesterol, 448–450
and dietary fiber, 506
Cholic acid and dietary calcium, colonic
    crypt epithelium, mice, 489, 492
Choline deficiency, 468–472, 476
Cirrhosis, 222, 224, 469
Clinical trials. *See* Breast cancer prevention,
    low-fat-diet phase III clinical trials,
    NCI
Clofibrate
    colon cancer, relation between dietary
        and serum cholesterol, 448
    liver cancer, dietary fat and carcinogen
        metabolism, 473–475
Clostridium, intestinal, 79, 81, 656, 657,
    662, 665
Cocoa butter, 180
Coconut oil, animal studies
    breast tumors, 270, 272
    colon cancer, 301–302, 305
Coffee and chemically induced breast tumor,
    rats, 275
Cohort studies, colon cancer, 75–76
Colon cancer
    calorie-restricted diets, 495–496,
        499–500
    dairy products, 836, 838, 839, 842–843,
        848–850
    bile acids, 840
    see also Intestinal microflora; *under* Cal-
        cium; *under* Fiber, dietary
Colon cancer, dietary fat and, 69–76,
    295–306, 311–312, 325
    amount and type, animal studies,
        295–306
    animal fat, 70, 71, 313–314
    animal protein, 71–72, 78
    azoxymethone-induced, 287–288, 296,
        299–304, 315
    beef fat, 299, 305, 315, 317–319
    calcium, 76, 82, 83
    carcinogen metabolic activation, 297,
        299, 300
    case-control studies, 72–74, 82, 83, 312
    cohort studies, 75–76
        spouses of colon cancer patients,
            75–76

correlational studies, 69–72
DMAB, 296, 298, 299
DMH, 296, 298, 299
epidemiologic data, 69–76, 311–312, 315
high socioeconomic status and, 311–312
Japanese migrants to Hawaii, 71, 75, 79, 80,
    325, 444, 506, 655–656
    methodologic issues, 5, 7, 18, 20, 25
    relation to experimental, 231, 234,
        239
    Seventh Day Adventists, 75, 79, 80,
        83, 312, 452
fat, *trans*, 287–288, 302–305
fecal bile acids, 72, 77–81, 305–306
    metabolism into mutagens/carcino-
        gens, 82–84
fecal steroids, 76–83
    colon cancer patients, 81–82
    population groups, 78–81
    and fiber. *See* Fiber, dietary
β-glucuronidase, 78, 79
heated and oxidized fats, mutagens, 194,
    199
initiation, 299–301
lard, 297, 298, 300, 301, 305
meat, 71, 73, 74, 312
MAM acetate, 296, 298, 299
MNU, 296, 298, 299
oils
    coconut, olive, safflower, 301–302,
        305
    corn, 297, 298, 300–305, 317, 318
    fish, 302–305
promotion, 299, 301–304
variable animal results, 311–327
    body weight, 320–322
    caloric intake effect, 323
    Crisco®, 317, 318
    DMH, 315, 316, 319–320, 322–324,
        326
    cf. human epidemiologic data,
        311–312, 325
    isocalorically balanced high-fat diet,
        317, 319, 320, 324, 325
    MNNG, 326
    NMU, 316, 323
    strain differences, 319–324
vegetables, 74, 75

Colon cancer, relation between dietary and serum cholesterol, 435–455
  bile acids, 449, 453–454
  colonic microflora, 453–454
  dietary cholesterol, 436–440, 450
    epidemiology, 436–438
    experimental, 437–440
    high, with hypocholesterolemia, increased risk, 453–454
  sex, 451–452
  serum or plasma cholesterol, 440–455
    clinical studies, 447–448
    drug and dietary intervention trials, 448–450, 455
    epidemiology, 440–447
    epidemiology, studies listed, 441–443
Colon carcinogenesis, experimental, role of macronutrients, 377, 389–394
  AOM, 389, 390, 392
  caloric intake, 394
  dietary fat, 389
  dietary protein, 392–393
  DMBA, 391
  DMH, 389, 390, 392–394
Colonic microflora. See Intestinal microflora
Communication, intercellular. See Gap junction-mediated intercellular communication (metabolic cooperation), breast tumor promotion
Complement, immune function and dietary fat, 563, 564, 573–574
Confounding factors, epidemiology, 9–10
Cooking oil, 179; see also specific oils
Corn oil
  breast tumor, chemically induced, rats, 267–270, 272–274
  calcium, dietary, effect on bile acid and fat, colonic crypt epithlium, mice, 490–492
  carcinogens, metabolic activation, 593–595, 597–600
  and colon cancer, animal studies, 297, 298, 300–305
    variable results, 317, 318
  liver cancer, dietary fat and carcinogen metabolism, 466, 468
  pancreatic cancer, enhancement by dietary fat, 340, 342, 344, 345, 349–350

  see also Carcinogenesis-toxicity testing, corn oil gavage test-compound effects (NTP), rodents
Coronary heart disease, 440, 448, 451, 452; see also Guidelines, dietary entries
Cottonseed oil and liver cancer, carcinogen metabolism, 463–464
Cream, 819, 822, 827, 830
Crisco®
  colon cancer, variable animal results, 317, 318
  liver cancer, and carcinogen metabolism, 462, 463
Cycasin, intestinal, 657–658
Cyclooxygenase, eicosanoids and, 687–689
Cyclopropenoid fatty acids, 463, 464
Cytochrome P-450, metabolic activation of carcinogens, 587, 589, 592, 594–596, 600

DAB, dietary fat and carcinogen metabolism, liver, 462, 463
Dairy products, changing patterns, U.S., 133, 138–140, 143–149, 815–833
  butter, 824, 829, 830, 833
  calcium, 825, 826
    hypertension, 826
    osteoporosis, 826
  change in contribution to total fat, 828–833
  cheese, 140, 143, 147, 149, 818–819, 821–823, 825, 827, 831
  cream, 819, 822, 827, 830
  disappearance data, 818, 837
  epidemiology, 815–817
  fat and energy content, various products, 827
  food supply data, U.S. since 1910, 133, 138–140, 143–149
  frozen deserts, 827, 830, 831, 833
  milk
    lowfat, 818–820, 822, 823, 827, 831
    whole, 818–820, 822, 825, 827, 830, 831
  mortality statistics, 815, 816
    site and year, 816
  nutrients, listed, 825
  per capita, 151, 820–822, 824, 828
  yogurt, 818–823, 825, 837

Dairy products, dietary fat and cancer, overview, 833–851
  breast cancer, 834–835, 837–838, 843, 845
    prolactin, 840
  carcinogenesis inhibition, 847–850
    nitrosamines, stomach, 847, 848
    calcium, 848, 849
    microflora, 849, 850
    yogurt, *Lactobacillus acidophilus*, 849–850
  colon cancer, 836, 838, 839, 842–843, 848–850
    bile acids, 840
  dietary guidelines, 845–847
  energy (calorie) intake, 843–845
    ad libitum feeding, 843–845
    restriction, 843, 844
  epidemiologic evidence, 834–839, 842
  experimental animal evidence, 835, 836, 839, 841, 843, 849
  inconsistencies/discrepancies in hypothesis, 837–845
    blood cholesterol, 842
    dietary cholesterol, 841–842
    polyunsaturated fatty acids, 841, 846, 847
    promoter, 840
    Seventh Day Adventists, 839
  obesity, 843, 845
  prostate cancer, 836–838, 840
  and protein, 842
Deep-fat frying, oil deterioration, 185–189
DEHP and liver cancer, 473–475
7-α-Dehydroxylation, intestinal microflora, 666, 667
Delayed-type hypersensitivity, 570
DEN and liver cancer, 474, 475
Deodorization, fats and oils, 167
Dermatitis, linoleic acid deficiency, 214–216
DES, 659
DHT, prostate carcinoma, 52–54, 56, 58
Diabetes, 221, 224
Diacylglycerol, breast tumorigenesis
endocrine–dietary fat interaction, 638–641
  gap junction-mediated intercellular communication, promotion, 615–618
Dietary modification and cancer, overview, 789–796

animal models
  caloric intakes, 794
  tumor data interpretation, 794–795
breast cancer, 25–26
dietary fat reduction, 792
dietary patterns, 790–792
EFA, 792
epidemiologic data, intrepretation, 794
food selection, 789–790
obesity, 789–790
polyunsaturated fatty acids, 792–793
  P/S ratio, 793
special food products, 793–794
trends in, U.S., 802–806, 811
USDA National Food Consumption Survey, 790, 791
see also Breast cancer prevention, low-fat-diet phase III clinical trials, NCI; Breast dysplasia, dietary-fat reduction, clinical trials, Canada; Dairy products *entries*; Guidelines, dietary *entries*; *under* National Cancer Institute (U.S.)
Diet, high-fat. *See* Fatty acid oxidation and triglyceride synthesis, adaptation to high-fat diet; Glucose metabolism adaptation to high-fat diet; *under* Cholesterol
Diglycerides, 155
Disappearance data, 127–128
  dairy products, 818, 837
  meat, 806, 809
DMAB, colon cancer and dietary fat, animal studies, 296, 298, 299
DMBA
  calorie-restricted diets and cancer, 495, 499–502
  and colon carcinogenesis, 391
  epidemiologic data, relation to experimental, 232–234, 238–240
  and fish oil, 290, 291
  see also Breast cancer, DMBA-induced *entries*
DMH and colon cancer, animal studies, 296, 298, 299, 389, 390, 392–394
  relation between dietary and serum cholesterol, 437, 449
  variable results, 315, 316, 319, 320, 322–324, 326

DMN, metabolic activation, 593–595, 599, 600

DNA
 binding, carcinogen activation, 588–591, 597–599
 methylation, liver cancer, 471–472
 single strand breaks, pancreatic carcinogenesis, enhancement by dietary fat, 334–336
 synthesis
  and hypolipidemic agents, liver cancer, 474, 475
  terminal duct lobular units, breast tumorigenesis, rats, 273
  ^{3}H-thymidine incorporation, breast cancer, fat–protein interaction, 421, 424–426

Dopamine, prolactin, and breast cancer, 411, 415, 416

DPH, hydrophobic probe, lymphocytes, 558, 575–577

Eggs and cholesterol, U.S. data since 1910, 147, 149, 152

Eicosanoids and cancer, 687–693
 arachidonic acid metabolism, 687, 692–693
 cell proliferation, 691
 cyclooxygenase, 687–689
 immune response effect, 689, 692
 leukotrienes, 687, 689
 metastasis, 691–692
 nonsteroidal anti-inflamatory agents, 689, 692
 platelets, 688
 production by breast and lung carcinomas, 690, 691
 prostaglandins, 687–693
 thromboxanes, 687–691
 see also specific eicosanoids

Eicosapentaenoic acid, 693
 and tumorigenesis, 289
 see also Fish (menhaden) oil

Emulsifiers, fats and oils, 171–172

Energy. See Calorie entries

Epidemiologic data, dietary fat and cancer, relation to experimental data, 231–243
 breast, 231, 232, 234–236, 238, 239, 241, 242

colon, 231, 234, 239
 fat amount and type, human populations, 234–238
  per capita statistics, 234–235
  percent calories from fat and carbohydrates, 235–236
 fat amount and type, tumorigenesis in animals, 232–234
  DMBA, 232–234, 238–240
 mechanism of action, 241–242
 non-fat dietary components, 240–241
 pancreas, 231, 232, 242
 PUFA, 232–234, 236–237, 241, 242
 timing and duration effect, 238–240
 metastases, 240
 see also specific cancers

Epidemiology, dietary fat and cancer, methodologic issues, 3–13
 assumptions of investigator, 4–5
 biological plausibility, 4
 breast cancer, 7, 10
 colon cancer, 5, 7, 18, 20, 25
 confounding and interacting factors, 9–10
 exposure distribution, 6–8
 inadequate research design, 8–9
 intervention methodology, 11–13
 listed, 3–4
 measurement sensitivity, 10–11
 single vs. multiple etiology, 5–6, 20

Epithelium. See Breast epithelium cultures, normal and neoplastic, fatty acid effects, rodents; under Calcium

Epoxides, metabolic activation, 21–22, 588–590, 593, 598–599

Erucic acid, 192–193

Escherichia coli, intestinal, 659

Eskimos, 238

ESR, 558

Essential fatty acids
 and BOP-induced pancreatic cancer, 394
 breast tumorigenesis
  chemically induced, rats, 267, 272
  endocrine-dietary fat interaction, 633, 636
 deficiency, and carcinogen activation, 593
 dietary modification, 792
 immune function and dietary fat, 556, 560, 563, 565–570, 572, 575–577

see also Polyunsaturated fatty acids,
 essential
Esterification, fats and oils, 170–171
Estrogens and breast cancer
 and DMBA, 381–382
  calorie-restricted diet, mice, 519–522,
   524
  endocrine–dietary fat interaction, 628–
   629, 632–634, 636
  receptors, 635
 enterohepatic circulation, and intestinal
  microflora, 668–672
 fat–protein interaction, defined two-generation studies, 415, 420
 obesity and, extra-ovarian production,
  33–38
  receptor status, 35, 37, 38
Estrogens and prostate carcinoma, 54–55,
 57–60
 androstenedione aromatization into estrone, 49–50, 58
Estrous cycle and breast tumorigenesis
 DMBA and calorie-restricted diet, mice,
  519, 523, 524
 endocrine–dietary fat interaction, 631,
  632
 fat–protein interaction, defined two-generation studies, 408, 411, 412,
  418–420, 424
Ether-soluble fecal mutagens, 674–675
Etiology, single vs. multiple, epidemiologic
 methodology issues, 5–6, 20
Eubacterium, intestinal microflora, 656, 659,
 664
Exercise, lack of, carcinogenesis-toxicity
 testing, rodent, 368
Exposure distribution, epidemiology, methodologic issues, 6–8

Familial polyposis, 5
Familial risk, prostate carcinoma, 55–56
FAO, 436, 438
Fats and oils, chemistry, 153–162
 components, 154–157
  triglycerides, 153–155
 definition, 153–154
 isomerism, geometric and positional (*cis*
  cf. *trans*), 161, 162, 164, 169,
  614-616

 saturated fatty acids, 157, 158
 unsaturated fatty acids, 158–162
  double bonds, 158–160
Fats and oils, nutritional aspects, 162–165
 dietary level of fat, 165
 essential fatty acids, 164–165; *see also*
  Essential fatty acids
 essential nutrient, 153, 163
 metabolism, 163–164
Fats and oils, processing, 165–174
 additives and processing aids, 172–174
 bleaching, 167
 crude fats and oils, 166
 deodorization, 167
 emulsifiers, 171–172
 esterification, 170–171
 fractionation, 167–168
 hexane, 165
 hydrogenation, 168–169
 interesterification, 169–170
 refining, 166
Fats and oils, products prepared from,
 178–183
 butter, 181–182
 food dressings/toppings/whiteners,
  182–183
 hard butters, 180–181
 margarine, 181
 medium chain triglycerides, 183
 salad and cooking oil, 179
 shortening, 179–180
Fats and oils, reactions, 174–178
 hydrolysis, 174–175
  oxidation, 175–176
 polymerization, 176
Fats, heated and oxidized, 176–178, 185–201
 charcoal broiling, 185, 195–196
  PAH, 185, 190–191, 195–197, 199
 chemical derivatives, 189–191
 deep-fat frying, oil deterioration, 185–189
 malonaldehyde, 185, 188, 190, 200
  TBA test, 188–189, 191
 mutagens and cancer, 194–201
  benzo(a)pyrene, 195–196
  breast, 194, 197, 199
  β-carotene, 198
  colon, 194, 199
  gastric cancer, 197, 199

Japan, Akita Prefecture, 198–199
N-nitrosamines, 200–201
retinoids, 197–198
nutritional considerations, 191–194
heart, liver, and kidney, effects of various fats, 192–194
vitamin E, 194, 200
peroxides, 185, 192, 195
Fatty acid(s)
de novo biosynthetic pathway, glucose metabolism adaptation to high-fat diet, 539–541
food supply data, U.S. since 1910, 141–146
free, 155, 156, 487
albumin as carrier, 541, 542
neutral, and experimental carcinogenesis, 249–242
short-chain, and dietary fiber, 507
trans, and animal tumorigenesis, 283–289, 291–292, 302–305
absence of linoleic acid, 285, 287
colon tumor, azoxymethane-induced, 287–288
DMBA-induced breast carcinogenesis, 284–287, 288
hydrogenation, 283–285
isomers, positional and geometric, 284
cf. other kinds of dietary fat, 285–288
see also Polyunsaturated fatty acids *entries*; Saturated fatty acids; Unsaturated fatty acids; specific fatty acids
Fatty acid oxidation and triglyceride synthesis, adaptation to high-fat diet, 541–545, 547
carnitine palmitoyl transferase, 542
G3P, 542
ketones, 541–543
malonyl CoA, 543
polyunsaturated fish oils, 542–544
respiratory quotient, 541
triglyceride synthesizing enzymes, 542–545
Fecal bile acids. *See under* Bile acids
Fecal mutagens and intestinal microflora, 672–676

ether-soluble, isolation, 674–675
structure, 676
Fecal steroids and colon cancer, 76–83
colon cancer patients, 81–82
population groups, 78–81
Fiber, dietary
cf. calorie-restricted diets and cancer, 508
and colon carcinogenesis, 69, 72, 74, 76, 79–81, 295, 299, 326, 504–509
bile acids, fecal, 507, 508
cholestyramine, 506
epidemiologic data, 504–507
Japanese in Hawaii, 506
microflora, 507
polysaccharides, 507
relation between dietary and serum cholesterol, 436, 437
short-chain fatty acids, 507
intestinal microflora, dietary fat, and cancer, 665, 667
NCI (U.S.), 780, 783
Fire point, fats and oils, 177–178
Fish, dietary, 133, 136–138, 143–149, 151, 805, 809
Fish (menhaden) oil, 213, 233, 242, 272, 693
and animal tumorigenesis, 283, 289–292
breast tumorigenesis, endocrine–dietary fat interaction, 624
carcinogens, metabolic activation, 594, 595, 598, 601
colon cancer and dietary fat, animal studies, 302–303, 305
fatty acid oxidation and triglyceride synthesis, adaptation to high-fat diet, 542–544
pancreatic cancer, enhancement by dietary fat, 349
perturbation of arachidonic acid cascade, 289–290
Flashpoint, fats and oils, 177–178
Fluorescence polarization, 575–577
Folic acid, 784–785
Food group sources, fats, food supply data, U.S. since 1910, 143–146
Food selection, 789–790
Food supply data, fat, U.S. since 1910, 127–149, 151–152

animal cf. vegetable sources, 132, 148
changes over time, 128–129
cholesterol, 146–149
    eggs, 146, 147, 152
dairy products, 133, 138–140, 143–149
    cheese, 140, 143, 147, 149
    per capita, 151
    see also Dairy products entries
disappearance data, 127–128
fats and oils, 133–136, 143–148, 152
    beef fat, 136, 143, 148, 152
    butter, 134, 143, 145, 148, 152
    lard vs. shortening, 134, 136, 143,
        145, 148, 152
    margarine, 134, 144–148, 152
    per capita consumption, 152
fatty acid levels, 141–146
    calories from, 141–142
    linoleic acid, 141, 142, 144, 146, 149
    oleic acid, 141, 142, 144, 145, 149
    saturated, 141–146, 149
food group sources, 133, 140–141,
    143–146
levels of fat, 129–130, 148
meat, poultry, fish, 133, 136–138,
    143–148
    per capita, 151
    pork cf. beef, 137–138, 143, 145–149
    see also Livestock and meat industry
        perspective (U.S.)
percentage of calories from fat, 131
USDA, 127–128
Fractionation, fats and oils, 167–168
Free fatty acids, 155, 156, 487
    albumin transport, 541, 542
Frozen deserts, 827, 830, 831, 833
Fructose-2,6-bisphosphate, glucose metabo-
    lism adaptation to high-fat diet,
    536–537
Frying, deep-fat, oil deterioration, 185–189
Fusobacterium, intestinal microflora, 656,
    657, 660

Gap junction-mediated intercellular commu-
    nication (metabolic cooperation),
    breast tumor promotion, 607–618
    epithelium cultures, fatty acid effects,
        719–722

growth regulatory molecules, small, 608,
    609
in vitro assay (HGPRT), 609–613
lipid effect, 612–616
    diacylglycerol, 615–618
    isomerism, geometric (cis, trans),
        614–616
    monounsaturated, 613–615
    protein kinase C, Ca^{2+}-activated,
        618, 638–641
    saturated, 612–615, 617
    unsaturated, 612–618
tumor promoters inhibiting, listed, 610
Gardner syndrome, 5
Gas chromatography, essential polyunsatu-
    rated fatty acids, 218–220
Gastric (stomach) cancer
    fats, heated and oxidized, mutagens, 197,
        199
    NCI (U.S.), 780
Gavage test. See Carcinogenesis-toxicity test-
    ing, corn oil gavage test-compound
    effects (NTP), rodents
Glucagon, 541, 543
Glucocorticoids, breast tumorigenesis, 629–
    630, 634–635
Glucokinase, 535
Glucose metabolism adaptation to high-fat
    diet, 531–541, 547
    adipose tissue, 533, 535, 540
    glycogen, 532–534
    hexokinase, 533, 535, 536
    insulin resistance, 532
    intracellular metabolism, 534–541
        de novo fatty acid biosynthetic path-
            way, 539–541
        glycolytic enzymes, 535–538
        muscle, 531, 533–537
        phosphofructokinase, 533, 535–537
        polyunsaturated fats, 539–540
        pyruvate dehydrogenase, 533, 538–539
        transport, 532–534
Glucose-6-phosphate, adaptation to high-fat
    diet, 535, 536, 542
β-Glucuronidase and colon cancer, 78, 79
    intestinal microflora, 657–660, 667, 671,
        677
Glutathione and liver cancer, 475–476

Glutathione-S-transferase, carcinogen metabolic activation, 591, 596, 599–601
Glycogen, glucose metabolism adaptation to high-fat diet, 532–534
Glycolytic enzymes, glucose metabolism adaptation to high-fat diet, 535–538
Graft-vs.-host reaction, 571
Growth hormone and breast tumorigenesis
   calorie-restricted diet, 520, 521
   endocrine–dietary fat interaction, 627–628, 631–632
Growth regulatory molecules, small, gap junction-mediated intercellular communication, 608, 609
Guidelines, dietary, heart disease and cancer reduction, 731–734, 749–765
   alcohol, 760
   Australia, 755–756
   Britain, 749–753
      World War II, low dietary fat levels, 759, 761
   Canada, 746, 753
   data base, 732, 760
   education, 763–764
   high-risk individuals, 762–763
   historical perspective, 732–734
   Ireland, 753
   Multiple Risk Factor Intervention Trial, 764
   Netherlands, 757–758
   New Zealand, 758
   Norway, 754–755
   obesity, 759
   removal vs. addition, 762
   saturated cf. polyunsaturated fat, 759
   Sweden, 755
   vitamin supplements, 760
   WHO, 756–757, 759
      FAO, 758
   see also Dietary modification and cancer, overview
Guidelines, dietary, heart disease and cancer reduction, U.S., 732, 734–749, 760–761
   AMA, 738, 744–745
   American Academy of Pediatrics, Canadian Pediatrics Society, 745–746
   American Cancer Society, 749

American Health Foundation, 745
American Heart Association, 735–736
American Institute for Cancer Research, 748
Basic Four Food Groups, 734–735, 738
Consensus Conference on Lowering Blood Cholesterol, 741–742
dairy products, 845–847
Dietary Goals for the U.S. (U.S. Senate), 736–739
Inter-Society Commission for Heart Disease Resources, 740
mortality, 732
NAS, Food and Nutrition Board, 742–744, 759
   RDAs, 742, 763–765
NAS, National Research Council, 747–748
NCI, 749
shift from nutritional deficiency to chronic disease, 760–761
Surgeon General's Report, 739–740
USDA/USDHHS, 740

Haloperidol, 520, 521
H-2 antigens, immune function and dietary fat, 557, 562–564
Ha-ras-1 oncogene, chemically induced breast tumor, rats, 266
Hawaii. See Japanese migrants to Hawaii
Heart
   disease, relation between dietary and serum cholesterol, 440, 448, 451, 452
   various fats, effects, 192–194
   see also Guidelines, dietary entries
Heating/cooking fats and oils, 176–178; see also Fats, heated and oxidized
Height, obesity, and breast cancer, 20, 21, 34, 38
Hexane, fat and oil processing, 165
Hexokinase, glucose metabolism adaptation to high-fat diet, 533, 535, 536
HGPRT assay, 609–613, 719–721
High-fat diet and colon cancer, variable animal results, 317, 319, 320, 324, 325
   see also Fatty acid oxidation and triglyceride synthesis, adaptation to high-fat diet; Glucose metabolism adap-

tation to high-fat diet; *under* Cholesterol
High-risk individuals, dietary guidelines for heart disease and cancer reduction, 762–763
Histamine release, mast cells, breast epithelium cultures, fatty acid effects, 704–705
HMG CoA reductase, cholesterol metabolism adaptation, high-fat diets, 545, 546
Hormone
  -dependence, chemically induced breast tumor, rats, 257, 274
  regulation, breast cancer, 411–420, 635–637; *see also* Estrogens and breast cancer
  sex, prostate carcinoma, 43, 49–52
  see also specific hormones
Hydrocortisone, breast epithelium cultures, fatty acid effects, 711–715
Hydrogenation, fats and oils, 168–169, 283–285
Hydrolysis, fats and oils, 174–175
Hyperplastic alveolar nodule, breast epithelium cultures, fatty acid effects, 708, 709
Hypersensitivity, delayed-type, 570
Hypertension and dairy products, 826

Immune response
  and DMBA-induced breast carcinogenesis, and dietary fat, 382–383
  calorie-restricted diet, 525–526
  eicosanoids and, 689, 692
Immune response, dietary fatty acid modulation, 555–580
  arachidonic acid, 572–574, 579
  B-cell responses, 565, 571–573, 576
    IgG 1 and 2, 572
    PFC responses, 572, 573
  complement, 563, 564, 573–574
  early postweaning diet, 566
  essential fatty acids, 556, 560, 563, 565–570, 575–577
  H-2 antigens, 557, 562–564
  Intralipid, 573, 574
  lymphocyte structural features, in vitro and in vivo, 556–561

antigens, 557–559, 575
Ca^{2+} influx, 576
cross-linking, 558, 574
DPH, hydrophobic probe, 558, 575–577
fluidity, 557–559, 575
membrane, 557, 560, 574–578
phospholipids, 560–561, 565, 576–579
receptors, 558, 559, 575
lytic susceptibility of tumor cells, 561–565
macrophages, 564, 565, 573–574
polyunsaturated cf. saturated, 556–558, 559–562, 570, 572, 575–579
cis cf. *trans*, 565
prostaglandins, 572–574, 578–579
T-cell responses, 565, 567–571, 576, 578–579
  blastogenesis, 568
  CTL, 562–563, 567–569
  DTH, 570
  GVH reaction, 571
  suppressor/helper, 568, 569
Immunoglobulins, dietary fat and, 572
Indomethacin, 689, 692, 714–716
INFOODS international data system, 782
Initiation
  breast tumorigenesis
    DMBA-induced, 381, 386
    endocrine–dietary fat interaction, 625
  colon cancer and dietary fat, animal studies, 299–301
  pancreatic cancer, enhancement by dietary fat, 344, 345, 348
Insulin
  and breast tumorigenesis
    endocrine–dietary fat interaction, 630, 631
    epithelium cultures, fatty acid effects, 711–715
  resistance, glucose metabolism adaptation to high-fat diet, 532
Intercellular communication. *See* Gap junction-mediated intercellular communication (metabolic cooperation), breast tumor promotion
Interesterification, fats and oils, 169–170

Intervention
    breast cancer, 27–28
        weight reduction, 37
    colon cancer, relation between dietary
        and serum cholesterol, 448–450,
        455
    epidemiology, methodologic issues, 11–13
    Multiple Risk Factor Intervention Trial,
        764
    see also Breast cancer prevention, low-
        fat-diet phase III clinical trials,
        NCI; Breast dysplasia, dietary-fat
        reduction, clinical trials, Canada;
Dietary modification and cancer, overview;
        Guidelines, dietary *entries*; National
        Cancer Institute (U.S.)
Intestinal microflora, 77, 79, 81, 655–678
    Ames *Salmonella* mutagenicity test, 658,
        660–662, 673
    animal tumor models, 676–678
    bacterial enzymes, 657–663
        azoreductase, 660, 666
        cycasin, 657–658
        β-glucuronidase, 657–660, 667, 671,
            677
        nitroreductase, 661–662, 667
        nitrosamines, 662–663
    bile acids, 666, 676
    breast cancer, enterohepatic circulation of
        estrogens, 668–672
        case-control studies, 669
        epidemiology, 668
    cholesterol metabolism, 453, 454, 666
    composition and distribution, 656–657,
        659, 662–665, 675–676
        anaerobes, 656–657
        Bacteroides, 656, 657, 659, 662–664,
            675–676
        Bifidobacterium, 656, 657, 664, 665
    dairy products, 849–850
    7-α-dehydroxylation, 666, 667
    fecal mutagens, 672–676
        epidemiology, 672–674
        ether-soluble, isolation, 674–675
        structure, 676
    fiber, dietary, 507, 665, 667
    omnivore (Western) cf. vegetarian diet,
        664–670, 672–674

    Japanese, 664, 666
    Seventh Day Adventists, 664–666,
        669, 673, 674
    oral antibiotics, 671–672, 677
    relation between dietary and serum cho-
        lesterol, 453, 454
    tryptophan, 663
    tyrosine, 663
Intralipid and immune function, 573, 574
Ireland, dietary guidelines, 753
Isomerism, geometric and positional (*cis*,
        trans), lipids, 161, 162, 164, 169
    gap junction-mediated intercellular com-
        munication, 614–616
    trans-fatty acids. *See under* Fatty acids
Israel, breast cancer, 18, 24

Japan
    breast cancer, 18, 19, 24–25, 38–39
    fats, heated and oxidized, Akita Prefec-
        ture, 198–199
    intestinal microflora, dietary fat, and can-
        cer, 664, 666
    prostate carcinoma, 46, 47
Japanese migrants to Hawaii
    breast cancer, 24, 39
    colon cancer, 71, 75, 79, 80, 325,
        655–656
        and dietary fiber, 506
        relation between dietary and serum
            cholesterol, 444

Ketones, adaptation to high-fat diet, 541–543
Kidney, various fats, effects, 192–194
Klebsiella, 665

Lactobacillus, 656, 665
    acidophilus, yogurt, 849–850
Lard, 192–193
    chemically induced breast tumor, rats,
        270, 271, 273, 274
    colon cancer, animal studies, 297, 298,
        300, 301, 305
    liver cancer, carcinogen metabolism,
        462, 463
    processing, 170
    vs. shortening, food supply data, U.S.
        since 1910, 134, 136, 143, 145,
        148, 152

Leukemia, corn oil gavage test, rodents, 363, 364, 366
Leukotrienes, 687, 689; *see also* Eicosanoids and cancer
Linoleic acid, 164, 165
    absence, *trans* fatty acids and tumorigenesis, 285, 287
    and breast cancer, 270, 272
        epithelium cultures, fatty acid effects, 700–703, 705–706
    carcinogenesis-toxicity testing, rodent corn oil gavage test, 366–367
    essential polyunsaturated fatty acids, 211, 213, 218
    deficiency, dermatitis, 214–216
    and fish oil, 290
    food supply data, U.S. since 1910, 141, 142, 144, 146, 149
Linolenic acid, 164, 168, 179
    essential polyunsaturated fatty acids, 211, 213, 217–218
Lipid peroxidation and liver cancer, 471, 472, 475, 476
Lipofuscin, 200
Liver
    cirrhosis, 222, 224
    fatty, 469
    various fats, effects, 192–194
Liver cancer, dietary fat and carcinogen metabolism, 461–477
    AAF, 463, 475
    aflatoxin, 463–464, 466, 468
    beef fat, 466, 468
    choline deficiency, 468–472, 476
    corn oil, 466, 468
    cottonseed oil, 463–464
        cyclopropenoid fatty acids, 463–464
    Crisco®, 462, 463
    DAB, 462, 463
    DEN, 474, 475
    DNA methylation, 471–472
    fatty liver and cirrhosis, 469
    glutathione, 475–476
    hypolipidemic agents, 472–476
    lard, 462, 463
    lipid peroxidation, 471, 472, 475, 476
    liver cell necrosis, 466–467
    MFOs, 465–466, 587–593, 596, 600

cytochromes P-450, 587, 589, 592, 594–596, 600
    phenobarbital, 466–468, 588, 592, 594–596, 599
    phosphatidylcholine, 465
    safflower oil, 465–466
    stage-specific effects, 467–468
Livestock and meat industry perspective (U.S.), 801–812
    breeding, 803, 810
    lean and "lite" products, 810
    NAS Dietary Guidelines, 801–802, 812
    red meat consumption patterns, 805–811
        measurement methodology, 805, 809
        cf. poultry and fish, 805, 809
        saturated fat, 807, 808, 811
    trends in animal products, 802–806
        changing to vegetable sources, 803–804
        per capita figures, 804–806, 811
        reduced fat content, 803
Lung cancer
    eicosanoid production, 690, 691
    and neutral fats and fatty acids, 250
    smoking and, 27
Lymphocytes. *See under* Immune response, dietary fatty acid modulation
Lytic susceptiblity, tumor cells, and dietary fat, 561–565

Macrophage function and dietary fat, 564, 565, 573–574
Malonaldehyde, heated and oxidized fats, mutagens, 185, 188, 190, 200
    TBA test, 189–191
Malonyl CoA, 543
MAM acetate, 296, 298, 299
Mammary
    alveolar lesions, breast epithelium cultures, fatty acid effects, 709, 711–716, 720
    tumor virus, breast epithelium cultures, fatty acid effects, 708, 712
    see also Breast *entries*
Margarine, 181
    food supply data, U.S. since 1910, 134, 144–148, 152
Mast cells, histamine release, breast epithelium cultures, fatty acid effects, 704–705

Mayonnaise, 182
Meat and colon cancer, 71–74, 312; *see also* Animal fat; Livestock and meat industry perspective (U.S.)
Membranes
   breast epithelium cultures, fatty acid effects, acid, 701–702
   colonic crypt epithelium, damage to, 487
   lymphocyte, dietary fatty acid modulation, 557, 560, 574–578
Menarche, age at, and breast cancer, 20, 21
Menhaden oil. *See* Fish (menhaden) oil
Menopause, obesity, and breast cancer, 35, 37, 39
Metabolic cooperation. *See* Gap junction-mediated intercellular communication (metabolic cooperation), breast tumor promotion
Metastasis, 240
   eicosanoids and, 691–692
Methodology. *See* Epidemiology, dietary fat and cancer, methodologic issues
3-Methylcholanthrene
   calorie-restricted diets, and cancer, 495, 498, 499
   metabolic activation, 593, 594, 598
Methylene chloride, corn oil gavage test, 357, 369
N-Methylnitrosurea. *See* MNU
α-Methylparatyrosine, 415–417
Microencapsulation cf. corn oil gavage, carcinogenesis-toxicity testing, rodent, 369
Microflora. *See* Intestinal microflora
Migrant studies. *See* Japanese migrants to Hawaii
Milk
   lowfat, 818–820, 822–823, 827, 831
   whole, 818–820, 822, 825, 827, 830, 831
Mitotic index. *See* Cell proliferation
Mixed function oxidases, liver microsomal, 587–593, 596, 600
   and cancer, 465–466
   cytochromes P-450, 587, 589, 592, 594–596, 600
   phenobarbital, 588, 592, 594–596, 599
MNNG, colon cancer, dietary fat and, variable animal results, 326

MNU (N-methylnitrosurea; NMU)
   breast cancer, 261–267, 269, 270, 272, 274, 275
   age-dependence, 266
   fat–protein interaction, 408, 418, 419, 430, 431
   Ha-*ras* oncogene, 266
   variable results, 316, 326
   colon cancer, 296, 298, 299
Monoglycerides, 155
Monounsaturated fatty acids, gap junction-mediated intercellular communication, breast tumor promotion, 613–615
Mormons, 70
   prostate carcinoma, 56
Mortality
   breast cancer, 19
   dietary guidelines for heart disease and cancer reduction, U.S., 732
   statistics, U.S., 815, 816
   site and year, 816
Muscle, glucose metabolism adaptation to high-fat diet, 531, 533–537

National Academy of Sciences (U.S.)
   Dietary Guidelines, 801–802, 812
   Food and Nutrition Board, 742–744, 759
   National Research Council, 747–748
National Cancer Advisory Board (U.S.), 95, 97, 98
National Cancer Institute (U.S.), 749
   Board of Scientific Counselors, 95–98
   Chemoprevention Branch, 774
   Diet and Cancer Branch, 773–786
      clinical trials, 783
      dietary fat, 778–780
      dietary fiber, 780, 783
      INFOODS, 782
      research directions, 744–778, 784–786
      research units, 783–784
      retinoids and carotenoids, 780–782
   Division of Cancer Prevention and Control, 93–97, 773
   Policy Advisory Committee, 99
   see also Breast cancer prevention, lowfat-diet phase III clinical trials, NCI

National Toxicology Program. *See* Carcinogenesis-toxicity testing, corn oil gavage test-compound effects (NTP),
rodents
Netherlands, dietary guidelines, 757–758
New Zealand, dietary guidelines, 758
Nigeria, prostate carcinoma, 52, 54, 55
Nitroreductase, intestinal microflora, dietary
fat, and cancer, 661–662, 667
Nitrosamines
fats, heated and oxidized, 200–201
intestinal microflora, dietary fat, and cancer, 662–663
stomach, dairy product inhibition, 847,
848
NMR, 576, 578
NMU. *See* MNU
Norway, dietary guidelines, 754–755
Nutrition Adjuvant Study, NCI (U.S.), 93,
107–111, 779–780

Obesity, 789–790
and breast cancer. *See* Breast cancer,
obesity and
dairy products, 843, 845
dietary guidelines for heart disease and
cancer reduction, 759
Oils. *See* Fats and oils *entries*; specific oils
Oleic acid, food supply data, U.S. since
1910, 141, 142, 144, 145, 149
Olive oil and colon cancer, animal studies,
301–302, 305
Organ cultures, breast epithelium, fatty acid
effects, 708–710, 714–715
Ornithine decarboxylase, 305–306
Osteoporosis prevention, dairy products, 826
Ovaries and breast tumorigenesis, endocrine–
dietary fat interaction, 625, 632, 634,
635
Overnutrition, carcinogenesis-toxicity testing, corn oil gavage test, rodents,
362–364, 366–369
Oxidation, fats and oils, 175–176; *see also*
Fats, heated and oxidized; Fatty acid
oxidation and triglyceride synthesis,
adaptation to high-fat diet

Pancreatic carcinogenesis, enhancement by
dietary fat, 331–342, 349–350

acinar cells, atypical nodules (AACN),
336, 338–339, 350
azaserine-induced, rats, 331–332,
342–349
AACN, 346–347, 349
AACN, baso- cf. acidophilic,
347–348
adenocarcinoma, 343–345
adenoma, 343, 345
AIN-76 diet (corn oil), 342, 344, 345
fish oil, 349
initiation cf. post-initiation, 344–345,
348
short- cf. long-term models, 346, 347
body weight, 340
BOP-induced, hamster, 331–342,
349–350
dietary fat and protein, 377, 394–395
EFA, 394
calorie consumption, 341
carcinogenesis-toxicity testing, corn oil
gavage test, rodent, 361–363, 369,
370
corn oil, 340, 349–350
DNA, ductular, single strand breaks,
334–336
epidemiologic data, relation to experimental, 231, 232, 242
protein levels, 333–334, 337–340, 342
Parenteral nutrition, immune function, and
dietary fat (Intralipid), 573, 574
Peptococcus, intestinal, 656, 664, 665
Peptostreptococcus, intestinal, 656, 659
Peroxides, and heated and oxidized fats, 185,
192, 195
Peroxisome structure and liver cancer,
473–476
Perphenazine and breast epithelium cultures,
fatty acid effects, 701
Phenobarbital, 466–468, 588, 592, 594–596,
599
Phosphatides, 155, 156
Phosphatidylcholine, liver cancer, dietary fat
and carcinogen metabolism, 465
Phosphofructokinase, adaptation to high-fat
diet, 533, 535–537
Phospholipids
breast tumorigenesis, endocrine–dietary
fat interaction, 638–639

lymphocytes, dietary fat and, 560–561, 565, 576–579
Pituitary
  breast tumorigenesis, endocrine–dietary fat interaction, 625, 634, 635
  insufficiency (pseudohypophysectomy), calorie-restricted diet and DMBA breast tumorigenesis, mice, 518–519
Plaque-forming cells and dietary fat, 572–573
Platelets, eicosanoids and, 688
Polycyclic aromatic hydrocarbons (PAH)
  charcoal broiling, 185, 190–191, 195–197, 199
  metabolic activation, 588
    bay regions, 589
  see also Benzo(a)pyrene
Polyenoic acids, metabolic activation, 592
Polymerization, fats and oils, 176
Polysaccharides, dietary fiber, 507
Polyunsaturated fatty acids (PUFA)
  chemically induced breast tumor, rats, 267, 272, 274
  carcinogens, metabolic activation, 592, 596, 597
  cf. dairy products, 841, 846, 847
  dietary modification, 792–793
  epidemiologic data, relation to experimental, 232–234, 236–237, 241, 242
  glucose metabolism adaptation to high-fat diet, 539–540
  P/S ratio, 701–703
  cf. saturated. See under Saturated fatty acids
Polyunsaturated fatty acids, essential, 211–225
  arachidonic acid, 211–212, 214, 222, 225
  deficiency, 220–225
    assay, 220–221
    in disease, 221, 223–225
    protein deficiency, 222–223
  gas chromatography, 218–220
  interaction, dietary, 216–217
  linoleic acid, 211, 213, 218
    deficiency, dermatitis, 214–216
  linolenic acid, 211, 213, 217–218

cf. nonessential, 212–214
prostaglandins, 212, 213
quantified requirement, 218–220
structural requirements, 211–214
thromboxanes, 212, 213
see also Essential fatty acids
Pork cf. beef, food supply data, U.S. since 1910, 137–138, 143, 145–149
Poultry, 133, 136–138, 143–148, 151, 805, 809
Processing. See Fats and oils, processing
Progesterone and breast tumorigenesis
  endocrine–dietary fat interaction, 629, 632, 636
  fat–protein interaction, defined two-generation studies, 415
Prolactin
  and colon cancer, 840
  and prostate carcinoma, 56–57
Prolactin and breast cancer, 840
  calorie intake, 843–845
  carcinogenesis inhibition, 847–850
  dietary guidelines, 845–847
  DMBA-induced, 382
    calorie-restricted diet, 519–522, 524
  endocrine–dietary fat interaction, 626–627, 632–634
    fibroadenomas, 627
    receptors, 636
  epithelium cultures, fatty acid effects, 701, 703–705, 711–715
  fat–protein interaction, defined two-generation studies, 411, 413–415, 417–419
  obesity, 843, 845
  protein, 842
Promotion
  breast tumorigenesis
    DMBA-induced, 381, 386
    endocrine–dietary fat interaction, 625
  colon cancer and dietary fat, animal studies, 299, 301–304
  dairy products, 840
  see also Gap junction-mediated intercellular communication (metabolic cooperation), breast tumor promotion

Prostaglandin endoperoxide synthase and carcinogen metabolic activation, 590–591, 593, 596
Prostaglandins, 687–693
    breast epithelium cultures, unsaturated fatty acid effects, 714–716
    and essential polyunsaturated fatty acids, 212, 213
        arachidonic acid, 211–212, 214, 222, 225
    immune function and dietary fat, 572–574, 578–579
    see also Arachidonic acid; Eicosanoids and cancer
Prostate cancer, 836–840
Prostate carcinoma, biochemical epidemiology, 43–60
    cf. BPH, 51, 53, 56–58
    case control studies, 49, 52–55
    dietary fat and, 43–44, 47–50
    diet–hormone interactions, 58–60
    high-risk populations, 55–56
    prolactin, 56–57
    prostatic fluid, 57–58
    risk, 44–47
        cf. breast cancer, 44, 45, 49–50
        familial, 55–56
        Hawaii, 46–48
        Japanese, 46, 47
        Mormons, 56
        Nigerians, 52, 54, 55
        Seventh Day Adventists, 48, 58, 60
        U.S. blacks, 49, 52, 54, 55, 59, 60
    sex hormones, 43, 49–52
Protein, dietary
    animal, and colon cancer, 71–72, 78
    and chemically induced breast tumor, 274, 384–387
    and colon carcinogenesis, 392–393
    deficiency, and essential polyunsaturated fatty acids, 222–223
    dairy products, 842
    pancreatic carcinogenesis, enhancement by dietary fat, 333, 334, 337–340, 342
Protein kinase C and breast tumorigenesis, 618, 638–641
Purified diets (AIN), 342, 344, 345, 378

Pyruvate dehydrogenase, glucose metabolism adaptation to high-fat diet, 533, 538–539

Rancidity, fat and oils, 175
Rapeseed oil, low erucic acid, 192–193
Recommended daily allowances (RDAs), U.S., 742, 763–765
Research design, epidemiology, methodologic issues, 8–9
Respiratory quotient, fatty acid oxidation and triglyceride synthesis, adaptation to high-fat diet, 541
Retinoids
    chemically induced breast tumor, rats, 275
    and colon cancer, 445, 451
    fats, heated and oxidized, mutagens, 197–198
    NCI (U.S.), 780–782
Reye's syndrome, 221, 224

Safflower oil
    colon cancer, animal studies, 301–302, 305
    liver cancer, dietary fat and carcinogen metabolism, 465–466
Salad oil, 179
Salmonella, Ames test, 199, 588, 599, 658, 660–662, 673
Saturated fatty acids, 157, 158
    food supply data, U.S. since 1910, 141–146, 149
    gap junction-mediated intercellular communication, breast tumor promotion, 612–617
    livestock/meat industry perspective, 807, 808, 811
    cf. polyunsaturated fats, 159, 161
        cis cf. trans, 565
        dietary guidelines for heart disease and cancer reduction, 759
        and DMBA-induced breast carcinogenesis, 384
        immune function and dietary fat, 559–562, 566–568, 570, 572, 575–579
        P/S ratio, 701, 702, 793
    cf. unsaturated, 159, 161

Selenium and breast cancer, 20, 274, 275
Seventh Day Adventists
    breast cancer, 18, 22
    and colon cancer, 75, 79–80, 83, 312,
        452
        intestinal microflora, 664–666, 669,
            673, 674
    dairy products, 839
Sex, colon cancer, relation between dietary
    and serum cholesterol, 451–452
Sex hormones, prostate carcinoma, 43,
    49–52
Sexual maturation, breast cancer, fat–protein
    interaction, defined two-generation
    studies, 408, 411, 412, 418–420, 424
SHBG, prostate carcinoma, 51, 53, 54
Shortening, 179–180
    colon cancer, dietary fat and, variable an-
        imal results, 317, 318
    vs. lard, food supply data, U.S. since
        1910, 134, 136, 143, 145, 148, 152
Smoking and lung cancer, 27
Smoking point, fats and oils, 177–178
Socioeconomic status, high, and colon can-
    cer, 311–312
Soybean oil and DMBA-induced breast carci-
    nogenesis, 382, 383
Spouses of colon cancer patients, 75–76
Staphylococcus, 656
Stearic acid, breast epithelium cultures, cf.
    unsaturated fatty acids, 700–703, 705,
    717–721
Steroids, fecal, and colon cancer, 76–83
    colon cancer patients, 81–82
    population groups, 78–81
Sterols, 156
Stomach (gastric) cancer
    fats, heated and oxidized, mutagens, 197,
        199
    NCI (U.S.), 780
Streptococcus, 656, 658
Sweden, dietary guidelines, 755

Tamoxifen, breast cancer Nutrition Adjuvant
    Study, 109
TBA test, heated and oxidized fats, muta-
    gens, 188–189, 191
T cells. See under Immune response, dietary
    fatty acid modulation

Teratogenicity, corn oil gavage test, 360, 369
Terminal duct lobular units, chemically in-
    duced breast tumor, rats, 260, 273
    DNA synthesis, 273
Terminal end buds, breast, 260, 421–423
Testosterone, prostate carcinoma, 51–54,
    56–60
Thromboxanes, 698–691
    and essential polyunsaturated fatty acids,
        212, 213
    see also Eicosanoids and cancer
^{3}H-Thymidine incorporation, DNA, breast
    cancer, fat–protein interaction, 421,
    424–426
Thymus, calorie-restricted diet and DMBA
    breast tumorigenesis, mice, 525–526
Thyroid hormone–dietary fat interaction,
    breast tumorigenesis, 630–631,
    634–635
Tobacco, 764
Tocopherols, 156, 166, 173
TPA, 609, 640
    breast epithelium cultures, fatty acid ef-
        fects, 717–721
Triglycerides, 153–155
    medium chain, 183
    see also Fatty acid oxidation and triglyc-
        eride synthesis, adaptation to high-
        fat diet
Tryptophan and intestinal microflora, 663
Tyrosine and intestinal microflora, 663

Ultraviolet-induced skin carcinogenesis,
    249–250
Underfeeding. See Calorie-restricted diet
    entries
United States
    breast cancer, 18–19
        Japan-Hawaii Cancer Study, 24, 39
        Mormons, Utah, 56, 70
    prostate carcinoma
        blacks, 49, 52, 54, 55, 59, 60
        Hawaii, 46–48
    USDA, meat grading standards, 803
    USDA National Food Consumption Sur-
        vey, 790, 791
    see also Food supply data, fat, U.S. since
        1910; Guidelines, dietary, heart
        disease and cancer reduction,

U.S.; Japanese migrants to Hawaii; National Cancer Institute *entries*
Unsaturated fatty acids, 158–162
  breast tumorigenesis, endocrine–dietary fat interaction, 624, 625, 638
  double bonds, C-to-C, 158–160
  gap junction-mediated intercellular communication, breast tumor promotion, 612–618
  monounsaturated, 613, 615
  /saturated fat ratio, breast epithelium cultures, fatty acid effects, 701, 702
  see also Polyunsaturated fatty acids *entries*
Utah, Mormons, 56, 70

Vegetable(s)
  and colon cancer, 74, 75
  fats, cf. animal fats, food supply data, U.S. since 1910, 132, 148

Vegetarian diet, intestinal microflora, dietary fat, and cancer, 664–670, 672–674
  Japanese, 664, 666
  see also Seventh Day Adventists
Virus, mammary tumor, 708, 712
Vitamins, 156, 157, 166, 181
  E, 191, 194, 200
    chemically induced breast tumor, rats, 274
Vivonex food supplement, 438

Weight. *See* Body weight; Breast cancer, obesity and
WHO, 436
  dietary guidelines, 758
  FAO, 436, 438
Women's Health Trial, NCI (U.S.), 93, 104–107, 779

Yogurt, 818–820, 822, 823, 825, 827
  Lactobacillus acidophilus, 849–850